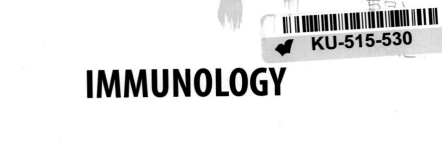
IMMUNOLOGY

Commissioning Editor: Inta Ozols
Development Editor: Louise Cook
Editorial Assistant: Nani Clansey
Project Manager: Jess Thompson
Design Manager: Jayne Jones
Illustration Manager: Bruce Hogarth
Illustrator: Cactus Illustration
Marketing Manager(s) (UK/USA): Ian Jordan and John Gore

Immunology

Seventh Edition

David Male MA PhD
Professor of Biology
Department of Biological Sciences
The Open University
Milton Keynes, UK

Jonathan Brostoff MA DM(Oxon) DSc(Med) FRCP (Lond) FRCPath FIBiol
Professor Emeritus of Allergy and Environmental Health
School of Biomedical and Health Sciences
King's College London
London, UK

David B Roth MD PhD
Irene Diamond Professor of Pathology
Investigator, Skirball Institute
Program in Molecular Pathogenesis
Chairman, Department of Pathology
New York University School of Medicine
New York, NY, USA

Ivan Roitt MA DSc (Oxon) Hon FRCP (Lon) FRCPath FRS
Emeritus Professor of Immunology
Royal Free and University College Medical School
University College
London, UK

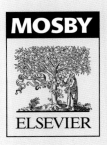

MOSBY

ELSEVIER

MOSBY
ELSEVIER
An imprint of Elsevier Limited

First edition published by Gower Medical Publishing Ltd., 1985
Second edition published by Gower Medical Publishing Ltd., 1989
Third edition published by Mosby-Year Book Europe Ltd., 1993
Fourth edition published by Mosby, an imprint of Times Mirror International Publishers, 1996
Fifth edition published by Mosby, an imprint of Times Mirror International Publishers, 1998
Sixth edition published by Elsevier Ltd., 2001
Seventh edition published by Elsevier Ltd., 2006

Main edition
ISBN: 978-0-323-03399-2
 Reprinted 2007, 2010, 2011

International edition
ISBN: 978-0-8089-2332-9
 Reprinted 2007, 2008, 2011

British Library Cataloguing in Publication Data
A catalogue record for this book is available from the British Library

Library of Congress Cataloging in Publication Data
A catalog record for this book is available from the Library of Congress

Notice
Medical knowledge is constantly changing. Standard safety precautions must be followed, but as new research and clinical experience broaden our knowledge, changes in treatment and drug therapy may become necessary or appropriate. Readers are advised to check the most current product information provided by the manufacturer of each drug to be administered to verify the recommended dose, the method and duration of administration, and contraindications. It is the responsibility of the practitioner, relying on experience and knowledge of the patient, to determine dosages and the best treatment for each individual patient. Neither the Publisher nor the author assume any liability for any injury and/or damage to persons or property arising from this publication.

The Publisher

Printed in China

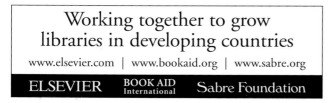

CONTENTS

PREFACE

Immunology as a distinctive subject developed in the middle of the 20th century as researchers started to understand how the adaptive immune system aids in defence against pathogens. For many years, text books reflected this view of immunology with short opening sections on innate defences, before giving detailed descriptions of how lymphocytes protect the body against infection. In the last few years, the neglected but critical elements of the innate immune system have come back into sharp focus and have been the subject of much research. Phagocytes and the evolutionarily ancient mechanisms for recognising pathogen, have been retained in mammals and indeed have developed alongside the adaptive immune system; it is only as we have started to understand how innate immunity operates, that we have started to recognise the importance of these systems. In the seventh edition of *Immunology*, we have included a new chapter on innate immunity, but equally important is the assimilation of descriptions of innate defences into other parts of the book. This truly reflects the way the immune system operates with the integration of ancient and recently-evolved immune defences.

The book is organised into five sections. The opening section describes the building blocks of the immune system, - cells, organs, complement and the major receptor molecules, including antibodies, T cell receptors and MHC molecules. The second section deals with the initiation of the immune response starting with innate defences, and leading on to antigen presentation, costimulation and cell activation pathways. The following three chapters discuss the principal effector arms of the immune response, TH2 responses with antibody production, TH1 responses and mononuclear phagocytes, and cytotoxicity, including cytotoxic T cells and NK cells. In this edition, material on individual cytokines has been incorporated into each of these chapters, rather than being treated as a separate subject. The final chapters in this section look into the regulation of the immune response, and there is a new chapter on the distinctive types of immune response that develop in different tissues of the body. Although it has long been recognised that immune responses in tissues vary, the underlying reasons for the differences are only just being elucidated.

Section three describes the immune responses that develop against different types of infection, and how immunodeficiency leads to increased susceptibility to particular infections. Indeed the diversity and complexity of the immune system can only be understood in relation to the diversity of the pathogens which it protects against. In recent years, the devious strategies employed by pathogens to evade immune responses, have provided some quite startling revelations, both on the adaptability of the pathogens and on the flexibility of the immune system. Ultimately the immune system can only be understood in relation to its principal function – defence against pathogens.

Section four describes immune responses against tissues, and section five hypersensitivity. These areas are of great clinical importance. One aim of this book is to provide readers with a sound understanding of the immune responses which underlie clinically important areas including hypersensitivity states and allergy, immunopathology, tumour immunotherapy and transplantation. In these sections, we have maintained what we believe to be an important feature of the book, namely a clear description of the scientific principles of clinical immunology, integrated with histology, pathology, and clinical examples. In this edition, the two chapters on tolerance and autoimmunity have been linked and rewritten, to reflect how the traditional system-based approach of clinical immunology and the cell-based approach of basic immunology are finally producing a coherent picture of how autoimmune disease develops.

Previously, we have included a final chapter which collates immunological techniques. In this edition the methods and techniques are distributed throughout the book, in methods boxes, in the most appropriate place. We hope that this will make it easier to locate relevant techniques if they are of interest, but allow the reader to pass over such material, if it is not.

A new feature of the book is the inclusion of in-text questions. These are designed to check that the reader understands the implications of the preceeding paragraphs or can relate that material to information in earlier chapters. Although the answers follow on immediately below the questions, we would suggest that readers pause to formulate an answer, before reading on through. Another useful learning aid is the critical thinking sections at the end of each chapter. A set of solutions to the problems is included at the end of the book, although some of the questions are open ended and would form a good basis for class discussion or tutorials. Finally, we have put a lot of care into the chapter summaries, ensuring that they really do distil the key aspects of each chapter, into a manageable overview. The summary boxes make an excellent revision guide for exams, in addition to setting the framework for each chapter.

In conjuction with the book, the *Immunology* seventh edition website provides access to the full set of illustrations and text on-line. Other ancillaries include a set of 16 animations, with a total of 90 minutes playing time, that were originally developed as one component of Immunology Interactive 3.0. The site also contains a question-bank and other ancillaries, to aid learning and enhance understanding of the subject.

The contributors to this volume include many experts in different areas of immunology, but we are particularly pleased to welcome David Roth as a new editor. We hope that David's contribution has further broadened our appreciation of how immunology is taught in other countries, in addition to his scientific input. Also, we would like to thank Jane Loughlin and Lindy van den Berghe for their critical reading of the text, suggestions for changes and contribution to the in-text questions. We greatly appreciate the hard work of our Publishers and their colleagues, particularly, Inta Ozols, Jess Thompson and Louise Cook from Elsevier.

Immunology bridges basic sciences and medicine and encompasses approaches from numerous fields, including biochemistry, genetics, cell biology, structural biology and molecular biology. For the past century, immunology has fascinated and inspired some of the greatest scientific thinkers of our time and numerous Nobel prizes have been awarded for fundamental discoveries in immunology, from Paul Ehrlich's work on antibodies (1908) to the studies of Zinkernagel and Doherty (1996) elucidating mechanisms of cell-mediated immunity. We wish our readers well in their study of immunology, a subject which continues to excite and surprise us, and which underpins many other areas of biology and biomedical sciences.

David Male
Jonathan Brostoff
David B Roth
Ivan Roitt
2006

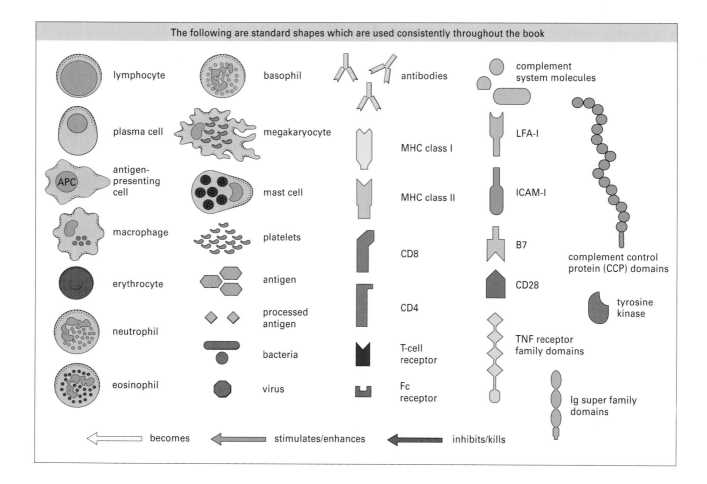

The following are standard shapes which are used consistently throughout the book

lymphocyte • basophil • antibodies • complement system molecules
plasma cell • megakaryocyte • MHC class I • LFA-I
antigen-presenting cell (APC) • mast cell • MHC class II • ICAM-I
macrophage • platelets • CD8 • B7 • complement control protein (CCP) domains
erythrocyte • antigen • CD4 • CD28 • tyrosine kinase
neutrophil • processed antigen • T-cell receptor • TNF receptor family domains
eosinophil • bacteria • Fc receptor • Ig super family domains
virus

becomes • stimulates/enhances • inhibits/kills

LIST OF CONTRIBUTORS

Arne Akbar
Professor of Immunology
Department of Immunology and
Molecular Pathology
Royal Free and University College
Medical School
Windeyer Institute of Medical Sciences
London, UK

Gregory J Bancroft
Reader in Immunology
Department of Infectious and Tropical
Diseases
London School of Hygiene and Tropical
Medicine
London, UK

Peter Beverley
Principal Reseach Fellow
The Edward Jenner Institute for Vaccine
Research
Compton
Berkshire, UK

Janette E Bradley
Chair of Parasitology
School of Biology
University of Nottingham
Nottingham, UK

Jonathan Brostoff
Professor Emeritus of Allergy and
Environmental Health
School of Biomedical and Health
Sciences
King's College London
London, UK

Warwick Britton
Professor of Medicine
Department of Medicine
Central Clinical School
University of Sydney
Sydney, NSW, Australia

Joanne E Cook
Postdoctoral Research Assistant
Department of Immunology and
Molecular Pathology
Royal Free and University College
Medical School
Windeyer Institute of Medical Sciences
London, UK

Andrew J T George
Professor of Molecular Immunology
Department of Immunology
Division of Medicine
Imperial College London
London, UK

Siamon Gordon
Professor of Cellular Pathology
Sir William Dunn School of Pathology
University of Oxford
Oxford, UK

Gillian M Griffiths
Professor of Experimental Pathology
Sir William Dunn School of Pathology
University of Oxford
Oxford, UK

Carlo E Grossi
Head of Department
Department of Experimental Medicine
Section of Human Anatomy
University of Genova
Genova, Italy

Frank Hay
Professor of Immunology and Society of
Apothecaries
Lecturer in the History of Medicine
Department of Biochemistry and
Immunology
St George's Hospital Medical School
London, UK

Roy Jefferis
Professor of Molecular Immunology
Division of Immunity and Infection
School of Medicine
University of Birmingham
Birmingham, UK

Robert I Lechler
Vice-Principal (Health)
Kings College London
London, UK

Jane Loughlin
Senior Lecturer in Cell Biology
Department of Biological Sciences
The Open University
Walton Hall
Milton Keynes
Bucks, UK

Peter Lydyard
Professor of Immunology
Department of Immunology and
Molecular Pathology
Division of Infection and Immunity
Royal Free and University College
Medical School
Windeyer Institute of Medical Sciences
London, UK

David Male
Professor of Biology
Department of Biological Sciences
The Open University
Walton Hall
Milton Keynes
Bucks, UK

Joseph C Marini
Principal Research Scientist
Clinical Pharmacology and Experimental
Medicine
Centocor Research and Development
Radnor
PA, USA

B Paul Morgan
Professor of Medical Biochemistry and Immunology
Department of Medical Biochemistry and Immunology
School of Medicine
University of Cardiff
Cardiff, UK

Anthony A Nash
Professor of Veterinary Pathology
Centre for Infectious Diseases
University of Edinburgh
Edinburgh, UK

Thomas A E Platts-Mills
Professor of Medicine
Asthma and Allergic Diseases Center
Charlottesville, VA, USA

Richard J Pleass
Lecturer of Parasite Immunology
Scholl of Biology
Institute of Genetics
Queens Medical Centre
University of Nottingham
Nottingham, UL

Ivan Roitt
Emeritus Professor of Immunology
Royal Free and University College Medical School
University College
London, UK

The late Fred S Rosen
Formerly Professor of Pediatrics
Harvard Medical School
The Centre for Blood Research
Boston , MA, USA

David B Roth
Irene Diamond Professor of Pathology
Investigator, Skirball Institute of Biomolecular Medicine
Program in Molecular Pathogenesis
Chairman, Departmental of Pathology
New York University School of Medicine
New York, NY, USA

P K Srivastava
Professor of Immunology
Director of the Center for Immunotherapy of Cancer and
Infectious Diseases
University of Connecticut School of Medicine
Farmington, CT, USA

John Trowsdale
Head of Division of Immunology
Cambridge University
Department of Pathology
Immunology Division
Cambridge, UK

Bruce D Walker
AIDS Research Center
Massachusetts General Hospital
Charlestown , MA, USA

Olwyn M R Westwood
MSc Programme Co-ordinator
School of Life Sciences
University of Surrey Roehampton
London, UK

D C Wraith
Professor of Experimental Pathology
Department of Pathology and Microbiology
University of Bristol
School of Medical Sciences
Bristol, UK

Components of the Immune System

Introduction to the Immune System

SUMMARY

- **The immune system has evolved to protect us from pathogens.** Intracellular pathogens infect individual cells (e.g. viruses), whereas extracellular pathogens divide extracellularly within tissues or the body cavities (e.g. many bacteria).

- **Phagocytes and lymphocytes are key mediators of immunity.** Phagocytes internalize pathogens and degrade them. Lymphocytes (B and T cells) bear receptors that recognize specific molecular components of pathogens and have specialized functions. B cells make antibodies, cytotoxic T lymphocytes (CTLs) kill virally infected cells, and helper T cells coordinate the immune response by direct cell–cell interactions and the release of cytokines.

- **Specificity and memory are two essential features of adaptive immune responses.** As a result the immune system mounts a more effective response on second and subsequent encounters with a particular antigen. Non-adaptive (innate) immune responses do not alter on repeated exposure to an infectious agent.

- **Antigens are molecules that are recognized by receptors on lymphocytes.** B cells usually recognize intact antigen molecules, whereas T cells recognize antigen fragments on the surface of other cells.

- **An immune response occurs in two phases – antigen recognition and antigen eradication.** In the first phase clonal selection involves recognition of antigen by particular clones of lymphocytes, leading to clonal expansion of specific clones of T and B cells and differentiation to effector and memory cells. In the effector phase, these lymphocytes coordinate an immune response, which eliminates the source of the antigen.

- **Vaccination depends on the specificity and memory of adaptive immunity.** Vaccination is based on the key elements of adaptive immunity, namely specificity and memory. Memory cells allow the immune system to mount a much stronger response on a second encounter with antigen.

- **Inflammation is a response to tissue damage.** It allows antibodies, complement system molecules, and leukocytes to enter the tissue at the site of infection, resulting in phagocytosis and destruction of the pathogens. Lymphocytes are also required to recognize and destroy infected cells in the tissues.

- **The immune system may fail (immunopathology).** This can lead to immunodeficiency, hypersensitivity, or autoimmune diseases.

- **Normal immune reactions can be inconvenient in modern medicine,** for example blood transfusion reactions and graft rejection.

THE IMMUNE SYSTEM PROTECTS US FROM PATHOGENS

A highly discriminatory immune system is fundamental to survival. How the immune system accomplishes this level of discrimination remains deeply enigmatic, but such questions are among the many that make immunology a fascinating discipline.

The immune system has evolved a powerful collection of defense mechanisms to protect against potential invaders that would otherwise take advantage of the rich source of nutrients provided by the vertebrate host. At the same time it:

- must be sophisticated enough to differentiate between the individual's own cells and those of harmful invading organisms and not attack the commensal flora that inhabit the gut, skin, and many other tissues to great benefit;
- should avoid rejecting tissue that is demonstrably foreign, namely the fetus.

This chapter provides an overview of the complex network of processes that form the immune system of higher vertebrates. It:

- illustrates how the components of the immune system fit together to allow students to rapidly grasp the 'big picture' before delving into the material in more depth in subsequent chapters;
- introduces the basic elements of the immune system and of immune responses, which are mediated principally by white blood cells or **leukocytes** (from the Greek for 'white cell') and are detailed in Chapters 2–18.

A description of cells and molecules important in immunology is given in Figs 1.1–1.4.

Over many millions of years, different types of immune defense, appropriate to the infecting pathogens, have evolved in different groups of organisms. In this book, we concentrate on the immune systems of mammals, especially humans. Because mammals are warm-blooded and long-lived, their immune systems have evolved particularly sophisticated systems for recognizing and destroying pathogens.

Q. Why do warm-blooded, long-lived animals require particularly complex immune defenses?
A. Infectious agents such as bacteria can divide rapidly in warm-blooded creatures. Animals have to remain healthy during their reproductive years to raise offspring.

Many of the immune defenses that have evolved in other vertebrates (e.g. reptiles, amphibians) and other phyla (e.g. sponges, worms, insects) are also present in some form in mammals and play crucial roles. Consequently the mammalian immune system consists of multi-layered, interlocking defense mechanisms that incorporate both primitive and recently evolved elements.

THE CELLS AND SOLUBLE MEDIATORS OF THE IMMUNE SYSTEM
Cells of the immune system
Immune responses are mediated by:
- a variety of cells; and
- the soluble molecules that these cells secrete (Fig. 1.1).

Although the leukocytes are central to all immune responses, other cells in the tissues also participate, by signaling to the lymphocytes and responding to the cytokines released by T cells and macrophages.

Phagocytes internalize antigens and pathogens and break them down
The most important long-lived phagocytic cells belong to the mononuclear phagocyte lineage. These cells are all derived from bone marrow stem cells, and their function is to:
- engulf particles, including infectious agents;
- internalize them; and
- destroy them.

For this purpose mononuclear phagocytes are strategically placed where they will encounter such particles. For example, the Kupffer cells of the liver line the sinusoids along which blood flows, while the synovial A cells line the synovial cavity (Fig. 1.2).

MONONUCLEAR PHAGOCYTES INCLUDE THE LONG-LIVED MONOCYTES AND MACROPHAGES – Leukocytes of the mononuclear phagocyte lineage are called **monocytes**. Monocytes migrate from the blood into the tissues, where they develop into tissue **macrophages**, which are very effective at presenting antigens to T cells (see Chapter 2, p. 21).

POLYMORPHONUCLEAR NEUTROPHILS ARE SHORT-LIVED PHAGOCYTES – Polymorphonuclear neutrophils (often just called **neutrophils** or **PMNs**) are another important group of phagocytes. Neutrophils constitute the majority

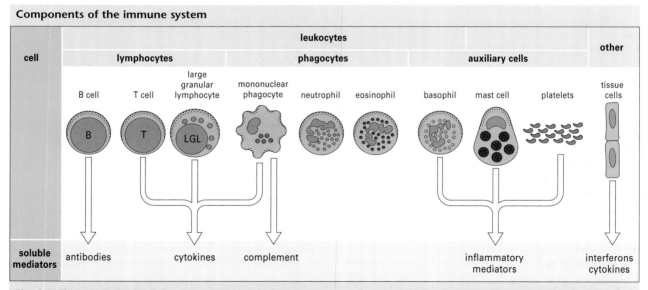

Fig. 1.1 The principal cells of the immune system and the mediators they produce are shown. Neutrophils, eosinophils, and basophils are collectively known as polymorphonuclear granulocytes (see Chapter 2). Cytotoxic cells include cytotoxic T lymphocytes (CTLs), natural killer (NK) cells (large granular lymphocytes [LGLs]), and eosinophils. Complement is made primarily by the liver, though there is some synthesis by mononuclear phagocytes. Note that each cell produces and secretes only a particular set of cytokines or inflammatory mediators.

Cells of the mononuclear phagocyte lineage

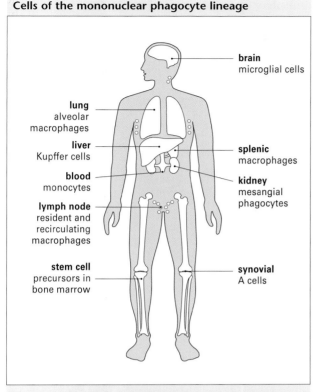

brain
microglial cells

lung
alveolar
macrophages

liver
Kupffer cells

blood
monocytes

lymph node
resident and
recirculating
macrophages

stem cell
precursors in
bone marrow

splenic
macrophages

kidney
mesangial
phagocytes

synovial
A cells

Fig. 1.2 Many organs contain cells belonging to the mononuclear phagocyte lineage. These cells are derived from blood monocytes and ultimately from stem cells in the bone marrow.

of the blood leukocytes and develop from the same early precursors as monocytes and macrophages.

Like monocytes, neutrophils migrate into tissues, particularly at sites of inflammation, However, neutrophils are short-lived cells that phagocytose material, destroy it, and then die.

B cells and T cells are responsible for the specific recognition of antigens

Lymphocytes are wholly responsible for the specific immune recognition of pathogens, so they initiate adaptive immune responses. All lymphocytes are derived from bone marrow stem cells, but T lymphocytes (T cells) then develop in the thymus, while B lymphocytes (B cells) develop in the bone marrow (in adult mammals).

B CELLS EXPRESS ANTIBODY – Each B cell is genetically programmed to express a surface receptor specific for a particular antigen. This antigen receptor molecule is called an **antibody**. If a B cell binds to its specific antigen, it will multiply and differentiate into **plasma cells** (see Fig. 1.13), which produce large amounts of the antibody, but in a secreted form.

Secreted antibody molecules are large glycoproteins found in the blood and tissue fluids. Because secreted antibody molecules are a soluble version of the original receptor molecule (antibody), they bind to the same antigen that initially activated the B cells.

T CELLS HAVE T CELL ANTIGEN RECEPTORS – There are several different types of T cell, and they have a variety of functions:
- one group interacts with mononuclear phagocytes and helps them destroy intracellular pathogens – these are called **type 1 helper T cells or TH1 cells**;
- another group interacts with B cells and helps them to divide, differentiate, and make antibody – these are the **type 2 helper T cells or TH2 cells**;
- a third group of T cells is responsible for the destruction of host cells that have become infected by viruses or other intracellular pathogens – this kind of action is called cytotoxicity and these T cells are therefore called **cytotoxic T lymphocytes (CTLs or Tc cells)**.

In every case, the T cells recognize antigens present on the surface of other cells using a specific receptor – the **T cell antigen receptor (TCR)** – which is quite distinct from, but related in structure to, the antigen receptor (antibody) on B cells.

T cells generate their effects either:
- by releasing soluble proteins, called **cytokines**, which signal to other cells; or
- by direct cell–cell interactions.

Cytotoxic cells recognize and destroy other cells that have become infected

Several cell types have the capacity to kill other cells should they become infected. Cytotoxic cells include CTLs, natural killer (NK) cells (large granular lymphocytes), and eosinophils. Of these, the CTL is especially important, but other cell types may be active against particular types of infection.

All of these cell types damage their different targets by releasing the contents of their intracellular granules close to them. Cytokines secreted by the cytotoxic cells, but not stored in granules, contribute to the damage.

LARGE GRANULAR LYMPHOCYTES ARE ALSO KNOWN AS NK CELLS – Lymphocytes known as large granular lymphocytes (LGLs) have the capacity to recognize the surface changes that occur on a variety of tumor cells and virally infected cells. LGLs damage these target cells, but use a different recognition system to CTLs. This action is sometimes called NK cell activity, so these cells are also described as NK cells.

EOSINOPHIL POLYMORPHS ENGAGE AND DAMAGE LARGE EXTRACELLULAR PARASITES – Eosinophils are a specialized group of leukocytes that have the ability to engage and damage large extracellular parasites, such as schistosomes.

Auxiliary cells control inflammation

The main purpose of inflammation is to attract leukocytes and the soluble mediators of immunity towards a site of infection. Inflammation is mediated by a variety of other cells including basophils, mast cells, and platelets.

BASOPHILS AND MAST CELLS RELEASE MEDIATORS OF INFLAMMATION – Basophils and mast cells have granules that contain a variety of mediators, which:
- induce inflammation in surrounding tissues; and
- are released when the cells are triggered.

Basophils and mast cells can also synthesize and secrete a number of mediators that control the development of immune reactions.

Mast cells lie close to blood vessels in all tissues, and some of their mediators act on cells in the vessel walls. Basophils are functionally similar to mast cells, but are mobile, circulating cells.

PLATELETS RELEASE MEDIATORS OF INFLAMMATION – Platelets are essential in blood clotting, but can also be activated during immune responses to release mediators of inflammation.

Soluble mediators of immunity

A wide variety of molecules are involved in the development of immune responses, including:
- antibodies and cytokines, produced by lymphocytes; and
- other molecules that are normally present in serum.

The serum concentration of a number of these proteins increases rapidly during infection and they are therefore called **acute phase proteins**.

One example of an acute phase protein is **C reactive protein (CRP)**, so-called because of its ability to bind to the C protein of pneumococci. This promotes the uptake of pneumococci by phagocytes, a process known as opsonization. Molecules such as antibody and CRP that promote phagocytosis are said to act as opsonins.

Another important group of molecules that can act as opsonins are components of the complement system.

Complement proteins mediate phagocytosis, control inflammation, and interact with antibodies in immune defense

The complement system is a group of about 20 serum proteins whose overall function is the control of inflammation (Fig. 1.3 and see Chapter 4). The components interact with each other, and with other elements of the immune system. For example:
- a number of microorganisms spontaneously activate the complement system, via the so-called '**alternative pathway**', which is an innate immune defense – this results in the microorganism being opsonized (i.e. coated by complement molecules, leading to its uptake by phagocytes);
- the complement system can also be activated by antibodies or by mannose binding lectin bound to the pathogen surface via the '**classical pathway**'.

Complement activation is a cascade reaction, where one component acts enzymatically on the next component in the cascade to generate an enzyme, which mediates the following step in the reaction sequence, and so on. (The blood clotting system also works as an enzyme cascade.)

Activation of the complement system generates protein molecules or peptide fragments, which have the following effects:

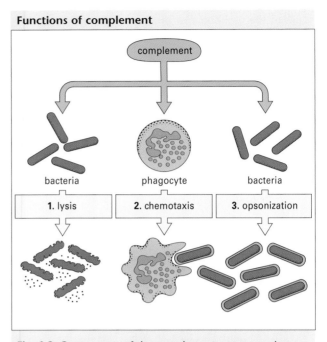

Functions of complement

Fig. 1.3 Components of the complement system can lyse many bacterial species (**1**). Complement fragments released in this reaction attract phagocytes to the site of the reaction (**2**). Complement components opsonize the bacteria for phagocytosis (**3**). In addition to the responses shown here, activation of the complement system increases blood flow and vascular permeability at the site of activation. Activated components can also induce the release of inflammatory mediators from mast cells.

- opsonization of microorganisms for uptake by phagocytes and eventual intracellular killing;
- attraction of phagocytes to sites of infection (chemotaxis);
- increased blood flow to the site of activation and increased permeability of capillaries to plasma molecules;
- damage to plasma membranes on cells, Gram-negative bacteria, enveloped viruses, or other organisms that have induced the activation, which in turn can result in lysis of the cell or virus and so reduce the infection;
- release of inflammatory mediators from mast cells.

Cytokines signal between lymphocytes, phagocytes, and other cells of the body

Cytokine is the general term for a large group of molecules involved in signaling between cells during immune responses. All cytokines are proteins or glycoproteins. The different cytokines fall into a number of categories, and the principal subgroups of cytokines are outlined below.

INTERFERONS LIMIT THE SPREAD OF CERTAIN VIRAL INFECTIONS – **Interferons (IFNs)** are cytokines that are particularly important in limiting the spread of certain viral infections:

- one group of interferons (IFNα and IFNβ) is produced by cells that have become infected by a virus;
- another type, IFNγ, is released by activated TH1 cells.

IFNs induce a state of antiviral resistance in uninfected cells (Fig. 1.4). They are produced very early in infection and are important in delaying the spread of a virus until such time as the adaptive immune response has developed.

INTERLEUKINS HAVE A VARIETY OF FUNCTIONS – The **interleukins (ILs)** are a large group of cytokines produced mainly by T cells, though some are also produced by mononuclear phagocytes or by tissue cells. They have a variety of functions. Many interleukins cause other cells to divide and differentiate.

COLONY STIMULATING FACTORS DIRECT THE DIVISION AND DIFFERENTIATION OF LEUKOCYTE PRECURSORS – **Colony stimulating factors (CSFs)** are cytokines primarily involved in directing the division and differentiation of bone marrow stem cells, and the precursors of blood leukocytes. The balance of different CSFs is partially responsible for the proportions of different immune cell types produced. Some CSFs also promote further differentiation of cells outside the bone marrow. For example, macrophage CSF (M-CSF) promotes the development of monocytes in bone marrow and macrophages in tissues.

CHEMOKINES DIRECT THE MOVEMENT OF LEUKOCYTES AROUND THE BODY – **Chemokines** are a large group of chemotactic cytokines that direct the movement of leukocytes around the body, from the blood stream into the tissues and to the appropriate location within each tissue. Some chemokines also activate cells to carry out particular functions.

OTHER CYTOKINES INCLUDE TNFα AND TNFβ, AND TGFβ – **Tumor necrosis factors** TNFα and TNFβ, and **transforming growth factor-β (TGFβ)**, have a variety of functions, but are particularly important in mediating inflammation and cytotoxic reactions.

EACH SET OF CELLS RELEASES A PARTICULAR BLEND OF CYTOKINES – Each set of cells releases a particular blend of cytokines, depending on the type of cell and whether, and how, it has been activated. For example:
- TH1 cells release one set of cytokines, which promote TH1 cell interactions with mononuclear phagocytes;
- TH2 cells release a different set of cytokines, which allow TH2 cells to activate B cells.

Some cytokines may be produced by all T cells, and some just by a specific subset.

Equally important is the expression of cytokine receptors. Only a cell that has the appropriate receptors can respond to a particular cytokine. For example:
- the receptors for interferons (see above) are present on all nucleated cells in the body;
- other receptors are much more restricted in their distribution.

In general, cytokine receptors are specific for their own individual cytokine, but this is not always so. In particular, many chemokine receptors respond to several different chemokines.

IMMUNE RESPONSES ARE ADAPTED TO DIFFERENT TYPES OF PATHOGEN

The environment contains a great variety of infectious agents, including bacteria, viruses, fungi, Protoctista, and multicellular parasites, which can enter the body and cause disease and, if they multiply unchecked, death.

The primary function of the immune system is to eliminate infectious agents and minimize the damage they cause. It ensures that most infections in normal individuals are short-lived and leave little permanent damage.

Infectious agents that cause damage are referred to as **pathogens**. However, even normally harmless organisms can pose a lethal threat to an individual who has a defect in a critical component of their immune system (see Chapters 16 and 17).

The immune system can fail to act or act inappropriately in a variety of ways, leading to immunopathological reactions. The paramount importance of immune defenses is underscored by the fact that individuals with genetic defects in various components of the immune system succumb to infections early in life (see Chapter 16).

Immune system responses vary and depend on the pathogen

Pathogens use many modes of transmission and reproduction, so the immune system has evolved many ways of responding to them.

The exterior defenses of the body (Fig. 1.5) present an effective barrier to most organisms. Very few infectious agents can penetrate intact skin. In contrast:
- many infectious agents gain access to the body across the epithelia of the gastrointestinal or urogenital tracts;

Interferons

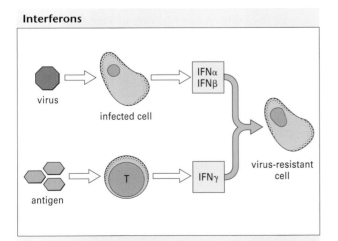

Fig. 1.4 Host cells that have been infected by virus secrete interferon-α (IFNα) and/or interferon-β (IFNβ). TH1 cells secrete interferon-γ (IFNγ) after activation by antigen. IFNs act on other host cells to induce resistance to viral infection. IFNγ has many other effects as well.

Exterior defenses

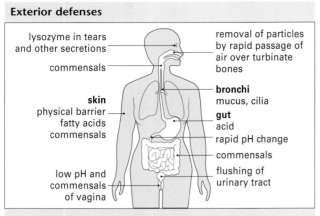

lysozyme in tears and other secretions

commensals

removal of particles by rapid passage of air over turbinate bones

bronchi
mucus, cilia

skin
physical barrier
fatty acids
commensals

gut
acid

rapid pH change

commensals

flushing of urinary tract

low pH and commensals of vagina

Fig. 1.5 Most infectious agents are prevented from entering the body by physical and biochemical barriers. The body tolerates a number of commensal organisms, which compete effectively with many potential pathogens.

- others, such as the virus responsible for the common cold, infect the respiratory epithelium of nasopharynx and lung;
- a small number of infectious agents infect the body only if they enter the blood directly (e.g. malaria and sleeping sickness).

Once inside the body, the site of the infection and the nature of the pathogen largely determine which type of immune response will be induced – most importantly (Fig. 1.6) whether the pathogen is:

Intracellular and extracellular pathogens

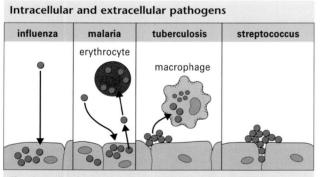

| influenza | malaria | tuberculosis | streptococcus |

erythrocyte

macrophage

Fig. 1.6 All infectious agents spread to infect new cells by passing through the body fluids or tissues. Many are intracellular pathogens and must infect cells of the body to divide and reproduce (e.g. viruses such as influenza viruses and malaria, which has two separate phases of division, either in cells of the liver or in erythrocytes). The mycobacteria that cause tuberculosis can divide outside cells or within macrophages. Some bacteria (e.g. streptococci, which produce sore throats and wound infections) generally divide outside cells and are therefore extracellular pathogens.

- an **intracellular pathogen** (i.e. invades the host cells to divide and reproduce); or
- an **extracellular pathogen** (i.e. does not invade the host cells);

Many bacteria and larger parasites live in tissues, body fluids, or other extracellular spaces, and are susceptible to the multitude of immune defenses, such as **antibodies** (see Chapter 3) and **complement** (see Chapter 4), that are present in these areas. Because these components are present in the tissue fluids of the body (the 'humors' of ancient medicine), they have been classically referred to as **humoral immunity**.

Some pathogens evade 'humoral immunity'

Many organisms (e.g. viruses, some bacteria, some parasites) evade these formidable defenses by being intracellular pathogens and replicating within host cells. To clear these infections, the immune system has developed ways to specifically recognize and destroy infected cells. This is largely the job of **cell-mediated immunity**.

Intracellular pathogens cannot, however, wholly evade the extracellular defenses (see Fig. 1.6) because they must reach their host cells by moving through the blood and tissue fluids. As a result they are susceptible to humoral immunity during this portion of their life cycle.

Any immune response involves:
- first, recognition of the pathogen or other foreign material; and
- second, a reaction to eliminate it.

Innate immune responses are the same on each encounter with antigen

Broadly speaking, immune responses fall into two categories – those that become more powerful following repeated encounters with the same antigen (**adaptive immune responses**) and those that do not become more powerful following repeated encounters with the same antigen (**innate immune responses**).

Innate immune responses (see Chapter 6) can be thought of as simple though remarkably sophisticated systems present in all animals that are the first line of defense against pathogens and allow a rapid response to invasion.

Innate immune response systems range from external barriers (skin, mucous membranes, cilia, secretions, and tissue fluids containing antimicrobial agents; see Fig. 1.5) to sophisticated receptors capable of recognizing broad classes of pathogenic organisms, for example:
- innate immune receptors on certain leukocytes recognize **pathogen-associated molecular patterns (PAMPs)**, which are common to many foreign invaders and are not normally present in the host (e.g. constituents of bacterial cell walls);
- components of the complement system (see Chapter 4), which are important soluble mediators of innate immunity, can be specifically activated by bacterial surface molecules.

The innate defenses are closely interlinked with adaptive responses.

Phagocytes internalize and kill invading organisms

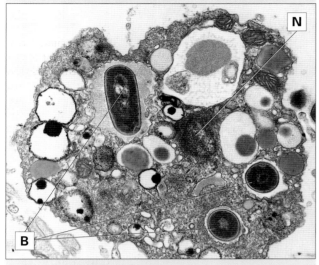

Fig. 1.7 Electron micrograph of a phagocyte from a tunicate (sea squirt) that has endocytosed three bacteria (B). (N, nucleus) (Courtesy of Dr AF Rowley)

PHAGOCYTES AND LYMPHOCYTES ARE KEY MEDIATORS OF IMMUNITY
Phagocytes are a first line of defense against infection

Phagocytes are found in all animals and are cells that ingest foreign substances. They form an important part of the innate immune system and include monocytes, macrophages, and neutrophils.

Phagocytes bind to invading organisms using a variety of receptors that recognize PAMPs and then internalize and kill the organism (Fig. 1.7). **Phagocytosis** describes the internalization (endocytosis) of large particles or microbes.

The primitive responses of phagocytes are highly effective, and people with genetic defects in certain phagocytic cells usually succumb to infections in infancy.

Lymphocytes have specialized functions

Adaptive immune responses are mediated by a specialized group of leukocytes, the **lymphocytes**, which includes T and B lymphocytes (T cells and B cells). These two classes of lymphocytes carry out very different protective functions:

- **B cells** are responsible for the humoral arm of the adaptive immune system, and thus act against extracellular pathogens;
- **T cells** are responsible for the cell-mediated arm of the adaptive immune system, and are mainly concerned with cellular immune responses to intracellular pathogens, such as viruses, and also with regulation of B cell responses.

B cells express their antigen receptor (**immunoglobulin** molecules) on their cell surface during their development and, when mature, secrete soluble immunoglobulin molecules (also known as antibodies) into the extracellular fluids.

Immunoglobulins are an essential component of humoral immunity, and, when bound to their cognate antigens, can activate the complement system and help phagocytes to take up antigens.

T cells recognize antigen via cell surface receptors (**T cell receptors**) and have a wide range of biological functions (Fig. 1.8):

- some are involved in the control of B cell development and antibody production;
- another group of T cells interacts with phagocytic cells to help them destroy pathogens they have taken up;
- a third set of T cells recognizes cells infected by virus and destroys them.

Functions of different types of lymphocyte

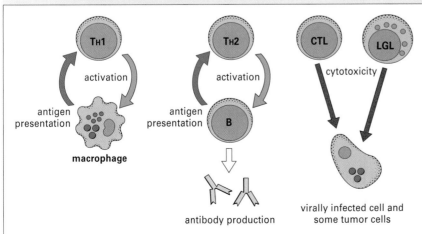

Fig. 1.8 Macrophages present antigen to TH1 cells, which then activate the macrophages to destroy phagocytosed pathogens. B cells present antigen to TH2 cells, which activate the B cells, causing them to divide and differentiate. Cytotoxic T lymphocytes (CTLs) and large granular lymphocytes (LGLs) recognize and destroy virally infected cells.

SPECIFICITY AND MEMORY ARE KEY FEATURES OF THE ADAPTIVE IMMUNE RESPONSE

In contrast to the innate immune response, which recognizes common molecular patterns such as PAMPs (see p. 140) in potential invaders, the adaptive immune system takes a highly discriminatory approach, with a very large repertoire of specific antigen receptors that can recognize virtually any component of a foreign invader (see Chapters 3 and 5). This use of highly specific antigen receptor molecules provides the following advantages:

- pathogens that lack stereotypical patterns (which might avoid recognition by the innate immune system) can be recognized;
- responses can be highly specific for a given pathogen;
- the **specificity** of the response allows the generation of immunological memory – related to its use of highly individual antigen receptors, the adaptive immune system has the capacity to 'remember' a pathogen.

These features underlie the phenomenon of specific immunity (e.g. diseases such as measles and diphtheria induce adaptive immune responses that generate life-long immunity following an infection).

Specific immunity can, very often, be induced by artificial means, allowing the development of vaccines (see Chapter 18).

ANTIGENS ARE MOLECULES RECOGNIZED BY RECEPTORS ON LYMPHOCYTES

Originally the term **antigen** was used for any molecule that induced B cells to produce a specific antibody (*anti*body *gen*erator). This term is now more widely used to indicate molecules that are specifically recognized by antigen receptors of either B cells or T cells.

Antigens, defined broadly, are molecules that initiate adaptive immune responses (e.g. components of pathogenic organisms), though purists may prefer the term **immunogen** in this context.

Antigens are not just components of foreign substances, such as pathogens. A large variety of 'self' molecules can serve as antigens as well, provoking autoimmune responses that can be highly damaging, and even lethal (see Chapter 20).

Antigens are the initiators and driving forces of all adaptive immune responses

The immune system has evolved to recognize antigens, destroy them, and eliminate the source of their production (e.g. bacteria, virally infected cells). When antigen is eliminated, immune responses switch off.

Both T cell receptors and immunoglobulin molecules (antibody) bind to their cognate antigens with a high degree of specificity. These two types of receptor molecules have striking structural relationships and are closely related evolutionarily, but bind to very different types of antigens and carry out quite different biological functions.

Antibody specifically binds to antigen

Soluble antibodies (also called immunoglobulins) are a group of serum molecules closely related to and derived from the antigen receptors on B cells.

All antibodies have the same basic Y-shaped structure, with two regions (variable regions) at the tips of the Y that bind to antigen. The stem of the Y is referred to as the constant region and is not involved in antigen binding (see Chapter 3).

The two variable regions contain identical antigen-binding sites that, in general, are specific for only one type of antigen. The amino acid sequences of the variable regions of different antibodies, however, are extremely variable. The antibody molecules in the body therefore provide an extremely large repertoire of antigen-binding sites. The way in which this great diversity of antibody variable regions is generated is explained in Chapter 3.

Each antibody binds to a restricted part of the antigen called an epitope

Pathogens typically have many different antigens on their surface. Each antibody binds to an **epitope**, which is a restricted part of the antigen. A particular antigen can have several different epitopes or repeated epitopes (Fig. 1.9). Antibodies are specific for the epitopes rather than the whole antigen molecule.

Q. Many evolutionarily related proteins have conserved amino acid sequences. What consequences might this have in terms of the antigenicity of these proteins?

A. Related proteins (with a high degree of sequence similarity) may contain the same epitopes and therefore be recognized by the same antibodies.

Fc regions of antibodies act as adapters to link phagocytes to pathogens

The constant region of the antibody (the Fc region, see Chapter 3) can bind to Fc receptors on phagocytes, so acting as an adapter between the phagocyte and the

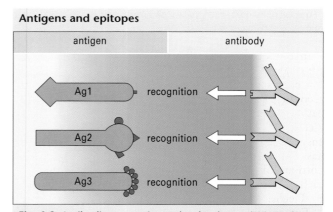

Antigens and epitopes

antigen	antibody

Ag1 — recognition ←

Ag2 — recognition ←

Ag3 — recognition ←

Fig. 1.9 Antibodies recognize molecular shapes (epitopes) on the surface of antigens. Each antigen (Ag1, Ag2, Ag3) may have several epitopes recognized by different antibodies. Some antigens have repeated epitopes (Ag3).

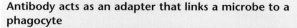

Antibody acts as an adapter that links a microbe to a phagocyte

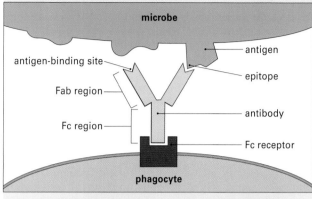

Fig. 1.10 The antibody binds to a region of an antigen (an epitope) on the microbe surface, using one of its antigen-binding sites. These sites are in the Fab regions of the antibody. The stem of the antibody, the Fc region, can attach to receptors on the surface of the phagocytes.

Opsonization

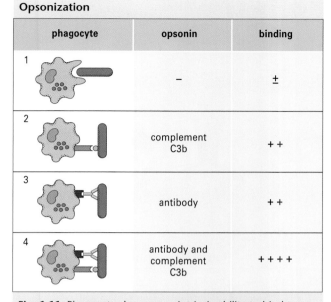

	phagocyte	opsonin	binding
1		–	±
2		complement C3b	+ +
3		antibody	+ +
4		antibody and complement C3b	+ + + +

Fig. 1.11 Phagocytes have some intrinsic ability to bind to bacteria and other microorganisms (**1**). This is much enhanced if the bacteria have been opsonized by complement C3b (**2**) or antibody (**3**), each of which cross-link the bacteria to receptors on the phagocyte. Antibody can also activate complement, and if antibody and C3b both opsonize the bacteria, binding is greatly enhanced (**4**).

pathogen (Fig. 1.10). Consequently, if antibody binds to a pathogen, it can link to a phagocyte and promote phagocytosis.

The process in which specific binding of an antibody activates an innate immune defense (phagocytosis) is an important example of collaboration between the innate and adaptive immune responses.

Other molecules (such as activated complement proteins) can also enhance phagocytosis when bound to microbial surfaces. The general process is termed **opsonization** (from the Latin, opsono, 'to prepare victuals for') to "render microorganisms delectable so that the white blood corpuscles pitch into them with an appetite" (GB Shaw).

Binding and phagocytosis are most effective when more than one type of adapter molecule (**opsonin**) is present (Fig. 1.11). Note that antibody can act as an adapter in many other circumstances, not just phagocytosis.

Peptides from intracellular pathogens are displayed on the surface of infected cells

Antibodies patrol only extracellular spaces and so only recognize and target for destruction extracellular pathogens. Intracellular pathogens (such as viruses) can escape antibody-mediated responses once they are safely ensconced within a host cell. The adaptive immune system has therefore evolved a specific method of displaying portions of virtually all cell proteins on the surface of each nucleated cell in the body so they can be recognized by T cells.

For example, a cell infected with a virus will present fragments of viral proteins (peptides) on its surface that are recognizable by T cells. The antigenic peptides are transported to the cell surface and presented to the T cells by **MHC molecules** (see Chapter 5). T cells use their antigen-specific receptors (T cell receptors – TCRs) to recognize the antigenic peptide–MHC molecule complex (Fig. 1.12).

Q. Why is it necessary to have a mechanism that transports antigen fragments to the host cell surface for cytotoxic T cells to recognize infected cells?

A. The T cell cannot 'see' what is going on inside an infected cell. Its antigen receptor can only interact with and recognize what is present on the surface of cells. Therefore antigen fragments need to be transported to the cell surface for recognition, and this is the key function of MHC molecules.

T cell responses require proper presentation of antigen by MHC molecules (**antigen presentation**). To activate T cell responses this must occur on the surface of specialized **antigen-presenting cells (APCs)**, which internalize antigens by phagocytosis or endocytosis. Several different types of leukocyte can act as APCs, including dendritic cells, macrophages, and B cells.

APCs not only display antigenic peptide–MHC complexes on their surface, but also express co-stimulatory molecules that are essential for initiating immune responses (see Chapter 7).

Co-stimulatory signals are upregulated by the presence of pathogens, which can be detected by the engagement of innate immune receptors that recognize PAMPs.

T cell recognition of antigen

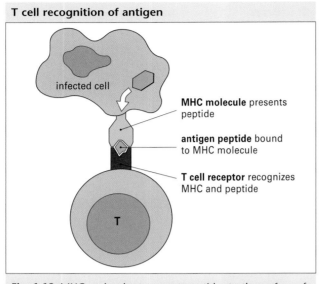

infected cell

MHC molecule presents peptide

antigen peptide bound to MHC molecule

T cell receptor recognizes MHC and peptide

T

Fig. 1.12 MHC molecules transport peptides to the surface of an infected cell where they are presented to T cells, which may recognize the MHC–peptide combination. If a cell is infected, MHC molecules present peptides derived from the pathogen, as well as the cell's own proteins.

T cells comprise the cell-mediated arm of the adaptive immune system

T cells recognize antigens only in the context of cell–cell interactions. A T cell must dock with an APC that bears the correct antigenic peptide presented by an MHC molecule. T cells therefore comprise the cell-mediated arm of the adaptive immune system. T cells function only in the context of intimate cell–cell contacts, which allow either:

- helper functions, such as control of antibody responses via contacts with APCs and B cells; or
- cytolytic functions, that is the recognition and lysis of virally infected cells requiring cell–cell contact.

These functions are carried out by different types of T cell, namely **helper T cells (TH)** and **cytotoxic T lymphocytes (CTLs or Tc cells)**.

ANTIGEN RECOGNITION AND ANTIGEN ERADICATION – THE TWO PHASES OF IMMUNE RESPONSES

Most immune responses to infectious organisms are made up of a variety of innate and adaptive components:

- in the earliest stages of infection, innate responses predominate;
- later the lymphocytes start to generate adaptive immune responses;
- after recovery, immunological memory remains within the population of lymphocytes, which can then mount a more effective and rapid response if there is a reinfection with the same pathogen at a later date.

The two major phases of any immune response are antigen recognition and a reaction to eradicate the antigen.

Lymphocytes are responsible for antigen recognition

In adaptive immune responses, lymphocytes are responsible for immune recognition, and this is achieved by **clonal selection**.

Antigen selects and activates specific clones of lymphocyte

Each lymphocyte is genetically programmed to be capable of recognizing just one particular antigen. However, the immune system as a whole can specifically recognize many thousands of antigens, so the lymphocytes that recognize any particular antigen are only a tiny proportion of the total.

How then is an adequate immune response to an infectious agent generated? The answer is that, when an antigen binds to the few lymphocytes that can recognize it, they are induced to proliferate rapidly. Within a few days there is a sufficient number to mount an adequate immune response. In other words, the antigen selects and activates the specific clones to which it binds (Fig. 1.13), a process called clonal selection. This operates for both B cells and T cells.

B cell clonal selection

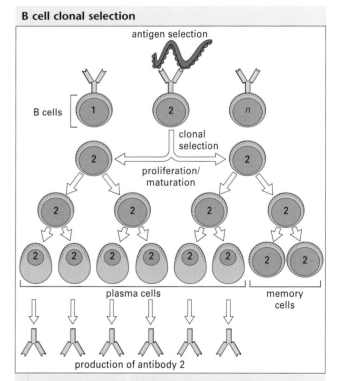

antigen selection

B cells

clonal selection

proliferation/ maturation

plasma cells

memory cells

production of antibody 2

Fig. 1.13 Each B cell expresses just one antibody (i.e. with specificity for a single particular antigen), which it uses as its antigen receptor. Antigen binds only to those B cells with the specific antibody (number 2 in this example), driving these cells to divide and differentiate into plasma cells and memory cells, all having the same specificity as the original B cell. Thus an antigen selects just the clones of B cells that can react against it.

How can the immune system 'know' which specific antibodies will be needed during an individual's lifetime? It does not know. The immune system generates antibodies (and T cell receptors) that can recognize an enormous range of antigens even before it encounters them. Many of these specificities, which are generated more or less at random (see Chapters 3 and 5), will never be called upon to protect the individual against infection.

Q. What advantage could there be in having an immune system that generates billions of lymphocytes that do not recognize any known infectious agent?
A. Many pathogens mutate their surface antigens. If the immune system could not recognize new variants of pathogens, it would not be able to make an effective response. By having a wide range of antigen receptors, at least some of the lymphocytes will be able to recognize any pathogen that enters the body.

Lymphocytes that have been stimulated, by binding to their specific antigen, take the first steps towards cell division. They:
- express new receptors that allow them to respond to cytokines from other cells, which signal proliferation;
- may start to secrete cytokines themselves;
- will usually go through a number of cycles of division before differentiating into mature cells, again under the influence of cytokines.

For example, proliferating B cells eventually mature into antibody-producing **plasma cells**.

Even when the infection has been overcome, some of the newly produced lymphocytes remain, available for restimulation if the antigen is ever encountered again. These cells are called **memory cells**, because they are generated by past encounters with particular antigens. Memory cells confer lasting immunity to a particular pathogen.

Antigen eradication involves effector systems

There are numerous ways in which the immune system can destroy pathogens, each being suited to a given type of infection at a particular stage of its life cycle. These defense mechanisms are often referred to as effector systems.

ANTIBODY BINDING RESULTING IN NEUTRALIZATION – In one of the simplest effector systems, antibodies can combat certain pathogens just by binding to them. For example, antibody to the outer coat proteins of some rhinoviruses (which cause colds) can prevent the viral particles from binding to and infecting host cells.

PHAGOCYTOSIS IS PROMOTED BY COMPLEMENT AND OPSONINS – More often antibody activates complement or acts as an opsonin to promote ingestion by phagocytes.

Phagocytes that have bound to an opsonized microbe, engulf it by extending pseudopodia around it. These fuse and the microorganism is internalized (endocytosed) in a phagosome. Granules and lysosomes fuse with the phagosome, pouring enzymes into the resulting phagolysosome, to digest the contents (Fig. 1.14). The mechanisms involved are described fully in Chapters 9 and 15.

Phagocytes have several ways of dealing with internalized opsonized microbes in phagosomes. For example:
- macrophages reduce molecular oxygen to form microbicidal reactive oxygen intermediates (ROIs), which are secreted into the phagosome;
- neutrophils contain lactoferrin, which chelates iron and prevents some bacteria from obtaining this vital nutrient.

CYTOTOXIC REACTIONS ARE DIRECTED AGAINST WHOLE CELLS – Cytotoxic reactions are effector systems directed against whole cells that are in general too large for phagocytosis.

The target cell may be recognized either by:
- specific antibody bound to the cell surface; or
- T cells using their specific TCRs.

In cytotoxic reactions the attacking cells direct their granules towards the target cell (in contrast to phagocytosis where the contents are directed into the phagosome). As a result granules are discharged into the extracellular space close to the target cell.

The granules of CTLs contain molecules called **perforins**, which can punch holes in the outer membrane of the target (see Fig. 10.12). (In a similar way, antibody bound to the surface of a target cell can direct complement to make holes in the cell's plasma membrane.)

Some cytotoxic cells can signal to the target cell to initiate programmed cell death – a process called **apoptosis**.

Q. What risks are associated with discharging granule contents into the extracellular space?
A. Cells other than the target cell may be damaged. This is minimized by close intercellular contact between the CTL and the target cell.

Phagocytosis

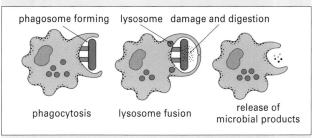

phagosome forming   lysosome   damage and digestion

phagocytosis   lysosome fusion   release of microbial products

Fig. 1.14 Phagocytes attach to microorganisms using cell surface receptors for microbial products or via antibody or complement C3b. Pseudopods extend around the microorganism and fuse to form a phagosome. Killing mechanisms are activated and lysosomes fuse with the phagosomes, releasing digestive enzymes that break down the microbe. Undigested microbial products may be released to the outside.

Termination of immune responses to avoid damaging host tissues

Although it is important to initiate immune responses quickly, it is also critical to terminate them appropriately once the threat has ended.

To clear the offending pathogen immune responses are often massive, with:

- millions of activated lymphocytes;
- proliferation of large clones of specific T and B cells;
- activation of huge numbers of inflammatory cells.

These responses, if left unchecked, can also damage host tissues.

A number of mechanisms are employed to dampen or terminate immune responses. One is a passive process – that is, simple clearance of antigen should lead to a diminution of immune responses.

Q. Why would removal of antigen lead to the decline in an immune response?

A. Antigen is required to stimulate B cell proliferation and differentiation, with the consequent production of antibody. Antigen combined with antibody activates several effector systems (e.g. complement). Antigen is also required to stimulate T cells with consequent production of cytokines. Therefore removal of antigen takes away the primary stimulus for lymphocyte activation.

Antigen elimination can be a slow process, however, so the immune system also employs a variety of active mechanisms to downregulate responses, as discussed in Chapter 11.

The innate and adaptive arms of the immune system interact and collaborate

Many examples of the intimate interconnections between the innate and adaptive arms of the immune defense network (some of which are outlined below) are explored in Chapters 3, 4, 6, and 9.

A key regulatory control for initiating immune responses

The recognition of PAMPs by innate immune receptors provides a key regulatory control for initiating immune responses (see Chapter 6). The innate immune system:

- senses 'danger' (e.g. by detecting the presence of bacterial cell wall material); and
- upregulates co-stimulatory molecules on the surface of APCs, allowing them to become potent activators of T cell (and, indirectly, B cell) responses.

This is a good example of collaboration between the innate and adaptive arms of the immune system.

Adaptive responses can augment innate immune defenses

In the example of antigen presentation given above (i.e. the presentation of bacterial antigens), the activated T cells release soluble signaling molecules (**cytokines**), which activate the phagocytes and cause them to destroy the pathogens they have internalized. Thus, the collaboration between T cells and APCs can be viewed as a two-way system (see Chapter 7).

Q. Can you think of another example where soluble factors from lymphocytes help in the destruction of pathogens?

A. Opsonization of pathogens by antibodies is another classic example of collaboration between innate and adaptive immune defenses.

Antibody can activate the complement system

Antibodies bound to bacterial surfaces can also stimulate activation of the complement system – an innate defense mechanism that enhances phagocytosis and drills holes in the outer phospholipid membrane of some types of bacteria, leading to their lysis (see Chapter 4).

Immune responses to extracellular and intracellular pathogens differ

In dealing with extracellular pathogens, the immune system aims to destroy the pathogen itself and neutralize its products.

In dealing with intracellular pathogens, the immune system has two options:

- T cells can destroy the infected cell (i.e. cytotoxicity); or
- T cells can activate the infected cell to deal with the pathogen itself (e.g. helper T cells release cytokines, which activate macrophages to destroy the organisms they have internalized).

Because many pathogens have both intracellular and extracellular phases of infection, different mechanisms are usually effective at different times. For example, the polio virus travels from the gut, through the blood stream to infect nerve cells in the spinal cord. Antibody is particularly effective at blocking the early phase of infection while the virus is in the blood stream, but to clear an established infection CTLs must kill any cell that has become infected.

Consequently, antibody is important in limiting the spread of infection and preventing reinfection with the same virus, while CTLs are essential to deal with infected cells (Fig. 1.15). These factors play an important part in the development of effective vaccines.

VACCINATION DEPENDS ON THE SPECIFICITY AND MEMORY OF ADAPTIVE IMMUNITY

The study of immunology has had its most successful application in vaccination (see Chapter 18), which is based on the key elements of adaptive immunity, namely specificity and memory. Memory cells allow the immune system to mount a much stronger response on a second encounter with antigen. Compared with the primary response, the secondary response is:

- faster to appear;
- more effective.

The aim in vaccine development is to alter a pathogen or its toxins in such a way that they become innocuous without losing antigenicity. This is possible because antibodies and T cells recognize particular parts of antigens (the **epitopes**), and not the whole organism or toxin.

Take, for example, vaccination against tetanus. The tetanus bacterium produces a toxin that acts on receptors

Reaction to extracellular and intracellular pathogens

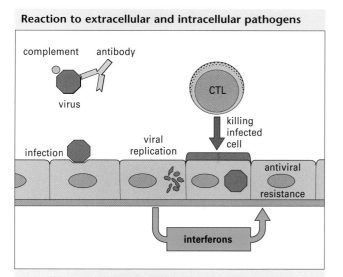

Fig. 1.15 Different immunological systems are effective against different types of infection, here illustrated as a virus infection. Antibodies and complement can block the extracellular phase of the life cycle and promote phagocytosis of the virus. Interferons produced by infected cells signal to uninfected cells to induce a state of antiviral resistance. Viruses can multiply only within living cells; cytotoxic T lymphocytes (CTLs) recognize and destroy the infected cells.

to cause tetanic contractions of muscle. The toxin can be modified by formalin treatment so that it retains its epitopes, but loses its toxicity. The resulting molecule (known as a toxoid) is used as a vaccine (Fig. 1.16).

Whole infectious agents, such as the poliovirus, can be attenuated so they retain their antigenicity, but lose their pathogenicity.

INFLAMMATION IS A RESPONSE TO TISSUE DAMAGE

Tissue damage caused by physical agents (e.g. trauma or radiation) or by pathogens results in the tissue response of **inflammation** (see p. 128), which has three principal components:

- increased blood supply to the infected area;
- increased capillary permeability due to retraction of the endothelial cells lining the vessels, permitting larger molecules than usual to escape from the capillaries;
- migration of leukocytes out of the venules into the surrounding tissues – in the earliest stages of inflammation, neutrophils are particularly prevalent, but in later stages monocytes and lymphocytes also migrate towards the site of infection or damage.

Q. What advantage could the inflammatory responses have in the defense against infection?

A. The inflammatory responses allow leukocytes, antibodies, and complement system molecules (all of which are required for the phagocytosis and destruction of pathogens) to enter the tissues at the site of infection. Lymphocytes are also required for the recognition and destruction of infected cells in the tissues.

Leukocytes enter inflamed tissue by crossing venular endothelium

The process of leukocyte migration is controlled by **chemokines** (a particular class of cytokines) on the surface of venular endothelium in inflamed tissues. Chemokines activate the circulating leukocytes causing them to bind to the endothelium and initiate migration across the endothelium (Fig. 1.17).

Once in the tissues, the leukocytes migrate towards the site of infection by a process of chemical attraction known as **chemotaxis**. For example, phagocytes will actively migrate up concentration gradients of certain (chemotactic) molecules.

Principle of vaccination

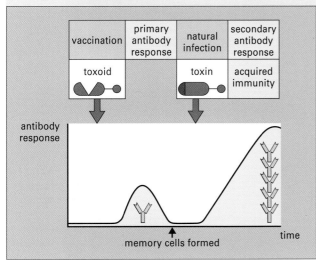

Fig. 1.16 Chemical modification of tetanus toxin produces a toxoid, which has lost its toxicity but retains many of its epitopes. A primary antibody response to these epitopes is produced following vaccination with the toxoid. If a natural infection occurs, the toxin restimulates memory B cells, which produce a faster and more intense secondary response against that epitope, so neutralizing the toxin.

Three phases in neutrophil migration across endothelium

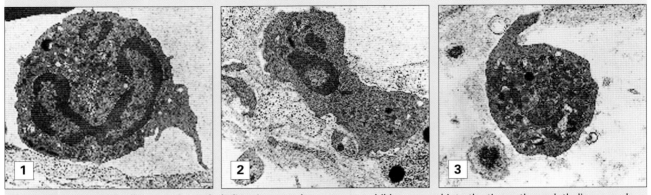

Fig. 1.17 A neutrophil adheres to the endothelium in a venule (**1**). It extends its pseudopodium between the endothelial cells and migrates towards the basement membrane (**2**). After the neutrophil has crossed into the tissue, the endothelium reseals behind (**3**). The entire process is referred to as diapedesis. (Courtesy of Dr I Jovis)

A particularly active chemotactic molecule is **C5a**, which is a fragment of one of the complement components (Fig. 1.18) and attracts both neutrophils and monocytes. When purified C5a is applied to the base of a blister in vivo, neutrophils can be seen sticking to the endothelium of nearby venules shortly afterwards. The cells then squeeze between the endothelial cells and move through the basement membrane of the microvessels to reach the tissues. This process is described more fully in Chapter 6.

THE IMMUNE SYSTEM MAY FAIL (IMMUNOPATHOLOGY)

Strong evolutionary pressure from infectious microbes has led to the development of the immune system in its

Chemotaxis

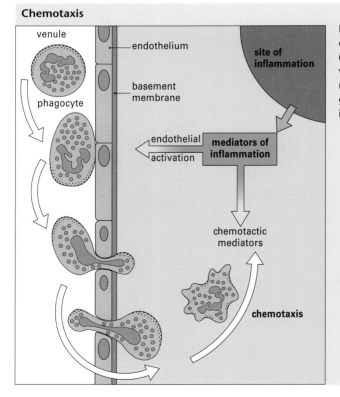

Fig. 1.18 At a site of inflammation, tissue damage and complement activation cause the release of chemotactic peptides (e.g. chemokines and C5a), which diffuse to the adjoining venules and signal to circulating phagocytes. Activated cells migrate across the vessel wall and move up a concentration gradient of chemotactic molecules towards the site of inflammation.

Failure of the immune system

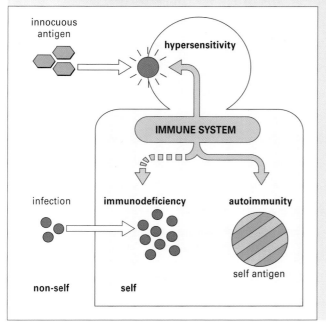

Fig. 1.19 The three principal ways in which the immune system can fail result in hypersensitivity (an overactive immune response to an antigen), immunodeficiency (an ineffective immune response to an infection), and autoimmunity (the immune system reacts against the body's own tissues).

present form. Deficiencies in any part of the system leave the individual exposed to a greater risk of infection, but other parts of the system may partly compensate for such deficiencies. However, there are occasions when the immune system is itself a cause of disease or other undesirable consequences.

In essence the immune system can fail in one of three ways (Fig. 1.19), resulting in autoimmunity, immunodeficiency, or hypersensitivity.

Inappropriate reaction to self antigens – autoimmunity

Normally the immune system recognizes all foreign antigens and reacts against them, while recognizing the body's own tissues as 'self' and making no reaction against them. The mechanisms by which this discrimination between 'self' and 'non-self' is established are described in Chapter 19.

When the immune system reacts against 'self' components, the result is an **autoimmune disease** (see Chapter 20), for example:
- rheumatoid arthritis (see p. 377);
- pernicious anemia (see p. 376).

Ineffective immune response – immunodeficiency

If any elements of the immune system are defective, the individual may not be able to fight infections adequately, resulting in **immunodeficiency** (see Chapters 16 and 17). Some immunodeficiency conditions:
- are hereditary and start to manifest shortly after birth;
- develop later in life, for example the acquired immune deficiency syndrome (AIDS).

Overactive immune response – hypersensitivity

Sometimes immune reactions are out of all proportion to the damage that may be caused by a pathogen. The immune system may also mount a reaction to a harmless antigen, such as a food molecule. Such immune reactions (**hypersensitivity**) may cause more damage than the pathogen or antigen (see Chapters 23–26). For example, molecules on the surface of pollen grains are recognized as antigens by particular individuals, leading to the symptoms of hay fever or asthma.

NORMAL IMMUNE RESPONSES CAN BE INCONVENIENT IN MODERN MEDICINE

Q. Can you think of an instance where an individual is treated to suppress an immune reaction that does not fall into one of the three categories of immunopathology described above?

A. Immunosuppression to prevent graft rejection.

The most important examples of normal immune reactions that are inconvenient in the context of modern medicine are:
- blood transfusion reactions (see Chapter 24);
- graft rejection (see Chapter 21).

In these cases it is necessary to carefully match the donor and recipient tissues so that the immune system of the recipient does not attack the donated blood or graft tissue.

Critical thinking: Specificity and memory in vaccination (see p. 493 for explanations)

The recommended schedules for vaccination against different diseases are strikingly different. Two examples are given in the table. For tetanus, the vaccine is a modified form of the toxin released by the tetanus bacterium. The vaccine for influenza is either an attenuated non-pathogenic variant of the virus, given intranasally, or a killed preparation of virus, given intra-dermally. Both vaccines induce antibodies that are specific for the inducing antigen.

Schedules for vaccination against tetanus and influenza A

pathogen	type of vaccine	recommended for	vaccination	effectiveness (%)
tetanus	toxoid	everyone	every 10 years	100
influenza A	attenuated virus	health workers and older people	annually	variable, 0–90

1 Why is it necessary to vaccinate against tetanus only every 10 years, though antibodies against the toxoid disappear from the circulation within a year?

2 Why is the vaccine against tetanus always effective, whereas the vaccine against influenza protects on some occasions but not others?

3 Why is tetanus recommended for everyone and influenza for only a restricted group of 'at-risk' individuals, even though influenza is a much more common disease than tetanus?

Cells, Tissues, and Organs of the Immune System

SUMMARY

- **Most cells of the immune system** derive from hemopoietic stem cells.

- **Phagocytic cells** are found in the circulation (monocytes and granulocytes) and reside in tissues (e.g. Kupffer cells in the liver).

- **Development and differentiation of different cell lineages** depend on cell interactions and cytokines.

- **Each cell type expresses characteristic surface molecules (markers)**, which identify them.

- **Eosinophils, basophils, mast cells, and platelets take part in the inflammatory response**.

- **NK cells recognize and kill virus-infected cells and certain tumor cells** through apoptosis.

- **Antigen-presenting cells** link the innate and adaptive immune systems and are required by T cells to enable them to respond to antigens.

- **Lymphocytes are heterogeneous** phenotypically, functionally, and morphologically.

- **B and T cells express antigen receptors**, which are required for the antigen recognition.

- **There are two major subpopulations of T cells**, which have helper and cytotoxic activities.

- **Cell surface immunoglobulin and signaling molecules** form the 'B cell receptor' complex.

- **B cells can differentiate into antibody-secreting plasma cells** following activation.

- **Lymphoid organs and tissues** are either primary (central) or secondary (peripheral).

- **Lymphoid stem cells develop and mature within the primary lymphoid organs** – the thymus and bone marrow – this process is called lymphopoiesis.

- **T cells developing in the thymus** are subject to positive and negative selection processes.

- **The diverse antigen repertoires found in mature animals** are generated during lymphopoiesis by recombination of gene segments encoding the T cell receptor (TCR) and immunoglobulin.

- **Mammalian B cells develop mainly in the fetal liver and from birth onwards in the bone marrow**. This process continues throughout life. B cells also undergo a selection process at the site of B cell generation.

- **Lymphocytes** migrate to, and function in, the secondary lymphoid organs and tissues.

- **Lymphoid organs and tissues protect different body sites** – the spleen responds to blood-borne antigens; the lymph nodes respond to lymph-borne antigens; and MALT protects the mucosal surface.

- **Systemic lymphoid organs** include the spleen and lymph nodes.

- **Mucosa-associated lymphoid tissue (MALT)** includes all the lymphoid tissues associated with mucosae. Peyer's patches are a major site of lymphocyte priming to antigens crossing mucosal surfaces of the small intestine.

- **Most lymphocytes recirculate around the body;** there is continuous lymphocyte traffic from the blood stream into lymphoid tissues and back again into the blood via the thoracic duct and right lymphatic duct.

MOST CELLS OF THE IMMUNE SYSTEM DERIVE FROM HEMATOPOIETIC STEM CELLS

There is great heterogeneity in the cells of the immune system, most of which originate from hematopoietic stem cells in the fetal liver and in the postnatal bone marrow.

Innate immune system cells are monocytes/macrophages, polymorphonuclear granulocytes, NK cells, mast cells, and platelets

Phagocytic cells of the innate immune system include:
- the monocytes/macrophages;

- the **polymorphonuclear granulocytes** (polymorpho-nuclear neutrophils [PMNs], basophils, and eosinophils), which are mainly involved in dealing with extracellular microbes; and
- natural killer (NK) cells, which are responsible for killing virus-infected cells.

Other cells that function in innate immune protection include mast cells and platelets (Fig. 2.1).

Cells of the innate system recognize microbes through their pathogen-associated molecular patterns (PAMP) receptors. PAMP receptors have broad specificity and a non-clonal distribution (see Chapter 6).

APCs link the innate and adaptive immune systems

A specialized group of cells termed antigen-presenting cells (APCs) link the innate and adaptive immune systems by producing molecules (cytokines), which:

- enhance innate immune cell function; and
- contribute to lymphocyte function (Fig. 2.2).

The main adaptive immune system cells are lymphocytes

Lymphocytes (T and B cells) recognize antigens through clonally expressed antigen receptors (see Chapters 3 and 5). T cells are produced in the thymus (see Fig. 2.1) and require antigen to be processed and presented to them by specialized APCs.

Whereas the cells of the innate immune system are found in the blood stream and in most organs of the body, lymphocytes are localized to specialized organs and tissues.

The lymphoid organs where the lymphocytes differentiate and mature from stem cells are the **primary lymphoid organs** and include:

- the thymus – the site of T cell development;
- the fetal liver and postnatal bone marrow – the sites of B cell development.

Cells of the T and B cell lineages migrate from the primary lymphoid organs to function in the **secondary lymphoid organs** – namely:

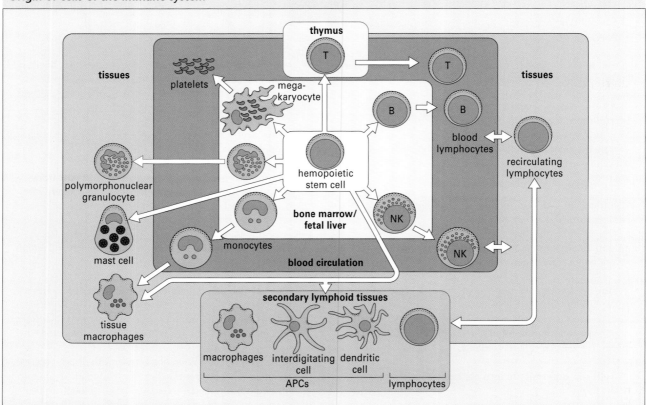

Origin of cells of the immune system

Fig. 2.1 All cells shown here arise from the hematopoietic stem cell. Platelets produced by megakaryocytes are released into the circulation. Polymorphonuclear granulocytes and monocytes pass from the circulation into the tissues. Mast cells are identifiable in all tissues. B cells mature in the fetal liver and bone marrow in mammals, whereas T cells mature in the thymus. The origin of the large granular lymphocytes with natural killer (NK) activity is probably the bone marrow. Lymphocytes recirculate through secondary lymphoid tissues. Interdigitating cells and dendritic cells act as antigen-presenting cells (APCs) in secondary lymphoid tissues.

Rapid Reference Box 2

adhesion molecules – cell surface molecules involved in the binding of cells to extracellular matrix or neighboring cells, where the principal function is adhesion rather than cell activation (e.g. integrins and selectins).

APCs (antigen-presenting cells) – a variety of cell types that carry antigen in a form that can stimulate lymphocytes.

dendritic cells – a set of cells that can be derived from either the lymphoid or mononuclear phagocyte lineages, are present in tissues, capture antigens, and migrate to the lymph nodes and spleen, where they are particularly active in presenting the processed antigen to T cells.

γδ T cells – the minor subset of T cells that express the gd form of the T cell receptor (TCR).

intercellular adhesion molecules (ICAMs) – cell surface molecules found on a variety of leukocytes and non-hematogenous cells that interact with integrins.

inflammation – a series of reactions that bring cells and molecules of the immune system to sites of infection or damage – this appears as an increase in blood supply, increased vascular permeability, and increased transendothelial migration of leukocytes.

LFA-1 (leukocyte functional antigen-1) – an integrin consisting of an α chain (CD11a) and a β chain (CD18) that acts as an intercellular adhesion molecule by binding to ICAM-1, ICAM-2, and ICAM-3. It has a role in leukocyte migration across vascular endothelium and in antigen presentation.

MHC (major histocompatibility complex) – a genetic region found in all mammals, encoding more than 100 genes. Class I and class II molecules are primarily responsible for transporting peptide antigens to the surface of a cell for recognition by T cells. Recognition of MHC class I and II molecules also underlies graft rejection.

Selected CD markers mentioned in this chapter

CD3 – a component of the T cell receptor complex.

CD4 – a marker of helper T cells.

CD5 – a marker of B-1 cells and marginal zone B cells.

CD8 – a marker of cytotoxic T lymphocytes (CTLs, Tc cells).

CD11a/CD18 – an integrin (LFA-1) found on most leukocytes.

CD11b/CD18 – an integrin (Mac-1) characteristic of mononuclear phagocytes.

CD16 – a low-affinity receptor for IgG, found on NK cells.

CD79 – a component of the B cell receptor complex.

Antigen-presenting cells (APCs) in the immune system

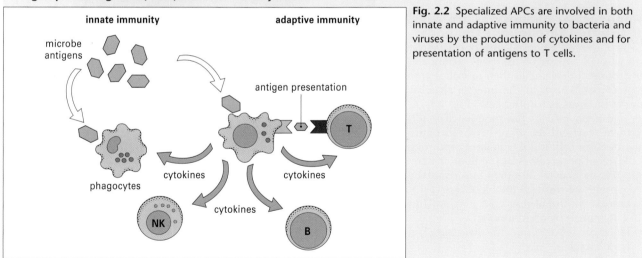

Fig. 2.2 Specialized APCs are involved in both innate and adaptive immunity to bacteria and viruses by the production of cytokines and for presentation of antigens to T cells.

- the spleen;
- lymph nodes; and
- mucosa-associated lymphoid tissues (MALT).

In the secondary lymphoid organs and tissues, the effector B and T cells account for the two major cell types participating in adaptive immune responses of humoral and cellular immunity, respectively.

As the cells of the immune system develop, they acquire molecules that are important for their function. These specific functional molecules are referred to as '**lineage markers**' because they identify the cell lineage, for example:

- myeloid cells – polymorphs and monocytes;
- lymphoid cells – T and B cells.

Other marker molecules include those involved in regulating cell proliferation and function and those involved in regulating the number of cells participating in the immune response. In both cases, these 'death receptors' mediate apoptosis of cells following their ligation.

PHAGOCYTIC CELLS ARE FOUND IN THE CIRCULATION AND IN THE TISSUES

Mononuclear phagocytes and polymorphonuclear granulocytes are the two major phagocyte lineages

Phagocytes belong to two major lineages:

- mononuclear phagocytes – monocytes/macrophages; and
- polymorphonuclear granulocytes.

The mononuclear phagocytes consist of circulating cells (the monocytes) and macrophages, which reside in a variety of organs (e.g. spleen, liver, lungs) where they display distinctive morphological features and perform diverse functions.

The other family of phagocytes, polymorphonuclear granulocytes, have a lobed, irregularly shaped (polymorphic) nucleus. On the basis of how their cytoplasmic granules stain with acidic and basic dyes they are classified into neutrophils, basophils, and eosinophils and have distinct effector functions:

- the neutrophils, also called polymorphonuclear neutrophils (PMNs), are most numerous and constitute the majority of leukocytes (white blood cells) in the blood stream (around 60–70% in adults);
- the primary actions of eosinophils and basophils, which can both function as phagocytes, involve granule exocytosis.

The mononuclear phagocytes and polymorphonuclear granulocytes develop from a common precursor (see below, Fig. 2.6).

Mononuclear phagocytes are widely distributed throughout the body

Cells of the mononuclear phagocytic system are found in virtually all organs of the body where the local microenvironment determines their morphology and functional characteristics (e.g. in the lung as alveolar macrophages and in the liver as Kupffer cells; Fig. 2.3).

The main role of the mononuclear phagocytes is to remove particulate matter of 'foreign' origin (e.g. microbes) or self origin (e.g. aged erythrocytes).

Myeloid progenitors in the bone marrow differentiate into pro-monocytes and then into circulating monocytes, which migrate through the blood vessel walls into organs to become macrophages.

The human blood monocyte:

- is large (10–18 μm in diameter) relative to the lymphocyte;
- has a horseshoe-shaped nucleus;
- contains azurophilic granules;
- possesses ruffled membranes, a well-developed Golgi complex, and many intracytoplasmic lysosomes (Fig. 2.4).

The lysosomes contain peroxidase and several acid hydrolases, which are important for killing phagocytosed microorganisms. Monocytes/macrophages actively phagocytose microorganisms or even tumor cells.

Microbial adherence, followed by ingestion, occurs through specialized receptors. These receptors (which include scavenger receptors, Toll-like receptors, and mannose receptors) attach mainly to sugars or lipids known as PAMPs on the microbial surface (see Chapter 6).

Kupffer cells

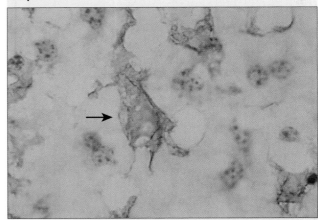

Fig. 2.3 Kupffer cells in the normal mouse liver stain strongly positive with antibody to F4/80 (arrow). Sinusoidal endothelial cells and hepatocytes are F4/80-negative. (Courtesy of Professor S Gordon and Dr DA Hume)

Morphology of the monocyte

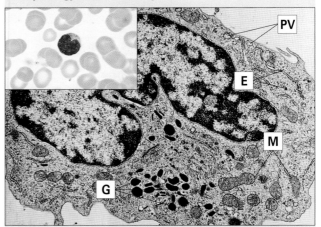

Fig. 2.4 Ultrastructure of a monocyte showing the horseshoe-shaped nucleus, pinocytotic vesicles (PV), lysosomal granules (G), mitochondria (M), and isolated rough endoplasmic reticulum cisternae (E). × 8000. (Courtesy of Dr B Nichols) Inset: Light microscope image of a monocyte from the blood. × 1200.

Coating microbes with complement components and/or antibodies (opsonization) enhances phagocytosis by monocytes/macrophages and is mediated by specialized complement receptors and antibody receptors (see Chapters 3 and 4).

Q. How do macrophages recognize microbes that have been coated with antibody?

A. Macrophages have Fc receptors that recognize the constant portion of the antibody molecule (see Figs 1.10 and 1.11).

There are three different types of polymorphonuclear granulocyte

Polymorphonuclear granulocytes (often referred to as **polymorphs** or **granulocytes**) consist mainly of neutrophils (PMNs). They:

- are released from the bone marrow at a rate of around 7 million per minute;
- are short-lived (2–3 days) relative to monocytes/macrophages, which may live for months or years.

Like monocytes, PMNs adhere to endothelial cells lining the blood vessels (marginate) and extravasate by squeezing between the endothelial cells to leave the circulation (see Fig. 1.17). This process is known as **diapedesis**. Adhesion is mediated by receptors on the granulocytes and ligands on the endothelial cells, and is promoted by chemo-attractants (**chemokines**) such as **interleukin-8 (IL-8)** (see Chapter 4 and Appendix 3).

Like monocytes/macrophages, granulocytes also have receptors for PAMPs, and PMNs play an important role in acute inflammation (usually synergizing with antibodies and complement) in providing protection against microorganisms. Their predominant role is phagocytosis and destruction of pathogens.

The importance of granulocytes is evident from the observation of individuals who have a reduced number of white cells or who have rare genetic defects that prevent polymorph extravasation in response to chemotactic stimuli (see Chapter 16). These individuals have a markedly increased susceptibility to infection.

NEUTROPHILS COMPRISE OVER 95% OF THE CIRCU-LATING GRANULOCYTES – Neutrophils have a characteristic multilobed nucleus and are 10–20 μm in diameter (Fig. 2.5). Chemotactic agents for neutrophils include:

- protein fragments released when complement is activated (e.g. C5a);
- factors derived from the fibrinolytic and kinin systems;
- the products of other leukocytes and platelets; and
- the products of certain bacteria (see Chapter 4).

Chemotactic stimuli result in neutrophil margination and diapedesis (see Fig. 1.17).

Neutrophils have a large arsenal of antibiotic proteins stored in two main types of granule:

- the primary (azurophilic) granules are lysosomes containing acid hydrolases, myeloperoxidase, and muramidase (lysozyme);
- the secondary granules (specific to neutrophils) contain lactoferrin and lysozyme (see Fig. 2.5).

The primary granules also contain the antibiotic proteins – defensins, seprocidins, cathelicidins, and bacterial permeability inducing (BPI) protein.

The lysosomes containing the antibiotic proteins fuse with vacuoles containing ingested microbes (termed **phagosomes**) to become **phagolysosomes** where the killing takes place.

Neutrophils can also release granules and cytotoxic substances extracellularly when they are activated by immune complexes through their Fc receptors. This may be an important pathogenetic mechanism in immune complex diseases (type III hypersensitivity, see Chapter 25).

Morphology of the neutrophil

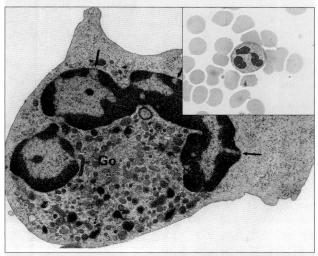

Fig. 2.5 At the ultrastructural level, the azurophilic (primary) granules are larger than the secondary (specific) granules with a strongly electron-dense matrix; the majority of granules are specific granules and contain a variety of toxic materials to kill microbes. A pseudopod (to the right) is devoid of granules. Arrows indicate nuclear pores. (Go, Golgi region) Inset: A mature neutrophil in a blood smear showing a multilobed nucleus. × 1500. (From Zucker-Franklin D, Grossi CE, eds. Atlas of blood cells: function and pathology, 3rd edn. Milan: Edi Ermes; 2003)

DIFFERENTIATION OF DIFFERENT CELL LINEAGES DEPENDS ON CELL INTERACTIONS AND CYTOKINES

Monocytes and neutrophils develop from a common precursor cell. **Myelopoiesis** (the development of myeloid cells) commences in the liver of the human fetus at about 6 weeks of gestation.

Studies in which colonies have been grown in vitro from individual stem cells have shown that the first progenitor cell derived from the hematopoietic stem cell (HSC) is the colony-forming unit (CFU), which can give rise to granulocytes, erythrocytes, monocytes, and megakaryocytes (CFU-GEMM).

CFU-GEMMs mature under the influence of colony-stimulating factors (CSFs) and several interleukins, including IL-1, IL-3, IL-4, IL-5, IL-6, and IL-7 (Fig. 2.6). These factors, which are relevant for the positive regulation of hemopoiesis, are:

- derived mainly from stromal cells (connective tissue cells) in the bone marrow;
- also produced by mature forms of differentiated myeloid and lymphoid cells.

Other cytokines, such as transforming growth factor-β (TGFβ) may downregulate hemopoiesis.

The CFU-granulocyte macrophage cells (CFU-GMs) are the precursors of both neutrophils and mononuclear phagocytes (see Fig. 2.6).

Development of granulocytes and monocytes

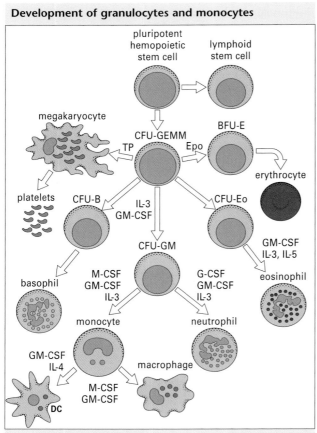

Fig. 2.6 Pluripotent hematopoietic stem cells generate colony-forming units (CFUs) that can give rise to granulocytes, erythrocytes, monocytes, and megakaryocytes (CFU-GEMMs). CFU-GEMMs therefore have the potential to give rise to all blood cells except lymphocytes. IL-3 and granulocyte–macrophage colony-stimulating factor (GM-CSF) are required to induce the CFU-GEMM stem cell to enter one of five pathways (i.e. to give rise to megakaryocytes, erythrocytes via burst-forming units, basophils, neutrophils, or eosinophils). IL-3 and GM-CSF are also required during further differentiation of the granulocytes and monocytes. Eosinophil (Eo) differentiation from CFU-Eo is promoted by IL-5. Neutrophils and monocytes are derived from the CFU-GM through the effects of G-CSF and M-CSF, respectively. Both GM-CSF and M-CSF, and other cytokines (including IL-1, IL-4, and IL-6), promote the differentiation of monocytes into macrophages. Thrombopoietin (TP) promotes the growth of megakaryocytes. (B, basophil; BFU-E, erythrocytic burst-forming unit; DC, dendritic cell; Epo, erythropoietin; G, granulocyte; M, monocyte)

EACH CELL TYPE EXPRESSES CHARACTERISTIC SURFACE MOLECULES
Monocytes express CD14 and significant levels of MHC class II molecules

CFU-GMs taking the monocyte pathway give rise initially to proliferating monoblasts. Proliferating monoblasts differentiate into pro-monocytes and finally into mature circulating monocytes (see Fig. 2.4). Circulating mono-

cytes are a replacement pool for the tissue-resident macrophages (e.g. lung macrophages).

CD34, like other early maturation markers in this lineage, is lost in mature neutrophils and monocytes/macrophages. Other markers may be lost as differentiation occurs along one pathway, but retained in the other. For example, the common precursor of monocytes and neutrophils, the CFU-GM cell, expresses **major histocompatibility complex (MHC) class II molecules**, but only monocytes continue to express significant levels of this marker.

Q. What is the functional significance of the expression of MHC molecules on monocytes?
A. Monocytes can present antigens to helper T cells, but neutrophils generally cannot.

Monocytes/macrophages and granulocytes have different functional molecules (e.g. monocytes express CD14 which is part of the receptor complex for the lipopolysaccharide of Gram-negative bacteria). In addition, monocytes acquire many of the same surface molecules as mature neutrophils (e.g. the adhesion molecules CD11a and b and antibody Fc receptors). Examples of the distinct and common functional molecules can be seen in the list of CD markers in Appendix 2.

Neutrophils express adhesion molecules and receptors involved in phagocytosis

CFU-GMs go through several stages to become neutrophils. As the CFU-GM cell differentiates along the neutrophil pathway, several distinct morphological stages are distinguished. Myeloblasts develop into promyelocytes and myelocytes, which mature and are released into the circulation as neutrophils.

The one-way differentiation of the CFU-GM into mature neutrophils is the result of acquiring specific receptors for growth and differentiation factors at progressive stages of development. Surface differentiation markers disappear or are expressed on the cells as they develop into granulocytes. For example, MHC class II molecules are expressed on the CFU-GM, but not on mature neutrophils.

Other surface molecules acquired during the differentiation process include:

- adhesion molecules (e.g. the leukocyte integrins CD11a, b, c, and d associated with CD18 β_2 chains); and
- receptors involved in phagocytosis including complement and antibody Fc receptors (see Appendix 4).

It is difficult to assess the functional activity of different developmental stages of granulocytes, but it seems likely that the full functional potential is realized only when the cells are mature.

There is some evidence that neutrophil activity, as measured by phagocytosis or chemotaxis, is lower in fetal than in adult life. However, this may be due, in part, to the lower levels of opsonins in the fetal serum, rather than to a characteristic of the cells themselves.

To become active in the presence of opsonins, neutrophils must interact directly with microorganisms and/or with cytokines generated by a response to antigen. This limitation could reduce neutrophil activity in early life.

Activation of neutrophils by cytokines and chemokines is also a prerequisite for their migration into tissues (see Chapter 9).

EOSINOPHILS, BASOPHILS, MAST CELLS, AND PLATELETS TAKE PART IN THE INFLAMMATORY RESPONSE
Eosinophils are thought to play a role in immunity to parasitic worms

Eosinophils comprise 2–5% of blood leukocytes in healthy non-allergic individuals. Human blood eosinophils usually have a bilobed nucleus and many cytoplasmic granules, which stain with acidic dyes such as eosin (Fig. 2.7). Although not their primary function, eosinophils appear to be capable of phagocytosing and killing ingested microorganisms.

The granules in mature eosinophils are membrane-bound organelles with crystalloid cores that differ in electron density from the surrounding matrix (see Fig. 2.7). The crystalloid core contains the **major basic protein (MBP)**, which:

- is a potent toxin for helminth worms;
- induces histamine release from mast cells;
- activates neutrophils and platelets; and
- of relevance to allergy, provokes bronchospasm.

Other proteins with similar effects are found in the granule matrix, for example:

- eosinophil cationic protein (ECP); and
- eosinophil-derived neurotoxin (EDN).

Release of the granules on eosinophil activation is the only way in which eosinophils can kill large pathogens (e.g. schistosomula), which cannot be phagocytosed. Eosinophils are therefore thought to play a specialized role in immunity to parasitic worms using this mechanism (see Fig. 15.15).

Basophils and mast cells play a role in immunity against parasites

Basophils are found in very small numbers in the circulation and account for less than 0.2% of leukocytes (Fig. 2.8).

The mast cell (Fig. 2.9), which is not found in the circulation, is indistinguishable from the basophil in a

Morphology of the basophil

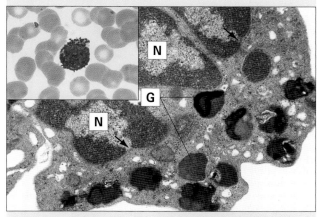

Fig. 2.8 Ultrastructural analysis shows a segmented nucleus (N) and the large cytoplasmic granules (G). Arrows indicate nuclear pores. × 11 000. (Adapted from Zucker-Franklin D, Grossi CE, eds. Atlas of blood cells: function and pathology, 3rd edn. Milan: Edi Ermes; 2003) Inset: This blood smear shows a typical basophil with its deep violet-blue granules. × 1000.

Morphology of the eosinophil

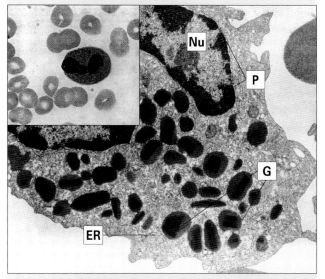

Fig. 2.7 The ultrastructure of a mature eosinophil shows granules (G) with central crystalloids. × 17 500. (ER, endoplasmic reticulum; Nu, nucleus; P, nuclear pores) Inset: A mature eosinophil in a blood smear is shown with a bilobed nucleus and eosinophilic granules. × 1000. (From Zucker-Franklin D, Grossi CE, eds. Atlas of blood cells: function and pathology, 3rd edn. Milan: Edi Ermes; 2003)

Histological appearance of human connective tissue mast cells

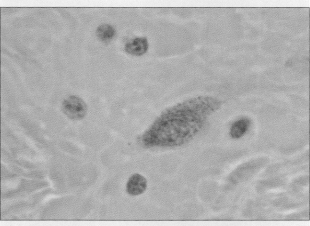

Fig. 2.9 This micrograph shows dark blue cytoplasm with purple granules. Alcian blue and safranin stain. × 600. (Courtesy of Dr TS Orr)

Some distinctive and common characteristics of basophils and mast cells

	basophils	mast cells
origin	bone marrow	bone marrow
site of maturation	bone marrow	connective tissues
presence in the circulation	yes	no
proliferative capacity	no	yes
life span	days	weeks to months
surface expression of FcεR1	yes	yes
granule content		
histamine	yes	yes
heparin	?	yes
cytokine production		
IL-4	yes	yes
IL-13	yes	yes

Fig. 2.10 Some distinctive and common characteristics of basophils and mast cells.

number of its characteristics, but displays some distinctive morphological features (Fig. 2.10).

The stimulus for mast cell or basophil degranulation is often an **allergen** (i.e. an antigen causing an allergic reaction). To be effective, an allergen must cross-link IgE molecules bound to the surface of the mast cell or basophil via its high-affinity Fc receptors for IgE (FcεRI) (see p. 77). Degranulation of a basophil or mast cell results in all contents of the granules being released very rapidly. This occurs by intracytoplasmic fusion of the granules, followed by discharge of their contents (Fig. 2.11).

Mediators such as histamine, released by degranulation, cause the adverse symptoms of allergy, but, on the positive side, also play a role in immunity against parasites by enhancing acute inflammation.

Platelets have a role in clotting and inflammation

Blood platelets (Fig. 2.12) are not cells, but cell fragments derived from megakaryocytes in the bone marrow. They contain granules, microtubules, and actin/myosin filaments, which are involved in clot contraction. Platelets are also involved in immune responses, especially in inflammation.

The adult human produces 10^{11} platelets each day. About 30% of platelets are stored in the spleen, but may be released if required.

Q. What circumstance might require the release of additional platelets into the circulation?

A. Severe blood loss.

Electron micrograph study of rat mast cells

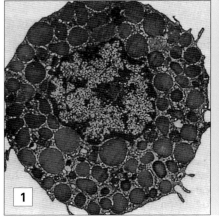 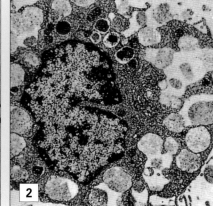

Fig. 2.11 Rat peritoneal mast cells show electron-dense granules (**1**). Vacuolation with exocytosis of the granule contents has occurred after incubation with anti-IgE (**2**). Transmission electron micrographs. × 2700. (Courtesy of Dr D Lawson)

Ultrastructure of a platelet

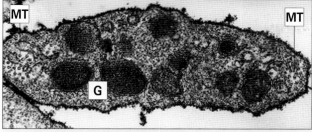

Fig. 2.12 Cross-section of a platelet showing two types of granule (G) and bundles of microtubules (MT) at either end. × 42 000. (Adapted from Zucker-Franklin D, Grossi CE, eds. Atlas of blood cells: function and pathology, 3rd edn. Milan: Edi Ermes; 2003)

Platelets express class I MHC products and receptors for IgG (CD32; FcγRII), which are important in platelet activation via IgG immune complexes. In addition, megakaryocytes and platelets carry:

- receptors for clotting factors (e.g. factor VIII); and
- other molecules important for their function, such as the GpIIb/IIIa complex (CD41) responsible for binding to fibrinogen, fibronectin, vitronectin (tissue matrix), and von Willebrand factor (another clotting factor).

Both receptors and adhesion molecules are important in the activation of platelets.

Following injury to endothelial cells, platelets adhere to and aggregate at the damaged endothelial surface. Release of platelet granule contents, which include de-novo synthesized serotonin and endocytosed fibrinogen, results in:

- increased capillary permeability;
- activation of complement (and hence attraction of leukocytes); and
- clotting.

NK CELLS KILL VIRUS-INFECTED AND TUMOR CELLS

NK cells account for up to 15% of blood lymphocytes and express neither T cell nor B cell antigen receptors. They are derived from the bone marrow and morphologically have the appearance of large granular lymphocytes (see Fig. 2.19).

Functional NK cells are found in the spleen, and cells found in lymph nodes that express CD56 but not CD16 (see below) might represent immature NK cells.

Most surface antigens detectable on NK cells by monoclonal antibodies are shared with T cells or monocytes/macrophages.

CD16 and CD56 are important markers of NK cells

Monoclonal antibodies to CD16 (FcγRIII) are commonly used to identify NK cells in purified lymphocyte populations. CD16 is involved in one of the activation pathways of NK cells and is also expressed by neutrophils, some macrophages, and some T cells.

On granulocytes, CD16 is linked to the surface membrane by a glycoinositol phospholipid (GPI) linkage, whereas NK cells, macrophages, and γδ T cells express the transmembrane form of the molecule.

The CD56 molecule, a homophilic adhesion molecule of the immunoglobulin superfamily (NCAM), is another important marker of NK cells.

The absence of CD3, but the presence of CD56 and CD16, are currently the most reliable markers for NK cells in humans, though both markers can also be found on a minority of T cells (mostly with CD3$^+$/CD8$^+$ phenotype).

Some markers of NK cells are given in Appendix 4. Resting NK cells also express the β chain of the IL-2 receptor, which is an intermediate affinity receptor of 70 kDa, and the signal transducing common γ chain of IL-2 and other cytokine receptors. Therefore, direct stimulation with IL-2 activates NK cells.

The function of NK cells is to recognize and kill (Fig. 2.13) through apoptosis:

- virus-infected cells; and
- certain tumor cells.

The mechanism of recognition is not fully understood, but involves both activating and inhibitory receptors.

Classical and non-classical MHC class I molecules (see Fig. 5.16) are ligands for the inhibitory receptors and this explains why normal body cells (all of which normally express MHC class I molecules) are not targeted by NK cells.

Downregulation or modification of MHC molecules in virus-infected cells and some tumors makes them susceptible to NK cell-mediated killing.

Q. What advantage is there for a virus in causing the loss of MHC class I molecules in the cell it has infected?

A. The infected cell can no longer be recognized by cytotoxic T cells (see Fig. 1.12).

An NK cell attached to a target cell

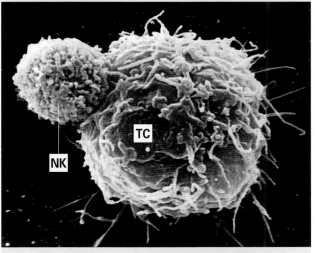

Fig. 2.13 An NK cell (NK) attached to a target cell (TC). × 4500. (Courtesy of Dr G Arancia and W Malorni, Rome)

NK cells are also able to kill targets coated with IgG antibodies via their receptor for IgG (FcγRIII, CD16). This property is referred to as **antibody-dependent cellular cytotoxicity (ADCC)**.

NK cells release interferon-γ (IFNγ) and other cytokines (e.g. IL-1 and GM-CSF) when activated, which might be important in the regulation of hemopoiesis and immune responses.

APCs LINK THE INNATE AND ADAPTIVE IMMUNE SYSTEMS

APCs are a heterogeneous population of leukocytes that are:
• important in innate immunity (see Fig. 2.2);
• play a pivotal role in the induction of functional activity of T helper (TH) cells.
In this regard, APCs are seen as the interface between the innate and adaptive immune systems.

Functionally, APCs are divided into those that both process and present foreign protein antigens to T cells – **dendritic cells (DCs)** – and a separate type of APC that passively presents foreign antigen in the form of immune complexes to B cells in lymphoid follicles – **follicular dendritic cells (FDCs**; Fig. 2.14).

APCs are found primarily in the skin, lymph nodes, and spleen, and within or underneath most mucosal epithelia. They are also present in the thymus, where they present self antigens to developing T cells (Fig. 2.15).

Langerhans' cells and IDCs are rich in class II MHC molecules

Langerhans' cells in the epidermis and in other squamous epithelia migrate as 'veiled cells', via the afferent lymphatics into the paracortex of the draining lymph nodes (see Fig. 2.15). Here, they interact with T cells and are termed interdigitating cells (IDCs; Fig. 2.16). These APCs are rich in class II MHC molecules, which are important for presenting antigen to TH cells.

Q. What function could the migration of Langerhans' cells to the lymph nodes from the mucosa or skin serve?

A. The migration of Langerhans' cells provides an efficient mechanism for carrying antigen from the skin and mucosa to the TH cells in the lymph nodes, and are rich in class II MHC molecules, which are important for presenting antigen to TH cells. Lymph nodes provide the appropriate environment for lymphocyte proliferation.

APCs are also present within the germinal centers (GCs) of secondary lymphoid follicles (i.e. they are the MHC class II molecule-positive germinal center DCs [GCDCs]). In contrast to FDCs, they are migrating cells, which on arrival in the GC interact with T cells and are probably involved in antibody class switching (see Chapter 8).

Thymic APCs (also called IDCs) are especially abundant in the medulla (see Fig. 2.15). The thymus is of crucial importance in the development and maturation of T cells, and it appears that IDCs play a role in deleting

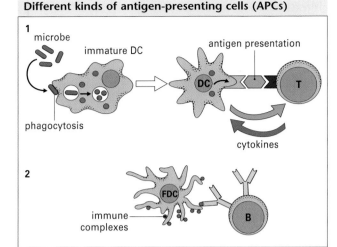

Different kinds of antigen-presenting cells (APCs)

Fig. 2.14 There are two main types of specialized APCs – dendritic cells (DCs) and follicular dendritic cells (FDCs). (1) Immature DCs are derived from bone marrow and interact mainly with T cells. They are highly phagocytic, take up microbes, process the foreign microbial antigens, and become mature APCs carrying the processed antigen on their surface with specialized MHC molecules. Specific T cells recognize the displayed antigen and, in the presence of cytokines produced by the mature DC, proliferate and also produce cytokines. (2) FDCs are not bone marrow derived and interact with B cells. In the B cell follicles of lymphoid organs and tissues they bind small immune complexes (IC, called iccosomes). Antigen contained within the IC is presented to specific B cells in the lymphoid follicles. This protects the B cell from cell death. The B cell then proliferates and with T cell help can leave the follicle and become a plasma cell or memory cell (see Fig. 2.48)

T cells that react against self antigen. This process is referred to as 'negative selection'.

Most APCs derive from one of two bone marrow precursors:
• a myeloid progenitor (DC1) that gives rise to myeloid DCs; and
• a lymphoid progenitor (DC2) that develops into plasmacytoid DCs (Fig. 2.17).
DCs are not the only APCs interacting with T cells because both macrophages and classical B cells are rich in membrane class II MHC molecules, especially after activation, and are thus able to process and present specific antigens to (activated) T cells (see Chapter 7).

Somatic cells other than immune cells do not normally express class II MHC molecules, but cytokines such as IFNγ and tumor necrosis factor-α (TNFα) can induce the expression of class II molecules on some cell types, and thus allow them to present antigen (e.g. epidermis and thyroid epithelium and endothelial cells). This induction of 'inappropriate' class II expression might contribute to the pathogenesis of autoimmune diseases and to prolonged inflammation (see Chapter 20).

Migration of antigen-presenting cells (APCs) into lymphoid tissues

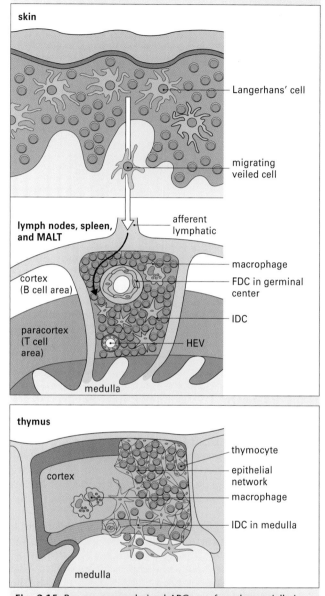

Fig. 2.15 Bone marrow-derived APCs are found especially in lymphoid tissues, in the skin, and in mucosa. APCs in the form of Langerhans' cells are found in the epidermis and are characterized by special granules (the tennis racquet-shaped Birbeck granules; not shown here). Langerhans' cells are rich in MHC class II molecules, and carry processed antigens. They migrate via the afferent lymphatics (where they appear as 'veiled' cells) into the paracortex of the draining lymph nodes. Here they make contact with T cells. These 'interdigitating dendritic cells (IDCs)', localized in the T cell areas of the lymph node, present antigen to T helper cells. Antigen is exposed to B cells on the follicular dendritic cells (FDCs) in the germinal centers of B cell follicles. Some macrophages located in the outer cortex and marginal sinus may also act as APCs. In the thymus, APCs occur as IDCs in the medulla. (HEV, high endothelial venule)

Ultrastructure of an interdigitating dendritic cell (IDC) in the T cell area of a rat lymph node

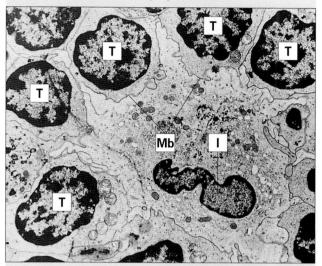

Fig. 2.16 Intimate contacts are made with the membranes of the surrounding T cells. The cytoplasm contains a well-developed endosomal system and does not show the Birbeck granules characteristic of skin Langerhans' cells. × 2000. (I, IDC nucleus; Mb, IDC membrane; T, T cell nucleus) (Courtesy of Dr BH Balfour)

FDCs lack class II MHC molecules and are found in B cell areas

Unlike the APCs that actively process and present protein antigens to T cells, FDCs have a passive role in presenting antigen in the form of immune complexes to B cells. They are therefore found in the primary and secondary follicles of the B cell areas of the lymph nodes, spleen, and MALT (see Fig. 2.15). They are a non-migratory population of cells and form a stable network (a kind of web) by establishing strong intercellular connections via desmosomes.

FDCs lack class II MHC molecules, but bind antigen via complement receptors (CD21 and CD35), which attach to complement associated with immune complexes (iccosomes; Fig. 2.18). They also express Fc receptors. These FDCs are not bone marrow derived, but are of mesenchymal origin.

LYMPHOCYTES ARE HETEROGENEOUS
Lymphocytes are phenotypically and functionally heterogeneous

Large numbers of lymphocytes are produced daily in the primary or central lymphoid organs (i.e. thymus and postnatal bone marrow). Some migrate via the circulation into the secondary lymphoid tissues (i.e. spleen, lymph nodes, and MALT).

The average human adult has about 2×10^{12} lymphoid cells and lymphoid tissue as a whole represents about 2% of total body weight. Lymphoid cells account for about 20% of the leukocytes in the adult circulation.

Myeloid and plasmacytoid dendritic cells

	myeloid DCs	**plasmacytoid DCs**
origin of precursor	myeloid (DC1)	lymphoid (DC2)
localization	diffuse – epidermis, mucosae, thymus, and T cell areas of secondary lymphoid organs and tissues	restricted to T cell areas of secondary lymphoid organs and tissues
myeloid markers	many	none
characteristic cytokines produced	mainly IL-8, IL-12	mainly type I interferons (on challenge with enveloped viruses)

Fig. 2.17 Myeloid and plasmacytoid dendritic cells (DCs).

Follicular dendritic cell

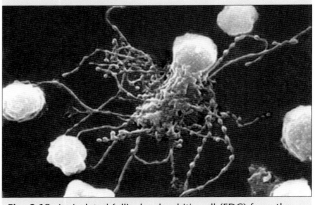

Fig. 2.18 An isolated follicular dendritic cell (FDC) from the lymph node of an immunized mouse 24 hours after injection of antigen. The FDC is of intermediate maturity with smooth filiform dendrites typical of young FDCs, and beaded dendrites, which participate in the formation of iccosomes (immune complexes) in mature FDCs. The adjacent small white cells are lymphocytes. (Electron micrograph kindly provided by Dr Andras Szakal; reproduced by permission of the Journal of Immunology)

Many mature lymphoid cells are long-lived, and persist as memory cells for many years.

Q. Given that there are roughly 10^9 lymphocytes/litre of blood and 10 litres of blood in an individual, and that roughly 2×10^9 new cells are produced each day, what can you infer about the location and life span of lymphocytes within an individual?

A. This implies that less than 1% of an individual's lymphocytes are in the circulation. This highly selective population of lymphocytes is mostly en route between tissues. The data also imply that many lymphocytes must die each day to maintain the overall balance of the lymphoid system, and that the average life span of a lymphocyte will be months to years. The actual values are, however, enormously variable, depending on the lymphocyte.

Lymphocytes are morphologically heterogeneous

In a conventional blood smear, lymphocytes vary in both size (from 6 to 10 μm in diameter) and morphology. Differences are seen in:
- nuclear to cytoplasmic (N:C) ratio;
- nuclear shape; and
- the presence or absence of azurophilic granules.

Two distinct morphological types of lymphocyte are seen in the circulation as determined by light microscopy and a hematological stain such as Giemsa (Fig. 2.19):
- the first type is relatively small, is typically agranular and has a high N:C ratio (Fig. 2.19[1]).
- the second type is larger, has a lower N:C ratio, contains cytoplasmic azurophilic granules, and is known as the large granular lymphocyte (LGL).

LGLs should not be confused with granulocytes, monocytes, or their precursors, which also contain azurophilic granules.

Most T cells express the αβ T cell receptor (see below) and, when resting, can show either of the above morphological patterns.

Most T helper (TH) cells (approximately 95%) and a proportion (approximately 50%) of cytotoxic T cells (Tc or CTL) have the morphology shown in Fig. 2.19(1).

The LGL morphological pattern displayed in Fig. 2.19(2) is shown by less than 5% of TH cells and by about 30–50% of Tc cells. These cells display LGL morphology with primary lysosomes dispersed in the cytoplasm and a well-developed Golgi apparatus, as shown in Fig. 2.19(3).

Most B cells, when resting, have a morphology similar to that seen in Fig. 2.19(1) under light microscopy.

B AND T CELLS EXPRESS ANTIGEN RECEPTORS
Lymphocytes express characteristic surface markers

Lymphocytes (and other leukocytes) express a large number of different functionally important molecules on their surfaces, which can be used to distinguish ('mark') cell subsets. Many of these cell markers can be identified by specific monoclonal antibodies (mAb) and can be used

Morphological heterogeneity of lymphocytes

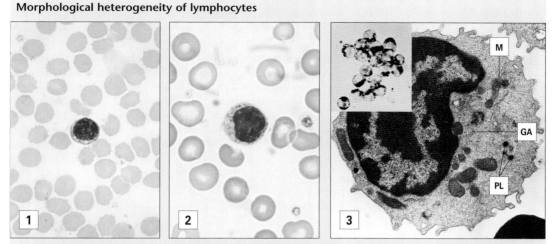

Fig. 2.19 (1) The small lymphocyte has no granules, a round nucleus, and a high N:C ratio. (2) The large granular lymphocyte (LGL) has a lower N:C ratio, indented nucleus, and azurophilic granules in the cytoplasm. Giemsa stain. (Courtesy of Dr A Stevens and Professor J Lowe) (3) Ultrastructure of the LGL shows characteristic electron-dense peroxidase-negative granules (primary lysosomes, PL), scattered throughout the cytoplasm, with some close to the Golgi apparatus (GA) and many mitochondria (M). ×10 000. (Adapted from Zucker-Franklin D, Grossi CE, eds. Atlas of blood cells: function and pathology, 3rd edn. Milan: Edi Ermes; 2003)

Main distinguishing markers of T and B cells

CD number	T cells	B cells
antigen receptor	TCR – (αβ or γδ)	immunoglobulin (Ig)
CD1	–	+
CD3	+ (part of the TCR complex)	–
CD4	+ (subset)	–
CD8	+ (subset)	–
CD19	–	+
CD20	–	+
CD23	+ (subset)	+
CD40	–	+
CD79a	–	+ (part of the BCR complex)
CD79b	–	+ (part of the BCR complex)
BCR, B cell receptor; TCR, T cell receptor		

Fig 2.20 Main distinguishing markers of T and B cells.

to distinguish T cells from B cells (Fig. 2.20 and see Appendix 2 for more CD markers).

Human lymphocytes can be identified in tissues and their function can be measured as separated populations. Immunofluorescence techniques to identify leukocytes are shown in Method Box 2.1.

Lymphocytes express a variety of cell surface molecules that belong to different families, which have prob-ably evolved from a few ancestral genes. These families of molecules are shared with other leukocytes and are distinguished by their structure. The major families include:
- the immunoglobulin superfamily;
- the integrin family;
- selectins;
- proteoglycans.

METHOD BOX 2.1
Identification of cell populations

Molecules on or in cells can be identified using fluorescent antibodies as probes. The antibodies can be applied to tissue sections or used in flow cytometry.

Immunofluorescence

Immunofluorescence detects antigen in situ. A section is cut on a cryostat from a deep-frozen tissue block. This ensures that labile antigens are not damaged by fixatives.

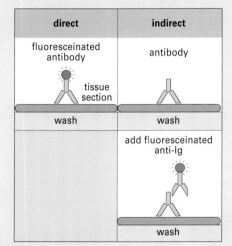

Fig. 1 Immunofluorescence.

Direct immunofluorescence

The test solution of fluoresceinated antibody, e.g. to CD3, is applied to the section in a drop, incubated, and washed off. Any bound antibody is then revealed under the microscope. Ultraviolet light is directed onto the section through the objective and as a result the field is dark and areas with bound fluorescent antibody on and in the T cells fluoresce.

Indirect immunofluorescence

Antibody applied to the section as a solution is visualized using fluoresceinated anti-immunoglobulin, to the mouse anti-human CD3 antibodies in this case.

Indirect complement amplified – an elaboration of indirect immunofluorescence

This is an elaboration of the indirect immunofluorescence for the detection of complement-fixing antibody. In the second step fresh complement is added, which becomes fixed around the site of antibody binding. Due to the amplification steps in the classical complement pathway (see Chapter 4) one antibody molecule can cause many C3b molecules to bind to the section – these are then visualized with fluoresceinated anti-C3.

Flow cytometry and cell sorting

Cells are stained with specific fluorescent reagents to detect surface molecules and are then introduced into the flow chamber of the flow cytometer. The cell stream passing out of the chamber is encased in a sheath of buffer fluid. The stream is illuminated by laser light and each cell is measured for size (forward light scatter) and granularity (90° light scatter), as well as for red and green fluorescence to detect two different surface markers. In a cell sorter the flow chamber vibrates the cell stream causing it to break into droplets, which are then charged and may be steered by deflection plates under computer control to collect different cell populations according to the parameters measured. Plot (**2.1**) shows peripheral blood mononuclear cells double stained with FITC-conjugated anti-CD3 antibody (x axis) and PE-labeled anti-CD8 antibody (y axis). Four populations can be seen, and the CD8 cells appear in the right upper quadrant. The CD8 cells are then selected (gated) and the isolated CD8 population is shown in plot (**2.2**).

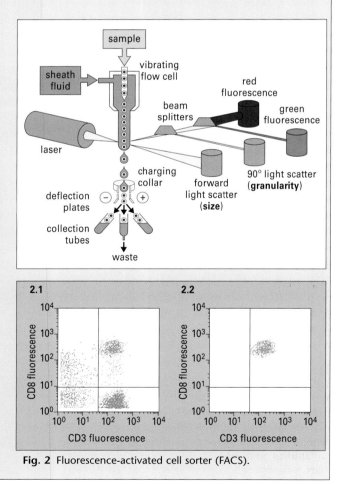

Fig. 2 Fluorescence-activated cell sorter (FACS).

METHOD BOX 2.1
Identification of cell populations *(Continued)*

ELISPOT assays
Individual B cells producing specific antibody or individual T cells secreting particular cytokines may be detected by enzyme linked immuno SPOT (ELISPOT) assay.

For detection of antibody-producing cells
The lymphocytes are plated onto an antigen-sensitized plate. Secreted antibody binds antigen in the immediate vicinity of cells producing the specific antibody. The spots of bound antibody are then detected chromatographically using enzyme coupled to anti-immunoglobulin and a chromogen.

For detection of cytokine-producing cells
The plates are coated with anti-cytokine and the captured cytokine is detected with enzyme-coupled antibody to a different epitope on the cytokine.

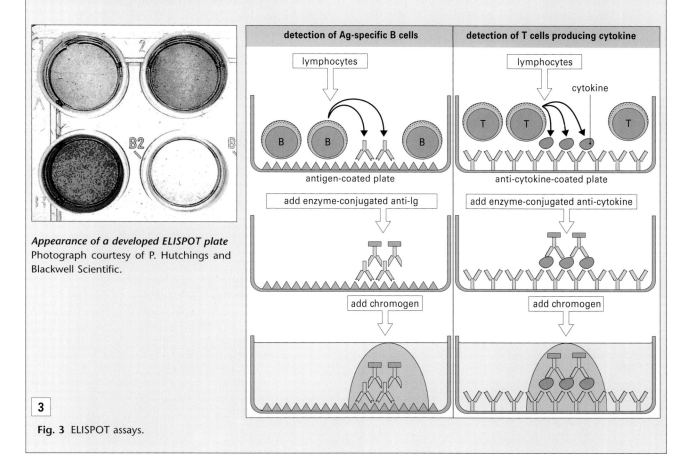

Appearance of a developed ELISPOT plate
Photograph courtesy of P. Hutchings and Blackwell Scientific.

3

Fig. 3 ELISPOT assays.

The **immunoglobulin superfamily** comprises molecules with structural characteristics similar to those of the immunoglobulins and includes CD2, CD3, CD4, CD8, CD28, MHC class I and II molecules, and many more.

The **integrin** family consists of heterodimeric molecules with α and β chains. There are several integrin subfamilies and all members of a particular subfamily share a common β chain, but each has a unique α chain:

- one integrin subfamily (**the β_2-integrins**) uses CD18 as the β chain, which can be associated with CD11a, CD11b, CD11c, or αd – these combinations make up the lymphocyte function antigens LFA-1, Mac-1

(CR3), p150,95, and $\alpha d\beta_2$ surface molecules respectively – and are commonly found on leukocytes.

- a second subfamily (**the β_1-integrins**) has CD29 as the β chain, which again is associated with various other peptides and includes the VLA (very late activation) markers.

The **selectins** (CD62, E, L, and P) are expressed on leukocytes (L) or activated endothelial cells and platelets (E and P). They have lectin-like specificity for a variety of sugars expressed on heavily glycosylated membrane glycoproteins (e.g. CD43).

The **proteoglycans**, typically CD44, have a number of glycosaminoglycan (GAG) binding sites (e.g. for chondroitin sulfate), and bind to extracellular matrix components (typically, hyaluronic acid).

Other families include:

- the tumor necrosis factor (TNF) and nerve growth factor (NGF) receptor superfamily;
- the C-type lectin superfamily;
- the family of receptors with seven transmembrane segments (tm7); and
- the tetraspanins, a superfamily with four membrane-spanning segments (tm4), for example CD20.

Marker molecules allow lymphocytes to communicate with their environment

The major function of the families of marker molecules described above is to allow lymphocytes to communicate with their environment. They are extremely important in cell trafficking, adhesion, and activation.

Markers expressed by lymphocytes can often be detected on cells of other lineages (e.g. CD44 is commonly expressed by epithelial cells).

Marker molecules allow lymphocytes to be isolated from each other

The presence of characteristic surface molecules expressed by cell populations allows them to be identified using fluorescent antibodies as probes. These can be applied to tissue sections to identify cell populations or be used in flow cytometry to enumerate and separate cells in suspension on the basis of their size and fluorescent staining (see Method Box 2.1). These techniques together with the expression of surface molecules allowing the cell populations to be isolated from each other using cell panning and immunomagnetic beads (Method Box 2.2) have allowed a detailed dissection of lymphoid cell populations.

METHOD BOX 2.2
Isolating cell populations

Density-gradient separation of lymphocytes on Ficoll Isopaque

Lymphocytes can be separated from whole blood using a density gradient. Whole blood is defibrinated by shaking with glass beads and the resulting clot removed. The blood is then diluted in tissue culture medium and layered on top of a tube half full of Ficoll. Ficoll has a density greater than that of lymphocytes, but less than that of red cells and granulocytes (e.g. neutrophils).

After centrifugation the red cells and polymorphonuclear neutrophils (PMNs) pass down through the Ficoll to form a pellet at the bottom of the tube while lymphocytes settle at the interface of the medium and Ficoll.

The lymphocyte preparation can be further depleted of macrophages and residual PMNs by the addition of iron filings. These are taken up by phagocytes, which can then be drawn away with a strong magnet. Macrophages can also be removed by leaving the cell suspension to settle on a plastic dish. Macrophages adhere to plastic, whereas the lymphocytes can be washed off.

Isolating cell populations using their characteristic surface molecules

The presence of characteristic surface molecules expressed by cell populations allows the cell populations to be isolated from each other using cell panning and immunomagnetic beads.

Isolation of lymphocyte subpopulations – panning

Cell populations can be separated on antibody-sensitized plates. Antibody binds non-covalently to the plastic plate (as for solid-phase immunoassay) and the cell mixture is applied to the plate. Antigen-positive cells (Ag$^+$) bind to the antibody and the antigen-negative cells (Ag$^-$) can be carefully washed off.

By changing the culture conditions or by enzyme digestion of the cells on the plate, it is sometimes possible to recover the cells bound to the plate.

Often the cells that have bound to the plate are altered by their binding (e.g. binding to the plate cross-links the antigen, which can cause cell activation). The method is therefore most satisfactory for removing a subpopulation from the population, rather than isolating it.

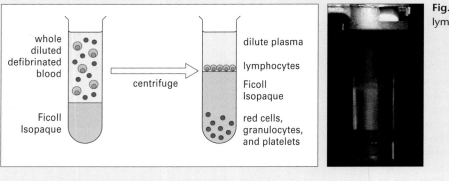

Fig. 1 Density-gradient separation of lymphocytes on Ficoll Isopaque.

METHOD BOX 2.2
Isolating cell populations *(Continued)*

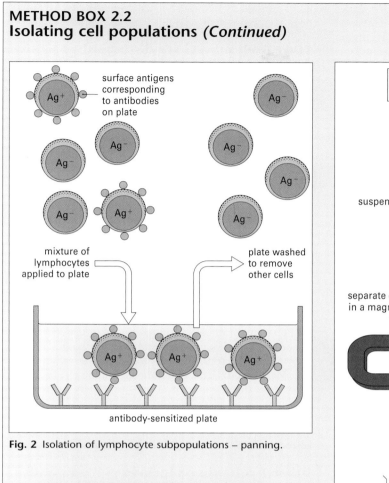

Fig. 2 Isolation of lymphocyte subpopulations – panning.

Examples of the application of this method include:

- separating T$_H$ and T$_C$ cell populations using antibodies to CD4 or CD8; and
- separating T cells from B cells using anti-Ig (which binds to the surface antibody of the B cell).

In reverse, by sensitizing the plate with antigen, antigen-binding cells can be separated from non-binding cells.

Cell separation by immunomagnetic beads
Direct method (shown in Fig. 3)
The beads are coated with a monoclonal antibody to the cellular antigen of interest, by either:

- direct binding to the bead; or
- binding the primary antibody to secondary antibody-coated beads.

The coated beads are then incubated with the cell suspension (or even whole blood) and the cells bound by the antibody on the beads (positively selected cells) are immobilized by applying a magnetic field to the tube. The non-immobilized cells (negatively selected) are removed from the tube and the positively selected cells are recovered following washing and dissociation from the antibody-coated beads.

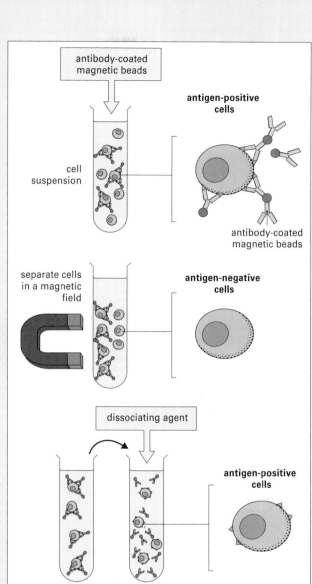

Fig. 3 Cell separation by immunomagnetic beads.

Indirect method
The monoclonal antibody to the target cellular antigen is first added to the cell suspension. Following incubation with the antibody, the cells are washed and mixed with beads coated with the appropriate secondary anti-Ig antibody. Cells bound to the magnetic beads (positively selected) are then immobilized with a magnetic field and the non-immobilized cells (negatively selected) removed. The positively selected cells are then washed and dissociated from the beads.

T cells can be distinguished by their different antigen receptors

The definitive T cell lineage marker is the T cell antigen receptor (TCR). The two defined types of TCR are:
- a heterodimer of two disulfide-linked polypeptides (α and β);
- a structurally similar heterodimer consisting of γ and δ polypeptides.

Both receptors are associated with a set of five polypeptides (the CD3 complex) and together form the TCR complex (TCR–CD3 complex; see Chapter 5).

Approximately 90–95% of blood T cells are $\alpha\beta$ T cells and the remaining 5–10% are $\gamma\delta$ T cells.

THERE ARE TWO MAJOR SUBPOPULATIONS OF T CELLS

$\alpha\beta$ T cells are subdivided into two distinct non-overlapping populations:
- one subset carries the **CD4 marker (CD4$^+$ T cells)** and mainly 'helps' or 'induces' immune responses (TH); and
- the other subset carries the **CD8 marker (CD8$^+$ T cells)** and is predominantly cytotoxic (Tc).

CD4$^+$ T cells recognize their specific antigens in association with MHC class II molecules, whereas CD8$^+$ T cells recognize antigens in association with MHC class I molecules (see Chapter 7). Thus, the presence of CD4 or CD8 limits (restricts) the type of cell with which the T cell can interact (Fig. 2.21).

A small proportion of $\alpha\beta$ T cells express neither CD4 nor CD8; these 'double negative' T cells might have a regulatory function.

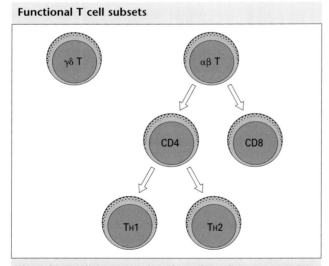

Functional T cell subsets

Fig. 2.21 T cells express either $\gamma\delta$ or $\alpha\beta$ T cell receptors (TCR). T cells are divided into CD4 and CD8 subsets and these subsets determine whether they see antigen (peptides) with MHC class II or I molecules, respectively. CD4$^+$ T cells can be further subdivided into TH1 and TH2 on the basis of their cytokine profiles.

In contrast, while most circulating $\gamma\delta$ cells are 'double negative', most $\gamma\delta$ T cells in the tissues express CD8.

CD4$^+$ T cell subsets are distinguished by their cytokine profiles

CD4$^+$ T cells can be further divided into functional subsets on the basis of the spectrum of the cytokines they produce:
- TH1 cells secrete IL-2 and IFNγ;
- TH2 cells produce IL-4, IL-5, IL-6, and IL-10 (see Fig. 11.9).

TH1 cells mediate several functions associated with cyto-toxicity and local inflammatory reactions. Consequently, they are important for combating intracellular pathogens including viruses, bacteria, and parasites.

Q. Which cell type do TH1 cells interact with to help combat intracellular pathogens?
A. Mononuclear phagocytes.

TH2 cells are more effective at stimulating B cells to proliferate and produce antibodies, and therefore function primarily to protect against free-living microorganisms (humoral immunity).

The number of cells producing a given cytokine can be measured using flow cytometry and antibodies that are allowed to penetrate the cells following permeabilization (see Method Box 2.1). The same technique can be used to determine the number of B cells producing a particular antibody.

The measurement of single cells secreting a particular cytokine or antibody can be achieved using an enzyme-linked method, namely ELISPOT (Method Box 2.1).

Other T cell subsets include $\gamma\delta$ T cells and NKT cells

$\gamma\delta$ T cells may protect the mucosal surfaces of the body

$\gamma\delta$ T cells are relatively frequent in mucosal epithelia, but form only a minor subpopulation of circulating T cells (around 5%). Most intraepithelial lymphocytes (IELs) are $\gamma\delta$ T cells and express CD8, a marker not found on most circulating $\gamma\delta$ T cells.

$\gamma\delta$ T cells have a specific repertoire of TCRs biased towards certain bacterial/viral antigens (**superantigens**, see Fig. 7.22).

Human blood $\gamma\delta$ T cells have specificity for low molecular mass mycobacterial products (e.g. ethylamine and isopentenyl pyrophosphate).

Current opinion is that $\gamma\delta$ T cells may play an important role in protecting the mucosal surfaces of the body.

Some $\gamma\delta$ T cells may recognize antigens directly (i.e. with no need for MHC molecule-mediated presentation).

$\gamma\delta$ T cells display LGL characteristics (see Fig. 2.19) and a dendritic morphology in lymphoid tissues (Fig. 2.22).

NKT cells may initiate T cell responses

NKT cells have T markers and also some NK cell markers. Characteristically they express CD3 and have a unique $\alpha\beta$ TCR (expressing an invariant Vα and Vβ11, see Chapter 5).

Dendritic morphology of γδ T cells in the tonsil

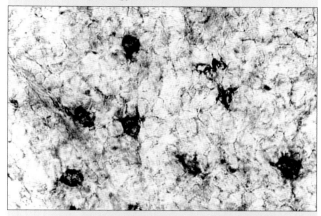

Fig. 2.22 The γδ T cell population is predominantly localized in the interfollicular T cell-dependent zones. Note the dendritic morphology of the cells. Anti-γδ T cell monoclonal antibody and immunoperoxidase. × 900. (Courtesy of Dr A Favre, from *Eur J Immunol* 1991;21:173, with permission)

Q. What markers would one normally use to distinguish T cells from NK cells?

A. CD16 and CD56 are used to distinguish NK cells. CD3 is characteristic of T cells.

NKT cells are thought to recognize glycolipid antigens presented by CD1d molecules (see Chapter 5), but not conventional MHC molecules. In response to antigen they are capable of producing large amounts of IFNγ and IL-4.

NKT cells are therefore thought to act as an interface between the innate and adaptive systems by initiating T cell responses.

NKT cells are also thought to regulate immune responses (especially dendritic cell function) through the production of cytokines (e.g. IL-10).

CELL SURFACE IMMUNOGLOBULIN AND SIGNALING MOLECULES FORM THE 'B CELL RECEPTOR' COMPLEX

About 5–15% of the circulating lymphoid pool are B cells, which are defined by the presence of surface immunoglobulin. Immunoglobulins are constitutively produced and are inserted into the B cell membrane, where they act as specific antigen receptors.

Most human B cells in peripheral blood express two immunoglobulin isotypes on their surface:
- IgM; and
- IgD (see Chapter 3).

On any B cell, the antigen-binding sites of these IgM and IgD isotypes are identical.

Fewer than 10% of the B cells in the circulation express IgG, IgA, or IgE, but B cells expressing IgG, IgA, or IgE are present in larger numbers in specific locations of the body (e.g. IgA-bearing cells in the intestinal mucosa).

Immunoglobulin associated with other 'accessory' molecules on the B cell surface forms the 'B cell antigen receptor complex' (BCR). These 'accessory' molecules consist of disulfide-bonded heterodimers of:
- Igα (CD79a); and
- Igβ (CD79b).

The heterodimers interact with the transmembrane segments of the immunoglobulin receptor (see Fig. 3.1), and, like the separate molecular components of the TCR/CD3 complex (see Fig. 5.2), are involved in cellular activation.

Other B cell markers include MHC class II antigens and complement and Fc receptors

Most B cells carry MHC class II antigens, which are important for cooperative (cognate) interactions with T cells. These class II molecules consist of I-A or I-E in the mouse and HLA-DP, DQ, and DR antigens in humans (see Fig. 5.18).

Complement receptors for C3b (CD35) and C3d (CD21) are commonly found on B cells and are associated with activation and, possibly, 'homing' of the cells. CD19/CD21 interactions with complement associated with antigen play a role in antigen-induced B cell activation via the antigen-binding antibody receptor.

Fc receptors for exogenous IgG (FcγRII, CD32) are also present on B cells and play a role in negative signaling to the B cell (see Chapter 11).

CD19 and CD20 are the main markers currently used to identify human B cells. Other human B cell markers are CD22 and CD72 to CD78.

Murine B cells also express CD72 (Lyb-2) together with B220, a high molecular weight (220 kDa) isoform of CD45 (Lyb-5).

CD40 is an important molecule on B cells and is involved in cognate interactions between T and B cells (see Fig. 8.8).

CD5⁺ B-1 cells and marginal zone B cells produce natural antibodies
CD5⁺ B-1 cells have a variety of roles

Many of the first B cells that appear during ontogeny express CD5, a marker originally found on T cells. These cells (termed B-1 cells) are found predominantly in the peritoneal cavity in mice, and there is some evidence for a separate differentiation pathway from 'conventional' B cells (termed **B-2 cells**).

CD5⁺ B-1 cells express their immunoglobulins from unmutated or minimally mutated germline genes and produce mostly IgM, but also some IgG and IgA. These so-called natural antibodies are of low avidity, but, unusually, they are polyreactive and are found at high concentration in the adult serum. CD5⁺ B-1 cells:
- respond well to TI (T-independent) antigens (i.e. antigens that can directly stimulate B cells without T cell help);
- may be involved in antigen processing and antigen presentation to T cells; and
- probably play a role in both tolerance and antibody responses.

Functions proposed for natural antibodies include:
- the first line of defense against microorganisms;
- clearance of damaged self components; and
- regulatory 'idiotype network' interactions within the immune system.

Characteristically, natural antibodies react against auto-antigens including:
- DNA;
- Fc of IgG;
- phospholipids; and
- cytoskeletal components.

CD5 has been shown to be expressed by B-2 cells when they are activated appropriately, so there is some controversy about whether CD5 represents an activation antigen on B cells. Current theories therefore support the notion for two different kinds of CD5+ B cells.

Although the function of CD5 on human B cells is unknown, it is associated with the BCR and may be involved in the regulation of B cell activation.

Marginal zone B cells are thought to protect against polysaccharide antigens

Much has been learned about **marginal zone B cells** over the past few years. These cells accumulate slowly in the marginal zone of the spleen – a process that takes between 1 and 2 years in humans.

Like B-1 cells, marginal zone B cells respond to thymus-independent antigens, and they are thought to be our main protection against polysaccharide antigens. They also produce natural antibodies, and together with B-1 cells have recently been termed 'innate-like B cells'.

B CELLS CAN DIFFERENTIATE INTO ANTIBODY-SECRETING PLASMA CELLS

Following B cell activation, many B cell blasts mature into **antibody-forming cells** (AFCs), which progress in vivo to terminally differentiated **plasma cells**.

Some B cell blasts do not develop rough endoplasmic reticulum cisternae. These cells are found in germinal centers and are named **follicle center cells** or **centrocytes**.

Under light microscopy, the cytoplasm of the plasma cells is basophilic due to the large amount of RNA being used for antibody synthesis in the rough endoplasmic reticulum. At the ultrastructural level, the rough endoplasmic reticulum can often be seen in parallel arrays (Fig. 2.23).

Plasma cells are infrequent in the blood, comprising less than 0.1% of circulating lymphocytes. They are normally restricted to the secondary lymphoid organs and tissues, but are also abundant in the bone marrow.

Antibodies produced by a single plasma cell are of one specificity and immunoglobulin class.

Immunoglobulins can be visualized in the plasma cell cytoplasm by staining with fluorochrome-labeled specific antibodies (Fig. 2.24).

Many plasma cells have a short life span, surviving for a few days and dying by apoptosis (Fig. 2.25). However, a subset of plasma cells with a long life span (months) has recently been described in the bone marrow.

Ultrastructure of the plasma cell

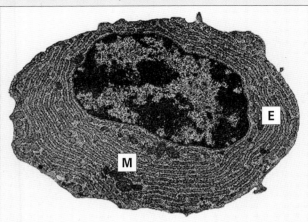

Fig 2.23 The plasma cell is characterized by parallel arrays of rough endoplasmic reticulum (E). In mature cells, these cisternae become dilated with immunoglobulins. Mitochondria (M) are also seen. × 5000. (Adapted from Zucker-Franklin D, Grossi CE, eds. Atlas of blood cells: function and pathology, 3rd edn. Milan: Edi Ermes; 2003)

Immunofluorescent staining of intracytoplasmic immunoglobulin in plasma cells

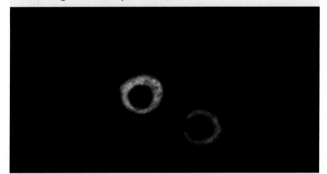

Fig. 2.24 Fixed human plasma cells, treated with fluoresceinated anti-human-IgM (green) and rhodaminated anti-human-IgG (red), show extensive intracytoplasmic staining. As the distinct staining of the two cells shows, plasma cells normally produce only one class or subclass (isotype) of antibody. × 1500. (Adapted from Zucker-Franklin D, Grossi CE, eds. Atlas of blood cells: function and pathology, 3rd edn. Milan: Edi Ermes; 2003)

LYMPHOID ORGANS AND TISSUES ARE EITHER PRIMARY OR SECONDARY

Lymphocytes, the effector cells of the adaptive immune response, are the major component of organs and tissues that collectively form the lymphoid system.

Plasma cell death by apoptosis

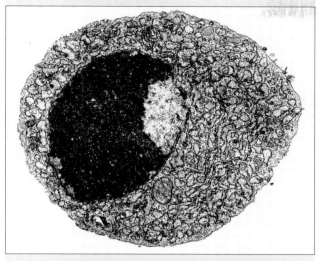

Fig. 2.25 Plasma cells are short-lived and die by apoptosis (cell suicide). Note the nuclear chromatin changes, which are characteristic of apoptosis. × 5000.

Major lymphoid organs and tissues

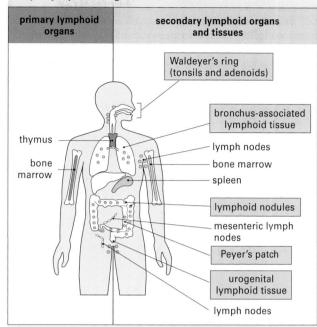

Fig. 2.26 Thymus and bone marrow are the primary (central) lymphoid organs. They are the sites of maturation for T and B cells, respectively. Cellular and humoral immune responses occur in the secondary (peripheral) lymphoid organs and tissues. Secondary lymphoid organs can be classified according to the body regions they defend. The spleen responds predominantly to blood-borne antigens. Lymph nodes mount immune responses to antigens circulating in the lymph, entering through the skin (subcutaneous lymph nodes) or through mucosal surfaces (visceral lymph nodes). Tonsils, Peyer's patches, and other mucosa-associated lymphoid tissues (MALT) (blue boxes) react to antigens that have entered via the surface mucosal barriers. Note that the bone marrow is both a primary and a secondary lymphoid organ because it gives rise to B and NK cells, but is also the site of B cell terminal differentiation (long-lived plasma cells).

Within the lymphoid organs, lymphocytes interact with other cell types of both hematopoietic and non-hematopoietic origin that are important for lymphocyte:
* maturation;
* selection;
* function; and
* disposal of terminally differentiated cells.

These other cell types are termed accessory cells and include:
* APCs;
* macrophages;
* reticular cells; and
* epithelial cells.

The lymphoid system is arranged into either discrete encapsulated organs or accumulations of diffuse lymphoid tissue, which are classified into primary (central) and secondary (peripheral) organs or tissues (Fig. 2.26).

In essence, lymphocytes:
* are produced, mature, and are selected in primary lymphoid organs; and
* exert their effector functions in the secondary lymphoid organs and tissues.

Tertiary lymphoid tissues are anatomical sites that under normal conditions contain sparse lymphocytes, if any, but may be selectively populated by these cells in pathological conditions (e.g. skin, synovium, and lungs).

LYMPHOID STEM CELLS DEVELOP AND MATURE WITHIN PRIMARY LYMPHOID ORGANS

In the primary lymphoid organs, lymphocytes (B and T cells):
* differentiate from lymphoid stem cells;
* proliferate;
* are selected; and
* mature into functional cells.

In mammals, T cells mature in the thymus and B cells mature in the fetal liver and postnatal bone marrow (see Chapter 8). Birds have a specialized site of B cell generation, the bursa of Fabricius.

In the primary lymphoid organs:
* lymphocytes acquire their repertoire of specific antigen receptors to cope with the antigenic challenges that individuals encounter during their lifetime;
* cells with receptors for **autoantigens** are mostly eliminated; and
* in the thymus, T cells also 'learn' to recognize appropriate **self MHC molecules**.

There is evidence that some lymphocyte development might occur outside primary lymphoid organs.

Thymus section showing the lobular organization

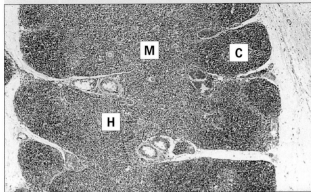

Fig. 2.27 This section shows the two main areas of the thymus lobule – an outer cortex of immature cells (C) and an inner medulla of more mature cells (M). Hassall's corpuscles (H) are found in the medulla. H&E stain. × 25. (Courtesy of Dr A Stevens and Professor J Lowe)

Q. Why do lymphocytes need to 'learn' what constitutes self MHC and self antigens?

A. Each individual is different and has a particular set of MHC molecules and particular variants of the many other molecules present in the body. The process of what constitutes immunological 'self' is different in each individual and therefore learning to recognize 'self' is a dialogue between T cells and APCs that takes place in each individual.

T CELLS DEVELOPING IN THE THYMUS UNDERGO SELECTION PROCESSES

The thymus in mammals is a bilobed organ in the thoracic cavity overlying the heart and major blood vessels. Each lobe is organized into lobules separated from each other by connective tissue trabeculae.

Within each lobule, the lymphoid cells (thymocytes) are arranged into:

• an outer tightly packed cortex, which contains the majority of relatively immature proliferating thymocytes; and

• an inner medulla containing more mature cells, implying a differentiation gradient from cortex to medulla (Fig. 2.27).

The main blood vessels that regulate cell traffic in the thymus are high endothelial venules (HEVs; see Fig. 2.29) at the corticomedullary junction of thymic lobules. It is through these veins that T cell progenitors formed in the fetal liver and bone marrow enter the **epithelial anlage** and migrate towards the cortex.

In the cortex of the thymus the T cell progenitors undergo proliferation and differentiation processes that lead to the generation of mature T cells through a corticomedullary gradient of migration.

A network of epithelial cells throughout the lobules plays a role in the differentiation and selection processes from fetal liver and bone marrow-derived prethymic cells to mature T cells.

The mature T cells probably leave the thymus through the same PCVs, at the corticomedullary junction from which the T cell progenitors entered (Fig. 2.28).

Cell migration to and within the thymus

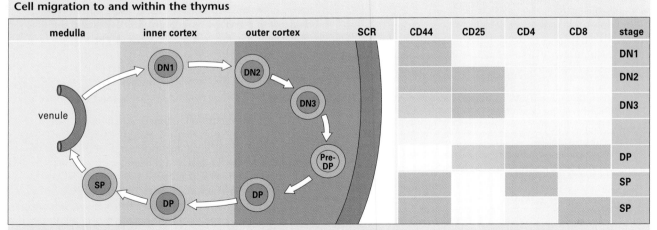

Fig. 2.28 T cell progenitors enter the thymic lobule through postcapillary venules (PCVs) at the corticomedullary junction. These double negative 1 (DN1) cells are CD4⁻, CD8⁻, CD25⁻, but CD44⁺. They move progressively towards the outer cortex and differentiate into DN2 (CD25⁺, CD44⁺) and DN3 cells (CD25⁺, CD44ˡᵒ). Thymocytes accumulate in the subcapsular region where they actively proliferate and differentiate into double positive (DP; CD4⁺, CD8⁺) cells. DP thymocytes reverse their polarity and move towards the medulla. In the course of this migration, thymocytes are selected and as single positive (SP; CD4⁺ or CD8⁺) cells ultimately leave the thymus, presumably via HEVs at the corticomedullary junction.

Three types of thymic epithelial cell have important roles in T cell production

At least three types of epithelial cell can be distinguished in the thymic lobules according to distribution, structure, function, and phenotype:

- the epithelial nurse cells are in the outer cortex;
- the cortical thymic epithelial cells (TECs) form an epithelial network; and
- the medullary TECs are mostly organized into clusters (Fig. 2.29).

These three types of epithelial cell have different roles for thymocyte proliferation, maturation, and selection:

- **nurse cells** in the outer cortex sustain the proliferation of progenitor T cells, mainly through cytokine production (e.g. IL-7);
- **cortical TECs** are responsible for the positive selection of maturing thymocytes, allowing survival of cells that recognize MHC class I and II molecules with associated peptides via TCRs of intermediate affinity;
- **medullary TECs** display a large variety of organ-specific self peptides.

Q. What is the significance of the presence of organ-specific self peptides in the thymus?

A. An individual needs to be tolerant of antigens that are expressed in other tissues, not just the thymus. By presenting a library of self molecules, the thymus can delete or tolerize lymphocytes that might otherwise react against self molecules once they had migrated into other tissues. Thus TECs, together with other APCs (interdigitating cells and macrophages), play a role in negative selection (i.e. the deletion of self-reactive T cells).

Hassall's corpuscles (see Fig. 2.27) are found in the thymic medulla. Their function is unknown, but they appear to contain degenerating epithelial cells rich in high molecular weight cytokeratins.

The mammalian thymus involutes with age (Fig. 2.30). In humans, atrophy begins at puberty and continues throughout life. Thymic involution begins within the cortex and this region may disappear completely, whereas medullary remnants persist.

Cortical atrophy is related to a sensitivity of the cortical thymocytes to corticosteroid, and all conditions associated

---

Schematic structure of the thymus

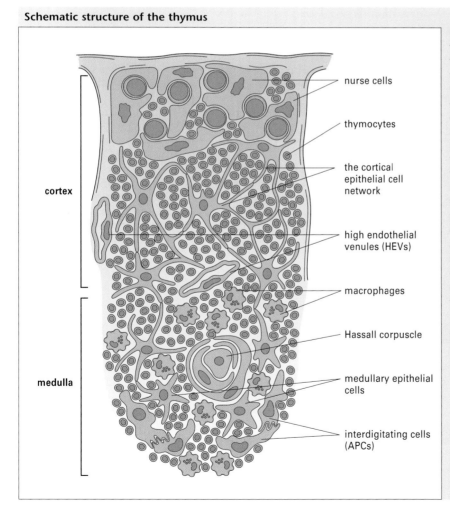

cortex

medulla

nurse cells

thymocytes

the cortical epithelial cell network

high endothelial venules (HEVs)

macrophages

Hassall corpuscle

medullary epithelial cells

interdigitating cells (APCs)

Fig. 2.29 A schematic representation of the cell types found in a fully developed thymic lobule. Subcapsular epithelial cells that produce IL-7 (nurse cells) sustain T lymphoblast proliferation in the outer cortex. Developing T cells interact with the cortical epithelial network where they are positively selected. Apoptotic cells are phagocytosed by macrophages present in the deep cortex and in the medulla. TCR[+] thymocytes co-expressing CD4 and CD8 undergo the process of negative selection by interacting with a variety of antigen-presenting cells (APCs), such as dendritic cells, interdigitating cells, macrophages, and epithelial cells. T cells that have survived the selection processes are exported from the thymus via high endothelial venules (HEVs) and lymphatic vessels. (From Zucker-Franklin D, Grossi CE, eds. Atlas of blood cells: function and pathology, 3rd edn. Milan: Edi Ermes; 2003)

Atrophic adult thymus

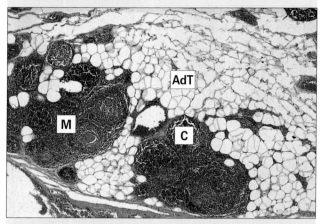

Fig 2.30 There is an involution of the thymus with replacement by adipose tissue (AdT). The cortex (C) is largely reduced and the less cellular medulla (M) is still apparent. (Courtesy of Dr A Stevens and Professor J Lowe)

with an acute increase in corticosteroids (e.g. pregnancy and stress) promote thymic atrophy.

It is conceivable that T cell generation within the thymus continues into adult life, albeit at a low rate. Evidence for de-novo T cell production in the thymus (recent thymic emigrants) has been shown in humans over the age of 76 years.

Stem cell migration to the thymus initiates T cell development

The thymus develops from the endoderm of the third pharyngeal pouch as an epithelial rudiment that becomes seeded with blood-borne stem cells. Relatively few stem cells appear to be needed to give rise to the enormous repertoire of mature T cells with diverse antigen receptor specificities.

From experimental studies, migration of stem cells into the thymus is not a random process, but results from chemotactic signals periodically emitted from the thymic rudiment. β_2-Microglobulin, a component of the MHC class I molecule, is one such putative chemoattractant.

In birds, stem cells enter the thymus in two or possibly three waves, but it is not clear that there are such waves in mammals.

Once in the thymus, the stem cells begin to differentiate into thymic lymphocytes (called thymocytes), under the influence of the epithelial microenvironment.

Whether or not the stem cells are 'pre-T cells' (i.e. are committed to becoming T cells before they arrive in the thymus) is controversial. Although the stem cells express CD7, substantial evidence exists that they are in fact multipotent. Granulocytes, APCs, NK cells, B cells, and myeloid cells have all been generated in vitro from hematopoietic precursors isolated from the thymus. This suggests that the prethymic bone marrow-derived cell entering the thymic rudiment is multipotent.

Epithelial cells, macrophages, and bone marrow-derived IDCs, molecules rich in MHC class II, are impor-

tant for the differentiation of T cells from this multipotent stem cell. For example, specialized epithelial cells in the peripheral areas of the cortex (the thymic nurse cells, see above) contain thymocytes within pockets in their cytoplasm. The nurse cells support lymphocyte proliferation by producing the cytokine IL-7.

The subcapsular region of the thymus is the only site where thymocyte proliferation occurs. Thymocytes develop into large, actively proliferating, self-renewing lymphoblasts, which generate the thymocyte population.

There are many more developing lymphocytes (85–90%) in the thymic cortex than in the medulla, and studies of function and cell surface markers have indicated that cortical thymocytes are less mature than medullary thymocytes. This reflects the fact that cortical cells migrate to, and mature in, the medulla.

Most mature T cells leave the thymus via HEVs at the corticomedullary junction, though other routes of exit may exist, including lymphatic vessels.

T cells change their phenotype during maturation

As with the development of granulocytes and monocytes, 'differentiation' markers of functional significance appear or are lost during the progression from stem cell to mature T cell.

Analyses of genes encoding $\alpha\beta$ and $\gamma\delta$ TCRs and other studies examining changes in surface membrane antigens suggest that there are multiple pathways of T cell differentiation in the thymus. It is not known whether these pathways are distinct, but it seems more likely that they diverge from a common pathway.

Only a small proportion (< 1%) of mature T lymphocytes express the $\gamma\delta$ TCR. Most thymocytes differentiate into $\alpha\beta$ TCR cells, which account for the majority (> 95%) of T lymphocytes in secondary lymphoid tissues and in the circulation.

Phenotypic analyses have shown sequential changes in surface membrane antigens during T cell maturation (Fig. 2.31). The phenotypic variations can be simplified into a three-stage model.

Stage I thymocytes are CD4⁻, CD8⁻

There are two phases of stage I (early) thymocytes. In the first phase, the TCR genes are in the germline configuration and the cells:
- express CD44 and CD25;
- are CD4⁻, CD8⁻ (i.e. double negative cells).

In this early first phase, cells entering the thymus via the HEVs in the corticomedullary junction express CD44, which allows them to migrate towards the outermost cortex, the zone of thymocyte proliferation. These cells are not fully committed to the T cell lineage, because outside the thymic environment they can give rise to other hematopoietic lineages. Surface expression of CD44 is downregulated once the cells are in the external cortex.

In the second phase the cells:
- become CD44⁻;
- are CD25⁺;
- remain double negative for CD4 and CD8;
- rearrange the β chain of the TCR;

Expression of human T cell markers during development

markers	prethymic	thymic cortex		thymic medulla	circulating T cells
		stage I	stage II	stage III	
TCR gene rearrange-ment		β			
		α			
expressed molecules					
TdT					
CD44					
CD25					
CD3		cyto	low	high	
γδ TCR			low	high	
αβ TCR			low	high	
CD4 + CD8					
CD1					
CD7					
CD5					
CD2					
CD38					

Fig. 2.31 Terminal deoxynucleotidyl transferase (TdT) is an enzyme in thymic stem cells. It decreases in stage II and is lost altogether in the medulla. Several surface glycoproteins appear during differentiation. CD1 is present on stage II cortical thymocytes and is lost in the medulla. CD2 and CD7 (the pan-T marker) appear very early in differentiation and are maintained through to the mature T cell stage. CD5 appears at an early stage and persists on mature T cells. CD3 is expressed first in the cytoplasm in stage I cells (cyto), and then on the surface simultaneously with the T cell receptor (TCR). In most stage II cells, both surface CD3 and the αβ TCR are expressed at low density, but these markers are present at high density on stage III cells. CD4 and CD8 are co-expressed on stage II cells (double positives). One of these molecules is lost during differentiation into mature stage III cells (single positives).

- express cytoplasmic but not surface TCR-associated CD3;
- are irreversibly committed to become T cells;
- continue to express CD7 together with CD2 and CD5.

Proliferation markers such as the transferrin receptor (CD71) and CD38 (a marker common to all early hematopoietic precursors) are also expressed at this stage.

Stage II thymocytes become CD4⁺, CD8⁺

Stage II (intermediate or common) thymocyte cells account for around 80% of thymocytes in the fully developed thymus. Characteristically they:
- are CD1⁺, CD44⁻, CD25⁻;
- become CD4+, CD8+ (double positives).

Genes encoding the TCR α chain are rearranged in these intermediate thymocytes; both chains of the αβ TCR are expressed at low density on the cell surface in association with polypeptides of the CD3/antigen receptor complex.

Stage III thymocytes become either CD4⁺ or CD8⁺

Stage III (mature) thymocytes show major phenotypic changes, namely:
- loss of CD1;
- cell surface CD3 associated with the αβ TCR expressed at a higher density;
- the distinction of two subsets of cells expressing either CD4 or CD8 (i.e. single positives).

Most stage III thymocytes:
- lack CD38 and the transferrin receptor;
- are virtually indistinguishable from mature, circulating T cells.

All stage III cells re-express the receptor CD44, which is thought to be involved in migration and homing to peripheral lymphoid tissues. L-selectin (CD62L) is also expressed at this time.

DIVERSE ANTIGEN REPERTOIRES ARE GENERATED BY RECOMBINATION OF GENE SEGMENTS ENCODING THE TCR
T cell receptor diversity is generated in the thymus

T cells have to recognize a wide variety of different antigens. The genes of the αβ and γδ TCR undergo **somatic recombination** during thymic development to produce functional genes for the different TCRs (see Chapter 5).

Q. How are receptors with different antigenic specificity distributed among the total population of T cells?
A. Each T cell has one specificity of receptor (i.e. the receptors are clonally distributed).

Q. Are there any differences in the mechanism by which TCRs are generated in CD4⁺ and CD8⁺ T cells?
A. Because CD4⁺ and CD8⁺ T cells do not differentiate until after TCR generation, the mechanism for generating diverse receptors is the same for both major T cell subsets.

TCR gene recombination takes place within the subcapsular and outer cortex of the thymus, where there is active cell proliferation. Through a random assortment of different gene segments, a large number of different TCRs are made and thymocytes that fail to make a functional receptor die.

The TCRs associate with peptides of the CD3 complex, which transduces activating signals to the cell.

'Alternative' forms of the T cell receptor during development

Studies in transgenic mice have shown that early in ontogeny T cells can express alternative forms of the TCR which may be involved in generating signals that drive development:

- TCRβ dimers can associate with CD3 in the absence of TCRα;
- TCRβ chains can be found on the cell surface as phosphoinositol linked proteins that do not associate with CD3;
- surface TCRβ chains can be associated with an incomplete CD3 complex;
- a 33-kDa glycoprotein linked to TCRβ chains in pre-T cells acts as a 'surrogate' chain (pre-Tα chain).

These pre-T cell antigen receptors, like the surrogate pre-B cell receptors (see Fig. 8.2), are probably involved in proliferation, maturation, and selection during the early phases of lymphocyte development.

POSITIVE AND NEGATIVE SELECTION OF DEVELOPING T CELLS IN THE THYMUS

The processes involved in the education of T cells are shown in Fig. 2.32, and self tolerance is discussed fully in Chapter 11.

Positive selection ensures only TCRs with an intermediate affinity for self MHC develop further

T cells:

- recognize antigenic peptides only when presented by self MHC molecules on APCs;
- show 'dual recognition' of both the antigenic peptides and the polymorphic part of the MHC molecules.

CD4, found on a subset of T cells, also recognizes the class II MHC molecule, but its non-polymorphic portion.

Positive selection (the first stage of **thymic education**) ensures that only those TCRs with an intermediate affinity for self MHC are allowed to develop further.

T cell differentiation within the thymus

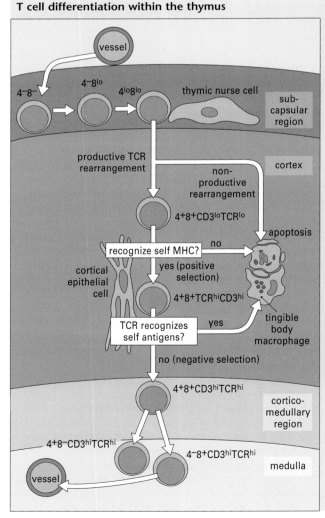

Fig. 2.32 In this model, pre-thymic T cells are attracted to and enter the thymic rudiment at the corticomedullary junction. They reach the subcapsular region where they proliferate as large lymphoblasts, which give rise to a pool of cells entering the differentiation pathway. Many of these cells are associated with epithelial thymic nurse cells. Cells in this region first acquire CD8 and then CD4 at low density. They also rearrange their T cell receptor (TCR) genes and may express the products of these genes at low density on the cell surface. Maturing cells move deeper into the cortex and adhere to cortical epithelial cells. These epithelial cells are elongated and branched, and thus provide a large surface area for contact with thymocytes. The TCRs on the thymocytes are exposed to epithelial MHC molecules through these contacts. This leads to positive selection. Those cells that are not selected undergo apoptosis and are phagocytosed by macrophages. There is an increased expression of CD3, TCR, CD4, and CD8 during thymocyte migration from the subcapsular region to the deeper cortex. Those TCRs with self reactivity are now deleted through contact with autoantigens presented by medullary thymic epithelial cells, interdigitating cells, and macrophages at the corticomedullary junction – a process called negative selection. Following this stage, cells expressing either CD4 or CD8 appear and exit to the periphery via specialized vessels at the corticomedullary junction. (Adapted from D Zucker-Franklin, CE Grossi, eds. Atlas of blood cells: function and pathology, 3rd edn. Milan: Edi Ermes; 2003)

There is evidence that positive selection is mediated by TECs acting as APCs.

T cells displaying very high or very low receptor affinities for self MHC undergo apoptosis and die in the cortex. Apoptosis is a pre-programmed 'suicide', achieved by activating endogenous nucleases that cause DNA fragmentation (Fig. 2.33).

T cells with TCRs that have intermediate affinities are rescued from apoptosis, survive, and continue along their pathway of maturation. A possible exception is provided by some T cells equipped with γδ receptors, which (like B cells) recognize native antigenic conformations with no need for APCs.

Negative selection ensures that only T cells that fail to recognize self antigen proceed in their development

Some of the positively selected T cells may have TCRs that recognize self components other than self MHC. These cells are deleted by a 'negative selection' process, which occurs:

- in the deeper cortex;
- at the corticomedullary junction; and
- in the medulla.

T cells interact with antigen presented by interdigitating cells, macrophages, and medullary TECs. The role of medullary TECs for negative selection has been emphasized recently by the finding that these cells express genes for virtually all tissue antigens in the body.

Only T cells that fail to recognize self antigen are allowed to proceed in their development. The rest undergo apoptosis and are destroyed. These, and all the other apoptotic cells generated in the thymus, are phagocytosed by (tingible body) macrophages (see Fig. 2.47) in the deep cortex.

T cells at this stage of maturation (CD4$^+$ CD8$^+$ TCR^{lo}) go on to express TCR at high density and lose either CD4 or CD8 to become 'single positive' mature T cells.

The separate subsets of CD4$^+$ and CD8$^+$ cells possess specialized homing receptors (e.g. CD44), and exit to the T cell areas of the peripheral (secondary) lymphoid tissues where they function as mature 'helper' and 'cytotoxic' T cells, respectively.

Q. Which subset of T cells functions as T$_H$ and which as T$_C$ cells?

A. CD4$^+$ T cells function mainly as T$_H$ cells whereas CD8$^+$ T cells are predominantly T$_C$ cells.

Less than 5% of thymocytes leave the thymus as mature T cells. The rest die as the result of:

- selection processes; or
- failure to undergo productive rearrangements of antigen receptor genes.

Adhesion of maturing thymocytes to epithelial and accessory cells is crucial for T cell development

Adhesion of maturing thymocytes to epithelial and other accessory cells is mediated by the interaction of complementary adhesion molecules, such as:

- CD2 with LFA-3 (CD58); and
- LFA-1 (CD11a, CD18) with ICAM-1 (CD54) (see Appendix 2).

These interactions induce the production of the cytokines IL-1, IL-3, IL-6, IL-7, and GM-CSF (see Appendix 3), which are required for T cell proliferation and maturation in the thymus.

Early thymocytes also express receptors for IL-2, which together with IL-7 sustains cell proliferation.

Negative selection may also occur outside the thymus in peripheral lymphoid tissues

Not all self-reactive T cells are eliminated during intrathymic development, probably because not all self antigens can be presented in the thymus. The thymic epithelial barrier that surrounds blood vessels may also limit access of some circulating antigens.

Given the survival of some self-reacting T cells, a separate mechanism is required to prevent them attacking the body. Experiments with transgenic mice have suggested that peripheral inactivation of self-reactive T cells (**peripheral tolerance**, see Chapter 19) could occur via several mechanisms as follows:

- downregulation of the TCR and CD8 (in cytotoxic cells) so that the cells are unable to interact with target autoantigens;
- **anergy**, due to the lack of crucial co-stimulatory signals provided by the target cells, followed by induction of apoptosis after interaction with autoantigen;
- regulatory T cells (Tregs).

Thymic cell apoptosis

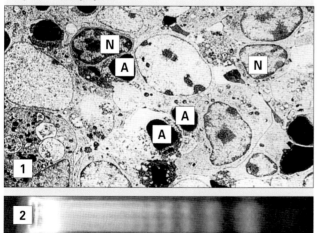

Fig. 2.33 (1) Fetal thymic lobes in culture were treated with anti-CD3 antibodies – this simulates activation via the TCR and therefore triggers programmed cell death (apoptosis). This electron micrograph shows the heavy condensation of nuclear chromatin in apoptotic nuclei (A) compared with the dispersed chromatin of normal cells (N). (Courtesy of Dr C Smith) (2) Analysis of the DNA from apoptotic cells by agarose gel electrophoresis shows the characteristically ordered, ladder-like pattern created by bands of digested DNA fragments.

Regulatory T cells are involved in peripheral tolerance

Tregs have been the subject of intensive research over the past few years, especially in the areas of autoimmunity and vaccine development.

In addition to NKT cells and γδ T cells regulating immune responses, there is now substantial evidence that separate CD4+ subsets also have this function. The general consensus is that there are two main types of Treg – naturally occurring and antigen induced.

Naturally occurring Tregs:
- constitutively express CD25 (the α chain of the low-affinity receptor for IL-2);
- constitute about 5–10% of the peripheral CD4+ T cells;
- express the unique transcription factor FoxP3;
- constitutively express the marker CTLA4;
- do not proliferate in response to antigenic challenge;
- are thought to produce their suppressive effects through cell contact (e.g. with APCs, TH1 or TH2 cells).

Antigen-induced Tregs:
- also express CD25;
- can develop from CD25−, CD4+ T cells;
- are believed to exert their suppressive effects through cytokines such as TGFβ and IL-10.

There is some evidence for extrathymic development of T cells

The vast majority of T cells require a functioning thymus for differentiation, but small numbers of cells carrying T cell markers that are often oligoclonal in nature have been found in athymic ('nude') mice. Although the possibility that these mice possess thymic remnants cannot be ruled out, there is accumulating evidence to suggest that bone marrow precursors can home to mucosal epithelia and mature without the need for a thymus to form:
- functional T cells with γδ TCRs; and
- probably also T cells with αβ TCRs.

The importance of extrathymic development in animals that are euthymic (i.e. that have a normal thymus) is at present unclear.

B CELLS DEVELOP MAINLY IN THE FETAL LIVER AND BONE MARROW

Unlike birds, which have a discrete organ for the generation of B cells (the bursa of Fabricius), in mammals B cells develop directly from lymphoid stem cells in the hematopoietic tissue of the fetal liver (Fig. 2.34). This occurs at 8–9 weeks of gestation in humans, and by about 14 days in the mouse. Later, the site of B cell production moves from the liver to the bone marrow, where it continues through adult life. This fetal liver-bone marrow migration of stem cells is also true for cells of other hematopoietic lineages such as erythrocytes, granulocytes, monocytes, and platelets.

B cell progenitors are also present in the omental tissue of murine and human fetuses and are the precursors of a self-replicating B cell subset, the B-1 cells (see above).

Hemopoiesis in fetal liver

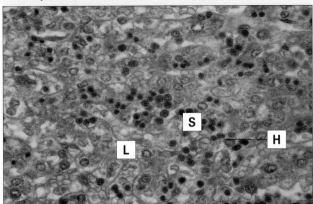

Fig. 2.34 Section of human fetal liver showing islands of hemopoiesis (H). Hematopoietic stem cells are found in the sinusoidal spaces (S) between plates of liver cells (L). (Courtesy of Dr A Stevens and Professor J Lowe)

B cell production in the bone marrow does not occur in distinct domains

B cell progenitors in the bone marrow are seen adjacent to the endosteum of the bone lamellae (Fig. 2.35). Each B cell progenitor at the stage of immunoglobulin gene re-arrangement may produce up to 64 progeny. The progeny migrate towards the center of each cavity of the spongy bone and reach the lumen of a venous sinusoid (Fig. 2.36).

In the bone marrow, B cells mature in close association with **stromal reticular cells**, which are found both adjacent to the endosteum and in close association with the central sinus, where they are termed **adventitial reticular cells**.

Where the B cells differentiate, the reticular cells have mixed phenotypic features with some similarities to fibroblasts, endothelial cells, and myofibroblasts. The reticular cells produce type IV collagen, laminin and the smooth muscle form of actin. Experiments in vitro have shown that reticular cells sustain B cell differentiation, possibly by producing the cytokine IL-7.

Adventitial reticular cells may be important for the release of mature B cells into the central sinus.

B cells are subject to selection processes.

Most B cells (> 75%) maturing in the bone marrow do not reach the circulation, but (like thymocytes) undergo a process of programmed cell death (apoptosis) and are phagocytosed by bone marrow macrophages.

Q. By analogy with T cell development, infer what determines whether a B cell will die during development in the bone marrow.

A. B cells with a non-productive rearrangement of the immunoglobulin genes do not survive and many self-reactive B cells are also eliminated through negative selection.

B cell–stromal cell interactions enhance the survival of developing B cells and mediate a form of selection that

Schematic organization of B cell development in the bone marrow

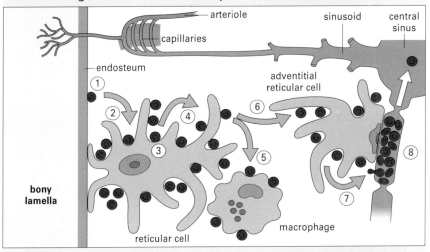

Fig. 2.35 The earliest B cell progenitors are found close to the endosteum (**1**) where they interact with stromal reticular cells (**2**). The stromal reticular cells prompt precursor B cell proliferation and maturation (**3** and **4**). During these processes, selection occurs, which implies B cell apoptosis and phagocytosis of apoptotic cells by macrophages (**5**). B cells that have survived selection mature further and interact with adventitial reticular cells (**6**), which may facilitate their ingress (**7**) into bone marrow sinusoids (**8**) and finally the central venous sinuses, from which they enter the general circulation. In this model, maturation and selection events follow a gradient from the periphery of the bone marrow tissue contained in the bony spaces towards the center.

rescues a minority of B cells with productive rearrangements of their immunoglobulin genes from programmed cell death.

Many self-reactive B cells are also eliminated through negative selection in the bone marrow.

From kinetic data, it is estimated that about 5×10^7 murine B cells are produced each day. As the mouse spleen contains approximately 7.5×10^7 B cells, a large proportion of B cells must die, probably at the pre-B cell stage, because of non-productive rearrangements of receptor genes or if they express self-reactive antibodies and are not rescued.

Immunoglobulins are the definitive B cell lineage markers
Lymphoid stem cells expressing terminal deoxynucleotidyl transferase (TdT) proliferate, differentiate, and undergo immunoglobulin gene rearrangements (see Chapters 3 and 8) to emerge as pre-B cells which express μ heavy chains in the cytoplasm. Some of these pre-B cells bear small numbers of surface μ chains, associated with 'surrogate' light chains $V_{pre\ B}$ and λ5 (see Fig. 8.2). **Allelic exclusion** of either maternal or paternal immunoglobulin genes has already occurred by this time. The proliferating pre-B cells are thought to give rise to smaller pre-B cells.

Once a B cell has synthesized light chains, which may be either κ- or λ-type, it becomes committed to the antigen-binding specificity of its surface IgM (sIgM) antigen receptor.

One B cell can therefore make only one specific antibody – a central tenet of the **clonal selection theory** for antibody production.

Surface immunoglobulin-associated molecules Igα and Igβ (CD79a and b) are present by the pre-B cell stage of development.

Developing B cells acquire characteristic surface molecules
A sequence of immunoglobulin gene rearrangements and phenotypic changes takes place during B cell ontogeny (see Chapter 8), similar to that described above for T cells.

Heavy-chain gene rearrangements occur in B cell progenitors and represent the earliest indication of B lineage commitment. This is followed by light-chain gene rearrangements, which occur at later pre-B cell stages.

B cells migrate to and function in the secondary lymphoid tissues
Early B cell immigrants into fetal lymph nodes (17 weeks in humans) are surface IgM+ and are B-1 cells. CD5+ B cell precursors are found in the fetal omentum.

Some CD5+ B cells are also found in the marginal zone of the spleen and mantle zone of secondary follicles in adult lymph nodes (see Fig. 2.44).

Following antigenic stimulation, mature B cells can develop into memory cells or antibody-forming cells (AFCs).

Bone marrow

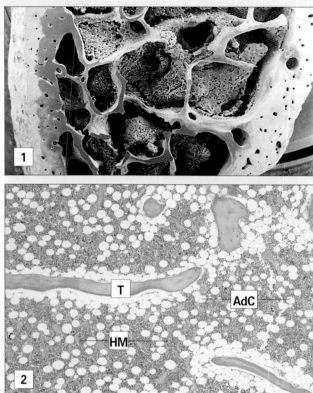

Fig. 2.36 (1) Low-power scanning electron micrograph showing the architecture of bone and its relationship to bone marrow. Within the cavities of spongy bone between the bony trabeculae, B cell lymphopoiesis takes place, with maturation occurring in a radial direction towards the center (from the endosteum to the central venous sinus). (2) The biopsy below shows hematopoietic bone marrow (HM) in the spaces between the bony trabeculae (lamellae) (T). Some of the space is also occupied by adipocytes (AdC). (Courtesy of Dr A Stevens and Professor J Lowe)

Surface immunoglobulins (sIg) are usually lost from plasma cells (the terminally differentiated form of an AFC) because their function as a receptor is no longer required. Like any other terminally differentiated hematopoietic cell, the plasma cell has a limited life span, and eventually undergoes apoptosis.

LYMPHOCYTES MIGRATE TO AND FUNCTION IN SECONDARY LYMPHOID ORGANS AND TISSUES

The generation of lymphocytes in primary lymphoid organs is followed by their migration into peripheral secondary tissues, which comprise:

- well-organized encapsulated organs, the **spleen** and **lymph nodes (systemic lymphoid organs)**; and
- non-encapsulated accumulations of lymphoid tissue.

Lymphoid tissue found in association with mucosal surfaces is called **mucosa-associated lymphoid tissue (MALT)**.

LYMPHOID ORGANS AND TISSUES PROTECT DIFFERENT BODY SITES

The systemic lymphoid organs and the mucosal system have different functions in immunity:

- the spleen is responsive to blood-borne antigens, and patients who have had their spleen removed are much more susceptible to pathogens that reach the blood stream;
- the lymph nodes protect the body from antigens that come from skin or from internal surfaces and are transported via the lymphatic vessels;
- the mucosal system protects mucosal surfaces.

Responses to antigens encountered via the spleen and lymph nodes result in the secretion of antibodies into the circulation and local cell-mediated responses.

The mucosal system is the site of first encounter (priming) of immune cells with antigens entering via mucosal surfaces, and lymphoid tissues are associated with surfaces lining:

- the intestinal tract – gut-associated lymphoid tissue (GALT);
- the respiratory tract – bronchus-associated lymphoid tissue (BALT); and
- the genitourinary tract.

The major effector mechanism at mucosal surfaces is secretory IgA antibody (sIgA), which is actively transported via the mucosal epithelial cells to the lumen of the tracts.

Q. More than 50% of the body's lymphoid tissue is in the MALT and IgA is the most abundant immunoglobulin in the body. What reason could explain this preponderance of immune defenses in mucosal tissues?

A. The mucosal surfaces present a large surface area, vulnerable to infectious agents. Most infectious agents enter the body by infecting and/or crossing mucosal surfaces.

SYSTEMIC LYMPHOID ORGANS INCLUDE THE SPLEEN AND LYMPH NODES
The spleen is made up of white and red pulp and a marginal zone

The spleen lies at the upper left quadrant of the abdomen, behind the stomach and close to the diaphragm. The adult spleen is around 13 × 8 cm in size and weighs approximately 180–250 g.

The outer layer of the spleen consists of a capsule of collagenous bundles of fibers, which enter the parenchyma of the organ as short trabeculae. These, together with a reticular framework, support two main types of splenic tissue:

- the **white pulp**; and
- the **red pulp**.

A third compartment, the **marginal zone**, is located at the outer limit of the white pulp.

White pulp of the spleen

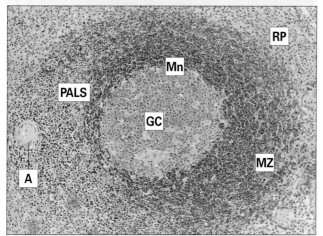

Fig. 2.37 Spleen section showing a white pulp lymphoid aggregate. A secondary lymphoid follicle, with germinal center (GC) and mantle (Mn), is surrounded by the marginal zone (MZ) and red pulp (RP). Adjacent to the follicle, an arteriole (A) is surrounded by the periarteriolar lymphoid sheath (PALS) consisting mainly of T cells. Note that the marginal zone is present only at one side of the secondary follicle. (Courtesy of Professor I Maclennan)

The white pulp consists of lymphoid tissue

The white pulp of the spleen consists of lymphoid tissue, the bulk of which is arranged around a central arteriole to form the periarteriolar lymphoid sheaths (PALS; Fig. 2.37). PALS are composed of T and B cell areas:

- the T cells are found around the central arteriole;
- the B cells may be organized into either primary 'unstimulated' follicles (aggregates of virgin B cells) or secondary 'stimulated' follicles (which possess a germinal center with memory cells).

The germinal centers also contain follicular dendritic cells (FDCs) and phagocytic macrophages. Macrophages and the FDCs present antigen to B cells in the spleen.

B cells and other lymphocytes are free to leave and enter the PALS via branches of the central arterioles, which enter a system of blood vessels in the marginal zone (see below). Some lymphocytes, especially maturing plasmablasts, can pass across the marginal zone via bridges into the red pulp.

The red pulp consists of venous sinuses and cellular cords

The venous sinuses and cellular cords of the red pulp contain:

- resident macrophages;
- erythrocytes;
- platelets;
- granulocytes;
- lymphocytes; and
- numerous plasma cells.

In addition to immunological functions, the spleen serves as a reservoir for platelets, erythrocytes, and granulocytes. Aged platelets and erythrocytes are destroyed in the red pulp in a process referred to as 'hemocatheresis'.

The functions of the spleen are made possible by its vascular organization (Fig. 2.38). Central arteries surrounded by PALS end with arterial capillaries, which open freely into the red pulp cords. Circulating cells can therefore reach these cords and become trapped. Aged platelets and erythrocytes are recognized and phagocytosed by macrophages.

Blood cells that are not ingested and destroyed can re-enter the blood circulation by squeezing through holes in the discontinuous endothelial wall of the venous sinuses, through which plasma flows freely.

The marginal zone contains B cells, macrophages, and dendritic cells

The marginal zone surrounds the white pulp and exhibits two major features, namely:

- a characteristic vascular organization; and
- unique subsets of resident cells (B cells, macrophages, and dendritic cells).

The blood vessels of the marginal zone form a system of communicating sinuses, which receive blood from branches of the central artery (see Fig. 2.38).

Most of the blood from the marginal sinuses enters the red pulp cords and then drains into the venous sinuses, but a small proportion passes directly into the venous sinuses to form a closed circulation.

Cells residing in the marginal zone comprise:

- various types of APC – metallophilic macrophages, marginal zone macrophages, dendritic cells;
- a subset of B cells with distinctive phenotype and function – they express IgM brightly with low or absent IgD and are long-lived recirculating cells (non-recirculating in the mouse);
- some B-1 cells.

Q. In humans, the marginal zone does not develop fully until 2 years of age. What is the functional consequence of this delay in development of the marginal zone?

A. Marginal zone B cells and B-1 cells respond strongly to **thymus-independent antigens**, including capsular polysaccharides of bacteria, and the main function of the marginal zone is to mount immune responses to bacteria that have reached the circulation (e.g. streptococci). Infants therefore have a reduced ability to respond to blood-borne infections with certain (encapsulated) bacteria.

Lymph nodes filter antigens from the interstitial tissue fluid and lymph

The lymph nodes form part of a network that filters antigens from the interstitial tissue fluid and lymph during its passage from the periphery to the thoracic duct and the other major collecting ducts (Fig. 2.39).

Lymph nodes frequently occur at the branches of the lymphatic vessels. Clusters of lymph nodes are strategically placed in areas that drain various superficial and deep regions of the body, such as the:

Vascular organization the spleen

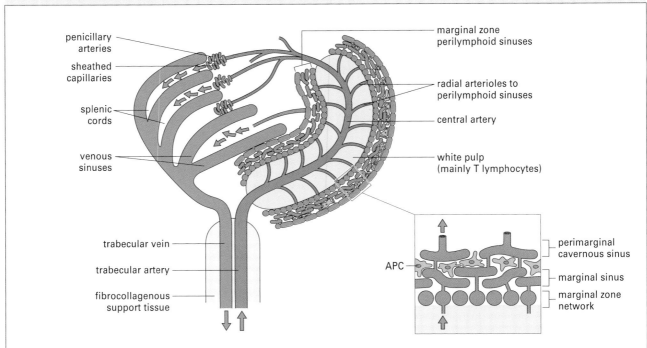

Fig. 2.38 The splenic artery branches to form trabecular arteries, which give rise to central arteries surrounded by periarteriolar lymphoid sheaths (PALS), which are the T cell areas of the white pulp. Leaving the PALS, the central arteries continue as penicillary arteries and sheathed capillaries, which open in the splenic cords of the red pulp. From the red pulp (where hemocatheresis takes place) the blood percolates through the wall of the venous sinuses. The central arterioles surrounded by PALS give collateral branches that reach a series of sinuses in the marginal zone. Most of the blood from the marginal sinuses enters the red pulp cords and then drains into the venous sinuses, but a proportion passes directly into the sinuses to form a closed circulation. (Courtesy of Dr A Stevens and Professor J Lowe)

- neck;
- axillae;
- groin;
- mediastinum; and
- abdominal cavity.

Lymph nodes protect the skin (superficial subcutaneous nodes) and mucosal surfaces of the respiratory, digestive, and genitourinary tracts (visceral or deep nodes).

Human lymph nodes are 2–10 mm in diameter, are round or kidney shaped, and have an indentation called the hilus where blood vessels enter and leave the node.

Lymph arrives at the lymph node via several afferent lymphatic vessels, and leaves the node through a single efferent lymphatic vessel at the hilus.

Lymph nodes consist of B and T cell areas and a medulla

A typical lymph node is surrounded by a collagenous capsule. Radial trabeculae, together with reticular fibers, support the various cellular components. The lymph node consists of:

- a **B cell area (cortex)**;
- a **T cell area (paracortex)**; and

- a central **medulla**, consisting of cellular cords containing T cells, B cells, abundant plasma cells, and macrophages (Figs 2.40–2.42).

The paracortex contains many APCs (interdigitating cells), which express high levels of MHC class II surface molecules. These are cells migrating from the skin (Langerhans' cells) or from mucosae (dendritic cells), which transport processed antigens into the lymph nodes from the external and internal surfaces of the body (Fig. 2.43). The bulk of the lymphoid tissue is found in the cortex and paracortex.

The paracortex contains specialized postcapillary vessels – **high endothelial venules (HEVs)** – which allow the traffic of lymphocytes out of the circulation into the lymph node (see 'Lymphocyte traffic' below and Fig. 2.54).

The medulla is organized into cords separated by lymph (medullary) sinuses, which drain into a terminal sinus – the origin of the efferent lymphatic vessel (see Fig. 2.42).

Scavenger phagocytic cells are arranged along the lymph sinuses, especially in the medulla. As the lymph passes across the nodes from the afferent to the efferent

The lymphatic system

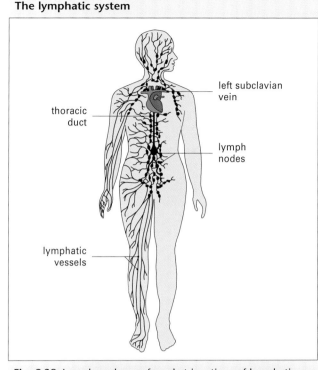

Fig. 2.39 Lymph nodes are found at junctions of lymphatic vessels and form a network that drains and filters interstitial fluid from the tissue spaces. They are either subcutaneous or visceral, the latter draining the deep tissues and internal organs of the body. The lymph eventually reaches the thoracic duct, which opens into the left subclavian vein and thus back into the circulation.

Lymph node section

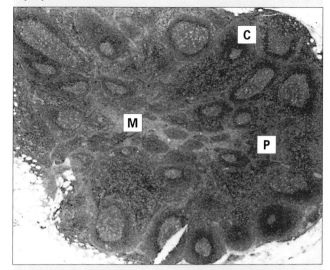

Fig. 2.40 The lymph node is surrounded by a connective tissue capsule and is organized into three main areas: the cortex (C), which is the B cell area; the paracortex (P), which is the T cell area; and the medulla (M), which contains cords of lymphoid tissue (T and B cell areas rich in plasma cells and macrophages). H&E stain. × 10. (Adapted from Zucker-Franklin D, Grossi CE, eds. Atlas of blood cells: function and pathology, 3rd edn. Milan: Edi Ermes; 2003)

lymphatic vessels, particulate antigens are removed by the phagocytic cells and transported into the lymphoid tissue of the lymph node.

The cortex contains aggregates of B cells in the form of primary or secondary follicles.

B cells are also found in the subcapsular region, adjacent to the marginal sinus. It is possible that these cells are similar to the splenic marginal zone B cells that intercept incoming pathogens primarily by mounting a rapid, IgM-based, T-independent response.

T cells are found mainly in the paracortex. Therefore, if an area of skin or mucosa is challenged by a T-dependent antigen, the lymph nodes draining that particular area show active T cell proliferation in the paracortex.

Q. How is antigen transported from the skin to the paracortex of the regional lymph nodes?
A. On Langerhans' cells/veiled cells in afferent lymph.

Further evidence for this localization of T cells in the paracortex comes from patients with congenital thymic aplasia (DiGeorge syndrome), who have fewer T cells in the paracortex than normal. A similar feature is found in neonatally thymectomized or congenitally athymic ('nude') mice or rats.

Histological structure of the lymph node

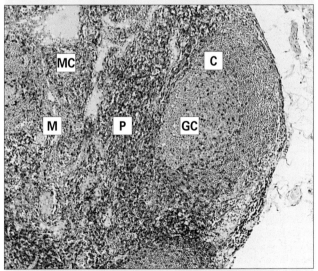

Fig. 2.41 Cortex (C), paracortex (P), and medulla (M) are shown. The section has been stained to show the localization of T cells. They are most abundant in the paracortex, but a few are found in the germinal center (GC) of the secondary lymphoid follicle, in the cortex, and in the medullary cords (MC). (Courtesy of Dr A Stevens and Professor J Lowe)

Schematic structure of the lymph node

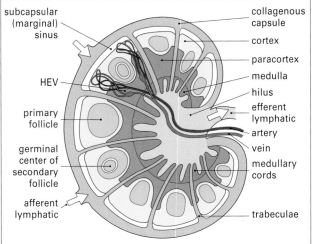

Fig. 2.42 Beneath the collagenous capsule is the subcapsular sinus, which is lined by endothelial and phagocytic cells. Lymphocytes and antigens from surrounding tissue spaces or adjacent nodes pass into the sinus via the afferent lymphatics. The cortex is mainly a B cell area. B cells are organized into primary or, more commonly, secondary follicles – that is, with a germinal center. The paracortex contains mainly T cells. Each lymph node has its own arterial and venous supply. Lymphocytes enter the node from the circulation through the highly specialized high endothelial venules (HEVs) in the paracortex. The medulla contains both T and B cells in addition to most of the lymph node plasma cells organized into cords of lymphoid tissue. Lymphocytes leave the node through the efferent lymphatic vessel.

Interdigitating cells in the lymph node paracortex

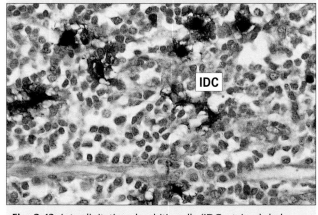

Fig. 2.43 Interdigitating dendritic cells (IDC; stained dark brown) form contacts with each other and with paracortical T cells. (Courtesy of Dr A Stevens and Professor J Lowe) (see also Fig. 2.16)

Structure of the secondary follicle

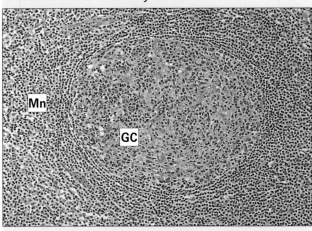

Fig. 2.44 A large germinal center (GC) is surrounded by the mantle zone (Mn).

Distribution of B cells in the lymph node cortex

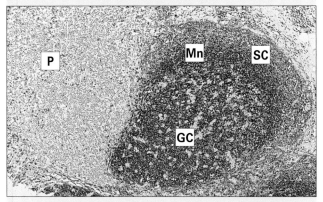

Fig. 2.45 Immunohistochemical staining of B cells for surface immunoglobulin shows that they are concentrated largely in the secondary follicle, germinal centre (GC), mantle zone (Mn), and between the capsule and the follicle – the subcapsular zone (SC). A few B cells are seen in the paracortex (P), which contains mainly T cells (see also Fig. 2.41).

Secondary follicles are made up of a germinal center and a mantle zone

Germinal centers in secondary follicles are seen in antigen-stimulated lymph nodes. These are similar to the germinal centers seen in the B cell areas of the splenic white pulp and of MALT.

Germinal centers are surrounded by a mantle zone of lymphocytes (Fig. 2.44). Mantle zone B cells (Fig. 2.45) co-express surface IgM, IgD, and CD44. This is taken as evidence that they are virgin and actively recirculating B cells.

In most secondary follicles, the thickened mantle zone or corona is oriented towards the capsule of the node. Secondary follicles contain:

• FDCs (Fig. 2.46);

Follicular dendritic cells in a secondary lymphoid follicle

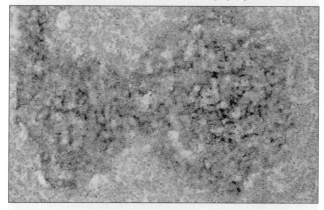

Fig. 2.46 This lymph node follicle is stained with enzyme-labeled monoclonal antibody to demonstrate follicular dendritic cells.

Germinal center macrophages

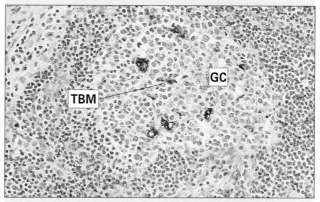

Fig. 2.47 Immunostaining for cathepsin D shows several macrophages localized in the germinal center (GC) of a secondary follicle. These macrophages, which phagocytose apoptotic B cells, are called tingible body macrophages (TBM). (Courtesy of Dr A Stevens and Professor J Lowe)

- some macrophages (Fig. 2.47); and
- a few CD4+ T cells.

All the cells in the secondary follicle together with specialized marginal sinus macrophages, appear to play a role in generating B cell responses and, in particular, in the development of B cell memory.

In the germinal centers B cells proliferate, are selected, and differentiate into memory cells plasma cell precursors

The germinal center consists of a dark zone and a light zone:

- the dark zone is the site where one or a few B cells enter the primary lymphoid follicle and undergo active proliferation leading to clonal expansion – these B cells are termed **centroblasts** and undergo a process of **somatic hypermutation**, which leads to the generation of cells with a wide range of affinities for antigen;
- in the light zone, B cells (**centrocytes**) encounter the antigen on the surface of FDCs (see Fig. 2.14) and only those cells with higher affinity for antigen survive.

Cells with mutated antibody receptors of lower affinity die by apoptosis and are phagocytosed by germinal center macrophages.

Selected centrocytes interact with germinal center CD4+ TH cells and undergo **class switching** (i.e.

Structure and function of the germinal center

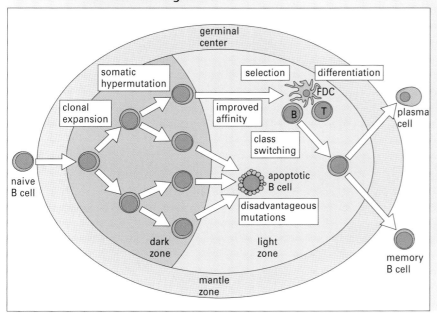

Fig. 2.48 One or a few B cells (founder cells) in the dark zone proliferate actively. This proliferation leads to clonal expansion and is accompanied by somatic hypermutation of the immunoglobulin V region genes. B cells with the same specificity, but different affinity, are therefore generated. In the light zone, B cells with disadvantageous mutations or with low affinity undergo apoptosis and are phagocytosed by macrophages. Cells with appropriate affinity encounter the antigen on the surface of the follicular dendritic cells (FDCs) and, with the help of CD4+ T cells, undergo class switching, leaving the follicle as memory B cells or plasma cells precursors.

53

replacement of their originally expressed immunoglobulin heavy chain constant region genes by another class – for instance IgM to IgG or IgA, see Chapter 8).

The selected germinal center B cells differentiate into **memory B cells** or **plasma cell** precursors and leave the germinal center (Fig. 2.48).

MALT INCLUDES ALL LYMPHOID TISSUES ASSOCIATED WITH MUCOSA

Aggregates of encapsulated and non-encapsulated lymphoid tissue are found especially in the lamina propria and submucosal areas of the gastrointestinal, respiratory, and genitourinary tracts (see Fig. 2.26).

The tonsils contain a considerable amount of lymphoid tissue, often with large secondary follicles and intervening T cell zones with HEVs. The three main kinds of tonsil that constitute Waldeyer's ring are:
- palatine tonsil;
- pharyngeal tonsil (called adenoids when diseased); and
- lingual tonsil (Fig. 2.49).

Aggregates of lymphoid tissue are also seen lining the bronchi and along the genitourinary tract.

The digestive, respiratory, and genitourinary mucosae contain dendritic cells for the uptake, processing, and transport of antigens to the draining lymph nodes.

Lymphoid tissues seen in the lamina propria of the gastrointestinal wall often extend into the submucosa and are found as either:
- solitary nodules (Fig. 2.50); or
- aggregated nodules such as in the appendix (Fig. 2.51).

Follicle-associated epithelium is specialized to transport pathogens into the lymphoid tissue

Peyer's patches are found in the lower ileum. The intestinal epithelium overlying Peyer's patches (follicle-associated epithelium – FAE) and other mucosa-associated

A solitary lymphoid nodule in the large intestine

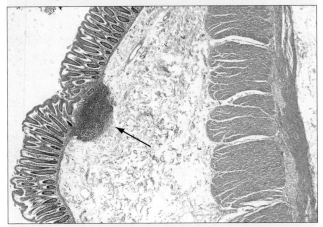

Fig. 2.50 This nodule is localized in the mucosa and submucosa of the intestinal wall (arrow). (Courtesy of Dr A Stevens and Professor J Lowe)

Lymphoid nodules in the human appendix

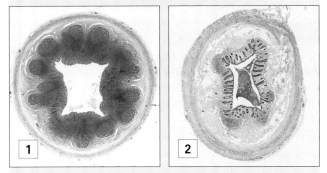

Fig. 2.51 (**1**) Appendix of a 10-year-old child showing large lymphoid nodules extending into the submucosa. (**2**) Appendix from a 36-year-old man. Note the dramatic reduction of lymphoid tissue, with the virtual disappearance of lymphoid follicles. This illustrates the atrophy of lymphoid tissues during ageing, which is not limited to the appendix. (Courtesy of Dr A Stevens and Professor J Lowe)

Structure of the lingual tonsil

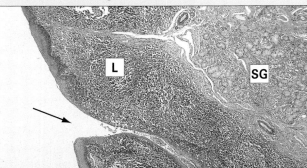

Fig. 2.49 The lingual tonsil, situated in the posterior one-third of the tongue, consists of accumulations of lymphoid tissue (L) with large secondary follicles associated with a mucosa that forms deep cleft-like invaginations (arrow). Mucus-containing salivary glands (SG) are seen around the tonsil. These are common features of all types of tonsil. (Courtesy of Dr A Stevens and Professor J Lowe)

lymphoid aggregates (e.g. the tonsils) is specialized to allow the transport of pathogens into the lymphoid tissue. This particular function is carried out by epithelial cells termed 'M' cells, which are scattered among other epithelial cells and so called because they have numerous microfolds on their luminal surface.

M cells contain deep invaginations in their basolateral plasma membrane, which form pockets containing B and T lymphocytes, dendritic cells, and macrophages (Fig. 2.52). Antigens and microorganisms are transcytosed into the pocket and to the organized mucosal lymphoid tissue under the epithelium (Fig. 2.53).

M cells are not exclusive to Peyer's patches, but are also found in epithelia associated with lymphoid cell accumulations at 'antigen sampling' areas in other mucosal sites.

Location of M cells

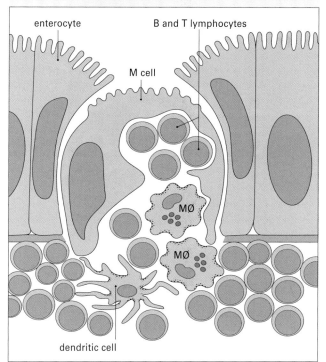

Fig. 2.52 The intestinal follicle-associated epithelium contains M cells. Note the lymphocytes and occasional macrophages (MØ) in the pocket formed by invagination of the basolateral membrane of the M cell. Antigens endocytosed by the M cell are passed via this pocket into the subepithelial tissues (not shown).

The dome area of Peyer's patches and the subepithelial regions of tonsils harbor B cells that display a phenotype and function similar to that seen for the splenic marginal zone B cells (see above).

Q. The major defense at mucosal surfaces is antibody of the IgA isotype. What characteristics of this antibody would be critical in this respect?
A. The IgA isotype antibody produced at the mucosal level is a specific secretory form that can traverse epithelial membranes and helps prevent the entry of infectious microorganisms. Resistance to digestion by enzymes in the gut would also be an important feature of secretory IgA in GALT. Transport of IgA across mucosal epithelium is described in detail in Chapter 3 (see Fig. 3.11).

Lamina propria and intraepithelial lymphocytes are found in mucosa

In addition to organized lymphoid tissue forming the MALT system, a large number of lymphocytes and plasma cells are found in the mucosa of the:
- stomach;
- small and large intestine;
- upper and lower respiratory airways; and
- several other organs.

Lymphocytes are found both in the connective tissue of the lamina propria and within the epithelial layer:
- lamina propria lymphocytes (LPLs) are predominantly activated T cells, but numerous activated B cells and plasma cells are also detected – these plasma cells secrete mainly IgA, which is transported across the epithelial cells and released into the lumen;

Mucosal lymphoid tissue

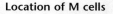

Fig. 2.53 Peyer's patches, as well as tonsils and other lymphoid areas of MALT, are sites of lymphocyte priming by antigens, which are internalized by M cells in the follicle-associated epithelium (FAE). The subepithelial region, the dome, is rich in APCs and also contains a subset of B cells similar to those found in the splenic marginal zone. Lymphoid follicles and intervening T-dependent zones are localized under the dome region. Lymphocytes primed by antigens in these initiation sites of the gut mucosa migrate to the mesenteric lymph nodes and then to the effector sites (the intestinal villi), where they are found both in the lamina propria (LPLs) and within the surface epithelium (IELs)

Patterns of lymphocyte traffic

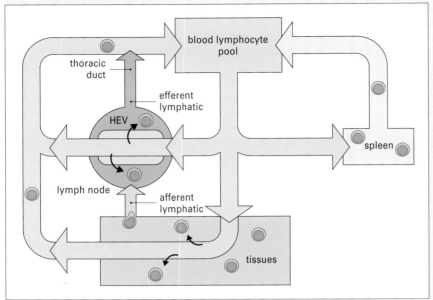

Fig. 2.54 The lymphocytes move through the circulation and enter the lymph nodes and MALT via the specialized endothelial cells of the postcapillary venules (i.e. high endothelial venules [HEVs]). They leave the lymph nodes and MALT through the efferent lymphatic vessels and pass through other nodes, finally entering the thoracic duct, which empties into the circulation at the left subclavian vein (in humans). Lymphocytes enter the white pulp areas of the spleen in the marginal zones, pass into the sinusoids of the red pulp, and leave via the splenic vein.

- intraepithelial lymphocytes (IELs) are mostly T cells – the population is different from the LPLs because it includes a high proportion of $\gamma\delta$ T cells (10–40%) and CD8$^+$ cells (70%).

Most LPL and IEL T cells belong to the CD45RO subset of memory cells. They respond poorly to stimulation with antibodies to CD3, but may be triggered via other activation pathways (e.g. via CD2 or CD28).

The integrin αE chain HML-1 (CD103) is not present on resting circulating T cells, but is expressed following phytohemagglutinin (PHA) stimulation. Antibodies to CD103 are mitogenic and induce expression of the low-affinity IL-2 receptor α chain (CD25) on peripheral blood T cells. αE is coupled with a β_7 chain to form an αE/β_7 heterodimer, which is an integrin expressed by IELs and other activated leukocytes. E-cadherin on epithelial cells is the ligand for αE/β_7. Binding of αE/β_7 to E-cadherin may be important in the homing and retention of αE/β_7-expressing lymphocytes in the intestinal epithelium.

IELs are known to release cytokines, including IFNγ and IL-5. One function suggested for IELs is immune surveillance against mutated or virus-infected host cells.

MOST LYMPHOCYTES RECIRCULATE AROUND THE BODY

Once in the secondary tissues the lymphocytes do not simply remain there; many move from one lymphoid organ to another via the blood and lymph (Fig. 2.54).

Lymphocytes leave the blood via high endothelial venules

Although some lymphocytes leave the blood through non-specialized venules, the main exit route in mammals is through a specialized section of the PCVs known as high

endothelial venules (HEVs; Figs 2.55 and 2.56). In the lymph nodes these are mainly in the paracortex, with fewer in the cortex and none in the medulla.

Some lymphocytes, primarily T cells, arrive from the drainage area of the node through the afferent lymphatics, not via HEVs – this is the main route by which antigen enters the nodes.

Besides lymph nodes, HEVs are also found in MALT and in the thymus (see Fig. 2.29).

Lymph node paracortex showing high endothelial venules (HEVs)

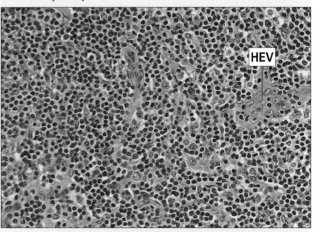

Fig. 2.55 Lymphocytes leave the circulation through HEVs and enter the node. H&E. × 200. (Courtesy of Dr A Stevens and Professor J Lowe)

Electron micrograph showing a high endothelial venule (HEV) in the paracortex of a lymph node

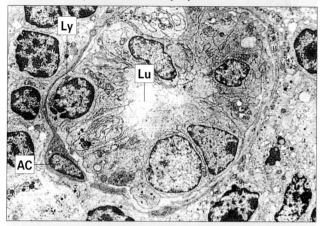

Fig. 2.56 A lymphocyte (Ly) in transit from the lumen (Lu) of the HEV can be seen close to the basal lamina. The HEV is partly surrounded by an adventitial cell (AC). × 1600.

Q. What types of molecule required for the movement of lymphocytes would you expect to be expressed on HEVs?
A. HEVs express a distinctive set of chemokines that signal lymphocytes to migrate into the lymphoid tissue. They also have a specialized set of adhesion molecules that allow the cells to attach to the endothelial cells, as they migrate.

HEVs are permanent features of secondary lymphoid tissues, but can also develop from normal endothelium at sites of chronic inflammatory reactions (e.g. in the skin and in the synovium). This, in turn, may direct specific T cell subsets to the area where HEVs have formed.

The movement of lymphocytes across endothelium is controlled by adhesion molecules (see Appendix 2) and chemokines (see Appendix 4). For example:
- the adhesion molecule MadCAM-1 is expressed on endothelial cells in intestinal tissues;
- VCAM-1 is present on endothelial cells in the lung and skin.

Homing molecules on lymphocytes selectively direct lymphocytes to particular organs by interaction with these adhesion molecules (see Chapter 6). In the case of the intestine, a critical role is played by $\alpha_4\beta_7$-integrins, which mediate adherence of lymphocytes to HEVs of Peyer's patches that express MadCAM-1.

Lymphocyte trafficking exposes antigen to a large number of lymphocytes

Lymphoid cells within lymph nodes return to the circulation by way of the efferent lymphatics, which pass via the thoracic duct into the left subclavian vein. About 1–2% of the lymphocyte pool recirculates each hour. Overall, this process allows a large number of antigen-specific lymphocytes to come into contact with their specific antigen in the microenvironment of the peripheral lymphoid organs.

Q. Why is it important that antigen can contact many lymphocytes?
A. Lymphoid cells are monospecific and only a limited number of lymphocytes are capable of recognizing any particular antigen. Lymphocyte recirculation and the movement of an antigen and APCs increase the opportunity for lymphocytes to encounter their specific antigen soon after infection.

Under normal conditions there is continuous lymphocyte traffic through the lymph nodes, but when antigen enters the lymph nodes of an animal already sensitized to that antigen there is a temporary shutdown in the traffic, which lasts for approximately 24 hours. Thus, antigen-specific lymphocytes are preferentially retained in the lymph nodes draining the source of antigen. In particular, blast cells do not recirculate but appear to remain in one site.

Antigen stimulation at one mucosal area elicits an antibody response largely restricted to MALT

One reason for considering MALT as a system distinct from the systemic lymphoid organs is that mucosa-associated lymphoid cells mainly recirculate within the mucosal lymphoid system. Thus, lymphoid cells stimulated in Peyer's patches pass via regional lymph nodes to the blood stream and then 'home' back into the intestinal lamina propria (Fig. 2.57 and see Fig. 2.53).

Specific recirculation is made possible because the lymphoid cells expressing homing molecules attach to adhesion molecules that are specifically expressed on endothelial cell adhesion molecules of the mucosal PCVs, but are absent from lymph node HEVs (see above).

Thus, antigen stimulation at one mucosal area elicits an antibody response largely, but not exclusively, restricted to mucosal tissues.

Lymphocyte circulation within the mucosal lymphoid system

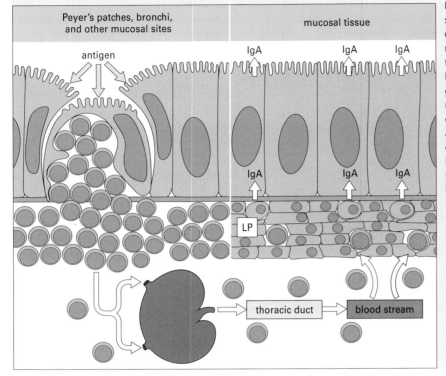

Fig. 2.57 Lymphoid cells that are stimulated by antigen in Peyer's patches (or the bronchi or another mucosal site) migrate via the regional lymph nodes and thoracic duct into the blood stream and hence to the lamina propria (LP) of the gut or other mucosal surfaces, which might be close to or distant from the site of priming. Thus lymphocytes stimulated at one mucosal surface may become distributed selectively throughout the MALT system. This is mediated through specific adhesion molecules on the lymphocytes and mucosal HEV.

FURTHER READING

Goldsby RA, Kindt TJ, Kuby J, Osborne BA. Kuby Immunology, 5th edn. Oxford: WH Freeman; 2003.

Janeway Jr CA, Travers P, Wolpert M, Schlomchik MJ. Immunobiology. London: Garland Publishing; 2004.

Lamm ME, Strober W, McGhee JR, Mayer L, eds. Mestecky J, Bienenstock J. Mucosal Immunology. San Diego: Academic Press; 2005.

Liu Y-J, Kanzler H, Soumelis V, Gilliet M. Dendritic cell lineage, plasticity and cross-regulation. Nature Immunology 2001;7:585–589.

Lydyard PM, Whelan A, Fanger MW. Instant Notes in Immunology, 2nd edn. London: Garland Science/Bios Scientific Publishing, 2004.

Playfair JHL, Chain BM. Immunology at a Glance, 7th edn. Oxford: Blackwell Scientific Publications; 2004.

Reddy KV, Yedery RD, Aranha C. Antimicrobial peptides: premises and promises. Int J Antimicrob Agents 2004;24:536–547.

Roitt IM, Delves P. Essential Immunology, 10th edn. Oxford: Blackwell Scientific Publications; 2001.

Shevach E. Regulatory/suppressor T cells in health and disease. Arthritis Rheum 2004;50:2721–2724.

Von Andrian UH, Mempel TR. Homing and cellular traffic in lymph nodes. Nature Rev Immunol 2003;3:867–878.

Critical thinking: Development of the immune system (see p. 493 for explanations)

Immunodeficiencies can tell us a lot about the way the immune system functions normally. Mice that congenitally lack a thymus (and have an associated gene defect that produces hairlessness), termed 'nude mice', are often used in research.

1 What effect would you expect this defect to have on numbers and types of lymphocytes in the blood? How would this affect the structure of the lymph nodes? What effect would this have on the ability of the mice to fight infections?

Occasionally adult patients develop a tumor in the thymus (thymoma) and it is necessary to completely remove the thymus gland.

2 What effect would you expect adult thymectomy to have on the ability of such patients to fight infections?

With the development of modern techniques in molecular biology, it is possible to produce animals that completely lack individual genes. Such animals are called 'gene knockouts'. Sometimes these knockouts can have quite surprising effects on development, and sometimes only minor effects. Others, like the immunodeficiencies, are very informative. Based on the information provided in Chapter 2, what effects would you expect the following 'knockouts' to have on the development of leukocytes and/or lymphoid organs?

3 RAG-1? (*RAG-1* and *RAG-2* genes are involved in the recombination processes that generate antigen receptors on B and T cells.)

4 Interleukin-7?

5 The β_7-integrin chain?

Antibodies

SUMMARY

- **Circulating antibodies (also called immunoglobulins) are soluble glycoproteins that recognize and bind antigens** present in serum, tissue fluids or on cell membranes. Their purpose is to help eliminate their specific antigens or microorganisms bearing those antigens. Immunoglobulins also function as membrane-bound antigen receptors on B cells, and play key roles in B cell differentiation.

- **All immunoglobulin isotypes, with the exception of IgD, are bifunctional** – they bind antigen and exhibit one or more effector functions. These biological activities are localized to sites that are distant from the antigen-binding sites.

- **Immunoglobulins are made up of a unit with four polypeptide chains** – two identical light chains and two identical heavy chains. The N terminal domains of each light and heavy chain are highly variable in sequence, are referred to as the variable regions (V_L and V_H, respectively), and form the antigen-binding sites of the antibody. The C terminal domains of the light and heavy chains together form the constant regions (C_L and C_H, respectively), which determine the effector functions of the immunoglobulin.

- **There are five classes of antibody in mammals** – IgG, IgA, IgM, IgD, and IgE.

- **Antigen-binding sites of antibodies are specific for the three-dimensional shape (conformation) of their target** – the antigenic determinant or epitope.

- **Antibody affinity** is a measure of the strength of the interaction between an antibody combining site and its epitope. The avidity (or functional affinity) of an antibody depends on its number of binding sites and its ability to engage multiple epitopes on the antigen – the more epitopes it binds, the greater the avidity.

- **Each immunoglobulin isotype (subclass) mediates a distinct set of effector functions.** In humans there are a number of different isotypes and these are determined by the constant (C) regions of their heavy chains.

- **Receptors for immunoglobulin constant regions (Fc receptors)** are expressed by mononuclear cells, neutrophils, natural killer cells, eosinophils, basophils, and mast cells. They interact with the Fc regions of different classes of immunoglobulin and promote activities such as phagocytosis, tumor cell killing, and mast cell degranulation.

- **A vast repertoire of antigen-binding sites is achieved by random selection and recombination** of a limited number of V, D, and J gene segments that encode the variable (V) domains. This process is known as VDJ recombination and generates the primary antibody repertoire.

- **Repeated rounds of somatic hypermutation and selection** act on the primary repertoire to generate antibodies with higher specificity and affinity for the stimulating antigen. Immunoglobulin class switching combines rearranged VDJ genes with various C region genes so that the same antigen receptor can serve a variety of effector functions.

IMMUNOGLOBULINS RECOGNIZE AND BIND ANTIGENS

The recognition of antigen is the hallmark of the specific adaptive immune response. Two distinct types of molecule are involved in this process:
- immunoglobulins (antibodies); and
- T cell antigen receptors (TCRs).

Structural and functional diversity are characteristic features of these molecules.

Antibody genes have diversified in different species by multiple gene duplications and subsequent divergence. In many species, including humans, diversity is further amplified by extensive gene recombination and somatic mutation during the lifetime of an individual.

Immunoglobulins function as membrane-bound antigen receptors on B cells and soluble circulating antibodies

Immunoglobulins are glycoproteins expressed as:
- membrane-bound receptors on the surface of B cells; or
- soluble molecules (secreted from plasma cells) and present in serum and tissue fluids.

Contact between the B cell receptor and the antigen it recognizes results in B cell activation and differentiation

Surface and secreted antibodies

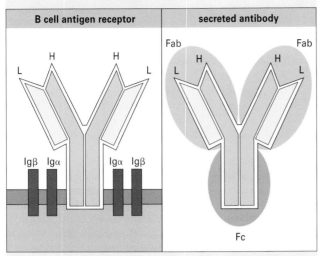

B cell antigen receptor	secreted antibody

Fig. 3.1 The B cell antigen receptor (left) consists of two identical heavy (H) chains and two identical light (L) chains. In addition, secondary components (Igα and Igβ) are closely associated with the primary receptor and are thought to couple it to intracellular signaling pathways. Circulating antibodies (right) are structurally identical to the primary B cell antigen receptors except they lack the transmembrane and intracytoplasmic sections. Many proteolytic enzymes cleave antibody molecules into three fragments – two identical Fab (antigen binding) fragments and one Fc (crystallizable) fragment.

to generate **plasma cells**, which secrete large amounts of antibody.

The secreted antibody has the same binding specificity as the original B cell receptor (Fig. 3.1).

Immunoglobulins are a family of glycoproteins

Immunoglobulins are a family of glycoproteins. In humans, five distinct **classes of immunoglobulin** molecule are recognized namely IgG, IgA, IgM, IgD, and IgE. They differ in:
* size;
* charge;
* amino acid sequence; and
* carbohydrate content.

The IgG class can be subdivided into four **subclasses** (IgG1, IgG2, IgG3, IgG4) and the IgA into two subclasses (IgA1, IgA2).

The classes and subclasses together represent nine **isotypes** – present in all normal individuals.

Each isotype is defined by the sequence of the constant region of its heavy chain.

Some antigens provoke an antibody response in each of the immunoglobulin isotypes, whereas responses to other antigens may be relatively restricted (e.g. IgG2 responses to carbohydrate antigens).

Rapid Reference Box 3

affinity – a measure of the binding strength between an antigenic determinant (epitope) and an antibody-combining site.

allotype – the protein of an allele that may be detectable as an antigen by another member of the same species.

antibody – a molecule produced in response to antigen that combines specifically with the antigen that induced its formation.

antigen – a molecule that reacts with antibody and the specific receptors on T and B cells.

avidity – the functional combining strength of an antibody with its antigen related to both the affinity of the reaction between the epitopes and paratopes, and the valencies of the antibody and antigen.

CD markers – cell surface molecules of leukocytes and platelets that are distinguishable with monoclonal antibodies and may be used to differentiate different cell populations (see Appendix 2).

cell-mediated immunity (CMI) – a term for immune reactions mediated by cells rather than by antibody or other humoral factors.

epitope – the part of an antigen that contacts the antigen-binding sites of an antibody or the T cell receptor.

idiotype – a single antigenic determinant on an antibody V region.

immunoglobulins – the serum antibodies, including IgG, IgM, IgA, IgE, and IgD.

isotype – refers to genetic variation within a family of proteins or peptides such that every member of the species will have each isotype of the family represented in its genome (e.g. immunoglobulin subclasses).

somatic mutation – a process occurring during B cell maturation and affecting the antibody gene region that permits refinement of antibody specificity.

recombination – a process by which genetic information is rearranged during meiosis; this process also occurs during the somatic rearrangements of DNA that occur in the formation of genes encoding antibody molecules and T cell receptors.

CD markers mentioned in this chapter
CD16 – FcγRIII (class of Fc receptor for IgG).
CD23 (CD23a and CD23b) – FcεRII (class of Fc receptor for IgE)
CD32 – FcγRII (class of Fc receptor for IgG).
CD64 – FcγRI (class of Fc receptor for IgG).

ALL IMMUNOGLOBULIN ISOTYPES (EXCEPT IgD) ARE BIFUNCTIONAL

Each immunoglobulin isotype is bifunctional (except serum IgD) – that is, they:
* recognize and bind antigen; and then
* promote the killing and/or removal of the immune complex formed through the activation of effector mechanisms.

One part of the antibody molecule determines its antigen specificity while another determines which effector functions will be activated. Effector functions include binding of the immunoglobulin to:

- receptors expressed on host tissues (e.g. phagocytic cells);
- the first component (C1q) of the complement system to initiate the classical pathway complement cascade (Fig. 3.2).

Immunoglobulin class and subclass depend on the structure of the heavy chain

The basic structure of each immunoglobulin molecule is a unit consisting of:

- two light polypeptide chains; and
- two heavy polypeptide chains.

The amino acid sequences of the two light chains are identical; so are the sequences of the two heavy chains.

Both light and both heavy chains are folded into discrete domains, and the type of heavy chain determines the class and subclass of the antibody:

- μ (IgM);
- γ1, γ2, γ3, and γ4 (IgG1, IgG2, IgG3, IgG4);
- α1 and α2 (IgA1, IgA2);
- δ (IgD);
- ε (IgE).

There are no subclasses of IgM, IgD, or IgE (Fig. 3.3).

Different immunoglobulin classes and subclasses activate different effector systems

The human IgG subclasses (IgG1–IgG4), which are are present in serum in the approximate proportions of 66, 23, 7, and 4%, respectively, appear to have arisen after the divergence of evolutionary lines leading to humans and the mouse. Consequently there is no direct structural or functional correlation between the four human and mouse IgG subclasses, despite their similar nomenclature.

The relative proportions of IgA1 and IgA2 vary between serum and external secretion, where IgA is present in a secretory form (see Fig. 3.3).

Q. What advantage might there be in having such a variety of different antibody classes?

A. Each class and subclass of antibody can act as an adapter for different types of immune effector system. Because different types of effector system are appropriate for dealing with each pathogen, the immune system can adjust the type of response that is generated according to the type of antibodies that are produced.

IgG is the predominant immunoglobulin in normal human serum

IgG accounts for 70–75% of the total serum immunoglobulin pool and consists of a monomeric four-chain molecule of mass 146–170 kDa.

IgM accounts for about 10% of the serum immunoglobulin pool

IgM accounts for approximately 10% of the serum immunoglobulin pool. It is a pentamer of a basic four-chain structure with a mass of ~970 kDa, formation of which is aided by the inclusion of the J (joining) polypeptide chain of mass ~15 kDa.

A transmembrane monomeric form (mIgM) is present as an antigen-specific receptor on mature B cells.

IgA is the predominant immunoglobulin in seromucous secretions

IgA accounts for approximately 15–20% of the serum immunoglobulin pool. In humans over 80% of serum IgA is a monomer of the four-chain unit, but in most mammals serum IgA is predominantly polymeric, occurring mostly as a dimer.

Antibodies act as adapter molecules for immune effector systems

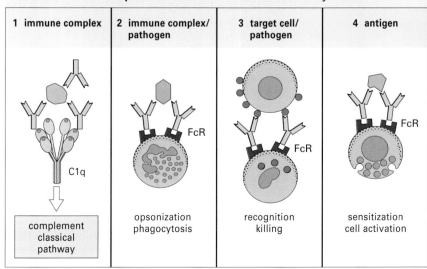

Fig. 3.2 Antibodies act as adapter molecules for different immune effector systems, linking antigens to receptor molecules (C1q and FcR) of the immune system. (1) Immune complexes can activate the complement classical pathway. (2) Antibodies bound to the surface of pathogens opsonize them for phagocytosis. (3) Antibodies bound to cells can promote their recognition and killing by NK cells. (Similarly recognition of some parasitic worms by eosinophils, mediated by antibodies, targets them for killing.) (4) Antibody bound to Fc receptors sensitizes cells so that they can recognize antigen, and the cell becomes activated if antigen binds to the surface antibody.

Physicochemical properties of human immunoglobulin classes

property	immunoglobulin type									
	IgG1	IgG2	IgG3	IgG4	IgM	IgA1	IgA2	sIgA	IgD	IgE
heavy chain	γ_1	γ_2	γ_3	γ_4	μ	α_1	α_2	α_1/α_2	δ	ϵ
mean serum conc. (mg/ml)	9	3	1	0.5	1.5	3.0	0.5	0.05	0.03	0.00005
sedimentation constant	7s	7s	7s	7s	19s	7s	7s	11s	7s	8s
mol. wt (kDa)	146	146	170	146	970	160	160	385	184	188
half-life (days)	21	20	7	21	10	6	6	?	3	2
% intravascular distribution	45	45	45	45	80	42	42	trace	75	50
carbohydrate (%)	2–3	2–3	2–3	2–3	12	7–11	7–11	7–11	9–14	12

Fig. 3.3 Each immunoglobulin class has a characteristic type of heavy chain. Thus IgG posesses γ chains; IgM, μ chains; IgA, α chains; IgD, δ chains; and IgE, ϵ chains. Variation in heavy chain structure within a class gives rise to immunoglobulin subclasses. For example, the human IgG pool consists of four subclasses reflecting four distinct types of heavy chain. The properties of the immunoglobulins vary between the different classes. In secretions, IgA occurs in a dimeric form (sIgA) in association with a protein chain termed the secretory component. The serum concentration of sIgA is very low, whereas the level in intestinal secretions can be very high.

IgA is the predominant immunoglobulin in seromucous secretions such as saliva, colostrum, milk, and tracheobronchial and genitourinary secretions.

Secretory IgA (sIgA) is comprised of a dimeric form of the basic unit together with the J chain and a secretory component, and has a total mass of ~385 kDa.

mIgD is an antigen-specific receptor on mature B cells

IgD accounts for less than 1% of the serum immunoglobulin pool.

A transmembrane monomeric form (mIgD) is present as an antigen-specific receptor on mature B cells. (B cells may have both mIgM and mIgD as their receptor, though on any one B cell these receptors will have the same antigen specificity.)

Basophils and mast cells are continuously saturated with IgE

Serum IgE levels are very low (< 0.05 μg/ml) relative to the other immunoglobulin isotypes, However, basophils and mast cells express an IgE-specific receptor of very high affinity with the result that they are continuously saturated with IgE.

IgE is a monomeric immunoglobulin of ~188 kDa.

IMMUNOGLOBULINS ARE MADE UP OF FOUR POLYPEPTIDE CHAIN UNITS

The basic four-chain structure of immunoglobulin molecules is illustrated by IgG1 (Fig. 3.4). This four-chain structure of antibody molecules was first demonstrated for rabbit IgG.

The **light chains** (25 kDa) are bound to the heavy chains (55 kDa) by interchain disulfide bridges and multiple non-covalent interactions.

The **heavy chains** are similarly bound to each other by interchain disulfide bridges and multiple non-covalent interactions.

Each segment of approximately 110 amino acids is folded to form a compact domain, which is stabilized through a covalent intrachain disulfide bond. Thus:

- the light chain has an intrachain disulfide bond in each of the VL and CL domains (Fig. 3.5 and see Fig. 3.4);
- there is one intrachain disulfide bond in each domain of the heavy chain.

Each disulfide bond encloses a peptide loop of 60–70 amino acid residues.

The amino acid sequence of immunoglobulin domains exhibits significant homology and this is reflected in a common conformational motif, referred to as the **immunoglobulin fold**. This characteristic fold defines the immunoglobulin superfamily members.

Q. What conditions are required to dissociate the heavy and light chains in an immunoglobulin molecule?

A. Because the heavy and light chains are linked by disulfide bonds, it is necessary to reduce these first before dissociating the chains under conditions of low pH.

VL and VH form antigen-binding sites and CL and CH determine effector functions

The light chains of most vertebrates have been shown to exist in two structurally distinct forms:

- kappa (κ); and
- lambda (λ).

These are isotypes, being present in all individuals.

Genetic variants (known as **allotype**s) of the κ chains exist in different individuals (see p. 79).

Either light chain type may combine with any of the heavy chain types, but in any individual immunoglobulin

The basic structure of IgG1

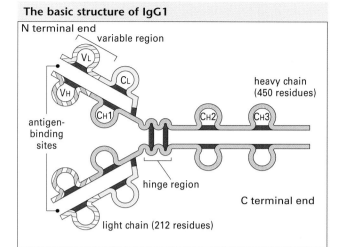

Fig. 3.4 The N terminal end of IgG1 is characterized by sequence variability (V) in both the heavy and light chains, referred to as the VH and VL regions, respectively. The rest of the molecule has a relatively constant (C) structure. The constant portion of the light chain is termed the CL region. The constant portion of the heavy chain is further divided into three structurally discrete regions: CH1, CH2, and CH3. These globular regions, which are stabilized by intrachain disulfide bonds, are referred to as 'domains'. The sites at which the antibody binds antigen are located in the variable domains. The hinge region is a segment of heavy chain between the CH1 and CH2 domains. Flexibility in this area permits the two antigen-binding sites to operate independently. There is close pairing of the domains except in the CH2 region (see Fig. 3.8). Carbohydrate moieties are attached to the CH2 domains.

Basic folding in the light chain

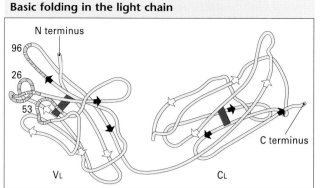

Fig. 3.5 The immunoglobulin domains in the light chain share a basic folding pattern with several straight segments of polypeptide chain lying parallel to the long axis of the domain. Light chains have two domains – one constant and one variable. Within each domain, the polypeptide chain is arranged in two layers, running in opposite directions, with many hydrophobic amino acid side chains between the layers. One of the layers has four segments (arrowed white), the other has three (arrowed black); both are linked by a single disulfide bond (red). Folding of the VL domains causes the hypervariable regions (see Fig. 3.6) to become exposed in three separate, but closely disposed, loops. One numbered residue from each hypervariable region is identified.

molecule both light chains and heavy chains are of the same type.

Amino sequence analysis of monoclonal mouse and human light chains has revealed two structurally distinct regions:

- the sequence of the ~110 N terminal residues was seen to be unique for each protein analysed;
- the C terminal sequence (~110 residues) was constant for a given isotype (κ or λ) and allotype.

Thus, the light chain variable (VL) and constant (CL) regions were defined and these regions correspond to the domains (see Fig. 3.5).

Similarly, the ~110 N terminal residues of heavy chains were seen to be unique for each protein analyzed whereas the remaining constant domains were characteristic for each immunoglobulin isotype.

The constant domains of the heavy chains are generally designated as CH1, CH2, CH3, and CH4, or according to the isotype of the constant domains.

Hypervariable regions form the antigen-combining site

Within the variable regions of both heavy and light chains, some polypeptide segments show exceptional variability and are termed **hypervariable regions**. These segments are located around amino acid positions 30, 50, and 95 (Fig. 3.6) and are referred to as Hv1, Hv2, and Hv3 or Lv1, Lv2, and Lv3, respectively.

X-ray crystallographic studies show that the hypervariable regions are intimately involved in antigen binding and hence in creating an interaction site that is complementary in shape, charge, and hydrophobicity to the epitope it binds. Consequently the hypervariable regions are also termed the complementarity determining regions (CDR1, CDR2, and CDR3).

The intervening peptide segments are called framework regions (FRs) and determine the fold that ensures the CDRs are in proximity to each other (see Fig. 3.6).

THE FIVE CLASSES OF ANTIBODY IN MAMMALS ARE IgG, IgA, IgM, IgD, AND IgE
The overall structure of an antibody depends on its class and subclass

X-ray crystallography has provided structural data on complete IgG molecules providing computer-generated α-carbon backbone and van der Waals surface models for this class of immunoglobulin (Fig. 3.7). Mobility around the hinge region allows for the generation of the Y- and T-shaped structures visualized by electron microscopy.

In IgG, there is extensive pairing between VH/VL and CH1/CL domains through extensive non-covalent interactions to form the IgG Fab region.

Amino acid variability in the variable regions of immunoglobulins

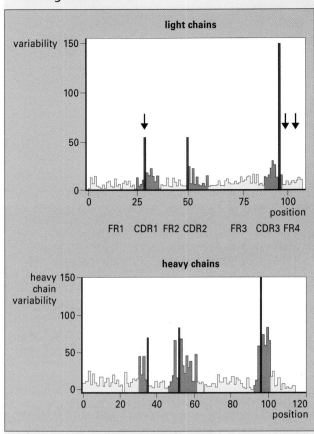

light chains

heavy chains

FR1 CDR1 FR2 CDR2 FR3 CDR3 FR4

Fig. 3.6 Variability is calculated by comparing the sequences of many individual chains and, for any position, is equal to the ratio of the number of different amino acids found at that position, to the frequency of the most common amino acid. The areas of greatest variability, of which there are three in the V_L domain, are termed the hypervariable regions. The areas shaded pink denote regions of hypervariability (CDR), and the most hypervariable positions are shaded red. The four framework regions (FR) are shown in yellow. (Courtesy of Professor EA Kabat)

Similarly, the C_H3 domains of the IgG Fc are paired.

The C_H2 domains are not paired, but bear an N-linked complex oligosaccharide moiety that is integral to the conformation of the IgG Fc.

Despite the structural similarities between V and C domains, there are significant differences in the manner in which they pair.

Each IgG subclass has a unique hinge region

Each of the four human IgG subclasses exhibits a unique profile of biological activities, despite the fact that there is over 95% sequence identity between their Fc regions.

The structures of the hinge regions are particularly distinct (Fig. 3.8) and contribute to the relative mobilities

Model of an IgG molecule

Fig. 3.7 A model of an IgG molecule showing the polypeptide backbones of the four chains as a ribbon. Heavy chains are shown in dark blue and dark green. The antigen-binding sites are at the tips of the arms of the Y-shaped molecule and are formed by domains from both the heavy and light chains. The extended, unfolded hinge region lies at the center of the molecule. Carbohydrate units are shown as ball and stick structures, covalently linked to the Fc region.

of the IgG Fab and IgG Fc moieties within the intact molecule and, presumably, the structural form of immune complexes.

The heavy chains bear N-linked oligosaccharides and although the oligosaccharide accounts for only 2–3% of the mass of IgG molecules it is crucial to the expression of effector functions.

Assembled IgM molecules have a 'star' conformation

IgM is present in human serum as a pentamer of the basic four-chain unit (see Fig. 3.8). Each heavy chain is comprised of a V_H and four C_H domains.

The subunits of the pentamer are linked by covalent disulfide bonds between adjacent C_H2 and C_H3 domains, and the C terminal 18-residue peptide sequence, referred to as the 'tailpiece'.

Assembly of the pentamer is further facilitated by incorporation of the J (joining) polypeptide chain. J chain is synthesized within plasma cells, has a mass of ~15 kDa and folds to form an immunoglobulin domain. It has four oligosaccharide moieties that account for approximately 12% of the mass.

In electron micrographs the assembled IgM molecule is seen to have a 'star' conformation with a densely packed central region and radiating arms (Fig. 3.9). Electron micrographs of IgM antibodies binding to poliovirus show molecules adopting a 'staple' or 'crab-like' configuration (see Fig. 3.9), which suggests that flexion readily occurs

Structural characteristics of various human immunoglobulins

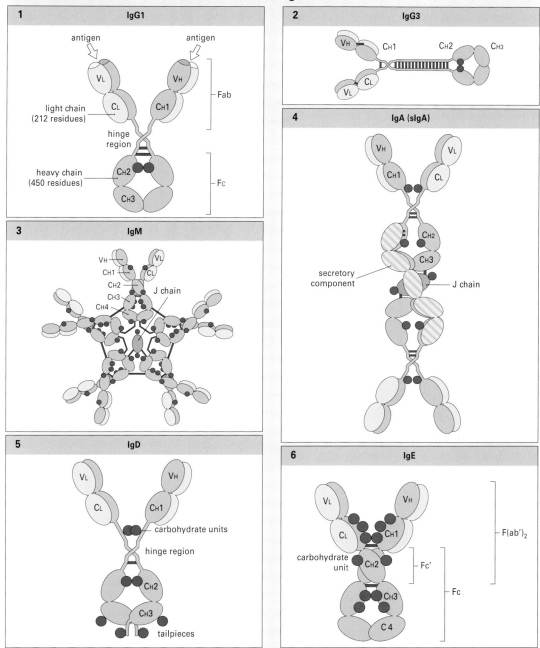

Fig. 3.8 Carbohydrate side chains are shown in blue. Inter heavy (H) chain disulfide bonds are shown in red, but interchain bonds between H and L chains are omitted. (**1**) A model of IgG1 indicating the globular domains of H and L chains. Note the apposition of the CH3 domains and the separation of the CH2 domains. The carbohydrate units lie between the CH2 domains. (**2**) Polypeptide chain structure of human IgG3. Note the elongated hinge region. (**3**) IgM H chains have five domains with disulfide bonds cross-linking adjacent CH3 and CH4 domains. The possible location of the J chain is shown. IgM does not have extended hinge regions, but flexion can occur about the CH2 domains. (**4**) The secretory component of sIgA is probably wound around the dimer and attached by two disulfide bonds to the CH2 domain of one IgA monomer. The J chain is required to join the two subunits. (**5**) This diagram of IgD shows the domain structure and a characteristically large number of oligosaccharide units. Note also the presence of a hinge region and short octapeptide tailpieces. (**6**) IgE can be cleaved by enzymes to give the fragments F(ab')₂, Fc, and Fc'. Note the absence of a hinge region.

between the CH2 and CH3 domains, though this region is not structurally homologous to the IgG hinge. Distortion of this region, known as **dislocation**, results in the 'staple' configuration of IgM required to activate complement.

sIgA is composed of IgA, J chain, and a secretory component

IgA is present in serum as a monomer of the basic four-chain structure. Each heavy chain is comprised of a VH and three CH domains.

The IgA1 and IgA2 subclasses differ substantially in the structure of their hinge regions:
- the hinge of IgA1 is extended and bears O-linked oligosaccharides;
- the hinge of of IgA2 is truncated.

Both heavy chains bear N-linked oligosaccharides.

IgA is the predominant antibody isotype in external secretions and exists as a complex secretory form. IgA is secreted by plasma cells as a dimer in which a heavy chain 'tailpiece' is disulfide linked to a J chain (see Fig. 3.8).

Electron micrographs of IgA dimers show double Y-shaped structures, suggesting that the monomeric subunits are linked end-to-end through the C terminal Cα3 regions (Fig. 3.10).

The dimeric form of IgA binds a **poly-Ig receptor** (Fig. 3.11) expressed on the basolateral surface of epithelial cells. The complex is internalized, transported to the apical surface, and released as the secretory form of IgA (sIgA), which has a mass of ~385 kDa and is comprised of:
- two units of IgA;
- J chain; and
- a secretory component (mass 70 kDa) (see Figs 3.8 and 3.11).

Secretory component results from enzymatic cleavage of the IgA–poly-Ig receptor complex. sIgA is relatively resistant to cleavage by enzymes in the gut.

The heavy chain of IgD bears three N-linked oligosaccharides

Serum IgD accounts for less than 1% of the total serum immunoglobulin. Each heavy chain is comprised of a VH domain and three CH domains with an extended hinge

Electron micrographs of IgM molecules

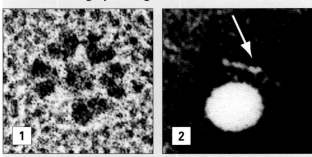

Fig. 3.9 (1) In free solution, deer IgM adopts the characteristic star-shaped configuration. ×195 000. (Courtesy of Drs E Holm Nielson, P Storgaard, and Professor S-E Svehag) (2) Rabbit IgM antibody (arrow) in 'crab-like' configuration with partly visible central ring structure bound to a poliovirus virion. × 190 000. (Courtesy of Dr B Chesebro and Professor S-E Svehag)

Electron micrographs of human dimeric IgA molecules

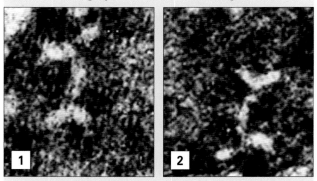

Fig. 3.10 The double Y-shaped appearance suggests that the monomeric subunits are linked end to end through the C terminal Cα3 domain. ×250 000. (Courtesy of Professor S-E Svehag)

Transport of IgA across the mucosal epithelium

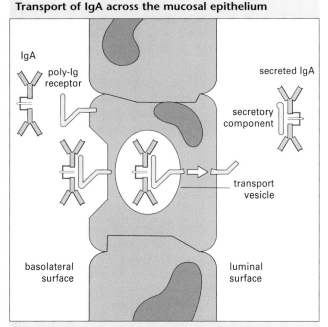

Fig. 3.11 IgA dimers secreted into the intestinal lamina propria by plasma cells bind to poly-Ig receptors on the internal (basolateral) surface of the epithelial cells. The sIgA–receptor complex is then endocytosed and transported across the cell while still bound to the membrane of transport vesicles. These vesicles fuse with the plasma membrane at the luminal surface, releasing IgA dimers with bound secretory component derived from cleavage of the receptor. The dimeric IgA is protected from proteolytic enzymes in the lumen by the presence of this secretory component.

region that is susceptible to proteolysis, at least on purification.

The heavy chain bears three N-linked oligosaccharides and the hinge region bears multiple O-linked oligosaccharides (see Fig. 3.8).

The heavy chain of IgE bears six N-linked oligosaccharides

It is estimated that serum IgE accounts for approximately 50% of total body IgE, with the rest being bound to mast cells and basophils through their high-affinity IgE Fcε receptor (FcεRI).

Each heavy chain is comprised of a V_H and four C_H domains and bears six N-linked oligosaccharides (see Fig. 3.8).

Immunoglobulins are prototypes of the immunoglobulin superfamily

The type of domain referred to as the immunoglobulin fold was first identified in antibodies. However, it also occurs in many other molecules that may or may not have an overt immune function. Examples include:
- the adhesion molecules ICAM-1 and VCAM-1 (see Chapter 6);
- the TCR (see Chapter 5);
- MHC molecules (see Chapter 5);
- cellular receptors for antibodies.

Such molecules are said to belong to the **immunoglobulin supergene family (IgSF)**.

The principal elements of the domain are two opposed β-pleated sheets, with stabilization by one or more disulfide bonds between the β-pleated sheets. This structure is sometimes referred to as a β **barrel**.

The immunoglobulin domain structure developed early in evolution and has been used and adapted in different molecules as vertebrates have radiated and diverged.

ANTIGEN-BINDING SITES OF ANTIBODIES ARE SPECIFIC FOR THE THREE-DIMENSIONAL SHAPE OF THEIR TARGET
Conformations of target antigen and receptor-binding site are complementary

Protein molecules are not rigid structures, but exist in a dynamic equilibrium between structures that differ in their ability to form a **primary interaction** with specific **ligands**.

Following a primary interaction, each 'partner' may influence the final **conformation** within the complex. This concept approximates to the 'induced fit' model of protein–protein interactions.

An examination of the interaction between the Fab fragment of the mouse D1.3 monoclonal antibody and hen egg white lysozyme (HEL) reveals the complementary surfaces of the epitope and the antibody's combining site. These surfaces extend beyond the hypervariable regions. In total, 17 amino acid residues on the antibody contact 16 residues on the lysozyme molecule (Fig. 3.12). All hypervariable regions in both the heavy and light chains contribute to the antibody-binding site, though the third hypervariable region in the heavy chain lying at the center of the combining site appears to be most important.

The Fab–lysozyme complex

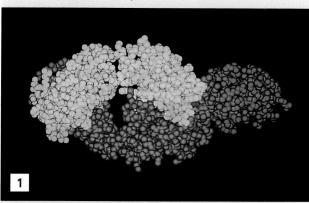

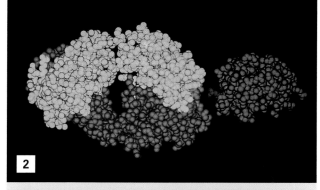

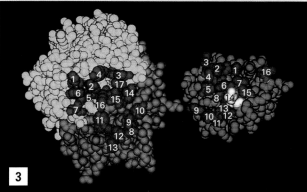

Fig. 3.12 (1) Lysozyme (green) binds to the hypervariable regions of the heavy (blue) and light (yellow) chains of the Fab fragment of antibody D1.3. (2) The separated complex with Glu121 visible (red). This residue fits into the center of the cleft between the heavy and light chains. (3) The same molecules rotated 90° to show the contact residues that contribute to the antigen–antibody bond. (Reprinted with permission from Poljak RJ, Science 1986;233:747–753. Copyright 1986 AAAS and reprinted with permission from Garcia KC et al, Science 1996;274:209–219. Copyright 1996 AAAS)

The binding site of this D1.3 monoclonal antibody may be regarded as 'classical'. The structures of other lysozyme–antibody complexes have been solved and show differing involvement of hypervariable and framework residues.

These studies are essential when engineering antibody molecules (e.g. when 'humanizing' an antibody to generate an antibody therapeutic, see Method Box 3.1).

ANTIBODY AFFINITY IS A MEASURE OF THE STRENGTH OF INTERACTION BETWEEN AN ANTIBODY-COMBINING SITE AND ITS EPITOPE

X-ray crystallographic studies of antibody Fab fragments show that the hypervariable regions are clustered at the end of the Fab arms to form a unique surface topography that is complementary to structures on the antigen. This complementary surface is called a **paratope** (corresponding to the antigenic determinant known as an **epitope**).

Proximal framework residues sometimes contribute to antigen binding, but their main role is to maintain the immunoglobulin fold and the integrity of the binding site.

Antibodies form multiple non-covalent bonds with antigen

The antigen–antibody interaction results from the formation of multiple non-covalent bonds. These attractive forces consist of:
- hydrogen bonds;
- electrostatic bonds;
- van der Waals forces; and
- hydrophobic forces.

Each bond is relatively weak in comparison with covalent bonds, but together they can generate a high-affinity interaction.

The strength of a non-covalent bond is critically dependent on the distance (d) between the interacting groups, being proportional to $1/d^2$ for electrostatic forces, and to $1/d^7$ for van der Waals forces.

Thus interacting groups must be in quite intimate contact before these attractive forces come into play.

For a paratope to combine with its epitope (see Fig. 3.12) the interacting sites must be complementary in shape, charge distribution, and hydrophobicity, and in terms of donor and acceptor groups capable of forming hydrogen bonds.

Close proximity of two protein surfaces can also generate repulsive forces (proportional to $1/d^{12}$) if electron clouds overlap.

In combination, the attractive and repulsive forces have a vital role in determining the specificity of the antibody molecule and its ability to discriminate between structurally similar molecules.

The great specificity of the antigen–antibody interaction is exploited in a number of widely used assays (Method Box 3.2)

All antigen–antibody interactions are reversible

The strength of the interaction between an antigen and an antibody is loosely referred to as **affinity**. It is the sum of the attractive and repulsive forces resulting from binding between the binding site of a monovalent Fab fragment and its epitope. (Note that true affinity is a thermo-

dynamic parameter and its determination is much more demanding, though not discussed here.)

The interaction between an antigen and an antibody will be reversible, so at equilibrium the Law of Mass Action can be applied and an equilibrium constant, K (the association constant), can be determined (Fig. 3.13).

Avidity is likely to be more relevant than affinity

Because each antibody unit of four polypeptide chains has two antigen-binding sites, antibodies are potentially multivalent in their reaction with antigen.

In addition, antigen can be:
- monovalent (e.g. small chemical groups, haptens); or
- multivalent (e.g. microorganisms).

The strength with which a multivalent antibody binds a multivalent antigen is termed **avidity** to differentiate it from the **affinity**, which is determined for a univalent antibody fragment binding to a single antigenic determinant.

The avidity of an antibody for its antigen is dependent on the affinities of the individual antigen-combining sites for the epitopes on the antigen. Avidity will be greater than the sum of these affinities if both antibody-binding sites bind to the antigen because all antigen–antibody bonds would have to be broken simultaneously for the complex to dissociate (Fig. 3.14).

In physiological situations, avidity is likely to be more relevant than affinity because antibodies are minimally divalent and most naturally occurring antigens are multivalent.

In practice we determine the association constant at equilibrium when the rate of formation of complex (ka) is equal to the spontaneous rate of dissociation (kd). The association or equilibrium constant is defined as K = ka/kd.

It has been suggested that B cell selection and stimulation during a maturing antibody response depend upon selection for the ability of antibodies to bind to antigens both:
- rapidly (kinetic selection); and
- tightly (thermodynamic selection).

Cross-reactive antibodies recognize more than one antigen

Antigen–antibody reactions can show a high level of specificity, but can also be **cross-reactive**, binding to a structurally related but different antigen.

The monoclonal antibodies to hen egg lysozyme (HEL) may therefore also bind the structurally homologous duck egg lysozyme (DEL), though the D1.3 antibody illustrated in Fig. 3.12 does not bind DEL (due to a single amino acid substitution within the epitope).

A polyclonal antiserum to HEL will contain populations of antibodies specific for HEL and others that cross-react with DEL (Fig. 3.15).

Antibodies recognize the conformation of antigenic determinants

Antibodies are capable of expressing remarkable specificity and are able to distinguish small differences in the

METHOD BOX 3.1
Recombinant antibodies for human therapy

Recombinant antibody therapeutics (rMAbs) are likely to become the largest family of disease-modifying drugs available to clinicians. Their efficacy results from specificity for the target antigen and biological activities (effector functions) activated by the immune complexes formed. Currently, 14 rMAbs are licensed and hundreds are in clinical trials or under development. Initial trials administered mouse monoclonal antibodies specific for human targets and provided 'proof of principle'.

Q. What problems could you envisage with the use of mouse antibodies to treat diseases in humans?
A. The antibodies might not interact appropriately with human Fc receptors. In the longer term an individual might mount an immune response against the non-self mouse antibodies.

However, individuals mounted immune responses against the non-self mouse antibodies and the development of these human anti-mouse antibody responses (HAMAs) meant that repeated dosing, which was required for chronic diseases, was not possible.
In response, scientists then produced:
- chimeric antibodies, in which the mouse V domains were linked to human antibody C domains;
- more recently, fully humanized antibodies.
This development of humanized antibodies has successively moderated, but not eliminated, such responses and sometimes human anti-human antibody (HAHA) responses are encountered.

Although such therapeutic antibodies are termed 'human', they are derived in a manner (phage display or Ig transgenic mice) that generates specificities that would ordinarily be eliminated by an individual's immune system because they are directed against self.

The success of antibodies such as infliximab (anti-TNFα) and rituximab (anti-CD20) has resulted in demands for their production in metric tonnes. The biopharmaceutical industry has met the challenge with the construction of new mammalian cell culture facilities (10 000–20 000-liter capacities) to produce rMAbs; however, productivity, cost, and potency remain to be optimized.

All antibody therapeutics that are currently licensed have been produced by mammalian cell culture using Chinese hamster ovary (CHO) cells or the mouse NSO or Sp2/0 plasma cell lines; other systems under development and evaluation include transgenic animals, fungi, and plants.

The efficacy of an antibody therapeutic is critically dependent on appropriate post-translational modifications (PTMs) and each production system offers a different challenge because PTMs show species, tissue, and site specificity. Essential PTMs are relevant not only to potency, but also to the potential immunogenicity of the product.

Further improvement of the potency of rMAbs depends on optimizing the 'downstream' biological effector functions activated in vivo by the immune complexes formed. This offers a considerable challenge due to the difficulty of monitoring events in vivo.

A number of genetically modified animal models are under development that might mimic human biology, for example

Production of Fv antibodies by phage display

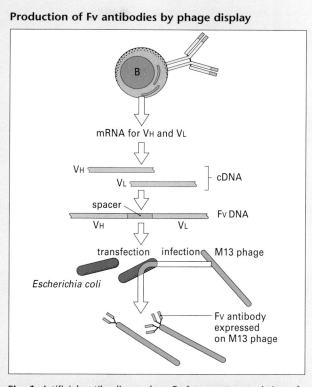

Fig. 1 Artificial antibodies such as Fv fragments, consisting of a hybrid of antibody VH and VL regions, can be generated by phage display. Antibody VH and VL genes are first amplified from B cell mRNA by the polymerase chain reaction. The genes are joined together with a spacer to give a gene for an Fv fragment. Bacteria are then transfected with the gene in a phagemid vector containing a leader sequence, a fragment of the gene expressing phage coat protein 3, and an M13 origin of replication, and then infected with M13 phage. The phages replicate and express the Fv on their tips. Phages displaying the right specificity are isolated by panning on antigen-coated plates, and amplified. The antigen-specific phage can be used to infect strains of bacteria that allow the secretion of the Fv protein into the culture medium.

transgenic and knockout mice that produce human antibodies and express human cellular IgG Fc receptors (FcγR).

At present we extrapolate from effector functions activated in vitro to presumed activity in vivo, for example complement-dependent cytotoxicity (CDC), antibody-dependent cellular cytotoxicity (ADCC), and the induction of apoptosis.

In recent years in-vitro studies have unequivocally established that essential effector functions are dependent on appropriate glycosylation of the antibody molecule.

Glycosylation has therefore been a focus of attention for the biopharmaceutical industry for the past several years because regulatory authorities require that a consistent human-type glycosylation is achieved for rMAbs, irrespective of the system in which they are produced.

METHOD BOX 3.2
Assays for antibodies and antigens

Immunoassays use labeled reagents for detecting either antibodies or antigens. They are very sensitive and economical in the use of reagents.

Solid-phase assays for antibodies using detection reagents labeled with radioisotopes (radioimmunoassay, RIA) or with enzymes (enzyme-linked immunosorbent assay, ELISA) are probably the most widely used of all immunological assays, because large numbers can be performed in a relatively short time.

Similar assays using fluorescent or chemiluminescent reagents to detect the bound antibody are also in common use.

Immunoassay for antibody

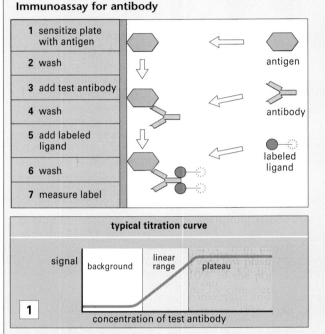

| 1 sensitize plate with antigen |
| 2 wash |
| 3 add test antibody |
| 4 wash |
| 5 add labeled ligand |
| 6 wash |
| 7 measure label |

typical titration curve

Fig. 1 (**1**) Antigen in saline is incubated on a plastic plate or tube, and small quantities become absorbed onto the plastic surface. (**2**) Free antigen is washed away. (The plate may then be blocked with excess of an irrelevant protein to prevent any subsequent non-specific binding of proteins.) (**3**) Test antibody is added, which binds to the antigen. (**4**) Unbound proteins are washed away. (**5**) The antibody is detected by a labeled ligand. The ligand may be a molecule such as staphylococcal protein A that binds to the Fc region of IgG – more often it is another antibody specific for the test antibody. By using a ligand that binds to particular classes or subclasses of test antibody it is possible to distinguish isotypes. (**6**) Unbound ligand is washed away. (**7**) The label bound to the plate is measured. A typical titration curve is shown in the graph. With increasing amounts of test antibody the signal rises from a background level through a linear range to a plateau. Antibody titers can only be detected correctly within the linear range. Typically the plateau binding is 20–100 times the background. The sensitivity of the technique is usually about 1–50 ng/ml of specific antibody. Specificity of the assay may be checked by adding increasing concentrations of free test antigen to the test antibody at step 3; this binds to the antibody and blocks it from binding to the antigen on the plate. Addition of increasing amounts of free antigen reduces the signal.

Enzyme-linked immunosorbent assay (ELISA)

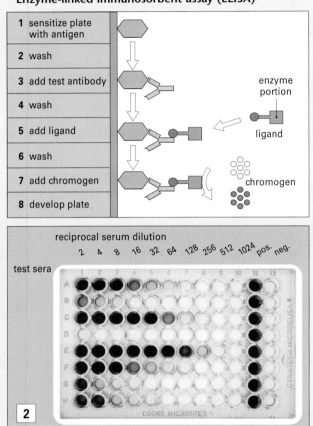

| 1 sensitize plate with antigen |
| 2 wash |
| 3 add test antibody |
| 4 wash |
| 5 add ligand |
| 6 wash |
| 7 add chromogen |
| 8 develop plate |

Fig. 2 The ELISA plate is prepared in the same way as the immunoassay up to step 4. In this system, the ligand is a molecule that can detect the antibody and is covalently coupled to an enzyme such as peroxidase. This binds the test antibody, and after free ligand is washed away (**6**) the bound ligand is visualized by the addition of chromogen (**7**) – a colorless substrate that is acted on by the enzyme portion of the ligand to produce a colored end-product. A developed plate (**8**) is shown in the lower panel. The amount of test antibody is measured by assessing the amount of colored end-product by optical density scanning of the plate.

METHOD BOX 3.2
Assays for antibodies and antigens (*Continued*)

Related assays are used to detect and quantitate antigens. Two examples are the competition immunoassay and the two-site capture immunoassay.

Assay of antigen

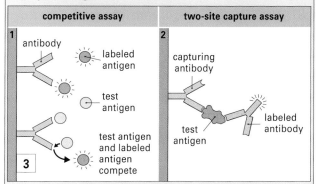

Fig. 3 (**1**) Competitive assay. The test antigen is placed together with labeled antigen onto a plate coated with specific antibody. The more test antigen present, the less labeled standard antigen binds. This type of assay is often used to measure antigens at relatively high concentrations, or hormones that have only a single site available for combination with antibody. (**2**) Two-site capture assay. The assay plate is coated with specific antibody, the test solution then applied, and any antigen present captured by the bound antibody. After washing away unbound material, the captured antigen is detected using a labeled antibody against another epitope on the antigen. Because the antigen is detected by two different antibodies, the second in excess, such assays are both highly specific and sensitive.

Calculation of antibody affinity

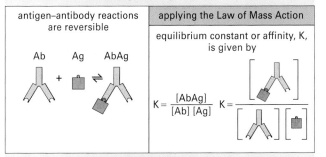

Fig. 3.13 All antigen–antibody reactions are reversible. The Law of Mass Action can therefore be applied, and the antibody affinity (given by the equilibrium constant, K) can be calculated. (Square brackets refer to the concentrations of the reactants)

Affinity and avidity

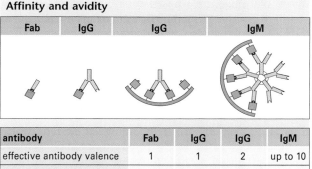

antibody	Fab	IgG	IgG	IgM
effective antibody valence	1	1	2	up to 10
antigen valence	1	1	n	n
equilibrium constant (L/mol)	10^4	10^4	10^7	10^{11}
advantage of multivalence	–	–	10^3-fold	10^7-fold
definition of binding	affinity	affinity	avidity	avidity
	intrinsic affinity		functional affinity	

Fig. 3.14 Multivalent binding between antibody and antigen (avidity or functional affinity) results in a considerable increase in stability as measured by the equilibrium constant, compared with simple monovalent binding (affinity or intrinsic affinity, here arbitrarily assigned a value of 10^4 L/mol). This is sometimes referred to as the 'bonus effect' of multivalency. Thus there may be a 10^3-fold increase in the binding energy of IgG when both valencies (combining sites) are used and a 10^7-fold increase when IgM binds antigen in a multivalent manner.

Specificity, cross-reactivity, and non-reactivity

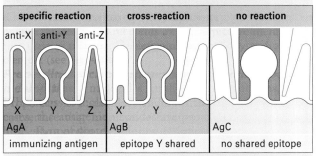

Fig. 3.15 Antiserum specificity results from the action of a population of individual antibody molecules (anti-X, anti-Y, anti-Z) directed against different epitopes (X, Y, Z) on the same or different antigen molecules. Antigen A (AgA) and antigen B (AgB) have epitope Y in common. Antiserum raised against AgA (anti-XYZ) not only reacts specifically with AgA, but cross-reacts with AgB (through recognition of epitopes Y and X'). The antiserum gives no reaction with AgC because there are no shared epitopes.

shape and chemical properties (e.g. charge, hydrophobicity) of epitopes. Small changes in the epitope, such as the position of a single chemical group, can therefore abolish binding (Fig. 3.16).

One consequence of this specificity is that many antibodies bind only to native antigens or to fragments of antigens that retain sufficient tertiary structure to permit the multiple interactions required for bond formation (Fig. 3.17).

Q. Consider an antibody that recognizes an antigen on the outer envelope of a virus. If the antigen mutated, what would be the effect on its ability to bind antibody?
A. It depends on the nature of the mutation. Only mutations that affect the structure of the epitope could affect binding. However, if the mutation caused a radical change in the epitope structure (e.g. charge change or the insertion of a bulky amino acid residue), then the ability to bind might be lost or the affinity of binding drastically reduced.

Q. What effect would it have on the virus if a mutation of the epitope prevented it from being recognized by the antibody?
A. Viruses that mutate to avoid recognition by antibody will be at a selective advantage because they will not be destroyed by the immune system or prevented from attaching to host cells. Many viruses, including influenza and HIV, mutate their surface molecules and so evade recognition by antibodies.

Analysis of antibodies to protein antigens reveals that specificity may be for epitopes:
- consisting of a single contiguous stretch of amino acids (**a continuous epitope**);
- dependent on the native conformation of the antigen and formed from two or more stretches of sequence that are separated in the primary structure (**discontinuous or conformational epitopes**).

Q. How might these differing characteristics of antigen be relevant when producing antibodies for immunological assays?
A. Antibodies specific for discontinuous epitopes may not bind denatured antigen, for example on immunoblots (Method Box 3.3), whereas antibodies to continuous epitopes bind denatured antigen more often.

EACH ISOTYPE (SUBCLASS) MEDIATES A DISTINCT SET OF EFFECTOR FUNCTIONS

Antibodies are bifunctional because they must both:
- form complexes with antigens to limit their spread;
- elicit host responses to facilitate antigen removal and destruction.

The nature of the constant region determines the effector function of the antibody and the various host responses elicited, such as complement-mediated lysis or phagocytosis.

In antibody–antigen complexes the antibody molecules are essentially aggregated such that the multiple Fc regions are able to engage and activate ligands or

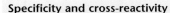

Specificity and cross-reactivity

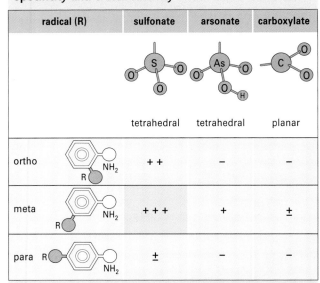

radical (R)	sulfonate	arsonate	carboxylate
	tetrahedral	tetrahedral	planar
ortho	+ +	−	−
meta	+ + +	+	±
para	±	−	−

Fig. 3.16 Antiserum raised to the meta isomer of aminobenzene sulfonate (the immunizing hapten) is mixed with ortho and para isomers of aminobenzene sulfonate, and also with the three isomers (ortho, meta, para) of two different, but related, antigens: aminobenzene arsonate and aminobenzene carboxylate. The antiserum reacts specifically with the sulfonate group in the meta position, but will cross-react (although more weakly) with sulfonate in the ortho position. Further, weaker cross-reactions are possible when the antiserum is reacted with either the arsonate group or the carboxylate group in the meta, but not in the ortho or para, position. Arsonate is larger than sulfonate and has an extra hydrogen atom, while carboxylate is the smallest of the three groups. These data suggest that an antigen's configuration is as important as the individual chemical groupings that it contains.

Configurational specificity

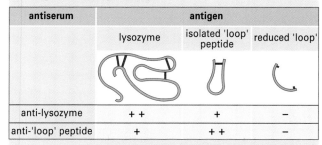

antiserum	antigen		
	lysozyme	isolated 'loop' peptide	reduced 'loop'
anti-lysozyme	+ +	+	−
anti-'loop' peptide	+	+ +	−

Fig. 3.17 The lysozyme molecule possesses an intrachain bond (red), which produces a loop in the peptide chain. Antisera raised against whole lysozyme (anti-lysozyme) and the isolated loop (anti-'loop' peptide) are able to distinguish between the two. Neither antiserum reacts with the isolated loop in its linear reduced form. This demonstrates the importance of tertiary structure in determining antibody specificity.

METHOD BOX 3.3
Assays to characterize antigens

The techniques of immunoprecipitation and immunoblotting (also known as western blotting) are both used to characterize antigens, giving information on their molecular mass and heterogeneity, and some limited information on their abundance.

These techniques may be useful for comparing the abundance of antigens, but are less well suited to the quantitation of antigens than the immunoassays described in Method Box 3.2.

Immunoblotting is a simple technique, but only antibodies that can recognize continuous epitopes can be used to detect the denatured antigens on the blots.

Immunoprecipitation is more often used where only antibodies that recognize undenatured antigens are available.

Immunoblotting

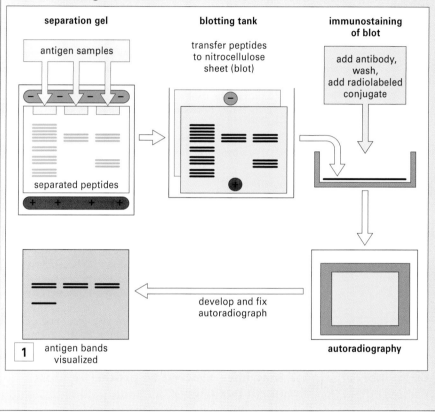

Fig. 1 In immunoblotting, antigen samples are first separated in an analytical gel (e.g. an SDS polyacrylamide gel or an isoelectric focusing gel). The resolved molecules are transferred electrophoretically to a nitrocellulose membrane in a blotting tank. The blot is then treated with antibody to the specific antigen and washed, and a radiolabeled conjugate to detect antibodies is bound to the blot. The principle is similar to that of a radioimmunoassay (RIA, see Method Box 3.2) or enzyme-linked immunosorbent assay (ELISA, see Method Box 3.2). After washing again, the blot is placed in contact with X-ray film in a cassette. The autoradiograph is developed and the antigen bands that have bound the antibody are visible. This immunoblotting technique can be modified for use with a chemiluminescent label or an enzyme-coupled conjugate (as in ELISA), where the bound material can be detected by treatment with a chromogen, which deposits an insoluble reagent directly onto the blot.

receptors (e.g. FcγR and C1q) (Fig. 3.18). Antibody is said to **opsonize** the antigen (bacterium, virus), making it a more attractive target for phagocytic cells.

IgM is the predominant antibody in the primary immune response

IgM is the first antibody formed in the primary immune response and is largely confined to the intravascular pool. It is frequently associated with the immune response to antigenically complex, blood-borne infectious organisms.

Once bound to its target, IgM is a potent activator of the classical pathway of complement.

Although the pentameric IgM antibody molecule consists of five Fcμ regions, it does not activate the classical pathway of complement in its uncomplexed form. However, when bound to an antigen with repeating identical epitopes, it forms a 'staple' structure (see Fig. 3.9), undergoing a conformational change referred to as **dislocation**, and the multiple Fcμ presented in this form are able to initiate the classical complement cascade.

IgG is the predominant antibody of secondary immune responses

IgG equilibrates between the intravascular and extravascular pools, so providing comprehensive systemic protection.

The four IgG subclasses are highly homologous in structure, but each has a unique profile of effector functions; thus, in activating the classical pathway of complement, complexes formed with:
- IgG1 and IgG3 antibodies are efficient;
- IgG2 antibodies are less effective;
- IgG4 antibodies are reported to be inactive.

METHOD BOX 3.3
Assays to characterize antigens
(Continued)

Immunoprecipitation

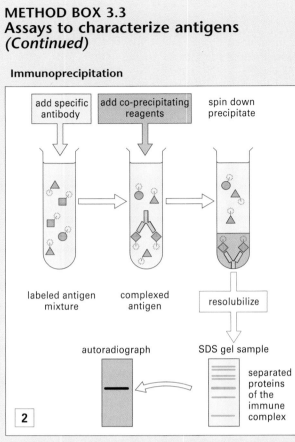

Fig. 2 In immunoprecipitation the antigens being tested are labeled with ^{125}I, and antibody is added that binds only to its specific antigen. The complexes are precipitated by the addition of co-precipitating agents, such as anti-immunoglobulin antibodies or staphylococcal protein A. The insoluble complexes are spun down and washed to remove any unbound labeled antigens. The precipitate is then resolubilized (e.g. in SDS), and the components are separated on analytical gels. After running, the fixed gels are autoradiographed, to show the position of the specific labeled antigen. Frequently the antigens are derived from the surface of radiolabeled cells, which are solubilized with detergents before the immunoprecipitation. It is also possible to label the antigens with biotin, and detect them at the end chromatographically using streptavidin (binds biotin) coupled to an enzyme such as peroxidase (see ELISA technique in Method Box 3.2).

The IgG subclasses also interact with a complex array of cellular Fc receptors (FcγR) expressed on various cell types (see Fig. 3.18 and below).

In humans, the newborn infant is not immunologically competent and the fetus must be protected by passive IgG antibody selectively transported across the placenta (Fig. 3.19). Transport is mediated by the neonatal Fc receptor (FcRn) – all IgG subclasses are transported. IgG subclasses are the only isotypes that are transported across the placenta, but the cord/maternal blood ratios differ,

being approximately 1.2 for IgG1 and approximately 0.8 for IgG4.

Q. How do you interpret these ratios with respect to IgG transport across the placenta?
A. IgG1 is transported more efficiently than IgG4. Also, because the ratio for IgG1 is >1, the antibody is moving up a concentration gradient; therefore it must be active transport.

In some species (e.g. the pig), maternal immunoglobulin is transferred to the offspring in the postnatal period through selective transport of IgG across the gastrointestinal tract via a homologous FcRn receptor.

IgA is characteristic of a secondary immune response
Serum IgA is characteristic of a secondary immune response. Immune complexes of IgA opsonize antigens and activate phagocytosis through cellular Fc receptors (FcαR).

A predominant role for IgA antibody is in its secretory form, affording protection of the respiratory, gastrointestinal, and reproductive tracts.

The IgA1 subclass predominates in:
- human serum (approximately 90% of total IgA); and
- secretions such as nasal mucus, tears, saliva, and milk (70–95% of total IgA).

In the colon, IgA2 predominates (approximately 60% of the total IgA). Many microorganisms that can infect the upper respiratory and gastrointestinal tracts have adapted to their environment by releasing proteases that cleave IgA1 within the extended hinge region, whereas the short hinge region of IgA2 is not vulnerable to these enzymes.

IgD is a transmembrane antigen receptor on B cells
IgD has no known effector functions as a serum protein. It functions as a transmembrane antigen receptor on mature B lymphocytes.

IgE may have evolved to protect against helminth parasites
Despite its low serum concentration, the IgE class:
- is characterized by its ability to bind avidly to circulating basophils and tissue mast cells through the high-affinity FcϵRI receptor (see below);
- sensitizes cells on mucosal surfaces such as the conjunctival, nasal, and bronchial mucosae.

IgE may have evolved to provide immunity against helminth parasites, but in developed countries it is now more commonly associated with allergic diseases such as asthma and hay fever.

Fc RECEPTORS ARE EXPRESSED BY MONONUCLEAR CELLS, NEUTROPHILS, NK CELLS, EOSINOPHILS, BASOPHILS, AND MAST CELLS
Antibodies sometimes protect just by binding to a pathogen, so preventing the pathogen from attaching to cells of the body and infecting them. More often, the biological and protective functions of antibodies are

Biological properties of human immunoglobulins

isotype	IgG1	IgG2	IgG3	IgG4	IgA1	IgA2	IgM	IgD	IgE
complement activation									
classical pathway	++	+	+++	–	–	–	+++	–	–
alternative pathway	varies with epitope density and antibody/antigen ratio								
lectin pathway	varies with glycosylation status								
Fc receptor binding									
FcγRI (monocytes)	+++	–	+++	++	–	–	–	–	–
FcγRIIa (monocytes, neutrophils, eosinophils, platelets)	+	±*	+	–	–	–	–	–	–
FcγRIIb (lymphocytes)	+	?	+	–	–	–	–	–	–
FcγRIII (neutrophils, eosinophils, macrophages, LGLs, NK cells, T cells)	+	–	+	±	–	–	–	–	–
FcεRI (mast cells, basophils)	–	–	–	–	–	–	–	–	+++
FcεRII (monocytes, platelets, neutrophils, B and T cells, eosinophils)	–	–	–	–	–	–	–	–	++
FcαR (monocytes, neutrophils, eosinophils, T and B lymphocytes)	–	–	–	–	+	+	–	–	–
FcμR (T cells, macrophages)	–	–	–	–	–	–	+	–	–
FcδR (T and B cells)	–	–	–	–	+	–	–	+	–
pIgR, poly-Ig receptor; mucosal transport	–	–	–	–	+	+	+	–	–
FcRn, placental transport and catabolism	+	+	+	+	–	–	–	–	–
products of microorganisms									
SpA, staphylococcal protein A	+	+	–	+					
SpG, streptococcal protein G	+	+	+	+	–	–	–	–	–

*dependent on the allotype of FcγRIIa; LGLs, large granular lymphocytes; NK cells, natural killer cells

Fig. 3.18 The biological functions of different antibody classes and subclasses depend on which receptors they bind to and the cellular distribution of those receptors.

mediated by acting as adapters that bind via their Fc region to Fc receptors on different cell types.

The three classes of Fc receptor for IgG are FcγRI, FcγRII, and FcγRIII

Three classes of cell surface receptor for IgG (FcγR) are defined in humans:

- FcγRI (CD64);
- FcγRII (CD32); and
- FcγRIII (CD16).

Each receptor is characterized by a glycoprotein α chain that binds to antibody and has extracellular domains homologous with immunoglobulin domains (Fig. 3.20) – that is, they belong to the immunoglobulin superfamily, as do receptors for IgA (FcαR) and IgE (FcεRI).

FcγRs are expressed constitutively on a variety of cell types and may be upregulated or induced by environmental factors (e.g. cytokines).

Biological activation results from cross-linking of the FcγR and consequent aggregation of **immunoreceptor tyrosine-based activation (ITAM)** or **immunoreceptor tyrosine-based inhibitory (ITIM)** motifs in the cytoplasmic sequences.

Phosphorylation of the ITAM motif triggers activities such as:

- phagocytosis;
- **antibody-dependent cell-mediated cytotoxicity (ADCC)**;
- mediator release; and
- enhancement of antigen presentation.

Immunoglobulins in the serum of the fetus and newborn child

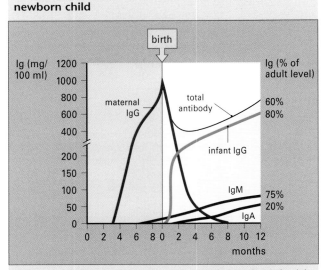

Fig. 3.19 IgG in the fetus and newborn infant is derived solely from the mother. This maternal IgG has disappeared by the age of 9 months, by which time the infant is synthesizing its own IgG. The neonate produces its own IgM and IgA; these classes cannot cross the placenta. By the age of 12 months, the infant produces 80% of its adult level of IgG, 75% of its adult IgM level, and 20% of its adult IgA level.

Fcγ receptors

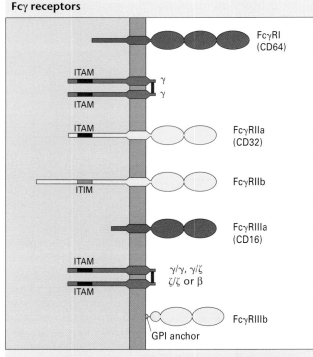

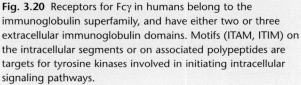

Fig. 3.20 Receptors for Fcγ in humans belong to the immunoglobulin superfamily, and have either two or three extracellular immunoglobulin domains. Motifs (ITAM, ITIM) on the intracellular segments or on associated polypeptides are targets for tyrosine kinases involved in initiating intracellular signaling pathways.

In contrast, phosphorylation of ITIM blocks cellular activation.

FcγRI is involved in phagocytosis of immune complexes and mediator release

FcγRI (CD64; 72 kDa) binds:
- monomeric IgG1 and IgG3 with high affinity (10^8–10^9 l/mol); and
- IgG4 with lower affinity (10^7–10^8 l/mol).

It has a more restricted cellular distribution than the other FcγRs, but is expressed on all cells of the mononuclear phagocyte lineage, and is involved in the phagocytosis of immune complexes, mediator release, etc.

The α chain contains three immunoglobulin domains in the extracellular portion and is associated with a γ chain that bears an ITAM motif in its cytoplasmic part.

FcγRII is expressed as FcγRIIa and FcγRIIb

FcγRII (CD32; 40 kDa) is expressed as structurally and functionally distinct FcγRIIa and FcγRIIb forms with wide but differing cellular distribution.

The α chains have:
- low affinity ($< 10^7$ l/mol) for monomeric IgG1 and IgG3;
- bind complexed (multivalent, aggregated) IgG with high avidity.

The FcγRIIa molecule:
- binds IgG1 and IgG3 only; and
- expresses an ITAM motif within its cytoplasmic tail.

It may also be associated with a γ chain and cross-linking results in cellular activation.

Polymorphism in the FcγRIIA gene results in the presence of histidine or arginine at position 131 in the extracellular domains – the His[131] allotype binds and is activated by immune complexes of IgG2.

The FcγRIIb molecule:
- expresses an ITIM motif within its cytoplasmic tail; and
- when cross-linked, blocks cellular activation, particularly on B cells (see Fig. 11.5).

FcγRIII is expressed as FcγRIIIa and FcγRIIIb

FcγRIII (CD16; 50–80 kDa) is expressed as structurally and functionally distinct FcγRIIIa and FcγRIIIb, which are extensively glycosylated and have differing cellular distributions.

FcγRIIIa is a transmembrane protein (like FcγRI, FcγRIIa, and FcγRIIb), whereas FcγRIIIb is GPI (glycosyl phosphatidyl inositol) anchored (see Fig. 3.20).

The α chains of FcγRIIIa:
- have a moderate affinity for monomeric IgG (approximately 3×10^7 l/mol); and
- may be associated with γ/ξ and/or β chains bearing ITAM motifs.

FcγRIIIa is expressed on monocytes, macrophages, NK cells, and some T cells.

The FcγRIIIb form:
- is selectively expressed on neutrophils; and
- has a low affinity for monomeric IgG ($<10^7$ l/mol).

It appears that engagement of FcγRIIIb can result in transmembrane signaling through its association with other membrane proteins bearing signaling motifs.

POLYMORPHISM IN THE FcγRIIIA AND FcγRIIIB GENES: FcγRIIIB-NA1 AND FcγRIIIB-NA2 FORMS – Polymorphism in the *FcγRIIIA* gene results in the presence of phenylalanine (Phe) or valine (Val) at position 158 in the extracellular domains; the Val[158] allotype is associated with more efficient NK cell activity.

Polymorphism in the *FcγRIIIB* gene results in multiple amino acid sequence differences, which affect the extent of glycosylation.

The consequent FcγRIIIb-NA1 and FcγRIIIb-NA2 forms are reported to differ in functional activity.

Q. What factors determine whether a particular IgG subclass will have a particular biological function (e.g. the ability to opsonize a bacterium for phagocytosis by a macrophage)?
A. The distribution of Fc receptors between different effector cells, the ability of each subclass of antibody to bind to these Fc receptors, and the affinity of binding.

IgG Fc interaction sites for several ligands have been identified

Application of site-directed mutagenesis, X-ray crystallography and nuclear magnetic resonance spectroscopy has allowed elucidation of the molecular topography of IgG Fc interaction sites for several ligands that bind overlapping non-identical sites at the CH2/CH3 interface, for example:

- staphylococcal protein A;
- streptococcal protein G;
- FcRn; and
- a monoclonal rheumatoid factor Fab fragment.

The interactions between maternal IgG and the MHC class I molecule-like FcRn expressed on the intestinal epithelium of the neonatal rat have now been studied at high resolution (Fig. 3.21) and are believed to mimic closely the binding of the human placental counterpart, hFcRn, with maternal IgG. Titration of IgG histidine residues in the binding site for FcRn may explain its:

- pH sensitivity;
- binding at pH 6.5 (the pH within vacuoles); and
- dissociating at pH 7.4 (the pH of blood).

Given the symmetry of the Fc region, the fragments used in the experiments above are functionally divalent and may form multimeric complexes.

If monomeric IgG were divalent for FcγR and C1q, however, it would not function properly because circulating monomeric IgG could form activating multimers. The interaction sites for these ligands (e.g. FcγR and C1q) have been 'mapped' to the CH2 domain next to the hinge.

The crystal structure of an IgG Fc/FcγRIII complex reveals an asymmetric interaction site embracing the CH2 domains of both heavy chains, thereby ensuring monovalency.

Site-directed mutagenesis indicates that common amino acid residues engage each of FcγRI, FcγRII, and FcγRIII, but care should be taken in extrapolating from isotype to isotype and from species to species.

For example, Glu318, Lys320, and Lys322 of the CH2 domain is widely quoted as the interaction motif for C1q activation, but this result was obtained for mouse

Neonatal rat intestinal Fc receptor FcRn

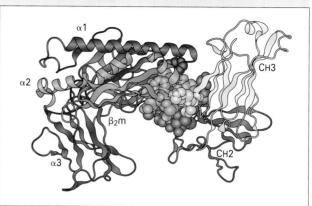
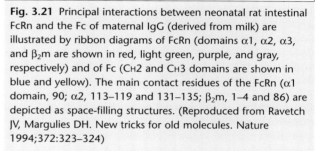

Fig. 3.21 Principal interactions between neonatal rat intestinal FcRn and the Fc of maternal IgG (derived from milk) are illustrated by ribbon diagrams of FcRn (domains α1, α2, α3, and β2m are shown in red, light green, purple, and gray, respectively) and of Fc (CH2 and CH3 domains are shown in blue and yellow). The main contact residues of the FcRn (α1 domain, 90; α2, 113–119 and 131–135; β2m, 1–4 and 86) are depicted as space-filling structures. (Reproduced from Ravetch JV, Margulies DH. New tricks for old molecules. Nature 1994;372:323–324)

IgG2b with guinea pig complement. This finding does not apply to the activation of human complement by human IgG1 – even though human IgG1 expresses the same Glu-x-Lys-x-Lys motif.

IgM–antigen complexes are very efficient activators of the classical complement system, but the mechanism by which IgM binds C1q appears different from that of IgG. The conformational change from a 'star' to a 'staple' conformation upon binding to multivalent antigen is thought to unveil a ring of occult C1q-binding sites that are not accessible in the star-shaped configuration (see Fig. 3.9).

Glycosylation is important for receptor binding to IgG

N-linked glycosylation of the IgG Cγ2 domain is essential for the binding and activation of FcγRI, FcγRII, FcγRIII, and C1q. The oligosaccharide is of a complex type, generating multiple glycoforms, and forms multiple noncovalent interactions with the polypeptide such that it appears to be sequestered within the protein structure and so inaccessible for direct interactions with the FcγRI, FcγRII, FcγRIII, and C1q ligands.

Fidelity of glycosylation has become an important issue in the production of monoclonal antibodies for therapy because glycosylation is a species- and tissue-specific post-translational modification (see Method Box 3.1).

Chinese hamster ovary (CHO) cells and mouse myeloma cells can produce appropriately glycosylated human IgG heavy chains, though the range of glycoforms is restricted. Recent studies have shown that the glycoforms thus produced do not express optimal effector functions (such as killing of tumor cells by ADCC; see

Chapter 10). These production cell lines, and other possible production platforms, are being engineered to produce optimal human glycoforms by transfecting in human glycosyltransferases and 'knocking-out' non-human glycosyltransferases.

The two classes of Fc receptor for IgE are FcεRI and FcεRII

Two classes of Fc receptor for IgE (FcεR) are defined in humans (Fig. 3.22):
- the high-affinity FcεRI (45 kDa), which is expressed on mast cells and basophils and is the 'classical' IgE receptor; and
- the low-affinity FcεRII (CD23; 45 kDa), which is expressed on leukocytes and lymphocytes.

The α chain of FcεRI is a glycoprotein and has two extracellular domains homologous to immunoglobulin domains; it is therefore a member of the immunoglobulin superfamily.

The low-affinity FcεRII is not a member of the immunoglobulin superfamily, but has substantial structural homology with several animal C-type lectins (e.g. mannose-binding lectin [MBL]).

Cross-linking of IgE bound to FcεRI results in histamine release

The high-affinity receptor (FcεRI) is present on the surface of mast cells and basophils as a complex with a β (33 kDa) and two γ (99 kDa) chains to form the αβγ₂ receptor unit (see Fig. 3.22).

FcεRI binds IgE with an affinity of approximately 10^{10} l/mol such that, although the serum concentration of IgE is very low, the receptors are permanently saturated. Cross-linking of the IgE bound to these receptors results

in the activation and release of histamine and other vasoactive and inflammatory mediators.

FcεRII is a type 2 transmembrane molecule

FcεRII is the low-affinity (CD23) receptor and is a type 2 transmembrane molecule (i.e. one in which the C termini of the polypeptides are extracellular, see Fig. 3.22). The two forms of human CD23 are:
- **CD23a**, which is expressed in antigen-activated B cells and influences IgE production; and
- **CD23b**, expression of which is induced in a wide range of cells by IL-4.

CD23a and CD23b differ by six or seven amino acids in their cytoplasmic N termini and contain different signaling motifs that modify their functions.

IgE receptors bind to IgE by different mechanisms

Decades of research and controversy surround the identification of the interaction site on IgE for the high-affinity FcεRI receptor.

Recent crystal structures of a Cε2Cε3Cε4 fragment and Cε3Cε4–FcεRI complex seem to have resolved the issue, and there is a striking structural homology between this site and the site on IgG Fc that binds FcγRIII.

One distinctive feature is that, unlike IgG binding to FcγRIII, binding of IgE to its receptor does not appear to depend on glycosylation of the immunoglobulin.

These studies should be interpreted with caution because the antibody fragments were not produced in mammalian cells.

Possible models for the interaction of IgE with the FcεRI and FcεRII receptors are illustrated in Fig. 3.22. The low-affinity IgE Fc receptor, FcεRII (CD23), is a C-type lectin and is therefore sensitive to glycosylation status.

A VAST REPERTOIRE OF ANTIGEN-BINDING SITES IS ACHIEVED BY RANDOM RECOMBINATION

How can a finite genome provide the information required for the vast repertoire of antibody molecules that an individual can synthesize? This question posed an intellectual and practical challenge for decades.

Ehrlich's side-chain hypothesis, put forward at the beginning of the 20th century (Fig. 3.23), proposed antigen-induced selection. His model is close to our present view of clonal selection, except that he placed receptors of several different specificities on the same cell and did not address the question of how the diverse receptors were generated.

Several decades later, Dreyer and Bennett realized that the existence of a constant region and a variable region implied that the antibody protein was encoded by at least two different genes, contrary to a central dogma of molecular biology ('one gene, one protein').

Shortly thereafter, Tonegawa performed the decisive experiments that proved the Dreyer and Bennett hypothesis and showed that somatic recombination events were able to take a limited amount of genetic material and create almost innumerable permutations, encoding a vast antigen receptor repertoire.

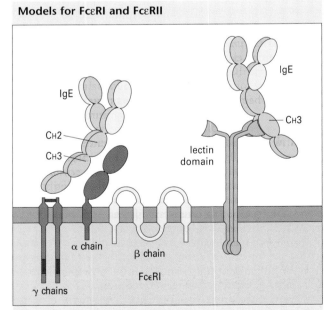

Models for FcεRI and FcεRII

Fig. 3.22 Models for the high-affinity IgE receptor (FcεRI), which binds to IgE via its α chain, and the low-affinity receptor (FcεRII), which binds using its lectin domains. Both receptors are shown with IgE bound.

Ehrlich's side-chain theory

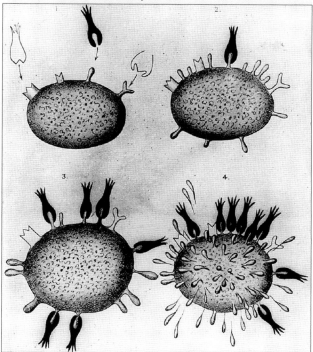

Fig. 3.23 Ehrlich proposed that the combination of antigen with a preformed B cell receptor (now known to be antibody) triggered the cell to produce and secrete more of those receptors. Although the diagram indicates that he thought a single cell could produce antibodies to bind more than one type of antigen, it is evident that he anticipated both the clonal selection theory and the idea that the immune system could generate receptors before contact with antigen.

Recently, however, it has been shown that functional heavy (H chain) antibodies devoid of light chains account for about half of the circulating immunoglobulins in the Camelidae family. This suggests new possibilities for using just VH domains as therapeutics.

Immunoglobulins show isotypic, allotypic, and idiotypic variation

Originally the immunoglobulin isotypes were defined serologically by the antigenic uniqueness of their constituent polypeptide chains, using antisera raised predominantly in rabbits. Allotypes were recognized using human sera from individuals that lacked the allotype.

Idiotypy (variation related to the specific structure of individual immunoglobulin domains and the antigen-binding site) was revealed with antisera raised to monoclonal IgG immunoglobulins isolated from the sera of patients with a B cell tumor. When adsorbed with polyclonal IgG, such an antiserum produced a reagent specific for the immunizing protein (the **idiotype**).

In the modern era, we identify the human immunoglobulin **isotypes** as products of defined immunoglobulin genes encoding the constant regions of heavy and light chains, and the **allotypes** as polymorphic variants of these genes.

The idiotype of an antibody molecule results from antigenic uniqueness reflecting the structural uniqueness of the VH and VL regions (Fig. 3.24).

Isotypes are the products of genes within the genome of all healthy members of a species

The human immunoglobulin heavy chain isotypes are encoded by μ, δ, $\gamma3$, $\gamma1$, $\alpha1$, $\gamma2$, $\gamma4$, $\alpha2$, and ε genes on chromosome 14. The single κ and multiple λ isotypes are encoded by Cκ and Cλ genes on chromosomes 2 and 22, respectively.

Q. Given that one human can produce more heavy chains and more light chains than there are genes in the entire human genome, what mechanism(s) could lead to the presence of the great diversity of immunoglobulin genes seen in different B cells, each encoding a specific antibody?
A. The antibody genes could be produced by splicing together different gene segments, with a different combination of segments used in different B cells.

Another mechanism could involve mutation of the original gene(s) with different mutations occurring in different B cells. In fact, both of these mechanisms take place in human B cells.

The two mechanisms occurring within individual B cells – gene segment recombination and gene mutation – described above, are termed **somatic recombination** and **somatic mutation** to distinguish them from the related processes that occur in germ cells.

In addition to somatic recombination and somatic mutation, which produce diverse heavy and light chains, the pairing of a unique VL domain with a unique VH domain to generate an antigen-binding site also generates diversity and became an established paradigm.

Variability of immunoglobulin structure

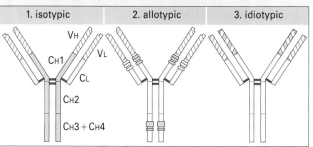

Fig. 3.24 All immunoglobulins have the basic four-chain structure. There are three types of immunoglobulin variability.
(**1**) Isotypic variation is present in the germline of all members of a species, producing the heavy (μ, δ, γ, ε, α) and light chains (Igκ, λ) and the V region frameworks (subgroups).
(**2**) Allotypic variation is intraspecies allelic variability.
(**3**) Idiotypic variation refers to the diversity at the antigen-binding site (paratope) and in particular relates to the hypervariable segments.

Allotypes result from genetic variation at a locus within the species

Immunoglobulin allotypes refer to proteins that are the product of polymorphic immunoglobulin genes (i.e. the result of genetic variation at a given locus within the species). The WHO-adopted nomenclature – for example G3m(g) – requires:

- definition of the heavy chain class;
- followed by the subclass;
- an m (indicating 'marker'); and
- the designated number or letter in brackets.

The sequence correlates have been determined. For example G1m(f) and G1m(z) allotypes are characterized by the presence of, respectively, an arginine or lysine residue at position 214 in the CH1 or Cγ1 domain of the heavy chains.

In humans allotypes are encountered within:

- IgG;
- IgA; and
- κ light chains.

Because all heavy chain genes are encoded within the same locus, they are inherited as a complex or **haplotype**. Studies of immunoglobulin haplotypes help in the identification of different population groups of humans.

Idiotypes result from antigenic uniqueness

The structural uniqueness of antibody variable regions can be reflected in antigenic uniqueness recognized by antisera raised in a heterologous species (e.g. rabbit).

However, in addition to antigenic uniqueness, cross-reactivity may be observed for two V regions that are highly homologous. The terms private and public (or cross-reactive and recurrent) idiotypes are used to describe this property. Idiotypes:

- may be specific for individual B cell or plasma cell clones (**private idiotypes**);
- are sometimes shared between different B cell clones (**public, cross-reacting, or recurrent idiotypes**).

Each therapeutic antibody is structurally unique and has the potential to provoke an immune response in recipients. This is a current concern for this very promising class of drugs.

Monoclonal antibodies have been developed as successful therapeutics, but their unique specificity is reflected in unique structure (idiotype) such that they are potentially immunogenic. In practice a variable proportion of patients produce **anti-idiotypic antibodies**, depending on the patient's genetic background, the disease treated, the dosing regimen, etc.

HEAVY CHAIN GENE RECOMBINATION PRECEDES LIGHT CHAIN RECOMBINATION

The revealed organization of mammalian genomes invalidated the earlier dogma of 'one gene, one polypeptide sequence' and replaced it with 'genes in pieces' as coding (exons) and non-coding (introns) DNA sequences were identified. Generally:

- an open reading frame is transcribed to nuclear RNA;
- the introns are 'spliced' out of nuclear RNA to yield a continuous messenger RNA (mRNA);
- protein is translated from continuous mRNA.

Germline DNA encoding immunoglobulin polypeptide chains shows a further level of complexity. Information for the variable domains is present in two or three libraries of gene segments termed **V, D, and J gene segments** that recombine at the level of the DNA. These gene segments are widely separated from exons encoding the constant regions.

Recombination between the V, D, and J gene segments generates a continuous sequence encoding the V domain. However, in the initial nuclear RNA transcript the information for the V and C domains is still widely separated.

The DNA encoding the leader to the end of the C gene, including introns, is transcribed into heterogeneous nuclear RNA (hnRNA).

The hnRNA is processed with the 'splicing out' of introns to yield the mRNA encoding the polypeptide V and C domains within a continuous RNA sequence that is translated into protein.

The primary antibody repertoire is:

- present in the B cell population and expressed as membrane-bound IgM and IgD acting as antigen receptors;
- generated through recombination of germline gene segments, with selection to eliminate B cells producing anti-self antibodies.

Immunoglobulin genes undergo rearrangement during B cell development

Immunoglobulin gene rearrangement is initiated at the heavy chain locus. If a 'productive' rearrangement occurs (i.e. generating a functional product), then rearrangement at the κ locus is initiated:

- if the κ rearrangement is productive, the assembled antibody is expressed as a membrane receptor;
- if recombination at the κ locus is not productive, rearrangement at the λ locus proceeds.

A number of **pseudogenes** (non-functional genes with high homology to the heavy chain genes) and **orphan genes** (putative genes with no known homology to known functional genes) have been identified as related to functional heavy and light chain genes.

A number of genes present within the VH, Vκ, and VL loci do not have 'open reading frames' and cannot be transcribed. They do not, therefore, contribute to the generation of antibody diversity.

Pseudogenes account for a large part of what is known as 'junk DNA' in eukaryotic genomes, and are thought to be derived by mutations in functional ancestral genes.

Rearrangement at the heavy chain VH locus precedes rearrangement at light chain loci

The germline human heavy chain locus, on chromosome 14 (Fig. 3.25), contains a library of 38 to 46 functional VH gene segments that encode the N terminal 95 residues of the VH region.

The C terminal residues of the VH region are encoded within 23 DH and six JH gene segments (see Fig. 3.25).

Productive rearrangement at the VH locus is an obligatory and early event in the generation of B cells that precedes rearrangement at light chain loci.

Heavy chain VDJ recombination in humans

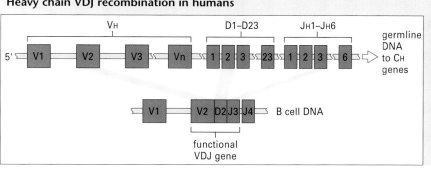

Fig. 3.25 The heavy chain gene loci recombine three segments to produce a VDJ gene, which encodes the VH domain. Of some 80 V genes, about 50 are functional and the others are pseudogenes. The V gene segment recombines with one of 23 DH segments and one of six JH segments to produce a functional VDJ gene in the B cell.

The first event is recombination between a JH gene segment and DH segments

DH segments:

- are highly variable, both in the number of codons and in the nucleotide sequence;
- may be read in three possible reading frames without generating stop codons; and
- can be used singly or in combinations.

Productive recombination between DH and JH gene segments signals recombination of this DJ sequence to a VH gene segment, forming a contiguous DNA sequence encoding the entire VH protein sequence (see Fig. 3.25).

The recombined VH, DH, and JH gene segments generate widely diverse hypervariable Hv3 (CDR3) sequences, which contribute greatly to the diversity of the primary antibody repertoire.

The heavy chain locus includes approximately 78 related pseudogenes, and orphan genes occur on chromosomes other than 14.

Rearrangement results in a Vκ gene segment becoming contiguous with a Jκ gene segment

The germline human κ light chain locus on chromosome 2 (Fig. 3.26) contains a library of 31 to 35 functional Vκ gene segments that encode the N terminal 95 residues of the Vκ region.

The C terminal residues of the Vκ region are encoded within five Jκ gene segments (see Fig. 3.26).

During B cell development, rearrangement of the DNA occurs such that one of the Vκ genes becomes contiguous with one of five Jκ genes.

Q. If there are 31 Vκ segments and five Jκ segments, what is the theoretical maximum number of rearrangements that could occur at this locus?

A. 155 (i.e. 31×5), but imprecise joining introduces additional diversity (see below).

The κ locus also includes over 30 related pseudogenes, and orphan genes are present on other chromosomes.

A leader or signal sequence (a short hydrophobic segment responsible for targeting the chain to the endoplasmic reticulum) precedes each Vκ segment. The leader sequence is cleaved in the endoplasmic reticulum, and the antibody molecule is then processed through the intracellular secretory pathway.

Recombination results in a Vλ gene segment becoming contiguous with a functional Jλ gene segment

The germline human λ light chain locus (Fig. 3.27) on chromosome 22 contains a library of 29 to 33 functional

κ chain production in humans

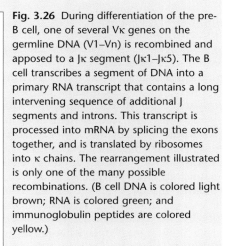

Fig. 3.26 During differentiation of the pre-B cell, one of several Vκ genes on the germline DNA (V1–Vn) is recombined and apposed to a Jκ segment (Jκ1–Jκ5). The B cell transcribes a segment of DNA into a primary RNA transcript that contains a long intervening sequence of additional J segments and introns. This transcript is processed into mRNA by splicing the exons together, and is translated by ribosomes into κ chains. The rearrangement illustrated is only one of the many possible recombinations. (B cell DNA is colored light brown; RNA is colored green; and immunoglobulin peptides are colored yellow.)

λ chain production in humans

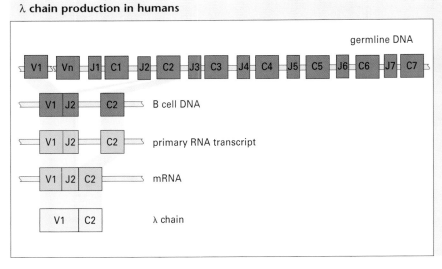

Fig. 3.27 During B cell differentiation, one of the germline Vλ genes recombines with a J segment to form a VJ combination. The rearranged gene is transcribed into a primary RNA transcript complete with introns (non-coding segments occurring between the genes), exons (which code for protein), and a poly A tail. This is spliced to form mRNA with loss of the introns, and then translated into protein.

Vλ gene segments that encode the N terminal 95 residues of the Vλ region.

There are 7 to 11 Jλ gene segments with each linked to a Cλ gene sequence (see Fig. 3.27) – the number of JλCλ sequences depends on the haplotype.

During the generation of B cells, unproductive rearrangement at the κ locus leads to recombination at the λ locus such that one of the Vλ genes becomes contiguous with one of four or five functional Jλ genes.

The number of possible λ chain variable regions that could be produced in this way is approximately 120 to 160. Imprecise joining introduces additional diversity (see below).

The λ locus also includes over 35 related pseudogenes, and orphan genes are present on other chromosomes.

Following recombination between Vλ and Jλ genes, there is still an intron (a non-coding intervening sequence) between the recombined VλJλ gene and the exon encoding the C region.

Recombination involves recognition of signal sequences by the V(DJ) recombinase

Recombination of germline gene segments is a key feature in the generation of the primary antibody repertoire. How is the recombination effected?

Each V, D, and J segment is flanked by **recombination signal sequences (RSS)**:

- a signal sequence found downstream (3′) of VH, VL, and DH gene segments consists of a heptamer CACAGTG or its analog, followed by a spacer of non-conserved sequence (12 or 23 bases), and then a nonamer ACAAAACC or its analog (Fig. 3.28);
- immediately upstream (5′) of a germline JL, DH, and JH segment is a corresponding signal sequence of a nonamer and a heptamer, again separated by an unconserved sequence (12 or 23 bases).

The heptameric and nonameric sequences following a VL, VH, or DH segment are complementary to those preceding the JL, DH, or JH segments (respectively) with which they recombine.

Recombination sequences in immunoglobulin genes

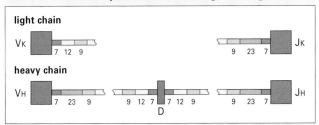

Fig. 3.28 The recombination sequences in the light chain genes (top) and heavy chain genes (bottom) consist of heptamers (7), 12 or 23 unconserved bases, and nonamers (9). The sequences of heptamers and nonamers are complementary and the nonamers act as signals for the recombination activating genes to form a synapsis between the adjoining exons. Similar recombination sequences are present in the T cell receptor V, D, and J gene segments (see Chapter 5).

The 12 and 23 base spacers correspond to either one or two turns of the DNA helix (see Fig. 3.28).

The recombination process is mediated by the protein products of the two **recombination-activating genes (RAG-1** and **RAG-2)**:

- a RAG-1–RAG-2 complex recognizes the RSS, bringing a 12-RSS and a 23-RSS together into a synaptic complex (Fig. 3.29);
- the RAG proteins initiate cleavage by introducing a nick in the area bordering the 5′ end of the signal heptamer and the coding region;
- the RAG proteins then convert this nick into a double-strand break, generating a hairpin at the coding end and a blunt cut at the signal sequence;
- the hairpinned coding end must be opened before the joining step, and usually undergoes further processing (the addition or deletion of nucleotides), resulting in an imprecise junction.

Stages of V(D)J recombination

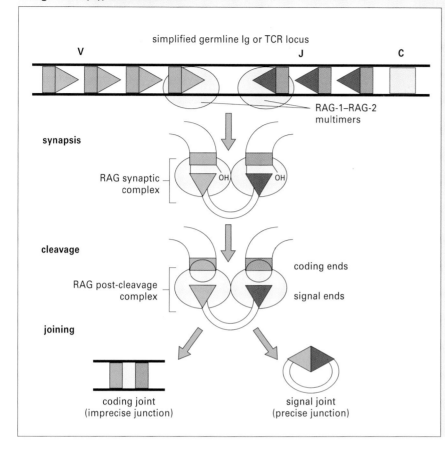

Fig. 3.29 The recombination-activating genes (RAG-1–RAG-2) bind to two recombination signal sequences (RSS) – one 12-RSS and one 23-RSS – bringing them into a synaptic complex. Synapsis stimulates cleavage: first, one DNA strand is nicked, and the resulting 3′ OH group attacks the opposite strand, leaving two hairpinned coding ends and two blunt signal ends. After cleavage, these ends are held in the RAG post-cleavage complex and joined by the non-homologous end-joining (NHEJ) factors. The coding joint forms the new variable region exon; the signal ends are joined together to form a signal joint, often (but not always) as an excised circular product that is lost from the cell. The signal joint has no known immunological function.

Signal ends, in contrast, are usually joined precisely to form circular signal joints that have no known immunological function and are lost from the cell (see Fig. 3.29)

The loss or addition of nucleotides during coding joint formation creates additional diversity in the junctions that is not encoded by the V, D, or J segments.

Furthermore, following cleavage, the enzyme terminal deoxynucleotidyl transferase may add random nucleotides to the exposed cut ends of the DNA. Nucleotides may therefore be inserted between D_H and J_H, and between V_H and D_H, without need of a template (Figs 3.30 and 3.31).

VARIABLE REGION GENES UNDERGO SOMATIC HYPERMUTATION

In the mid-20th century, following the elucidation of the structure of DNA, it was believed that the function of tissues, the cells that constitute them, and therefore the integrity of the individual depended on accurate replication of DNA sequences. The enormous size and sequence variability of the antigen-specific antibody repertoire, however, made the 'one gene, one polypeptide chain' dogma untenable.

Light chain diversity created by variable recombination

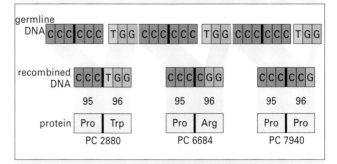

Fig. 3.30 The same Vκ21 and J1 sequences of the germline create three different amino acid sequences in the proteins PC2880, PC6684, and PC7940 by variable recombination. PC2880 has proline and tryptophan at positions 95 and 96, caused by recombination at the end of the CCC codon. Recombination one base down produces proline and arginine in PC6684. Recombination two bases down from the end of Vκ21 produces proline and proline in PC7940.

Heavy chain diversity created by variable recombination and N region diversity

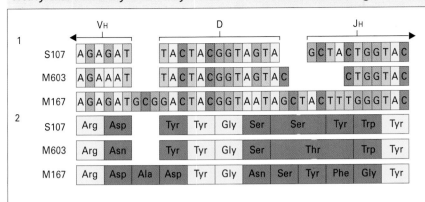

Fig. 3.31 The DNA sequence (**1**) and amino acid sequence (**2**) of three heavy chains of anti-phosphorylcholine are shown. Variable recombination between the germline, V, D, and J regions, and N region insertion causes variation (orange) in amino acid sequences. In some cases (e.g. M167) there appear to be additional inserted codons. However, these are in multiples of three, and do not alter the overall reading frame.

A period of intense intellectual and experimental activity followed as seemingly opposing germline and somatic mutation models were explored. Introduction of a theory of somatic mutation for immunoglobulin genes to account for a structural diversity that could not be accommodated within the genome led to a schism between immunologists and classical geneticists.

In due time, the argument proved unnecessary because it became evident that nature actually employs both types of process to form the antibody repertoire.

Libraries of germline gene segment sequences recombine, with a degree of junctional diversity, to generate the primary antibody repertoire, but this process does not account for the sequence diversity observed for antibodies that are generated during a secondary immune response.

It is now established that in germinal centers the recombined DNA encoding variable light and heavy chain sequences undergoes repeated rounds of random mutation (**somatic hypermutation**) to generate B cells expressing structurally distinct receptors (Fig. 3.32). Survival and expansion of these B cells requires that their receptors engage antigen presented to them by follicular dendritic cells in the lymphoid tissues:

- a majority will acquire a deleterious mutation and, in the absence of a survival signal, die;
- a minority bind antigen with increased affinity and compete with those of lower affinity (i.e. antibodies characteristic of the primary response).

This process, called **affinity maturation**, is dependent on both T cells and germinal centers.

Athymic mice lacking T cells do not form germinal centers and show no affinity maturation.

Diversity is generated at several different levels

Antibody diversity therefore arises at several levels:

- first there are the multiple V genes recombining with D and J segments;
- the imprecision with which joining of the segments occurs produces further variation;
- as virtually any light chain may pair with any heavy chain, the combinatorial binding of heavy and light chains amplifies the diversity enormously (Fig. 3.33).

Mutations in the DNA of two heavy chain genes

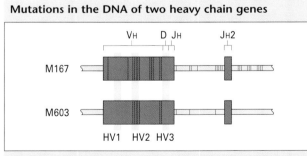

Fig. 3.32 DNA of two IgG antibodies to phosphorylcholine are illustrated. Both antibodies share the T15 idiotype. Black lines indicate positions where the sequence has mutated from the germline sequence. There are large numbers of mutations in both the introns and exons of both genes, but particularly in the second hypervariable region (HV2). By comparison, there are no mutations in the regions encoding the constant genes, implying that the mutational mechanism is highly localized.

Seven mechanisms for the generation of antibody diversity

1. multiple germline V genes
2. VJ and VDJ recombinations
3. N–nucleotide addition
4. gene conversion
5. recombinational inaccuracies
6. somatic point mutation
7. assorted heavy and light chains

Fig. 3.33 Because each mechanism can occur with any of the others, the potential for increased diversity multiplies at each step of immunoglobulin production.

The structures of the first and second hypervariable regions (CDR-1 and CDR-2) of the primary antibody repertoire are encoded entirely by germline gene segments whereas CDR-3 diversity is generated by recombination events.

Different species have different strategies for generating diversity

Current understanding of the mechanisms for generating antibody diversity results primarily from studies in the mouse and human, species that show remarkable similarities in gene organization and expression. However, other species have evolved additional solutions to the problem of generating antibody diversity from a relatively small amount of genetic information. As a result, whereas mouse and human employ recombination among multiple germline genes together with somatic mutation:

- sharks rely on a large number of antibody genes and do not use somatic recombination (Fig. 3.34); and
- chickens have a very small number of antibody genes that undergo a very high level of gene conversion (Fig. 3.35).

Shark immunoglobulin VH loci

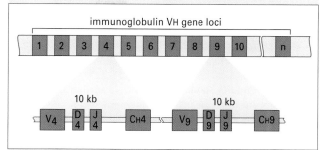

Fig. 3.34 In the shark there is a series of about 200 heavy chain gene clusters, each with a single V, D, J, and C gene segment. The fourth and ninth clusters are shown expanded. VH, DH, and JH segments are closely linked and occur within approximately 1.3 kb. Together with the CH segment, they occupy only about 10–15 kb. The arrangement of genes within a cluster appears to be encoded in the germline rather than by somatic rearrangement mechanisms, which may account for the lack of interindividual variation associated with the immune response of this species. (Based on data of Dr JJ Marchalonis and Dr GW Litman)

Genetic basis of antibody diversity in chickens

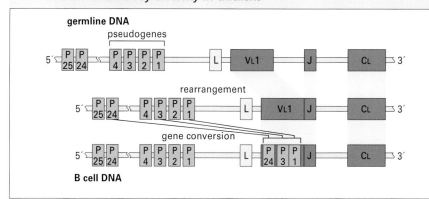

Fig. 3.35 The chicken germline immunoglobulin light chain locus has less than 30 kb of DNA. A single functional V gene (VL) lies 2 kb upstream from a single JC unit, with an adjacent cluster of 25 pseudogenes (P) in a 19-kb region. Rearrangement occurs briefly during early B cell development. Antibody diversity is achieved by gene conversion between P and the rearranged sequence. The arrangement shown (P1, P3, and P24) is illustrative; converted segments do not necessarily lie in order in the V gene segment.

FURTHER READING

Almogren A, Senior BW, Loomes LM, Kerr MA. Structural and functional consequences of cleavage of human secretory and human serum immunoglobulin A1 by proteinases from *Proteus mirabilis* and *Neisseria meningitidis*. Infect Immun 2003;71:3349–3356.

Burton D, Woof JM. Human antibody effector function. Adv Immunol 1992;51:1–84.

Glennie MJ, van de Winkel JG. Renaissance of cancer therapeutic antibodies. Drug Discov Today 2003;8:503–510.

Gould HJ, Sutton BJ, Beavil AJ, et al. The biology of IgE and the basis of allergic disease. Annu Rev Immunol 2003;21:579–628.

Jefferis R, Lund J, Pound JD. IgG-Fc-mediated effector functions: molecular definition of interaction sites for effector ligands and the role of glycosylation. Immunol Rev 1998;163:59–76.

Jefferis R, Lund J. Interaction sites on human IgG-Fc for FcγR: current models. Immunol Lett 2002;82:57–65.

Jung D, Alt FW. Unraveling V(D)J recombination; insights into gene regulation. Cell 2004;116:299–311.

Montiero RC, van de Winkel JG. IgA Fc receptors. Annu Rev Immunol 2003;21:177–204.

Padlan EA. X-ray crystallography of antibodies. Adv Protein Chem 1996;49:57–133.

Ravetch JV, Bolland S. IgG Fc receptors. Annu Rev Immunol 2001;19:275–290.

Rudd PM, Elliott T, Cresswell P, et al. Glycosylation and the immune system. Science 2001;291:2370–2376.

Woof JM, Burton D. Human antibody-Fc receptor interactions illuminated by crystal structures. Nat Rev Immunol 2004;4:89–99.

INTERNET REFERENCES

IMGT, the International ImMunoGeneTics Information System® http://imgt.cines.fr

- An integrated knowledge resource for the immunoglobulins (IG), T cell receptors (TR), major histocompatibility complex (MHC), immunoglobulin superfamily and related proteins of the immune system of human and other vertebrate species.

Mike Clark's Immunoglobulin Structure/Function Home Page http://www.path.cam.ac.uk/~mrc7/mikeimages.html

- Provides a wealth of information, of his own generation and through access to many other related sites.

National Center for Biotechnology Information (NCBI) http://www.ncbi.nlm.nih.gov/

- Established in 1988 as a national resource for molecular biology information, NCBI creates public databases, conducts research in computational biology, develops software tools for analyzing genome data, and disseminates biomedical information – all for the better understanding of molecular processes affecting human health and disease.

Roy Jefferis Home Page http://medweb.bham.ac.uk/immunity infection/research/RoyJefferis/home.html

- Provides a basic introductory course and information on the influence of glycosylation on antibody structure and function

V BASE http://www.mrc-cpe.cam.ac.uk/COMPILATION.php?menu=901

- Compiled using all available human germline V gene sequences (V, D, or J) taken from the literature and from the EMBL/Genbank databases.
- Currently, 961 sequences from 145 different publications make up the V BASE database.

Critical thinking: The specificity of antibodies (see p. 493 for explanations)

The human rhinovirus HRV14 is formed from four different polypeptides: one of them (VP4) is associated with viral RNA in the core of the virus, while the other three polypeptides (VP1–VP3) make up the shell of the virus – the capsid.

1 When virus is propagated in the presence of neutralizing antiviral antiserum it is found that mutated forms of the virus develop. Mutations are detected in VP1, VP2, or VP3, but never in VP4. Why should this be so?

The most effective neutralizing antibodies are directed against the protein VP1 – this is termed an immunodominant antigen. Two different monoclonal antibodies against VP1 were developed and used to induce mutated forms of the virus. When the sequences of the mutated variants were compared with the original virus, it was found that only certain amino acid residues became mutated (see table below).

antibody	amino acid number	residue in wild type	observed mutations
VP1-a	91	Glu	Ala, Asp, Gly, His, Asn, Val, Tyr
VP1-a	95	Asp	Gly, Lys
VP1-b	83	Gln	His
VP1-b	85	Lys	Asn
VP1-b	138	Glu	Asp, Gly
VP1-b	139	Ser	Pro

2 What can you tell about the epitopes that are recognized by the two different monoclonal antibodies?
3 When the binding of the antibody VP1-a is measured against the different mutant viruses, it is found that it binds with high affinity to the variant with glycine (Gly) at position 138, with low affinity to the variant with Gly at position 95, and does not bind to the variant with lysine (Lys) at position 95. How can you explain these observations?

Complement

SUMMARY

- **Complement is central to the development of inflammatory reactions** and forms one of the major immune defense systems of the body.

- **Complement activation pathways have evolved to label pathogens for elimination.** The classical pathway links to the adaptive immune system. The alternative and lectin pathways provide non-specific 'innate' immunity, and the alternative pathway is linked to the classical pathway.

- **The complement system is controlled to protect the host.** C1 inhibitor controls the classical and lectin pathways. C3 and C5 convertase activity are controlled by decay and enzymatic degradation.

- **The membrane attack pathway results in the formation of a transmembrane pore.** Regulation of the membrane attack pathway reduces the risk of 'bystander' damage to adjacent cells.

- **Many cells express one or more membrane receptors for complement products.** Receptors for fragments of C3 are widely distributed on different leukocyte populations. Receptors for C1q are present on phagocytes, mast cells, and platelets The plasma complement regulator fH binds leukocyte surfaces.

- **Complement has a variety of functions.** Its principal functions are chemotaxis including opsonization and cell activation, lysis of target cells, and priming of the adaptive immune response.

- **Complement deficiencies illustrate the homeostatic roles of complement.** Classical pathway deficiencies result in tissue inflammation. Deficiencies of mannan-binding lectin (MBL) are associated with infection in infants. Alternative pathway and C3 deficiencies are associated with bacterial infections. Terminal pathway deficiencies predispose to Gram-negative bacterial infections. C1 inhibitor deficiency leads to hereditary angioedema. Deficiencies in alternative pathway regulators produce a secondary loss of C3.

COMPLEMENT IS CENTRAL TO THE DEVELOPMENT OF INFLAMMATORY REACTIONS

The complement system was discovered at the end of the 19th century as a heat-labile component of serum that augmented (or 'complemented') its bactericidal properties.

Complement is now known to comprise some 16 plasma proteins, together constituting nearly 10% of the total serum proteins, and forming one of the major immune defense systems of the body (Fig. 4.1). The functions of the complement system include:
- the triggering and amplification of inflammatory reactions;
- attraction of phagocytes by chemotaxis;
- clearance of immune complexes;
- cellular activation;
- direct microbial killing; and
- an important role in the development of antibody responses.

In evolutionary terms the complement system is very ancient and antedates the development of the adaptive immune system: even starfish and worms have a functional complement system.

The importance of complement in immune defense is readily apparent in individuals who lack particular components – for example, children who lack the component **C3** are subject to overwhelming bacterial infections.

Like most elements of the immune system, when overactivated or activated in the wrong place the complement system can cause harm.

Complement is involved in the pathology of many diseases, provoking a search for therapies that control complement activation.

COMPLEMENT ACTIVATION PATHWAYS HAVE EVOLVED TO LABEL PATHOGENS FOR ELIMINATION

One major function of complement is to label pathogens and other foreign or toxic bodies for elimination from the host. The complement activation pathways have evolved to serve this purpose, and the multiple ways in which activation can be triggered, together with intrinsic amplification mechanisms, ensure efficient:
- recognition; and
- clearance.

Role of complement in inflammation

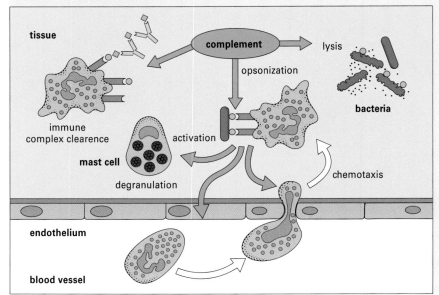

Fig. 4.1 Complement has a central role in inflammation causing chemotaxis of phagocytes, activation of mast cells and phagocytes, opsonization and lysis of pathogens, and clearance of immune complexes.

Complement activation pathways

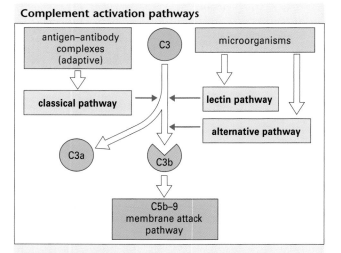

Fig. 4.2 Each of the activation pathways generates a C3 convertase, which converts C3 to C3b, the central event of the complement pathway. C3b in turn activates the terminal lytic membrane attack pathway. The first stage in the classical pathway is the binding of antigen to antibody. The alternative pathway does not require antibody and is initiated by the covalent binding of C3b to hydroxyl and amine groups on the surface of various microorganisms. The lectin pathway is also triggered by microorganisms in the absence of antibody, with sugar residues on the pathogen surface providing the binding sites. The alternative and lectin pathways provide non-specific 'innate' immunity, whereas the classical pathway represents a more recently evolved link to the adaptive immune system.

Moreover, there are several different ways to activate the complement system, so providing a large degree of flexibility in response (Fig. 4.2).

The first activation pathway to be discovered, now termed the **classical pathway**, is initiated by antibodies bound to the surface of the target. Although an efficient means of activation, it requires that the host has previously encountered the target microorganism in order for an antibody response to be generated.

The **alternative pathway**, described in the 1950s, provides an antibody-independent mechanism for complement activation on pathogen surfaces.

The **lectin pathway**, the most recently described activation pathway, also bypasses antibody to enable efficient activation on pathogens.

All three pathways – classical, alternative, and lectin pathways:
- involve the activation of C3, which is the most abundant and most important of the complement proteins;
- comprise a proteolytic cascade in which complexes of complement proteins create enzymes that cleave other complement proteins in an ordered manner to create new enzymes, thereby amplifying and perpetuating the activation cascade.

Thus a small initial stimulus can rapidly generate a large effect. Fig. 4.3 summarizes how each of the pathways is activated.

All activation pathways converge on a common **terminal pathway** – a non-enzymatic system for causing membrane disruption and lytic killing of pathogens.

The immune defense and pathological effects of complement activation are mediated by the fragments and complexes generated during activation:
- the small chemotactic and proinflammatory fragments **C3a** and **C5a**;

Rapid Reference Box 4

alternative pathway – the activation pathways of the complement system involving C3 and factors B, D, P, H, and I, which interact in the vicinity of an activator surface to form an alternative pathway C3 convertase (C$\overline{\text{3bBb}}$).

amplification loop – the alternative complement activation pathway that acts as a positive feedback loop when C3 is split in the presence of an activator surface.

anaphylatoxins – complement peptides (C3a and C5a) that cause mast cell degranulation and smooth muscle contraction.

bystander lysis – complement-mediated lysis of cells in the immediate vicinity of a complement activation site that are not themselves responsible for the activation.

C1–C9 – the components of the complement pathways responsible for mediating inflammatory reactions, opsonization of particles, and lysis of cell membranes.

C3 convertases – the enzyme complexes C$\overline{\text{3bBb}}$ and C$\overline{\text{4b2a}}$ that cleave C3.

classical pathway – the pathway by which antigen–antibody complexes can activate the complement system, involving components C1, C2, and C4, and generating a classical pathway C3 convertase (C$\overline{\text{4b2a}}$).

complement – a group of serum proteins involved in the control of inflammation, the activation of phagocytes, and the lytic attack on cell membranes.

complement receptors (CR1–CR4) – a set of four cell surface receptors for fragments of complement C3.

decay accelerating factor (DAF) – a cell surface molecule on mammalian cells that limits activation and deposition of complement C3b.

lectin pathway – a pathway of complement activation, initiated by mannan-binding lectin (MBL), that intersects the classical pathway.

membrane attack complex (MAC) – the assembled terminal complement components C5b–C9 of the lytic pathway that becomes inserted into cell membranes.

zymogen – pro-enzyme that requires proteolytic cleavage to become active; the enzymatically active form is distinguished from its precursor by a bar drawn above.

Summary of the activators of the classical, lectin, and alternative pathways

	immunoglobulins	microorganisms			other
		viruses	**bacteria**	**other**	
classical pathway	immune complexes containing IgM, IgG1, IgG2, or IgG3	HIV and other retroviruses, vesicular stomatitis virus		*Mycoplasma* spp.	polyanions, especially when bound to cations PO$_4^{3-}$ (DNA, lipid A, cardiolipin) SO$_4^{2-}$ (dextran sulfate, heparin, chondroitin sulfate)
lectin pathway		HIV and other retroviruses	many Gram-positive and Gram-negative organisms		arrays of terminal mannose groups
alternative pathway	immune complexes containing IgG, IgA, or IgE (less efficient than the classical pathway)	some virus-infected cells (e.g. by Epstein–Barr virus)	many Gram-positive and Gram-negative organisms	trypanosomes, *Leishmania* spp., many fungi	dextran sulfate, heterologous erythrocytes, complex carbohydrates (e.g. zymosan)

Fig. 4.3 Summary of the activators of the classical, lectin, and alternative complement activation pathways.

- the large opsonic fragments **C3b** and **C4b**; and
- the lytic **membrane attack complex (MAC)**.

The details of complement activation, the nomenclature, and the ways in which the pathways are controlled are shown in Fig. 4.4.

The classical pathway links to the adaptive immune system

The classical pathway is activated by antibody bound to antigen and requires Ca²⁺

Only surface-bound IgG and IgM antibodies can activate complement, and they do so via the classical pathway. Surface binding is the key:

- IgM is the most efficient activator, but unbound IgM in plasma does not activate complement;
- among IgG subclasses, IgG1 and IgG3 are strong complement activators, whereas IgG4 does not activate because it is unable to bind the first component of the classical pathway.

Q. What occurs when IgM binds to the surface of a bacterium that allows it to activate complement?

A. A transition occurs from a flat planar molecule to a staple form, which exposes binding sites for the first component of the complement system, C1 (see Fig. 3.9).

Overview of the complement activation pathways

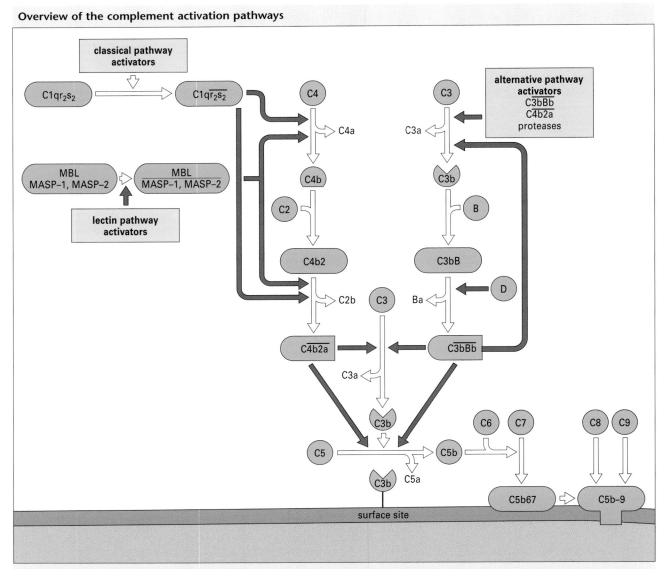

Fig. 4.4 The proteins of the classical and alternative pathways are assigned numbers (e.g. C1, C2). Many of these are zymogens (i.e. pro-enzymes that require proteolytic cleavage to become active). The cleavage products of complement proteins are distinguished from parent molecules by suffix letters (e.g. C3a, C3b). The proteins of the alternative pathway are called 'factors' and are identified by single letters (e.g. factor B, which may be abbreviated to fB or just 'B'). Components are shown in green, conversion steps as white arrows, and activation/cleavage steps as red arrows. The classical pathway is activated by the cleavage of C1r and C1s following association of C1qr$_2$s$_2$ with classical pathway activators (see Fig. 4.3), including immune complexes. Activated C1s cleaves C4 and C2 to form the classical pathway C3 convertase C$\overline{4b2a}$. Cleavage of C4 and C2 can also be effected via MASP-1 and MASP-2 of the lectin pathway, which are associated with mannan-binding lectin (MBL). The alternative pathway is activated by the cleavage of C3 to C3b, which associates with factor B and is cleaved by factor D to generate the alternative pathway C3 convertase C$\overline{3bBb}$. The initial activation of C3 happens to some extent spontaneously, but this step can also be effected by classical or alternative pathway C3 convertases or a number of other serum or microbial proteases. Note that C3b generated in the alternative pathway can bind more factor B and generate a positive feedback loop to amplify activation on the surface. Note also that the activation pathways are functionally analogous, and the diagram emphasizes these similarities. For example, C3 and C4 are homologous, as are C2 and factor B. MASP-1 and MASP-2 are homologous to C1r and C1s, respectively. Either the classical or alternative pathway C3 convertases may associate with C3b bound on a cell surface to form C5 convertases, C$\overline{4b2a3b}$ or C$\overline{3bBb3b}$, which split C5. The larger fragment C5b associates with C6 and C7, which can then bind to plasma membranes. The complex of C5b67 assembles C8 and a number of molecules of C9 to form a membrane attack complex (MAC), C5b–9.

The first component of the pathway, **C1**, is a complex molecule comprising a large recognition unit termed **C1q** and two molecules each of **C1r** and **C1s**, the enzymatic units of the complex (Fig. 4.5). Assembly of the C1 complex is Ca^{2+}-dependent, and the classical pathway is therefore inactive if Ca^{2+} ions are absent.

C1 activation occurs only when several of the head groups of C1q are bound to antibody

C1q in the C1 complex binds through its globular head groups to the Fc regions of the immobilized antibody and undergoes changes in shape that trigger autocatalytic activation of the enzymatic unit C1r. Activated C1r then cleaves C1s at a single site in the protein to activate it.

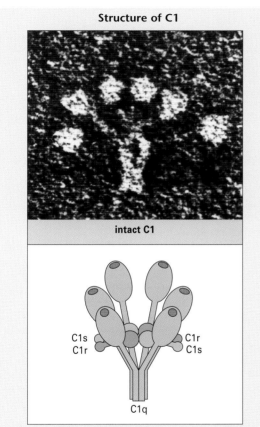

Structure of C1

intact C1

C1s
C1r

C1r
C1s

C1q

Fig. 4.5 Electron micrograph of a human C1q molecule demonstrates six subunits. Each subunit contains three polypeptide chains, giving 18 in the whole molecule. The receptors for the Fc regions of IgG and IgM are in the globular heads. The connecting stalks contain regions of triple helix and the central core region contains collagen-like triple helix. The lower panel shows a model of intact C1 with two C1r and two C1s pro-enzymes positioned within the ring. The catalytic heads of C1r and C1s are closely apposed and conformational change induced in C1q following binding to complexed immunoglobulin causes mutual activation/cleavage of each C1r unit followed by cleavage of the two C1s units. The cohesion of the entire complex is dependent on Ca^{2+}. (Electron micrograph, reproduced by courtesy of Dr N Hughes-Jones)

Because C1 activation occurs only when several of the head groups of C1q are bound to antibody, only surfaces that are densely coated with antibody will trigger the process. This limitation reduces the risk of inappropriate activation on host tissues.

C1s enzyme cleaves C4 and C2

The C1s enzyme has two substrates – C4 and C2 – which are the next two proteins in the classical pathway sequence. (Note that the complement components were named chronologically, according to the order of their discovery, rather than according to their position in the reaction.) C1s cleaves the abundant plasma protein **C4** at a single site in the molecule:

- releasing a small fragment, **C4a**; and
- exposing a labile thioester group in the large fragment **C4b**.

Through the highly reactive thioester, C4b becomes covalently linked to the activating surface (Fig. 4.6).

C4b binds the next component, **C2**, in a Mg^{2+}-dependent complex and presents it for cleavage by C1s in an adjacent C1 complex:

- the fragment **C2b** is released; and
- **C2a** remains associated with C4b on the surface.

C4b2a is the classical pathway C3 convertase

The complex of C4b and C2a (termed **$\overline{C4b2a}$** – the classical pathway C3 convertase) is the next activation enzyme. C2a in the $\overline{C4b2a}$ complex cleaves **C3**, the most abundant of the complement proteins:

- releasing a small fragment, **C3a**; and

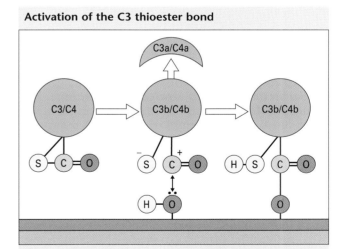

Activation of the C3 thioester bond

C3a/C4a

C3/C4

C3b/C4b

C3b/C4b

S C O

S C O

H S C O

H O

O

Fig. 4.6 The α chain of C3 contains a thioester bond formed between a cysteine and a glutamine residue, with the elimination of ammonia. Following cleavage of C3 into C3a and C3b, the bond becomes unstable and susceptible to nucleophilic attack by electrons on -OH and $-NH_2$ groups, allowing the C3b to form covalent bonds with proteins and carbohydrates – the active group decays rapidly by hydrolysis if such a bond does not form. C4 also contains an identical thioester bond, which becomes activated similarly when C4 is split into C4a and C4b.

- exposing a labile thioester group in the large fragment **C3b**.

As described above for C4b, C3b covalently binds the activating surface.

C4b2a3b is the classical pathway C5 convertase

Some of the C3b formed will bind directly to $\overline{C4b2a}$, and the trimolecular complex formed, $\overline{C4b2a3b}$ (the classical pathway C5 convertase), can bind **C5** and present it for cleavage by C2a:

- a small fragment, **C5a**, is released; and
- the large fragment, **C5b**, remains associated with the $\overline{C4b2a3b}$ complex.

Cleavage of C5 is the final enzymatic step in the classical pathway.

The ability of C4b and C3b to bind surfaces is fundamental to complement function

C3 and C4 are homologous molecules that contain an unusual structural feature – an internal thioester bond between a glutamine and a cysteine residue that, in the intact molecule, is buried within the protein.

When either C3 or C4 is cleaved by the convertase enzyme, a conformational change takes place that exposes the internal thioester bond in C3b and C4b, making it very unstable and highly susceptible to attack by nucleophiles such as hydroxyl groups (-OH) and amine groups ($-NH_2$) in membrane proteins and carbohydrates. This reaction creates a covalent bond between the complement fragment and the membrane ligand, locking C3b and C4b onto the surface (see Fig. 4.6).

The exposed thioester remains reactive for only a few milliseconds because it is susceptible to hydrolysis by water. This lability restricts the binding of C3b and C4b to the immediate vicinity of the activating enzyme and prevents damage to surrounding structures.

The alternative and lectin pathways provide non-specific 'innate' immunity

The lectin pathway is activated by microbial carbohydrates

The lectin pathway differs from the classical pathway only in the initial recognition and activation steps. Indeed, it can be argued that the lectin pathway should not be considered a separate pathway, but rather a route for classical pathway activation that bypasses the need for antibody.

The C1 complex is replaced by a structurally similar multimolecular complex, comprising the C1q-like recognition unit **mannan-binding lectin (MBL)** and several **MBL-associated serine proteases (MASPs)**, which provide enzymatic activity. As in the classical pathway, assembly of this initiating complex is Ca^{2+}-dependent.

C1q and MBL are members of the collectin family of proteins characterized by globular head regions with binding activities and long collagenous tail regions with diverse roles (see Fig. 6.23).

MBL binds the simple carbohydrates mannose and *N*-acetyl glucosamine present in the cell walls of diverse pathogens, including bacteria, yeast, fungi, and viruses. Binding induces shape changes in MBL that in turn induce autocatalytic activation of the MASPs. These enzymes can cleave C4 and C2 to continue activation exactly as in the classical pathway.

The lectin pathway is not the only means of activating the classical pathway in the absence of antibody. Mitochondria and other products of cell damage can directly bind C1q, triggering complement activation and aiding the clearance of the dead and dying tissue.

Alternative pathway activation is accelerated by microbial surfaces and requires Mg^{2+}

The alternative pathway of complement activation also provides antibody-independent activation of complement on pathogen surfaces. This pathway is in a constant state of low-level activation (termed 'tickover').

C3 is hydrolyzed at a slow rate in plasma and the product, $C3(H_2O)$, has many of the properties of C3b, including the capacity to bind a plasma protein **factor B (fB)**, which is a close relative of the classical pathway protein C2. Formation of the complex between C3b (or $C3(H_2O)$) and fB is Mg^{2+}-dependent, so the alternative pathway is inactive in the absence of Mg^{2+} ions. (The differences in the ion requirements of the classical and alternative pathway are exploited in laboratory tests for complement activity.)

The $C\overline{3bBb}$ complex is the C3 convertase of the alternative pathway

Once bound to $C3(H_2O)$ or C3b, fB can bind and activate a plasma enzyme termed **factor D (fD)**. fD cuts fB in the C3bB complex:

- releasing a fragment, **Ba**;
- while the residual portion, **Bb**, becomes an active protease.

The $C\overline{3bBb}$ complex is the C3 cleaving enzyme (C3 convertase) of the alternative pathway. C3b generated by this convertase can be fed back into the pathway to create more C3 convertases, thus forming a positive feedback amplification loop (Fig. 4.7). Activation may occur in plasma or, more efficiently, on surfaces.

Q. What physiological advantages and problems can you see in a system with a positive feedback loop (i.e. where the presence of C3b leads to the production of an enzyme $C\overline{3bBb}$ that generates more C3b)?

A. The positive feedback amplification and 'always on' features of the alternative pathway are well suited to pathogen surveillance. For example, a small initial stimulus could produce the deposition of large amounts of C3b on a pathogen surface, thereby facilitating its phagocytosis. If unregulated, however, the system will continue to activate until all available C3 has been consumed. Self cells would also be subjected to complement activation and could be damaged or destroyed.

Specific features of host cell surfaces, including their surface carbohydrates and the presence of complement regulators (see below), act to rescue the host cell from being destroyed, and such surfaces are non-activating.

On an activating surface such as a bacterial membrane, amplification will occur unimpeded and the surface will

Regulation of the amplification loop

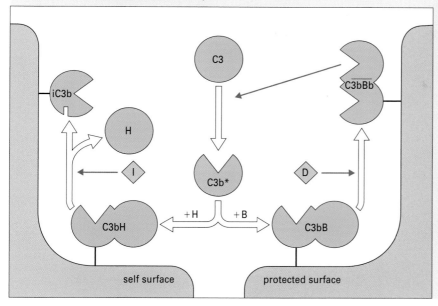

Fig. 4.7 Alternative pathway activation depends on the presence of activator surfaces. C3b bound to an activator surface recruits factor B, which is cleaved by factor D to produce the alternative pathway C3 convertase C3bBb, which drives the amplification loop, by cleaving more C3. However, on self surfaces the binding of factor H is favored and C3b is inactivated by factor I. Thus the binding of factor B or factor H controls the development of the alternative pathway reactions. In addition, proteins such as membrane cofactor protein (MCP) and decay accelerating factor (DAF) also limit complement activation on self cell membranes (see Fig. 4.9).

rapidly become coated with C3b (see Fig. 4.7). In a manner analogous to that seen in the classical pathway, C3b molecules binding to the C3 convertase will change the substrate specificity of the complex, creating a C5 cleaving enzyme, C3bBbC3b.

Cleavage of C5 is the last proteolytic step in the alternative pathway and the C5b fragment remains associated with the convertase.

The alternative pathway is linked to the classical pathway

The alternative pathway is inexorably linked to the classical pathway in that C3b generated through the classical pathway will feed into the alternative pathway to amplify activation. It therefore does not matter whether the initial C3b is generated by the classical, lectin, or alternative pathway – the amplification loop can ratchet up the reactions if they take place near an activator surface.

THE COMPLEMENT SYSTEM IS CONTROLLED TO PROTECT THE HOST

Control of the complement system is required to prevent the consumption of components through unregulated amplification and to protect the host. Complement activation poses a potential threat to host cells, because it could lead to cell lysis. To defend against this threat a family of regulators has evolved alongside the complement system to prevent uncontrolled activation and protect cells from attack.

C1 inhibitor controls the classical and lectin pathways

In the activation pathways, the regulators target the enzymes that drive amplification:

- activated C1 is controlled by a plasma serine protease inhibitor (**serpin**) termed **C1 inhibitor (C1inh)**, which removes C1r and C1s from the complex, switching off classical pathway activation;
- C1inh also regulates the lectin pathway in a similar manner, removing the MASP enzymes from the MBL complex to switch off activation.

C3 and C5 convertase activity are controlled by decay and enzymatic degradation

The C3 and C5 convertase enzymes are heavily policed with plasma and cell membrane inhibitors to control activation. In the plasma:

- **factor H (fH)** and a related protein **factor H-like 1 (fHL-1)** destroy the convertase enzymes of the alternative pathway;
- **C4 binding protein (C4bp)** performs the same task in the classical pathway.

On membranes, two proteins, **membrane cofactor protein (MCP)** and **decay accelerating factor (DAF)**, collaborate to destroy the convertases of both pathways (Fig. 4.8).

The regulators of the C3 and C5 convertases are structurally related molecules that have arisen by gene duplication in evolution. These duplicated genes are tightly linked in a cluster on chromosome 1, termed the **regulators of complement activation (RCA) locus**. This locus also encodes several of the complement receptors (see below).

Control of the convertases is mediated in two complementary ways

THE FIRST CONTROL IS DECAY ACCELERATION – The convertase complexes are labile, with a propensity to dissociate within a few minutes of creation. The regulators

C3 and C5 convertase regulators

	number of SCR domains	dissociation of C3 and C5 convertases		cofactor for factor I on		localization
		classical pathway	alternative pathway	C4b	C3b	
C4b binding protein (C4bp)	52 or 56 in 7or 8 chains	+	–	+	–	plasma
factor H (fH)	20	–	+	–	+	plasma
decay accelerating factor (DAF) (CD55)	4	+	+	–	–	blood cells, endothelia, epithelia
membrane cofactor protein (MCP) (CD46)	4	–	–	+	+	blood cells (not erythrocytes), endothelia, epithelia
complement receptor 1 (CR1) (CD35)	30	+	+	+	+	erythrocytes, B cells, follicular dendritic cells, macrophages

SCR, short consensus repeat

Fig. 4.8 The five proteins listed are widely distributed and control aspects of C3b and C4b dissociation or breakdown. Each of these proteins contains a number of short consensus repeat (SCR) domains. They act either by enhancing the dissociation of C3 and C5 convertases or by acting as cofactors for the action of factor I on C3b or C4b.

fH, fHL-1, and C4bp from the fluid phase and DAF on cell membranes bind the convertase complex and markedly accelerate decay, knocking out:
- C2a from the classical pathway convertase; and
- Bb from the alternative pathway enzyme (Fig. 4.9).

Very recently, genetic defects in fH have been implicated in patients with the non-diarrheal form of hemolytic uremic syndrome (HUS).

Point mutations in fH inhibit binding to host cells and weaken defense against complement, resulting in the hemolysis, platelet dysfunction, and renal damage that typify the syndrome.

THE SECOND CONTROL MECHANISM IS FACTOR I COFACTOR ACTIVITY – **Factor I (fI)** is a fluid-phase enzyme that, in the presence of an appropriate cofactor, can cleave and irreversibly inactivate C4b and C3b (see Fig. 4.9). MCP is a cofactor for fI cleavage of both C4b and C3b, whereas:
- C4bp specifically catalyzes cleavage of C4b; and
- fH/fHL-1 catalyzes cleavage of C3b.

It is interesting to note that, whereas the plasma regulators contain both activities in a single molecule, the two membrane regulators each contain only one activity.

Efficient regulation of the convertases on membranes therefore requires the concerted action of:
- DAF to dissociate the complex; and
- MCP to irreversibly inactivate it by catalyzing cleavage of the central component.

The alternative pathway also has a unique positive regulator, **properdin**, which stabilizes the C3 convertase and markedly increases its life span.

The two processes by which C3 convertase regulators inactivate the enzymes

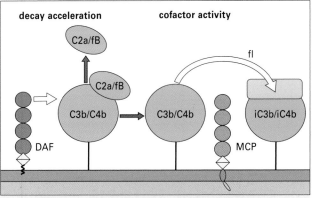

Fig. 4.9 DAF binds the enzyme complex, displacing the enzymatically active component (C2a or Bb). Membrane cofactor protein (MCP) binds the C3b/C4b unit released after decay and acts as a cofactor for factor I (fI) cleavage of C3b or C4b, resulting in the irreversible inactivation of the convertase.

Complement receptor 1 (CR1) is often included in the list of membrane regulators of C3 convertase activity, and, indeed, CR1 is a powerful regulator with both decay accelerating and cofactor activities in both pathways. Nevertheless, it is excluded from the above discussion because CR1 is primarily a receptor for complement-coated particles and does not have a role in protecting the host cell.

THE MEMBRANE ATTACK PATHWAY RESULTS IN THE FORMATION OF A TRANSMEMBRANE PORE

The **terminal or membrane attack pathway** involves a distinctive set of events whereby:

- a group of five globular plasma proteins associate with one another; and,
- in the process, acquire membrane-binding and pore-forming capacity to form the membrane attack complex (MAC).

The MAC is a transmembrane pore (Fig. 4.10). Cleavage of C5 creates the nidus for MAC assembly to begin. While still attached to the convertase enzyme, C5b binds first **C6** then **C7** from the plasma. Conformational changes occurring during assembly of this trimolecular **C5b67** complex:

- cause release from the convertase; and
- expose a labile hydrophobic site.

The membrane attack pathway

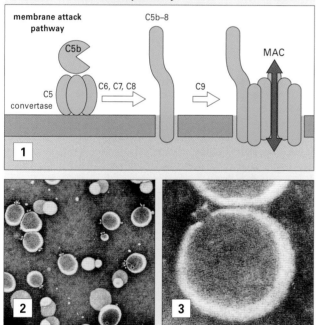

Fig. 4.10 (1) C5b, while still attached to the C5 convertase, binds C6 and C7 from the fluid phase. The trimolecular C5b–7 complex dissociates from the convertase and binds the target cell membrane. Binding of C8 and multiple copies of C9 generates a rigid protein-lined transmembrane channel, the membrane attack complex (MAC). (**2** and **3**) Electron micrographs of the MAC. The complex consists of a cylindrical pore in which the walls of the cylinder, formed by C9, traverse the cell membrane. In these micrographs the human C5b–9 complex has been incorporated into a lecithin liposomal membrane. × 234 000. (Courtesy of Professor J Tranum-Jensen and Dr S Bhakdi)

The complex can stably associate with a membrane through the labile hydrophobic site, though the process is inefficient and most of the C5b67 formed is inactivated in the fluid phase.

Membrane-bound C5b67 recruits **C8** from the plasma, and, finally, multiple copies of **C9** are incorporated in the complex to form the MAC.

The latter stages of assembly are accompanied by major conformational changes in the components with globular hydrophilic plasma proteins unfolding to reveal amphipathic regions that penetrate into and through the lipid bilayer.

The fully formed MAC creates a rigid pore in the membrane, the walls of which are formed from multiple (up to 12) copies of C9 arranged like barrel staves around a central cavity.

The MAC is clearly visible in electron microscopic images of complement-lysed cells as doughnut-shaped protein-lined pores, first observed by Humphrey and Dourmashkin 40 years ago (see Fig. 4.10). The pore has an inner diameter approaching 10 nm:

- allowing the free flow of solutes and electrolytes across the cell membrane; and
- because of the high internal osmotic pressure, causing the cell to swell and sometimes burst.

Metabolically inert targets such as aged erythrocytes are readily lyzed by even a small number of MAC lesions, whereas viable nucleated cells resist killing through a combination of ion pump activities and recovery processes that remove MAC lesions and plug membrane leaks.

Even in the absence of cell killing, MAC lesions may severely compromise cell function or cause cell activation.

Regulation of the membrane attack pathway reduces the risk of 'bystander' damage to adjacent cells

Although regulation in the activation pathways is the major way in which complement is controlled, there are further failsafe mechanisms to protect self cells from MAC damage and lysis.

First, the membrane binding site in C5b67 is labile. If the complex does not encounter a membrane within a fraction of a second after release from the convertase, the site is lost through:

- hydrolysis; or
- binding of one of the fluid-phase regulators of the terminal pathway – **S protein** (also termed **vitronectin**) or **clusterin** – both of which are multifunctional plasma proteins with diverse roles in homeostasis.

C8, an essential component of the MAC, also behaves as a regulator in that binding of C8 to C5b–7 in the fluid phase blocks the membrane binding site and prevents MAC formation.

The net effect of all these plasma controls is to limit MAC deposition to membranes in the immediate vicinity of the site of complement activation, so reducing risk of 'bystander' damage to adjacent cells.

Complexes that do bind are further regulated on host cells by **CD59**, a membrane protein that locks into the MAC as it assembles and inhibits binding of C9, thereby preventing pore formation (Fig. 4.11). CD59 is a broadly

Role of CD59 in protecting host cells from complement damage

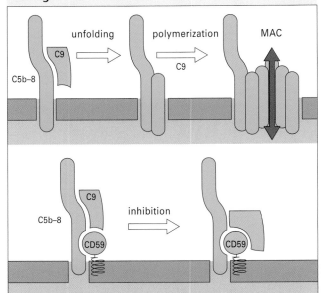

Fig. 4.11 The upper diagram models assembly of the MAC in the absence of the regulator CD59 – C9 binds C5b–8, unwinds, and traverses the membrane and recruits further C9 molecules, which in turn unfold and insert to form the MAC. In the lower diagram, CD59 binds the C5b–8 complex and prevents the unfolding and insertion of C9, which is essential for the initiation of MAC pore formation.

expressed, glycolipid-anchored protein that is structurally unrelated to the complement regulators described above.

IMPORTANCE OF CD59 IN PROTECTING HOST CELLS FROM COMPLEMENT DAMAGE – The importance of CD59 in protecting host cells from complement damage is well illustrated in the hemolytic disorder paroxysmal nocturnal hemoglobinuria (PNH), in which erythrocytes and other circulating cells are unable to make glycolipid anchors and as a consequence lack CD59 (and also DAF). The 'tickover' complement activation that occurs on all cells without much consequence is then sufficient in the absence of CD59 to cause low-grade hemolysis and hemolytic crises.

MANY CELLS EXPRESS ONE OR MORE MEMBRANE RECEPTORS FOR COMPLEMENT PRODUCTS
Receptors for fragments of C3 are widely distributed on different leukocyte populations

Many cells express one or more membrane receptors for complement products (Fig. 4.12). An understanding of the receptors is essential because the majority of the effects of complement are mediated through these molecules. The best characterized of the complement receptors are those binding fragments of C3.

CR1, CR2, CR3, and CR4 bind fragments of C3 attached to activating surfaces

Four different receptors, termed complement receptors 1, 2, 3, and 4 (CR1, CR2, CR3, and CR4), bind fragments of C3 attached to activating surfaces:

- **CR1**, expressed on erythrocytes and leukocytes, binds the largest fragment C3b (and also C4b), an interaction that is crucial to the processing of immune complexes (see below);
- **CR2**, expressed mainly on B cells and follicular dendritic cells (FDCs), binds fragments derived from fI-mediated proteolysis of C3b – iC3b and C3d;

These interactions aid the B cell response to complement-coated particles.

Both CR1 and CR2 are structurally related to the C3 convertase regulators fH, C4bp, MCP, and DAF, and are encoded in the RCA cluster on chromosome 1.

CR3 and **CR4**:
- belong to the integrin family of cell adhesion molecules;
- are expressed on the majority of leukocytes;
- bind the iC3b fragment, aiding adhesion of leukocytes to complement-coated particles and facilitating phagocytic ingestion of these particles.

Receptors for C3a and C5a mediate inflammation

C3a, the small fragment released during activation of C3, binds to a receptor (**C3aR**) expressed abundantly on eosinophils and basophils, and at much lower levels on neutrophils and many other cell types.

The C5a fragment released from C5 during activation is closely related to C3a and binds a distinct, but structurally related, receptor, the C5a receptor (**C5aR**), which is present on a wide variety of cell types, including all leukocytes.

The receptors for C3a and C5a are members of the large receptor family of seven-transmembrane segment receptors that associate with heterotrimeric G proteins. Receptors for chemokines belong to this same family and in many ways C3a and C5a behave like chemokines.

Together, C3aR and C5aR are important in orchestrating inflammatory responses (see below).

Receptors for C1q are present on phagocytes, mast cells, and platelets

Receptors for C1q are less well characterized than C3 receptors, but are increasingly recognized as important in homeostasis.

Receptors for the collagen tails (**cC1qR**):
- can recognize C1q attached through its globular head regions to complement-coated particles;
- are present on leukocytes, platelets, and some other cell types; and
- likely play roles in enhancing phagocytosis of C1q-labeled particles.

Receptors for the globular heads (**C1qRp**):
- bind C1q in an orientation that mimics antibody binding;
- are expressed principally on phagocytic cells, mast cells, and platelets; and
- may collaborate with cC1qR to mediate cell activation events.

Cell receptors for complement components and fragments

ligand	receptor	structure	function	location
C1q	cC1qR (C1q receptor enhancing phagocytosis)	acidic 100-kDa transmembrane glycoprotein	binds collagenous tail of C1q, enhances phagocytosis	myeloid cells, endothelia, platelets
	C1qRp (receptor for C1q globular heads)	acidic 33-kDa glycoprotein	binds globular heads of C1q, possible role in phagocytosis	all blood cells
C3, C4, and C5 fragments	CR1 (complement receptor 1 – CD35)	SCR-containing transmembrane glycoprotein, 30 SCRs	binds C3b and C4b, cofactor and decay accelerating activities, roles in immune complex handling	erythrocytes, B cells, FDCs, macrophages
	CR2 (complement receptor 2 – CD21)	SCR-containing transmembrane glycoprotein, 15 or 16 SCRs	binds C3d and iC3b, role in regulating B cell response to antigen	B cells, FDCs, some T cells, basophils, epithelia
	CR3 (complement receptor 3 – CD11b/CD18)	integrin family member, heterodimer	binds iC3b, roles in cell adhesion	myeloid cells, some B cells and NK cells
	CR4 (complement receptor 4 – CD11c/CD18)	integrin family member, heterodimer	binds iC3b, roles in cell adhesion	myeloid cells, FDCs, activated B cells
	C3aR (receptor for the C3a anaphylatoxin)	G protein-coupled 7-transmembrane spanning receptor	binds C3a, mediates cell activation	widely distributed on blood and tissue cells
	C5aR (receptor for the C5a anaphylatoxin – CD88).	G protein-coupled 7-transmembrane spanning receptor	binds C5a, mediates cell activation and chemotaxis	myeloid cells, smooth muscle, endothelia, epithelia

Fig. 4.12 Summary of information on the cell surface receptors for complement components and fragments and their biological roles. (FDC, follicular dendritic cell)

The bulk of C1q in the circulation is, however, already complexed with C1r and C1s to form intact C1, and in this complex C1q does not interact with its receptors. This ensures that C1q receptors are activated only in specific circumstances, such as during complement activation when free C1q is available.

The plasma complement regulator fH binds leukocyte surfaces

The plasma complement regulator fH binds leukocyte surfaces in a specific and saturable manner, suggesting the presence of an fH receptor, which remains uncharacterized.

It has been suggested that surface-bound fH plays important roles in modulating leukocyte activation as well as in protecting cells from complement attack. Indeed, a fascinating disease, atypical hemolytic uremic syndrome, which is typified by hemolysis, platelet destruction, and renal damage that may progress to renal failure, appears to be caused in many cases by loss of the surface binding capacity of fH. Uncontrolled complement activation due to the production of a mutant fH lacking the membrane binding site has been demonstrated in patients.

COMPLEMENT HAS A VARIETY OF FUNCTIONS

The principal functions of complement are:
- chemotaxis;
- opsonization and cell activation;
- lysis of target cells; and
- priming of the adaptive immune response.

C5a is chemotactic for macrophages and polymorphs

Polymorphs and macrophages express receptors for C3a and C5a. These small (~10 kDa) fragments (i.e. C3a and C5a) diffuse away from the site of activation, creating a chemical gradient along which the motile cells migrate to congregate at the site of activation (Fig. 4.13).

Binding of C3a and C5a to their receptors also causes cell activation:
- increasing adhesive properties;
- triggering extravasation; and
- priming phagocytes to release proinflammatory molecules including enzymes, vasoactive amines, reactive oxygen intermediates, and inflammatory cytokines.

Actions of anaphylatoxins

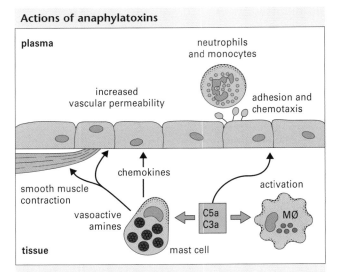

Fig. 4.13 C5a and C3a both act on mast cells to cause degranulation and release of vasoactive amines, including histamine and 5-hydroxytryptamine, which enhance vascular permeability and local blood flow. The secondary release of chemokines from mast cells causes cellular accumulation, and C5a itself acts directly on receptors on monocytes and neutrophils to induce their migration to sites of acute inflammation and subsequent activation.

C3a and C5a also enhance adhesion molecule expression on phagocytes, increasing cell stickiness, and may cause increased expression of the C3 fragment receptors CR1 and CR3.

Q. What effect would increased expression of CR1 and CR3 have on phagocytes?

A. It would enhance their ability to phagocytose particles coated with C3b and iC3b.

C3a and C5a activate mast cells and basophils

Tissue mast cells and basophils also express C3aR and C5aR, and binding of ligand triggers massive release of:

- histamine; and
- cytokines (see Fig. 4.13).

Together, these products cause local smooth muscle contraction and increased vascular permeability to generate the swelling, heat, and pain that typify the inflammatory response. These effects mirror on a local scale the more generalized and severe reactions that can occur in severe allergic or anaphylactic reactions, and for this reason C3a and C5a are sometimes referred to as **anaphylatoxins**.

The actions of C3a and C5a are limited temporally and spatially by the activity of a plasma enzyme, carboxypeptidase-N, which cleaves the carboxy terminal amino acid, arginine, from both of these fragments. The products, termed C3a-desArg and C5a-desArg (-desArg = without arginine), respectively, are either completely biologically inert (C3a-desArg) or have much reduced activity (C5a-desArg).

The retention in C5a-desArg of some chemotactic activity enables the recruitment of phagocytes even from distant sites, making C5a and its metabolite the most important complement-derived chemotactic factor.

C3b and iC3b are important opsonins

Complement activation and amplification cause complement fragments to efficiently coat activator surfaces of targets such as bacteria or immune complexes. Phagocytes and other cells carrying receptors for these complement fragments are then able to bind the target, triggering ingestion and cell activation. The key players here are the surface-bound fragments of C3 and the family of C3 fragment receptors described above.

The amplification inherent in the system ensures that bacteria and other activating surfaces rapidly become coated with C3b and its breakdown product **iC3b** (i.e. the process of **opsonization**; Fig. 4.14).

Phagocytes lured by the complement-derived chemotactic factors described above and activated to increase expression of CR1 and CR3 (receptors for C3b and iC3b, respectively) will bind the activating particle and engulf it for destruction in the phagosome system.

Opsonization, binding, and phagocytosis

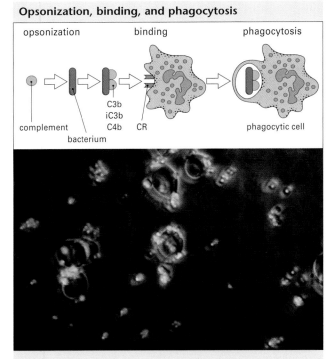

Fig. 4.14 A bacterium is sensitized by the covalent binding of C3b, iC3b, and C4b, which allow it to be recognized by complement receptors (CR) on neutrophils and mononuclear phagocytes. This promotes phagocytosis and activation of the phagocyte. In primates, erythrocytes also express CR1, which allows them to bind opsonized bacteria and immune complexes. In the lower panel fluoresceinated bacteria that have been opsonized with antibody and complement are seen adhering to human erythrocytes. (Courtesy of Professor GD Ross)

Q. In addition to C3b and iC3b, what other complement components can act as opsonins?
A. C1q via its interaction with C1q receptors and C4b by binding to CR1.

The importance of complement opsonization for defense against pathogens is illustrated in individuals deficient in complement components. C3 deficiency (see below) in particular is always associated with repeated severe bacterial infections that without adequate prophylaxis inevitably lead to early death.

C3b disaggregates immune complexes and promotes their clearance

Immune complexes containing antigens derived either from pathogens or from the death of host cells form continuously in health and disease. Because they tend to grow by aggregation and acquisition of more components, they can cause disease by precipitating in capillary beds in the skin, kidney, and other organs, where they drive inflammation.

Complement activation on the immune complex via the classical pathway efficiently opsonizes the immune complex and helps prevent precipitation in tissues:
- first, coating with C3b masks the foreign antigens in the core of the immune complex, blocking further growth;
- second, coating with C3b disaggregates large immune complexes by disrupting interactions between antigen and antibody;
- third, C3b (and C4b) on immune complexes interacts with CR1 on erythrocytes, taking the immune complex out of the plasma – the **immune adherence phenomenon**.

Immune complex adherence to erythrocytes provides an efficient means of handling and transporting the hazardous cargo to sites of disposal (i.e. the resident macrophages in spleen and liver). Here the immune complex is:
- released from the erythrocyte; and
- captured by complement and immunoglobulin receptors on the macrophage, internalized, and destroyed.

The MAC damages some bacteria and enveloped viruses

Assembly of the MAC creates a pore that inserts into and through lipid bilayers, breaching the membrane barrier (see Fig. 4.10). The consequences of MAC attack vary from target to target:
- for most pathogens, opsonization is the most important antibacterial action of complement;
- for Gram-negative bacteria, particularly organisms of the genus *Neisseria*, MAC attack is a major component of host defense, and individuals deficient in components of the MAC (e.g. patients with C6 deficiency, which is the second most common deficiency of complement) are susceptible to neisserial meningitis.

Gram-negative bacteria are protected by a double cell membrane separated by a peptidoglycan wall. Precisely how MAC traverses these protective structures to damage the inner bacterial membrane and causes osmotic lysis of these organisms remains unclear.

The MAC:
- may also play roles in the efficient dispatching of other pathogens, including some viruses;
- can also damage or destroy host cells – in some instances, such as autoimmunity, the host cell is itself the target and complement is directly activated on the cell, leading to MAC attack.

Q. What term is applied to the deposition of MACs on cells near to but not directly the cause of complement activation, and what mechanism normally limits this process?
A. This event is called **bystander lysis** and is normally limited by the presence of CD59 and fluid phase regulators, and the inefficiency of C5b6 deposition.

Erythrocytes have only a limited capacity to resist and repair damage and can be lysed, as is seen in autoimmune hemolytic anemias and some other hemolytic disorders. Although nucleated host cells may escape lysis by MAC, the insertion of pores in the membrane is not without consequence. Ions, particularly Ca^{2+}, flow into the cell and cause activation events with diverse outcomes that may contribute to disease.

Immune complexes with bound C3b are very efficient in priming B cells

Complement is a key component of the innate immune response. However, it has recently become apparent that complement also plays important roles in adaptive immunity and acts as a bridge between these two arms of immunity. This realization arose from studies in complement-depleted and complement-deficient mice in which antibody responses to foreign particles were markedly reduced. At least three linked mechanisms contribute to this effect (Fig. 4.15):
- first, immature B cells directly bind foreign particles through the B cell receptor (BCR) recognizing specific antigen in the particle, and through CR2 recognizing attached C3d – this co-ligation triggers B cell maturation, with the mature cells migrating to the lymphoid organs;
- second, while in the lymph nodes, mature B cells encounter opsonized antigen and, in the presence of B cell help, are induced to become activated and to proliferate;
- finally, in the lymphoid organs FDCs capture antigen through attached C3 fragments and use this bait to select the correct activated B cells and switch them on to further maturation and proliferation to form plasma cells and B memory cells (see Chapters 8 and 11).

The overriding principle of this 'adjuvant' effect of C3 opsonization is that simultaneous engagement of CR2 and BCR on the B cell, by recruiting signaling molecules to form an activation complex on the B cell surface, efficiently triggers the B cell response. As a consequence, complement-opsonized particles may be 1000-fold as active as the unopsonized particle in triggering antibody production.

Complement plays important roles in adaptive immunity

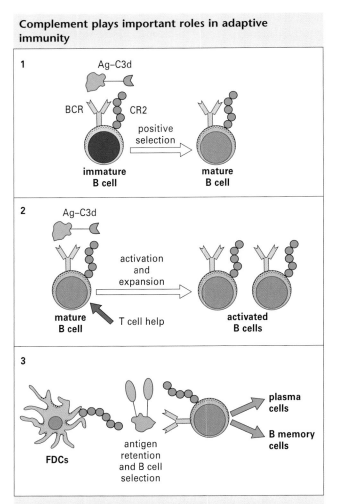

Fig. 4.15 C3 fragments bound to antigen (Ag) bind complement receptors on B cells and follicular dendritic cells (FDCs), enhancing B cell development at multiple stages in the process. (**1**) B cells bind Ag through the B cell receptor (BCR) and bind Ag-attached C3d through CR2. The combined signals, delivered through these receptors and their co-receptors, markedly enhance positive selection of Ag-reactive B cells and subsequent maturation. (**2**) Binding of C3d-opsonized Ag to mature B cells in the lymphoid follicles (with appropriate T cell help) triggers B cell activation and proliferation. (**3**) In the spleen and bone marrow, C3-opsonized Ag binds complement receptors on FDCs to retain Ag on the FDC, where it is efficiently presented to activated B cells. Ligation of BCR and C3d on the activated B cell triggers differentiation to plasma cells and B memory cells.

COMPLEMENT DEFICIENCIES ILLUSTRATE THE HOMEOSTATIC ROLES OF COMPLEMENT

Genetic deficiencies of each of the complement components and many of the regulators have been described and provide valuable 'experiments of nature' illustrating the homeostatic roles of complement. In general, complement deficiencies are rare, though some deficiencies are much more common in some racial groups.

A variety of assays (Method Box 4.1) are available for detecting:
- the activity of different complement pathways;
- the functional activity of individual components;
- the total amount of individual components (functional or non-functional).

The consequences of a deficiency in part of the complement system depend upon the pathway(s) affected (Fig. 4.16).

METHOD BOX 4.1

A variety of assays are available for detecting:
- the activity of different complement pathways;
- the functional activity of individual components;
- the total amount of individual components (functional or non-functional).

Measuring classical and alternative pathway activity

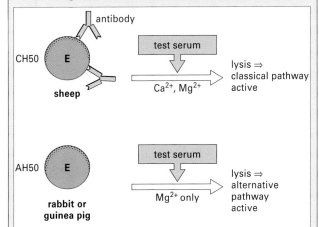

Fig. 1 Classical pathway activity is measured using antibody-sensitized sheep erythrocytes in a buffer containing both Ca^{2+} and Mg^{2+} ions. Alternative pathway activity is measured using rabbit erythrocytes in a buffer containing Mg^{2+} ions but no Ca^{2+} ions. In both assays, standards and samples diluted in the specific buffer are incubated with the relevant target cell and the amount of hemolysis is measured. The results are converted mathematically to standardized hemolytic units (CH50 for classical pathway, AH50 for alternative pathway).

Functional activity of individual components is measured in similar hemolytic assays by assessing the capacity of the test serum to restore hemolytic activity to sera depleted of individual components – for example, C6 activity would be tested using C6-depleted serum in a classical pathway assay.

The total amount of an individual component is measured using specific antisera in techniques such as nephelometry, radial immunodiffusion, and rocket immunoelectrophoresis.

Complement system deficiencies

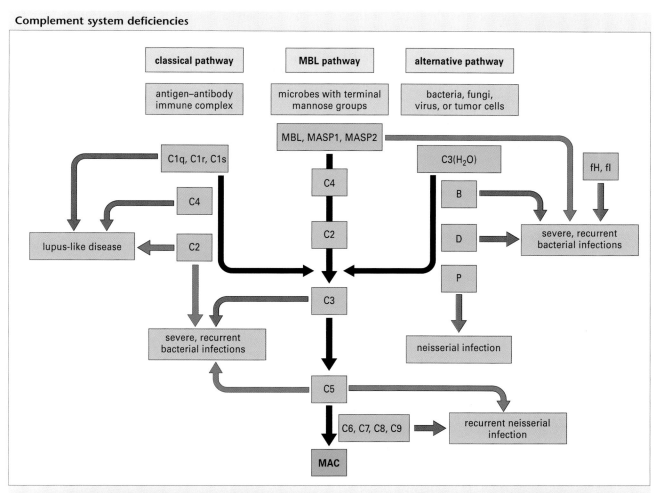

Fig. 4.16 A summary of the clinical consequences of the various complement deficiencies. Black arrows denote pathway, red arrows show strong effects, and blue arrows indicate weak effects.

Classical pathway deficiencies result in tissue inflammation

Deficiency of any of the components of the classical pathway (C1, C4, and C2) predisposes to a condition that closely resembles the autoimmune disease systemic lupus erythematosus (SLE), in which immune complexes become deposited in the kidney, skin, and blood vessels.

Deficiency of any of the C1 subunits (C1q, C1r, or C1s) invariably causes severe disease with typical SLE features including skin lesions and kidney damage. The disease usually manifests early in childhood and few patients reach adulthood.

C4 deficiency also causes severe SLE. Total deficiency of C4 is extremely rare because C4 is encoded by two separate genes (*C4A* and *C4B*), but partial deficiencies of C4 are relatively common and are associated with an increased incidence of SLE.

C2 deficiency is the commonest complement deficiency in Caucasians. Although it predisposes to SLE, the majority of C2-deficient individuals are healthy.

The large majority of cases of SLE are, however, not associated with complement deficiencies, and autoimmune SLE is discussed below and on p. 376.

The historical view of immune complex disease in classical pathway deficiency was based upon defective immune complex handling.

Q. Why would a deficiency in the classical pathway lead to impaired handling of immune complexes?

A. Classical pathway activation and opsonization of immune complexes helps prevent precipitation in tissues and aids the carriage of immune complexes on erythrocytes. Classical pathway deficiencies would therefore result in a failure to maintain solubilization and permit the resultant precipitation of immune complexes in the tissues where they drive inflammation.

Although these mechanisms of immune complex handling undoubtedly contribute, a new perspective has recently developed that takes a different view of the role of complement in waste management.

Cells continually die by apoptosis in tissues and are removed silently by tissue macrophages. Complement contributes to this essential process because the apoptotic cell binds C1q and activates the classical pathway. In C1 deficiencies, apoptotic cells accumulate in the tissues and eventually undergo necrosis, which releases toxic cell contents and causes inflammation.

This recent observation, emerging from studies in complement deficiencies, has altered the way we think of the handling of waste in the body and moved complement to center-stage in this vital housekeeping role.

Deficiencies of MBL are associated with infection in infants

MBL is a complex multi-chain **collectin**. Each chain comprises a collagenous stalk linked to a globular carbohydrate recognition domain.

The plasma level of MBL is extremely variable in the population, and governed by a series of single nucleotide polymorphisms in the *MBL* gene, either in the promoter region or in the first exon, encoding part of the collagenous stalk:

- mutations in the promoter region alter the efficiency of gene transcription;
- mutations in the first exon disrupt the regular structure of the collagenous stalk, destabilizing complexes containing mutated chains, perhaps disrupting association with the MASP enzymes.

At least seven distinct haplotypes arise from mixing of these mutations, four of which yield very low plasma MBL levels. As a consequence, at least 10% of the population have MBL levels below 0.1 µg/ml and are considered to be MBL deficient.

MBL deficiency is associated in infants with increased susceptibility to bacterial infections. This tendency disappears as the individual ages and the other arms of immunity mature.

In adults, MBL deficiency is of little consequence unless there is an accompanying immunosuppression – for example, people with HIV infection who are MBL deficient appear to have more infections than those who have high levels of MBL.

Alternative pathway and C3 deficiencies are associated with bacterial infections

Deficiencies of either fB or fD prevent complement amplification through the alternative pathway amplification loop, markedly reducing the efficiency of opsonization of pathogens. As a consequence, deficient individuals are susceptible to bacterial infections and present with a history of severe recurrent infections with a variety of pyogenic (pus-forming) bacteria. Only a few families with each of these deficiencies has been identified, but the severity of the condition makes it imperative to identify affected families so that prophylactic antibiotic therapy can be initiated.

C3 is the cornerstone of complement, essential for all activation pathways and for MAC assembly, and is also the source of the major opsonic fragments C3b and iC3b. Individuals with **C3 deficiency** present early in childhood with a history of severe, recurrent bacterial infections affecting the respiratory system, gut, skin, and other organs. Untreated, all die before adulthood. When given broad-spectrum antibiotic prophylaxis, patients do reasonably well and survival into adulthood becomes the norm.

Terminal pathway deficiencies predispose to Gram-negative bacterial infections

Deficiencies of any of the terminal complement components (C5, C6, C7, C8, or C9) predisposes to infections with Gram-negative bacteria, particularly those of the genus *Neisseria*. This genus includes the meningococci responsible for meningococcal meningitis and the gonococci responsible for gonorrhea.

Q. Why should these deficiencies be specifically associated with infection by Gram-negative bacteria and not with all bacterial infections?
A. Gram-negative bacteria have an outer phospholipid membrane, which may be targeted by the lytic pathway. Gram-positive bacteria have a thick bacterial cell wall on the outside.

Individuals with terminal pathway deficiencies usually present with meningitis, which is often recurrent and often accompanied by septicemia. Any patients with second or third episodes of meningococcal infection without obvious cause should be screened for complement deficiencies because prophylactic antibiotic therapy can be life-saving. Terminal pathway-deficient patients should also be intensively immunized with the best available meningococcal vaccines.

It is likely that terminal pathway deficiencies are relatively common and underascertained in most countries:

- in Caucasians and most other groups investigated, C6 deficiency is the most common;
- in the Japanese population, C9 deficiency is very common, with an incidence of more than 1 in 500 of the population.

C1 inhibitor deficiency leads to hereditary angioedema

Deficiency of the classical pathway regulator C1inh is responsible for the syndrome **hereditary angioedema (HAE)**. C1inh regulates C1 and MBL in the complement system and also controls activation in the kinin pathway that leads to the generation of bradykinin and other active kinins (Fig. 4.17).

HAE is relatively common because the disease presents even in those heterozygous for the deficiency (i.e. it is an autosomal dominant disease).

The halved C1inh synthetic capacity in those with HAE cannot maintain plasma levels in the face of continuing consumption of C1inh, which is a **suicide inhibitor** that is consumed as it works. As a consequence, the plasma levels measured are often only 10–20% of normal, even in periods of health.

Episodes of angioedema are often triggered in the skin or mucous membranes by minor trauma – occasionally stress may be sufficient to induce an attack. Swelling, which may be remarkable in severity, rapidly ensues as

Pathogenesis of hereditary angioedema

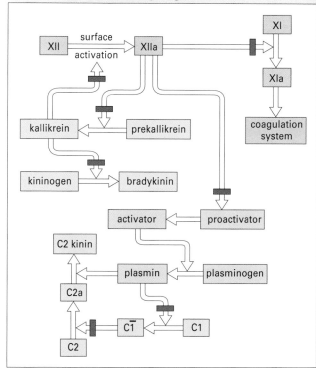

Fig. 4.17 C1 inhibitor (C1inh) is involved in the inactivation of elements of the kinin, plasmin, complement, and clotting systems, all of which may be activated following the surface-dependent activation of factor XII. The points at which C1inh acts are shown in red. Uncontrolled activation of these pathways results in the formation of bradykinin and C2 kinin, which induce edema.

Hereditary angioedema

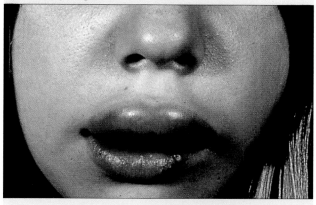

Fig. 4.18 The clinical appearance of hereditary angioedema, showing the local transient swelling that affects mucous membranes.

unregulated activation of the kinin and complement systems occurs in the affected area, inducing vascular leakiness. Swelling of mucous membranes in the mouth and throat may block the airways, leading to asphyxia (Fig. 4.18).

Episodes of angioedema are transient and usually wane over the course of a few hours without therapy. Emergency treatment for life-threatening attacks involves the infusion of a purified C1inh concentrate. Prophylactic treatment involves the induction of C1inh synthesis using anabolic steroids, or minimizing consumption of C1inh using protease inhibitors.

Although the majority of cases of HAE involve a mutation that prevents synthesis of C1inh by the defective gene (type I), in about 15% of cases the mutation results in the production of a functionally defective protein (type II). In type II HAE, the plasma levels of C1inh may be normal or even high, but its function is markedly impaired, leading to disease.

A similar syndrome to type II HAE can develop later in life. Acquired angioedema is, in most or all cases, associated with autoantibodies that:
• target C1inh;
• may arise in an otherwise healthy individual or may be associated with other autoimmune diseases, particularly SLE.

Occasionally, acquired angioedema occurs in association with some lymphoproliferative disorders – whether autoantibodies are involved in these cases remains unclear.

Deficiencies in alternative pathway regulators produce a secondary loss of C3

fH or fI deficiency predisposes to bacterial infections

fH and fI collaborate to control activation of the alternative pathway amplification loop. Deficiency of either leads to uncontrolled activation of the loop and complete consumption of C3, which is the substrate of the loop. The resultant **acquired C3 deficiency** predisposes to bacterial infections and yields a clinical picture identical to that seen in primary C3 deficiency.

Properdin deficiency causes severe meningococcal meningitis

Properdin is a stabilizer of the alternative pathway C3 convertase that increases efficiency of the amplification loop. **Properdin deficiency** is inherited in an X-linked manner and is therefore seen exclusively in males. Boys deficient in properdin present with severe meningococcal meningitis, often with septicemia. The first attack is often fatal and survivors do not usually have recurrent infections because the acquisition of anti-meningococcal antibody enables a response via the classical pathway in the next encounter. Diagnosis is nevertheless important to identify affected relatives before they get disease – administration of meningococcal vaccine and antibiotic prophylaxis will prevent infection.

FURTHER READING

Barrington R, Zhang M, Fischer M, Carroll MC. The role of complement in inflammation and adaptive immunity. Immunol Rev 2001;180:5–15.

Campbell RD, Law SKA, Reid KBM, et al. Structure, organization, and regulation of the complement genes. Annu Rev Immunol 1988;6:161–195.

Carroll MC. The complement system in B cell regulation. Mol Immunol 2004;41:141–146.

Cole DS, Morgan BP. Beyond lysis: how complement influences cell fate. Clin Sci 2003;104:455–466.

Colten HR, Rosen FS. Complement deficiencies. Annu Rev Immunol 1992;10:809–834.

Davis AE 3rd. The pathogenesis of hereditary angioedema. Transfus Apher Sci 2003;39:195–203.

Dodds AW, Ren XD, Willis AC, et al. The reaction mechanism of the internal thioester in the human complement component C4. Nature 1996;379:177–179.

Frank MM, Fries LF. The role of complement in inflammation and phagocytosis. Immunol Today 1991;12:322–326.

Gerard C, Gerard NP. C5a anaphylatoxin and its seven transmembrane-segment receptor. Annu Rev Immunol 1994;12:775–808.

Holmskov U, Malhotra R, Sim RB, et al. Collectins: collagenous C-type lectins of the innate immune defense system. Immunol Today 1994;14:67–74.

Hourcade D, Holers VM, Atkinson JP. The regulators of complement activation (RCA) gene cluster. Adv Immunol 1989;45:381–416.

Jack DL, Klein NJ, Turner MW. Mannose-binding lectin: targeting the microbial world for complement attack and opsonophagocytosis. Immunol Rev 2001;180:86–99.

Lambris JD, Reid KBM, Volanakis JE. The evolution, structure, biology and pathophysiology of complement. Immunol Today 1999;20:207–211.

Liszewski MK, Farries TC, Lublin DM, et al. Control of the complement system. Adv Immunol 1996;61:201–283.

Manderson AP, Botto M, Walport MJ. The role of complement in the development of systemic lupus erythematosus. Annu Rev Immunol 2004;22:432–456.

Moffitt MC, Frank MM. Complement resistance in microbes. Springer Semin Immunopathol 1994;15:327–344.

Morgan BP. Complement regulatory molecules: application to therapy and transplantation. Immunol Today 1995;16:257–259.

Morgan BP. Complement in inflammation. In: Rey K, ed. Physiology of inflammation. Oxford: Oxford University Press; 2001:131–145.

Morgan BP, Harris CL. Complement therapeutics; history and current progress. Mol Immunol 2003;40:159–170.

Morgan BP, Meri S. Membrane proteins that protect against complement lysis. Springer Semin Immunopathol 1994;15:369–396.

Morgan BP, Walport MJ. Complement deficiency and disease. Immunol Today 1991;12:301–306.

Muller-Eberhard HJ. The membrane attack complex of complement. Annu Rev Immunol 1986;4:503–528.

Nonaka M, Yoshizaki F. Evolution of the complement system. Mol Immunol 2004;40:879–902.

Reid KB, Turner MW. Mammalian lectins in activation and clearance mechanisms involving the complement system. Springer Semin Immunopathol 1994;15:307–326.

Walport MJ. Complement: first of two parts. N Engl J Med 2001;344:1058–1066.

Walport MJ. Complement: second of two parts. N Engl J Med 2001;344:1140–1144.

Critical thinking: Complement deficiency (see p. 494 for explanations)

A family has been identified in which three of the seven children have had repeated upper respiratory tract infections since early childhood. Of these, one has developed bacterial meningitis, and another a fatal septicemia. In all of the children the levels of antibodies in the serum are within the normal range. When an assay for hemolytic complement (CH50) is carried out, however, the three affected children are all found to be deficient in this functional assay.

1 Why would a deficiency in complement cause the children to be particularly susceptible to bacterial infections?

Measurements are made of individual complement components of the classical and alternative pathways to determine which of the components is defective. The results are shown in the table.

complement component	normal concentration (μg/ml)	levels in affected children (μg/ml)
C4	600	480–520
C2	20	15–22
C3	1300	10–80
factor B (fB)	210	not detectable
factor H (fH)	480	200–350
factor I (fI)	35	not detectable

2 Using knowledge of the complement reaction pathways, how can you explain the apparent combined deficiencies in C3, fB, and fI?

3 What is the fundamental deficiency in this family and how would you treat the affected children?

T Cell Receptors and MHC Molecules

SUMMARY

- **The T cell antigen receptor (TCR) is located on the surface of T cells and plays a critical role in the adaptive immune system.** Its major function is to recognize antigen and transmit a signal to the interior of the T cell, which generally results in activation of T cell responses.

- **TCRs are similar in many ways to immunoglobulin molecules.** Both are made up of pairs of subunits (α and β or γ and δ), which are themselves members of the immunoglobulin superfamily, and both recognize a wide variety of antigens via N terminal variable regions. Both the $\alpha\beta$ TCR and the $\gamma\delta$ TCR are associated with CD3, forming TCR complexes.

- **The two types of TCR may have distinct functions.** In humans and mice, the $\alpha\beta$ TCR predominates in most peripheral lymphoid tissues, whereas cells bearing the $\gamma\delta$ TCR are enriched at mucosal surfaces. Critical signaling functions are performed by the invariant chains of the TCR, the CD3 complex.

- **Like immunoglobulins, TCRs are encoded by several sets of genes,** and a large repertoire of TCR antigen-binding sites is generated by V(D)J recombination during T cell differentiation. Unlike immunoglobulins, TCRs are never secreted and do not undergo class switching or somatic hypermutation.

- **Recognition by the $\alpha\beta$ TCR requires the antigen to be bound to a specialized antigen-presenting structure known as a major histocompatibility complex (MHC) molecule.** Unlike immunoglobulins, TCRs recognize antigen only in the context of a cell–cell interaction.

- **Class I and class II MHC molecules bind to peptides derived from different sources.** Class I MHC molecules bind to peptides derived from cytosolic (intracellular) proteins, known as endogenous antigens. Class II MHC molecules bind to peptides derived from extracellular proteins that have been brought into the cell by phagocytosis or endocytosis (exogenous antigens).

- **Class I and class II MHC present peptide antigens to the TCR in a cell–cell interaction** between an antigen-presenting cell (APC) and a T cell.

- **HLA-A, HLA-B, and HLA-C gene loci encode class I MHC molecules**

- **HLA-DP, HLA-DQ, AND HLA-DR gene loci encode class II MHC molecules.**

- **An individual's MHC haplotype affects susceptibility to disease.**

- **CD1 is an MHC class 1-like molecule that presents lipid antigens.**

THE TCR PLAYS A CRITICAL ROLE IN THE ADAPTIVE IMMUNE SYSTEM

As discussed in Chapter 1, the immune system of higher vertebrates can be divided into two components – humoral immunity and cell-mediated immunity.

Humoral immunity, of which antibodies are a key component, provides protection via the extracellular fluids. Antibodies deal quite effectively with extracellular pathogens:
- targeting them for phagocytosis or complement-mediated lysis;
- neutralizing receptors on the surface of bacteria and viruses; and
- inactivating circulating toxins.

If antibodies were our only defense, however, pathogens could escape immune surveillance simply by hiding within cells. In fact, many pathogens – all viruses, some bacteria, and certain parasites – do just that, carrying out substantial portions of their life cycles within host cells. Remarkably, some bacteria even thrive within macrophages after being phagocytosed. These considerations highlight the need for a second arm of the immune response – **cell-mediated immunity** – of which T cells are critical operatives.

T cells recognize antigen via specialized cell surface antigen receptors – T cell receptors (TCRs) – which are structurally and evolutionarily related to antibodies.

TCRs recognize antigen via variable regions generated through **V(D)J recombination** (see Chapter 3), much like immunoglobulins, but are much more restrictive in their antigen recognition capabilities.

TCRs recognize peptides displayed by MHC molecules

T cells generally recognize fragments of degraded proteins (peptides), which must be bound to ('presented by') specialized antigen-presenting molecules termed **major histocompatibility complex (MHC) molecules**.

MHC molecules can display a wide range of peptides derived from intracellular proteins on the cell surface, thereby alerting the immune system to the presence of intracellular invaders.

Because MHC molecules are expressed only on the surface of antigen-presenting cells (APCs), engagement of the TCR occurs only in the context of intimate cell–cell interactions.

When a primed T cell bearing an appropriate TCR (capable of recognizing, for example, a particular viral peptide) comes into contact with an infected cell, it can rapidly kill that cell and thereby limit the spread of the viral infection.

The requirement for cell–cell interaction also allows T cells to provide critical regulatory functions. T cells, for example, can couple signals from the innate immune system, such as those arising from 'professional' APCs (e.g. dendritic cells) with adaptive (T and B cell) responses, providing a critical layer of integration, coordination, and regulation.

TCRs ARE SIMILAR TO IMMUNOGLOBULIN MOLECULES

The TCR was identified much later than immunoglobulin, even though early theoretical considerations strongly suggested that T cells must bear cell surface antigen receptors. It is now clear that there are two varieties of TCR, termed $\alpha\beta$ and $\gamma\delta$, and that both molecules:

- resemble immunoglobulins in several significant ways (Fig. 5.1);
- are made up of heterodimers (either α and β or γ and δ subunits), which are disulfide-linked;

- are integral membrane proteins with large extracellular domains and short cytoplasmic tails.

The extracellular portions are responsible for antigen recognition and contain variable N terminal regions, like antibodies. Both α and β (or γ and δ) subunits contribute to the antigen-binding sites.

THE TWO TYPES OF TCR MAY HAVE DISTINCT FUNCTIONS

The two types of TCR tend to populate different tissue sites and are thought to perform distinct functions.

The $\alpha\beta$ heterodimer is the antigen recognition unit of the $\alpha\beta$ TCR

The $\alpha\beta$ TCR is the predominant receptor found in the thymus and peripheral lymphoid organs of mice and humans. It is a disulfide-linked heterodimer of α (40–50 kDa) and β (35–47 kDa) subunits and its structural features have been determined by X-ray crystallography (Fig. 5.2).

Each polypeptide chain of the $\alpha\beta$ TCR contains two extracellular immunoglobulin-like domains of approximately 110 amino acids, anchored into the plasma membrane by a transmembrane domain that has a short cytoplasmic tail.

Q. How can receptors that lack intracytoplasmic domains signal to the cell? Give some examples.

A. They signal by associating with other membrane molecules that do have intracytoplasmic domains. For example, immunoglobulin associates with Igα and Igβ (see Fig. 3.1), and FcγRI associates with its γ chain dimer (see Fig. 3.20).

The extracellular portions of the α and β chains fold into a structure that resembles the antigen-binding portion (Fab) of an antibody (see Fig. 3.12). Indeed, as in antibodies, the amino acid sequence variability of the TCR resides in the N terminal domains of the α and β (and also the γ and δ) chains.

The regions of greatest variability correspond to immunoglobulin hypervariable regions and are also known as **complementarity determining regions**

Similarities and differences between T cell receptors and immunoglobulins

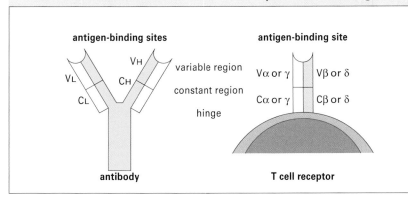

Fig. 5.1 TCRs are very similar to Fab fragments of B cell receptors. Both receptor types are composed of two different peptide chains and have variable regions for binding antigen, constant regions, and hinge regions. The principal differences are that TCRs remain membrane-bound and contain only a single antigen-binding site.

The T cell antigen receptor

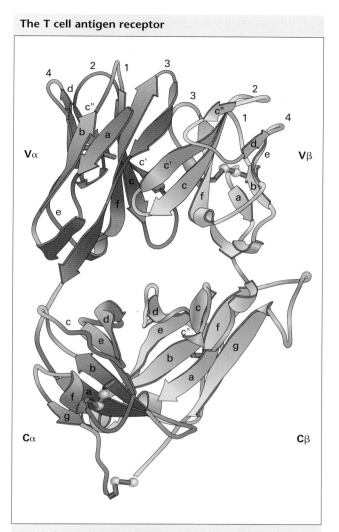

Fig. 5.2 Three-dimensional structure of an αβ TCR – only extracellular domains are shown. The α chain is colored blue (residues 1–213), and the β chain is colored green (residues 3–247). The β strands are represented as arrows and labeled according to the standard convention used for the immunoglobulin fold. The disulfide bonds (yellow balls for sulfur atoms) are shown within each domain and for the C terminal interchain disulfide. The complementarity determining regions (CDRs) lying at the top of the diagram are numerically labeled (1–4) for each chain. These form the binding site for antigen/MHC molecule. (Adapted from Garcia KC, Degano M, Stanfield RL, et al. Science 1996;274:209–219. Copyright AAAS)

Rapid Reference Box 5

CDRs (complementarity determining regions) – the sections of an antibody or T cell receptor V region responsible for antigen or antigen–MHC molecule binding.

H-2 – the mouse MHC.

histocompatibility – the ability to accept grafts between individuals.

HLA – the human MHC.

ITAMs (immunoreceptor tyrosine activation motifs) and ITIMs (immunoreceptor tyrosine inhibitory motifs) – target sequences for phosphorylation by kinases involved in cell activation or inhibition.

MHC (major histocompatibility complex) – a genetic region found in all mammals whose products are primarily responsible for the rapid rejection of grafts between individuals; it functions in the signaling between lymphocytes and cells expressing antigen.

MHC class I and II molecules – molecules coded within the MHC – class I molecules have one MHC-encoded peptide complexed with β_2-microglobulin; class II molecules have two MHC-encoded peptides, which are non-covalently associated.

MHC restriction – a characteristic of many immune reactions in which cells cooperate most effectively with other cells that share an MHC haplotype.

RAG-1 and RAG-2 – recombination activating genes, required for recombination of V, D, and J gene segments during the generation of functional antigen receptor genes.

V, D, and J genes – variable (V), joining (J), and diversity (D) genes.

of the extracellular portion of the receptor and the transmembrane domain (shown as the C terminal residue in the α and β chain in Fig. 5.2).

One remarkable feature of the transmembrane portion of the receptor is the presence of positively charged residues in both the α and β chains. Unpaired charges would be unfavorable in a transmembrane segment. Indeed, these positive charges are neutralized by assembly of the complete TCR complex, which contains additional polypeptides bearing complementary negative charges (see below).

The CD3 complex associates with the antigen-binding αβ or γδ heterodimers to form the complete TCR

The αβ or γδ heterodimers must associate with a series of polypeptide chains collectively termed the **CD3 complex** for the antigen-binding domains of the TCR to form a complete, functional receptor that is stably expressed at the cell surface and is capable of transmitting a signal upon binding to antigen.

The four members of the CD3 complex (γ, δ, ε, and ζ) are sometimes termed the **invariant chains** of the TCR because they do not show variability in their amino acid sequences. (The γ and δ chains of the CD3 complex should not be confused with the quite distinct antigen-binding variable chains of the TCR that bear the same names.)

(CDRs). They are clustered together to form an antigen-binding site analogous to the corresponding site on antibodies (see Fig. 5.2). Note, however, that:

- the CDR3 loops from both the α and β chains lie at the center of the antigen-binding site.

These CDR3 loops make contact with antigen, which in the case of the TCR, is a peptide (see below).

The disulfide bond that links the α and β chains is in a peptide sequence located between the constant domain

The CD3 chains are assembled as heterodimers of γε and δε subunits with a homodimer of ζ chains, giving an overall TCR stoichiometry of $(\alpha\beta)_2$, γ, δ, ε_2, ζ_2. Current data suggest that the TCR complex exists as a dimer (Fig. 5.3).

The CD3 γ, δ, and ε chains are the products of three closely linked genes, and similarities in their amino acid sequences suggest that they are evolutionarily related.

Indeed, all three are members of the immunoglobulin superfamily, each containing an external domain followed by a transmembrane region and a substantial, highly conserved, cytopasmic tail of 40 or more amino acids.

As with the transmembrane domains of the variable chains of the TCR, the membrane-spanning regions of these CD3 chains contain charged amino acids.

It is thought that the negatively charged residues in the transmembrane region of the CD3 chains interact with (and neutralize) the positively charged amino acids in the αβ polypeptides, leading to the formation of a stable TCR complex (Fig. 5.3).

The CD3 ζ gene is on a different chromosome from the CD3 γδε gene complex, and the ζ protein is structurally unrelated to the other CD3 components. The ζ chains possess:

- a small extracellular domain (nine amino acids);
- a transmembrane domain carrying a negative charge; and
- a large cytoplasmic tail.

An alternatively spliced form of CD3ζ, called CD3η, possesses an even larger cytoplasmic tail (42 amino acids longer at the C terminus).

The cytoplasmic portions of ζ and η chains contain ITAMs

These ζ and η chains may associate in all three possible combinations (ζζ, ζη, or ηη) and play a critical role in signal transduction through the TCR. The cytoplasmic portions of these subunits contain particular amino acid sequences called **immunoreceptor tyrosine-based activation motifs (ITAMs)**, and each chain contains three of these motifs.

Q. Which other group of cell surface molecules contains ITAMs?

A. The Fcγ receptors, either as an intrinsic intracellular domain of the receptor, or because they associate with signaling molecules that have ITAMs (see Fig 3.20).

The conserved tyrosine residues in the ITAM motifs are targets for phosphorylation by specific protein kinases. When the TCR is bound to its cognate antigen–MHC complex, the ITAM motifs become phosphorylated within minutes in one of the first steps in T cell activation (see Fig. 7.21).

ITAMs:

- are essential for T cell activation, and mutational substitution of the tyrosines in the motif prevents activation;
- play critical roles in B cell activation, and are present in the B cell receptor chains, Igα and Igβ (see Fig. 3.1 and Chapter 8).

CD3ζ also functions in another signaling pathway, associating with the low-affinity FcγRIIIa receptor (CD16), which is involved in the activation of macrophages and natural killer (NK) cells (see Fig. 3.20).

Other subunits of the CD3 complex (γ, δ, ε), though lacking in ITAMs, may also become phosphorylated following TCR engagement. Phosphorylation of the CD3γ chain downregulates TCR expression on the cell surface via a mechanism involving increased receptor internalization.

The γδ TCR structurally resembles the αβ TCR but may function differently

The overall structure of the γδ TCR is similar to that of its αβ counterpart. Each chain is organized into:

- extracellular V and C domains;

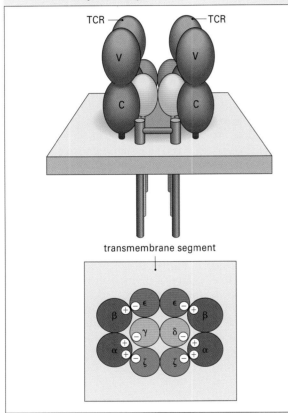

The T cell receptor complex

transmembrane segment

Fig. 5.3 The TCR α and β (or γ and δ) chains each comprise an external V and C domain, a transmembrane segment containing positively charged amino acids, and a short cytoplasmic tail. The two chains are disulfide linked on the membrane side of their C domains. The CD3 γ, δ, and ε chains comprise an external immunoglobulin-like C domain, a transmembrane segment containing a negatively charged amino acid, and a longer cytoplasmic tail. A dimer of ζζ, ηη, or ζη is also associated with the complex. Several lines of evidence support the notion that the TCR–CD3 complex exists at the cell surface as a dimer. The transmembrane charges are important for the assembly of the complex. A plausible arrangement that neutralizes opposite charges is shown.

- a transmembrane segment containing positively charged amino acids; and
- a short cytoplasmic tail.

One indication that the two types of T cell (i.e. T cells with αβ TCRs and T cells with γδ TCRs) might perform different functions comes from their anatomic distribution:

- in humans and mice, αβ TCRs are present on more than 95% of peripheral blood T cells and on the majority of thymocytes;
- T cells bearing γδ TCRs are relatively rare in spleen, lymph nodes, and peripheral blood but predominate at epithelial surfaces – they are common in skin and in the epithelial linings of the reproductive tract and are especially numerous in the intestine, where they are found as **intraepithelial lymphocytes**.

It is further believed that there are distinct subsets of γδ T cells that can perform different functions.

Antigen recognition by γδ T cells is unlike that of their αβ counterparts

The fact that γδ T cells are rare in anatomic locations known to support the classical mechanisms of antigen presentation and lymphocyte clonal expansion suggests the possibility that γδ cells might not need to rely upon normal antigen presentation mechanisms for their activation.

Several lines of evidence support the hypothesis that γδ T cells can recognize antigen in an MHC-independent fashion, for example:

- γδ T cells can be found in normal numbers in MHC class I and class II-deficient mice;
- their cognate antigens are not necessarily peptides, and do not require classical processing – indeed, some murine γδ T cells have been found to recognize proteins directly, including MHC molecules and viral proteins, in a manner that requires neither antigen processing nor presentation by MHC.

γδ T cells therefore appear to be able to follow a different paradigm for T cell recognition of antigen than that employed by αβ T cells.

γδ T cells recognize at least two classes of ligand:

- molecules that signal the presence of cellular stress; and
- small organic molecules that serve as signifiers of infection.

For example, human intraepithelial γδ T cells have been found to respond to MHC class I-related antigens (MICA and MICB) expressed on the surface of stressed cells.

In addition, some human γδ T cells recognize small, non-peptidic, organic compounds secreted by mycobacteria, such as monoethylphosphate and isopentenyl pyrophosphate. These ligands are secreted by a number of bacteria and may also be produced by some eukaryotic pathogens.

The γδ T cell arm of the adaptive immune system therefore appears to share some key characteristics of innate immune responses.

γδ T CELLS HAVE A VARIETY OF BIOLOGICAL ROLES – γδ T cells:

- are essential for primary immune responses to certain viral and bacterial pathogens in mouse models, but in many cases their contribution to the primary response

can be substituted for by αβ T cells, and they rarely contribute to memory responses;
- interact with a variety of lymphocytes, and have been implicated in stimulating immunoglobulin class switch recombination by B cells in response to T-dependent antigens;
- provide regulatory signals to αβ T cells and have been implicated in shaping immune responses (e.g. γδ cells appear to be involved in downregulating inflammation and in this role may be responding to epithelial cells stressed by inflammatory processes rather than to specific antigens borne by pathogens).

The unique ability of γδ T cells to, on the one hand, sense tissue damage and, on the other, to recognize antigens without the normal constraints of antigen processing/MHC restriction (see below), may allow them to fill several key biological roles such as immunoregulation. In particular, γδ T cells may downregulate potentially damaging inflammatory responses, providing immuno-protection:

- when MHC function is compromised by, for example, viral infections that downregulate MHC;
- in early life when αβ T cell function is immature and when the antigen processing and antigen sampling systems have not yet matured.

TCRs ARE ENCODED BY SEVERAL SETS OF GENES

The general arrangement of the genes encoding the α, β, γ, and δ chains of the TCR is remarkably similar to that of the immunoglobulin heavy chain genes (see Chapter 3, p. 81), suggesting a common origin from a primordial rearranging antigen receptor locus.

Fig. 5.4 illustrates the murine TCR genes, which are similar to those of humans. All four TCR gene families have been strongly conserved across more than 400 million years of evolution of the jawed vertebrates, which suggests a strong selective pressure for the preservation of both αβ and γδ T cell functions.

The nomenclature of the TCR genes is simple – the TCRA locus encodes the α gene, TCRB the β gene, and so on. Interestingly, the TCRD locus is nested within the TCRA cluster.

The α and γ loci have sets of V and J gene segments (analogous to immunoglobulin light chain loci), whereas the β and δ loci have V, D, and J gene segments (analogous to immunoglobulin heavy chains).

TCR variable region gene diversity is generated by V(D)J recombination

As with antibody genes, a highly diverse repertoire of TCR variable region genes is generated during T cell differentiation by a process of somatic gene rearrangement termed V(D)J recombination (see Chapter 3). Variable (V), joining (J), and sometimes diversity (D) gene segments are joined together to form a completed variable region gene.

Junctional diversity (imprecise joining of V, D, and J with loss and/or addition of nucleotides) contributes an enormous amount of variability to the TCR repertoire in

Murine T cell receptor genes

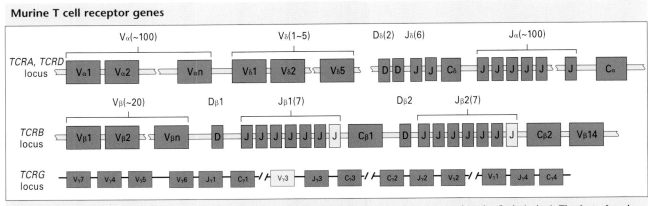

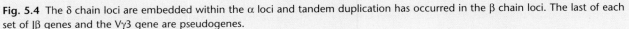

Fig. 5.4 The δ chain loci are embedded within the α loci and tandem duplication has occurred in the β chain loci. The last of each set of Jβ genes and the Vγ3 gene are pseudogenes.

addition to the variation that results from combinatorial assortment of the various gene segments. There is minor variation in detail for each locus (see Fig. 5.4).

TCRA recombination entails joining of V to J gene segments

As in the kappa light chain (IgK locus), joining of a Vα segment to a Jα segment produces a complete variable region gene. The large number of Jα segments contributes to the ultimate diversity of TCRα specificities.

The TCRB locus includes two sets of D, J, and C genes

Most of the Vβ genes are grouped together, but one (Vβ14) is present at the extreme 3′ end of the locus. The tandem duplication of Dβ, Jβ, and Cβ must have occurred early in mammalian evolution because it is present in both mice and humans. Extensive diversity is generated by recombination because not only are VDJ arrangements possible, but also VJ and VDDJ combinations.

The D segments are used in all three reading frames, further contributing to β chain diversity.

The arrangement of the TCRG locus differs in mice and in humans

The murine γ locus bears a striking similarity to the antibody light chain locus, with four Cγ genes (including a pseudogene), each associated with one J gene and from one to four Vγ genes. There are no D genes.

In humans there are eight Vγ genes, followed by three Jγ and the first Cγ, then two additional Jγ genes before Cγ2.

The TCRD locus possesses only five Vδ, two Dδ, and six Jδ genes

The TCRD locus was discovered during studies on the TCRA locus and possesses only five Vδ, two Dδ, and six Jδ genes. Despite this relative paucity of genetic material, more than 1000 different δ chains can be generated.

Q. How may the great number of δ chains be generated when there is only a limited number of V, D, and J gene segments in the TCRD locus?
A. As described in Chapter 3, the two D region segments can be used in all three possible reading frames, and imprecise joining of the VD and DJ junctions produces further diversity.

The mechanism of V(D)J recombination is the same in both T cells and B cells

The TCR genes are flanked by recombination signal sequences, just like their immunoglobulin cousins (see Fig. 3.29), and the same recombination machinery (the RAG proteins) operates in both B and T cells. Indeed, experiments have shown that TCR Dβ and Jγ genes can rearrange appropriately even if transfected into B cells.

Analysis of the amino acid sequences of many different TCRs shows that the greatest diversity lies within the third CDR (CDR3), which is also the case for B cell receptors. Addition of N regions (non-templated nucleotides added to the junctions by terminal deoxynucleotidyl transferase, TdT) is much more pronounced in TCRs, however. It is important to note, too, that neither somatic hypermutation nor class switching occur in T cells.

Q. Why is it that, unlike B cells, T cells have not evolved a class switching mechanism?
A. Class switching is irrelevant because there is no secreted form of the TCR and hence no interaction analogous to that of immunoglobulin and FcR.

RECOMBINATION YIELDS GREAT DIVERSITY – Hunkapiller and Hood have calculated that it is possible to construct about:
- 4.4×10^{13} different forms of TCR Vβ; and
- 8.5×10^{12} forms of TCR Vα.

They estimate that if only 1% of the sequences coded for viable proteins this would still give 2.9×10^{22} receptors. Even if 99% of these viable receptors were rejected due

RECOGNITION BY THE αβ TCR REQUIRES ANTIGEN TO BE BOUND TO AN MHC MOLECULE

to autoreactivity or other defects, recombination would still yield 2.9×10^{20} possible murine TCRs. This would seem to be more than enough potential diversity, given that the thymus produces fewer than 10^9 thymocytes over the lifetime of a mouse.

TCR V genes used in the responses against different antigens

A major area of research in recent years has been to determine which sets of TCR V genes are used in the responses against different antigens. Because T cells recognize antigenic peptides bound to a particular MHC molecule this depends on:
- the antigen; and
- the MHC molecules expressed by an individual.

Once the TCRs have been generated, T cells are subjected to thymic selection and may be further selected by interactions with APCs in the periphery. For these reasons, even if TCRs are generated by random recombination of gene segments, the expressed repertoire will be skewed toward the use of particular gene segments. Furthermore, the preference for different V gene segments by distinct T cell subsets may reflect their ontogeny. For example:
- γδ T cells residing in mouse skin (dendritic epidermal cells or DECs) express only the Vγ3 and Vδ1 segments;
- intraepithelial lymphocytes from the gut express Vγ5 almost exclusively (in combination with Vδ4–7).

It is thought that these populations arise at distinct stages of intrathymic T cell development, and they appear to have distinct functions.

RECOGNITION BY THE αβ TCR REQUIRES ANTIGEN TO BE BOUND TO AN MHC MOLECULE

Intracellular pathogens and neoplasia present a special challenge to the immune system. The immediate problem is one of detection. The immune system has therefore evolved an elegant means of recognizing pathogens that have invaded or been taken into the host cell, as well as tumor antigens produced within the cytosol:
- proteins from within the cell are digested into short peptide fragments;
- the short peptide fragments are displayed on the cell surface through binding to specialized antigen-presenting molecules termed **MHC class I** proteins;
- in a similar fashion, peptides derived from proteins ingested from the extracellular environment by phagocytosis are presented by **MHC class II** molecules;
- the peptide–MHC complexes serve as ligands for TCRs.

This antigen processing and presentation pathway, upon which both activation and regulation of the immune response rests, is a complex and fascinating subject (see Chapter 7).

In humans the MHC is known as the HLA

The proteins responsible for presenting antigens to T cells, MHC class I and class II proteins, were originally discovered as histocompatibility (transplantation) anti-gens. Histocompatibility refers to the ability to accept tissue grafts from an unrelated donor.

The major histocompatibility complex locus (MHC) comprises over 100 separate genes and was discovered when it was recognized that both donor and recipient had to possess the same MHC haplotype to avoid graft rejection.

The principal moieties that determine rejection were identified as MHC class I and class II molecules (see below), but we know now that that the main purpose of the MHC is not to prevent graft rejection. The remaining genes in the MHC (sometimes called class III) are very diverse. Some encode:
- complement system molecules (C4, C2, factor B);
- cytokines (e.g. tumor necrosis factor);
- enzymes;
- heat-shock proteins; and
- other molecules involved in antigen processing.

There are no functional or structural similarities between these other gene products.

All mammalian species possess the MHC, though details of the complex vary from one species to the next. In humans the locus is known as the **HLA** (an abbreviation for **human leukocyte antigen**); in mice it is known as the **H-2 locus** (Fig. 5.5).

MHC molecules provide a sophisticated surveillance system for intracellular antigens

From a cell's perspective, there are two types of antigen that must be dealt with:
- antigens that are **intrinsic** to the cell (antigenic peptides from viruses or other pathogens that inhabit the cell);
- antigens that are **extrinsic** to the cell.

Q. How are antigens taken up by APCs?
A. They are internalized by phagocytosis or pinocytosis, either by directly binding to receptors on the surface of the APC (see Fig. 1.11) or following opsonization by antibody and/or complement (see Fig. 4.14).

MHC class I molecules handle intrinsic antigens, while MHC class II molecules handle extrinsic antigens. In both cases, the antigenic peptides are produced by proteolytic processing of proteins.

In general:
- MHC class I molecules present antigen to cytotoxic T cells, which are important in controlling viral infections by lysing infected cells;
- MHC class II molecules present antigen to helper T cells, which aid B cells in generating antibody responses to extracellular protein antigens.

MHC class I molecules consist of an MHC-encoded heavy chain bound to a β₂-microglobulin

The overall structure of the extracellular portion of an MHC class I molecule is depicted in Fig. 5.6. It comprises a glycosylated heavy chain (45 kDa) non-covalently associated with β₂-microglobulin (12 kDa), which is a polypeptide that is also found free in serum.

Organization of the murine and human MHCs

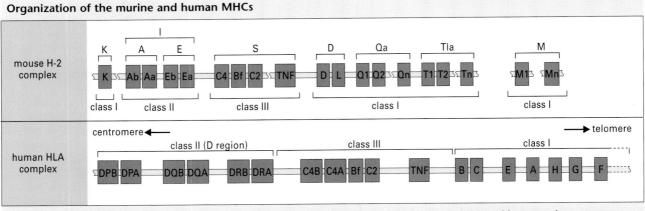

Fig. 5.5 Diagram showing the locations of subregions of the murine and human MHCs and the positions of the major genes within these subregions. The human organization pattern, in which the class II loci are positioned between the centromere and the class I loci, occurs in every other mammalian species so far examined. The regions span 3–4 Mbp of DNA.

A model of an MHC class I molecule

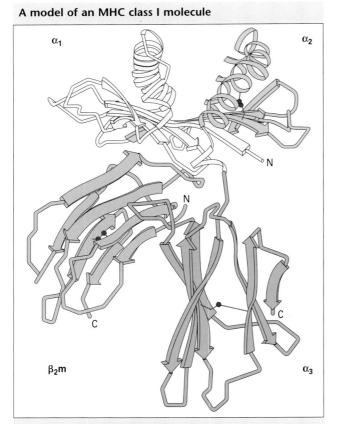

Fig. 5.6 The peptide backbone of the extracellular portion of HLA-A2 is shown. The three globular domains (α_1, α_2, and α_3) of the heavy chain are shown in green or turquoise and are closely associated with the non-MHC-encoded peptide, β_2-microglobulin (β_2m, gray). β_2-Microglobulin is stabilized by an intrachain disulfide bond (red) and has a similar tertiary structure to an immunoglobulin domain. The groove formed by the α_1 and α_2 domains is clearly visible.

The class I heavy chain consists of:
- three extracellular domains, designated α_1 (N terminal), α_2, and α_3;
- a transmembrane region; and
- a cytoplasmic tail.

The three extracellular domains each comprise about 90 amino acids:
- the α_2 and α_3 domains both have intrachain disulfide bonds enclosing loops of 63 and 86 amino acids, respectively;
- the α_3 domain is structurally homologous to the immunoglobulin constant region domain (C) and contains a site that interacts with CD8 on cytotoxic T cells.

The extracellular portion of the class I heavy chain is glycosylated, the degree of glycosylation depending on the species and haplotype.

The predominantly hydrophobic transmembrane region comprises 25 amino acid residues and traverses the lipid bilayer, most probably in an α-helical conformation.

The hydrophilic cytoplasmic domain, 30 to 40 residues long, may be phosphorylated in vivo.

β_2-Microglobulin is essential for expression of MHC class I molecules

β_2-Microglobulin:
- is non-polymorphic in humans, but dimorphic in mice (because of a single amino acid change at position 85);
- like the α_3 domain, has the structure of an immunoglobulin constant region domain;
- associates with a number of other class I-like molecules, such as the products of the *CD1* genes on chromosome 1 in humans (see below) and the Fc receptor, which mediates the uptake of IgG from milk in neonatal rat intestinal cells. These class I-like molecules, which have a structural similarity to the products of the MHC class I genes, are encoded by genes located in the class I loci and are referred to as **class Ib molecules**.

- is essential for the expression of all class I molecules at the cell surface – mutant mice lacking β$_2$-microglobulin do not express MHC class I molecules and are severely defective in presenting intrinsic antigens to T cells.

Heavy chain α$_1$ and α$_2$ domains form the antigen-binding groove

X-ray crystallography has shown that the α$_1$ and α$_2$ domains constitute a platform of eight antiparallel β strands supporting two antiparallel α helices (Fig. 5.7). The disulfide bond in the α$_2$ domain connects the N terminal β strand to the α helix of the α$_2$ domain. A long groove separates the α helices of the α$_1$ and α$_2$ domains.

The original crystal structure of the HLA-A2 molecule revealed diffuse extra electron density in the groove, suggesting the presence of bound peptide antigen. This interpretation was supported by the observation that the majority of polymorphic residues and T cell epitopes on class I molecules are located in or near the groove.

VARIATIONS IN AMINO ACID SEQUENCE CHANGE THE SHAPE OF THE BINDING GROOVE – Comparison of the structures of HLA-A2 and HLA-Aw68 have further refined our understanding of the structural basis for the binding of peptide to class I antigens.

The differences between HLA-A2 and HLA-Aw68 result from amino acid side-chain differences at 13 positions:
- six in α$_1$;
- six in α$_2$; and
- one (residue 245, which contributes to interactions with CD8) in α$_3$.

Ten of the twelve differences between HLA-A2 and HLA-Aw68 are at positions lining the floor and side of the peptide-binding groove (see Fig. 5.7). These differences give rise to dramatic differences in the shape of the groove and on the antigen peptides that it will bind.

Seen in detail, the peptide-binding groove forms a number of ridges and pockets with which amino acid side chains can interact. Typically the groove of an MHC class I molecule will accommodate peptides of eight or nine residues.

Amino acid variations within the peptide-binding groove can vary the positions of the pockets, providing the structural basis for differences in peptide-binding affinity that in turn govern exactly what is presented to a T cell (Fig. 5.8).

MHC class II molecules resemble MHC class I molecules in their overall structure

The products of the MHC class II genes are:
- A and E in the mouse;
- DP, DQ, and DR in humans.

These products are heterodimers of heavy (α) and light (β) glycoprotein chains, and both chains are encoded in the MHC:
- the α chains have molecular weights of 30–34 kDa;
- the β chains range from 26 to 29 kDa, depending on the locus involved.

A number of lines of evidence indicate that the α and β chains have the same overall structures. An extracellular portion comprising two domains (α$_1$ and α$_2$ or β$_1$ and β$_2$)

The antigen-binding site of the MHC class I molecule HLA-A2

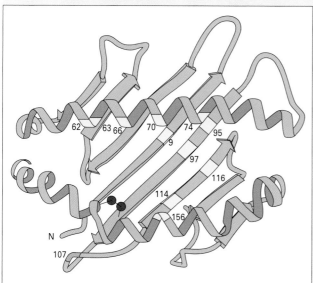

Fig. 5.7 The view of the peptide antigen-binding groove in HLA-A2 as 'seen' by the TCR. The α$_1$ and α$_2$ domains each consist of four antiparallel β strands followed by a long helical region. The domains pair to form a single eight-stranded β sheet topped by α helices. The locations of the most polymorphic residues are highlighted. Residues around the binding site are highly polymorphic. For example, HLA-2 and HLA-Aw68 differ from each other by 13 amino acid residues. Ten of these differences occur around the antigen-binding site (yellow). (Modified from Bjorkman et al. Nature 1987;329:512–516, with additional data from Parham P. Nature 1989;342:617–618)

Peptide-binding grooves of HLA-Aw68 and HLA-A2

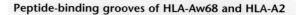
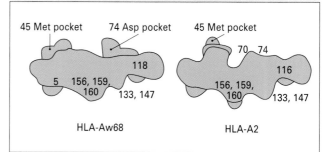

Fig. 5.8 The shapes of the antigen-binding groove on each molecule are illustrated. Differences in amino acids around the groove create different antigen-binding sites. For example, residues around position 45 produce a methionine-binding pocket in both molecules, but the aspartate-binding pocket around residue 74 is present only in HLA-Aw68.

is connected by a short sequence to a transmembrane region of about 30 residues and a cytoplasmic domain of about 10 to 15 residues.

The α_2 and β_2 domains are similar to the class I α_3 domain and β_2-microglobulin, possessing the structural characteristics of immunoglobulin constant domains.

The β_1 domain contains a disulfide bond, which generates a 64 amino acid loop.

The difference in molecular weights of the class II α and β chains is due primarily to differential glycosylation:
• the α_1, α_2, and β_1 domains are N-glycosylated;
• the β_2 domain is not N-glycosylated.
The β_2 domain does, however, contain a binding site for CD4, and MHC class II molecules on APCs interact with CD4 on T cells in a manner analogous to the interaction of MHC class I molecules with CD8. CD4 and CD8 are important elements in the recruitment of kinases that signal T cell activation.

Despite the differences in length and organization of the polypeptide chains, the overall three-dimensional structure of MHC class II molecules is very similar to that of MHC class I molecules (Fig. 5.9).

MHC CLASS I AND CLASS II MOLECULES BIND TO PEPTIDES DERIVED FROM DIFFERENT SOURCES
The MHC class II binding groove accommodates longer peptides than MHC class I

The structures of MHC class I and class II molecules reflect their functional differences.

The binding groove of MHC class II molecules is more open than that of MHC class I molecules, to accommodate longer peptides (Figs 5.10 and 5.11):
• MHC class I molecules bind short fragments of eight to ten amino acids; whereas
• MHC class II molecules bind peptides of 13 to 24 amino acids.
The structural features of the class II antigen-binding site have been illuminated by determination of the crystal structure of HLA-DR1 complexed with an influenza virus peptide. Pockets clearly visible within the peptide-binding site accommodate five side chains of the bound peptide and explain the peptide specificity of HLA-DR1.

The precise topology of the MHC peptide-binding groove depends partly on the nature of the amino acids within the groove, and thus varies from one haplotype to the next.

Which peptide can bind to a particular MHC molecule depends on the nature of the side chains of the peptide and their complementarity with the MHC molecule's binding groove. Some amino acid side chains of the peptide stick out of the groove and are available to contact the TCR.

Peptides are held in MHC molecule binding grooves by characteristic anchor residues
It is possible to purify and sequence peptides that have been generated by a cell and then bound by MHC molecules at the cell surface. These peptides include:

Comparison of the extracellular domains of class I and class II molecules

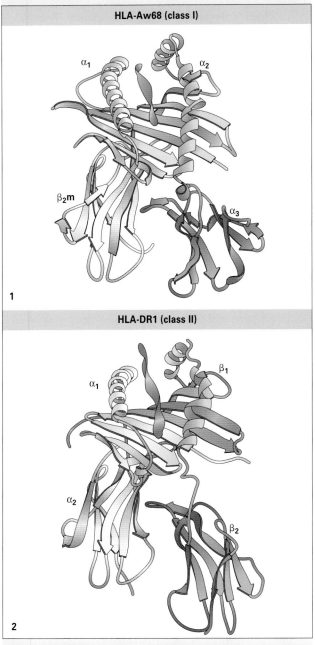

Fig. 5.9 Ribbon diagrams of the extracellular domains of class I HLA-Aw68 (**1**) and class II HLA-DR1 (**2**) MHC molecules. The binding cleft is shown with a resident peptide. These diagrams emphasize the similarity in the three-dimensional structures of class I and class II molecules. (Redrawn from Stern LJ. Structure 1994;2:245–251. Copyright 1994 with permission from Elsevier)

• foreign peptides from internalized antigens or viral particles; and
• self molecules produced within the cell or endocytosed from extracellular fluids.

Peptide-binding sites of class I (H-2K^b) and class II (HLA-DR1) MHC molecules

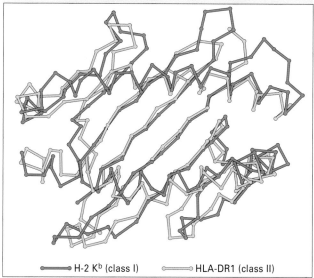

===== H-2 K^b (class I)   ○====○ HLA-DR1 (class II)

Fig. 5.10 The peptide binding sites of class I (H-2K^b) and class II (HLA-DR1) MHC molecules are shown as α carbon atom traces in a top view of the peptide-binding clefts. The similarities between the two sites can clearly be seen, but there are also some differences, some of which account for the difference in peptide length preference between class I (8–10 amino acid residues) and class II (>12 amino acid residues). (Redrawn from Stern LJ. Structure 1994;2:245–251. Copyright 1994 with permission from Elsevier)

Peptides bind non-covalently within the antigen-binding groove

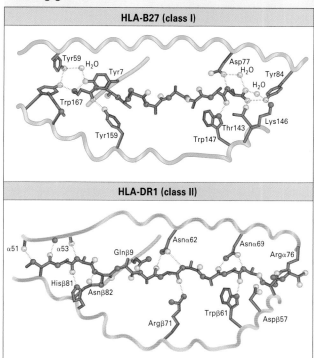

Fig. 5.11 The hydrogen bonds made by the main chain of a bound peptide with class I (HLA-B27) or class II MHC molecules (HLA-DR1) are shown. The major difference between the two hydrogen-bonding patterns is the clustering of conserved class I hydrogen bonds at the ends of the peptide. By contrast, conserved class II hydrogen bonds are distributed throughout the length of the peptide. (Redrawn from Stern LJ. Structure 1994;2:245–251. Copyright 1994 with permission from Elsevier)

Self peptides eluted from MHC class I molecules have been purified and sequenced.

For MHC class I molecules, interactions at the N and C terminals confine the peptide to the binding groove

A number of peptides bound by particular MHC molecules have been sequenced, and characteristic residues identified – one at the C terminus and another close to the N terminus of the peptide. These characteristic motifs distinguish sets of binding peptides for different MHC class I molecules (Fig. 5.12).

The significance of the conserved residues has become clear by analysis of the three-dimensional structures of several MHC class I molecules, which have generated a clear picture of the peptide residing in the binding groove:

- the ends of the peptide-binding groove are closed;
- the peptide is an extended (not α-helical) chain of nine amino acids and the N and C terminals are buried at the ends of the groove;
- some of the side chains extend into the pockets formed within the variable region of the class I heavy chain;
- numerous hydrogen bonds are formed between residues in the class I molecule and those of the peptide along its length;
- in particular, tyrosine residues commonly found at the N terminus of the peptide and a conserved lysine in the

MHC class I molecule binding groove stabilize peptide binding (see Fig. 5.11);
- the centers of the peptides bulge out of the groove, so presenting different structures to TCRs.

This picture is consistent with the characteristic motifs found at the ends of peptides eluted from class I molecules.

For MHC class II molecules, peptides may extend beyond the ends of the binding groove

The binding groove of the MHC class II molecule:

- also incorporates a number of binding pockets, though the locations are somewhat different from that on class I molecules;
- is not closed at the ends, so bound peptides extend out of the ends of the groove.

Consistent with this observation, peptides eluted from MHC class II molecules tend to be longer (over 15 residues).

Conserved anchor residues in peptides eluted from MHC class II molecules have been identified (Fig. 5.13), but these are more difficult to detect than those of class I

Allele-specific motifs in peptides eluted from MHC class I molecules

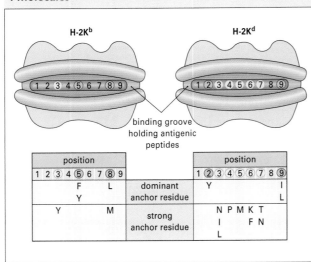

position										position								
1	2	3	4	⑤	6	7	⑧	9		1	②	3	4	5	6	7	8	⑨
				F			L		dominant anchor residue		Y							I
				Y														L
Y							M		strong anchor residue						N	P M	K T	
																I		F N
																L		

Fig. 5.12 Class I MHC molecules from either H-2K^b or H-2K^d haplotypes were immunoprecipitated. Peptides bound to these molecules were purified and sequenced. Amino acid residues commonly found at a particular position are classified as 'dominant' anchor residues. Residues that are fairly common at a site are shown as 'strong'. Positions for which no amino acid is shown could be occupied by several different amino acids with equal frequency. The one-letter amino acid code is used. The diagram represents the class I MHC molecule binding groove, viewed from above with anchor positions of each haplotype highlighted.

Allele-specific motifs in peptides eluted from MHC class II molecules

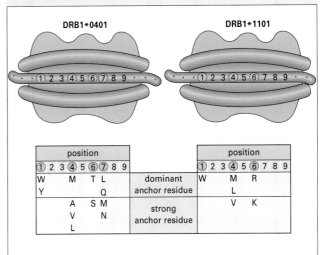

position										position								
①	2	3	④	5	⑥	⑦	8	9		①	2	3	④	5	⑥	7	8	9
W			M		T	L			dominant anchor residue	W			M		R			
Y						Q							L					
A			S		M				strong anchor residue				V		K			
V					N													
L																		

Fig. 5.13 HLA-DR molecules of two haplotypes (DRB1*0401 and DRB1*1101) were purified and incubated with a library of peptides (generated in phage M13). After multiple rounds of selection, peptides that bound effectively to the MHC class II molecules were identified and sequenced. Residues having a frequency greater than 20% are shown as 'dominant' anchor residues. Other fairly common residues are shown as 'strong'. Note that the binding site on MHC class II molecules accommodates longer peptides than that on MHC class I molecules. (Data abstracted from Hammer J, Valsasnini P, Tolba K, et al. Cell 1993;74:197–203)

peptides because of the ragged ends and the more even distribution of bonds tethering the peptide to the MHC class II molecule binding groove (see Fig. 5.11).

Peptides binding MHC class II are less uniform in size than those binding MHC class I molecules

A major difference between MHC class I and class II molecules occurs at the ends of the peptide-binding groove:
- for MHC class I molecules, interactions at the N and C terminals confine the peptide to the cleft;
- for MHC class II molecules, peptides may extend beyond the ends of the cleft.

The peptides that bind to MHC class I molecules come from proteins synthesized within the cell, which are broken down and transported to the endoplasmic reticulum. The mechanism of antigen processing is explained fully in Chapter 7, but it should be noted here that the internal antigen processing pathways generally produce peptides of an appropriate size to occupy the MHC class I molecule antigen-binding groove.

Peptides that bind to MHC class II molecules come from proteins that have been internalized by the cell and then degraded. These peptides are less uniform in size than those that bind to MHC class I molecules and may be

trimmed once they have found their way to the MHC class II molecule.

The MHC class II molecule antigen processing pathway is quite distinct from the MHC class I molecule pathway (see Chapter 7).

CLASS I AND CLASS II MHC MOLECULES PRESENT PEPTIDE ANTIGENS TO THE TCR IN A CELL–CELL INTERACTION

Once the structures of the TCR and the MHC–peptide complex had been established, the next question was to determine how they interacted.

The first crystallographic data were derived using a co-crystal of a mouse MHC class I molecule bound to an endogenous cellular peptide and αβ TCR (Fig. 5.14). This structure showed that the axis of the TCR was roughly aligned with the peptide-binding groove on the MHC molecule, but set at 20–30° askew. This means that:
- the first and second CDRs of the TCR α and β chains (see Fig. 5.1) are positioned over residues near the N and C terminals of the presented polypeptide; and
- the third CDRs of each chain, lying at the center of the TCR binding site, are positioned over the central residues of the peptide that protrude from the groove.

Interaction of a T cell receptor and MHC–peptide complex

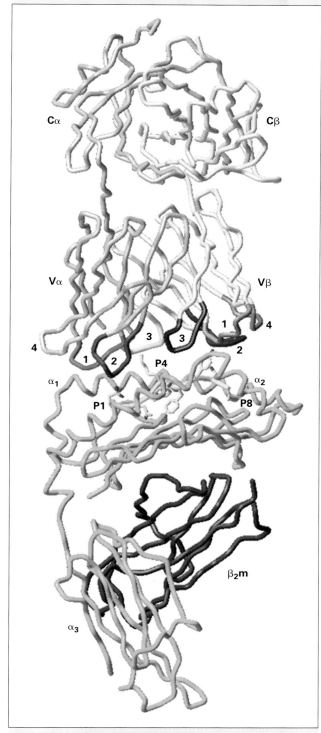

Fig. 5.14 The structure of an MHC class I molecule (H-2K^b) complexed to an octapeptide (yellow tube) is shown bound to an αβ TCR. The six CDRs that contact the peptide (1, 2, 3, 3, 1, 2) are highlighted in deeper colors. Residues from αHV4 (pink) and βHV4 (orange) are not positioned to take part in the intermolecular interactions. (Illustration kindly provided by Dr Christopher Garcia, from Science 1996;274:209–219. Copyright 1996 AAAS)

Residues from each of the CDRs are positioned to interact with residues from the MHC molecule.

Q. What advantage is there in having CDR3 segments at the center of the TCR binding site?
A. CDR3 demonstrates the greatest diversity of the TCR CDRs (because it is generated by gene recombination, see Fig. 3.6). It is therefore better suited than CDR1 and CDR2 for interactions with diverse antigenic peptides.

The molecular structure therefore underpins the experimental findings that T cells recognize antigenic peptides bound to particular MHC molecules.

This arrangement of TCR and MHC–antigen is broadly comparable to those found with the small number of receptors so far analyzed by X-ray crystallography.

Aggregation of TCRs initiates T cell activation

Although basic models of T cell activation by antigen–MHC show one receptor being triggered by one complex (e.g. Fig. 1.9), this is simplistic.

Each T cell may express 10^5 receptors and each APC has a similar number of MHC molecules. If a T cell engages an APC, only a tiny proportion of the MHC–antigen complexes on its surface will be of the correct type to be recognized by the T cell.

What, then, is the minimum signal for T cell activation? In practice:

• only a few peptide–MHC–TCR interactions are needed – perhaps 100 specific interactions, involving about 0.1% of the MHC molecules on the APC;
• moreover, the interactions can take place over a period of time – it is not necessary for all 100 TCRs to be engaged simultaneously.

The model of the TCR shown in Fig. 5.3 suggests that it can form a dimeric structure clustered around the signaling molecules of the CD3 complex.

Interestingly, there is some evidence that MHC molecules can also dimerize, and that TCRs bound to MHC–peptide complexes tend to form dimers or aggregates. These observations have led to the view that T cell activation requires the cooperative aggregation of specific TCRs with MHC–peptide complexes.

The auxiliary molecules CD4 and CD8 are also important in T cell activation, and the presence of CD4 or CD8 can help stabilize the interaction of the TCR and MHC–peptide. In addition, kinases associated with these molecules are brought into proximity with CD3 so they can phosphorylate the ζζ dimer that initiates activation (Fig. 5.15) The ensuing steps are described in Chapter 7 (see Fig. 7.21).

Antigenic peptides can induce or antagonize T cell activation

The affinity of TCRs for antigen peptide–MHC, expressed as an association constant, is typically of the order of 10^{-5} to 10^{-6} M, which is much lower than the affinity of antibody for an epitope on an antigen commonly generated by an immune response.

The role of CD4 and CD8 in T cell activation

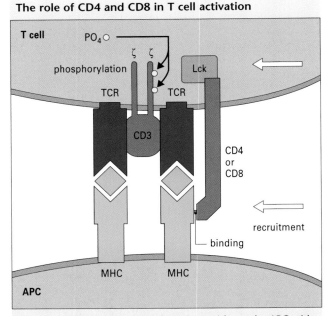

Fig. 5.15 After aggregation of MHC–peptide on the APC with the TCR, either CD4 or CD8 can join the complex. CD4 binds to MHC class II molecules and CD8 to MHC class I molecules. The kinase Lck is attached to the intracytoplasmic portion of CD4 or CD8. Binding of the CD4 or CD8 molecules to specific sites of the MHC molecules brings the kinase into proximity with the ITAMs on the CD3 $\zeta\zeta$ dimer (see Fig. 5.3). The kinase phosphorylates the motifs, as the first step in T cell activation.

The affinity of antigen–MHC for the TCR is especially important because it determines the degree to which the T cell becomes activated. Peptides that activate a T cell are called **agonist peptides**. By changing one or two amino acids in an agonist peptide, it is possible to generate peptides that antagonize the normal activation by the original peptide. The **antagonist peptides** typically have a lower affinity for the TCR than the original agonist peptide and are thought to act by either:

- interfering with the binding of the agonist peptide to the MHC molecule; or
- binding less effectively to the TCR.

Occasionally, a modified peptide will be more effective than the agonist in activating the T cell. These **strong agonist (or superagonist) peptides** produce higher affinity binding in the TCR–MHC–peptide complex.

The distinctions between these three different types of peptide (agonist, antagonist, and strong agonist) have biological ramifications. Researchers are attempting, for example, to use antagonist peptides to block adverse immune responses.

Understanding TCR affinity could provide insight into how T cells become tolerant to self antigens during development (see Chapter 19).

What constitutes T cell specificity?

Finally we should consider the question of what constitutes T cell specificity. When the specificity of

lymphocytes was first explained in Chapter 1, it was stated that each lymphocyte binds to just one antigen using its receptor. Although this is a useful starting point for understanding immune responses, it is not strictly true.

In Chapter 3 it was seen that immunoglobulins could bind to different antigens if they had epitopes that were sufficiently similar. This chapter has shown that antigenic peptides can be mutated and still bind and trigger T cell activation.

One question, then, is how far a peptide can be mutated and still bind to its own TCR. In some cases it has been possible to individually change each amino acid in a peptide without destroying its ability to bind to the MHC molecule or the TCR.

Provided the peptide can form part of the TCR–MHC–peptide complex and provide sufficient binding energy, its precise amino acid sequence does not matter. This is a very important observation.

Later, when we consider how antigenic peptides from microorganisms can trigger autoimmune diseases (see Chapter 20), we learn that one possible mechanism is that a self peptide and a foreign peptide are sufficiently similar to bind to the same T cell, so causing a breakdown in self tolerance. One conclusion from the work cited above is that such peptides do not have to be identical to be cross-reactive.

THE OVERALL ORGANIZATION OF THE MHC LOCI DIFFERS BETWEEN SPECIES

The number of gene loci for MHC class I and class II molecules varies between species and between different haplotypes within each species, and many polymorphic variants have been described at each of the loci.

Much of the original work on the MHC was done using mice and what has been learned from these studies has been broadly applicable to humans.

The three principal human MHC class I loci are HLA-A, HLA-B, and HLA-C

The human MHC class I region contains three principal class I loci – called HLA-A, HLA-B, and HLA-C. Each locus encodes the heavy chain of a classical MHC class I molecule and the whole region:

- extends over 1.8 million bases of DNA; and
- includes 118 genes (Fig. 5.16).

Closer analysis of this region has revealed multiple additional MHC class I genes.

HLA-E, HLA-F, HLA-G, and HLA-H are class Ib genes

The *HLA-E*, *HLA-F*, *HLA-G*, and *HLA-H* genes also encode MHC class I proteins, and are called class Ib genes. They are much less polymorphic than the A, B, and C locus gene products, and recent work has ascribed various functions to them. For example, *HLA-E* and *HLA-G* gene products can bind to antigenic peptides, but are involved in recognition by NK cells (see p. 207).

Genes within the human MHC class I region

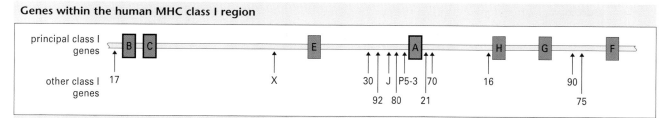

Fig. 5.16 The human MHC class I region lies telomeric to the MHC class II region (see Fig. 5.5). In addition to the genes encoding the classic transplantation antigens (*HLA-A, HLA-B*, and *HLA-C*), several other principal class I-like genes have been identified (*HLA-E, HLA-F*, and *HLA-G*). Mutations in the *HLA-H* gene are associated with hemochromatosis, a disorder that causes the body to absorb excessive amounts of iron from the diet. A number of other non-classical class I genes and pseudogenes are present, mostly with unknown functions.

Mice have two or three MHC class I loci

The mouse MHC (H-2) has two or three MHC class I loci, but the number of MHC class I genes varies between haplotypes (Fig. 5.17).

MHC class I genes involved in antigen presentation to T cells are located in H-2K, H-2D, and H-2L loci.

The organization of the H-2K region is similar in all strains that have been studied. It contains two class I genes, termed K and K2:

- the *H-2K* gene encodes the H-2K antigen expressed on most cell types and recognized serologically; whereas
- the *H-2K2* gene exhibits varied patterns of expression, depending on the strain.

The numbers of genes in the H-2D and H-2L loci are variable (see Fig. 5.17).

Qa, Tla, and M genes encode MHC class Ib molecules

The Qa, Tla, and M genes of the mouse MHC class I region (see Figs 5.5 and 5.17) encode class Ib molecules, of which the functions are mostly unknown:

- the Qa locus comprises about 200 kb of DNA distal to H-2D/L and encodes the serologically detectable molecules Qa-1, 2, 3, 4, and 5, and encompasses a cluster of eight (BALB/c) to ten (B10) MHC class I genes;
- Qa-1b corresponds to HLA-E, which is involved in NK cell recognition (see Fig. 10.4);
- the Tla region, although defined initially as encoding the TL (thymus leukemia) antigen, has subsequently been shown to contain the largest number of class I genes and the greatest number of differences in organization between the B10 and BALB/c haplotypes;
- the M region contains a number of new MHC class I genes, termed M1–M7.

The class Ib genes exhibit a low degree of polymorphism.

Human MHC class II genes are located in the HLA-D region

The human MHC class II region spans about 1000 kb of DNA, and the order and orientation of the various loci are similar to that of the homologous loci in the mouse MHC class II region (see below).

The HLA-D region encodes at least six α and ten β chain genes for MHC class II molecules (Fig. 5.18). Three loci (DR, DQ, and DP) encode the major expressed prod-

Genes within the murine class I region

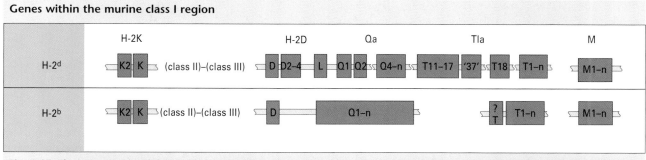

Fig. 5.17 The organization of the MHC class I region of two haplotypes, BALB/c (H-2^d) and B10 (H-2^b), is shown. The class II region lies between the H-2K and H-2D regions. The brackets denote gaps added to align alleles between the two haplotypes. H-2^d and H-2^b haplotypes have different numbers of class I genes in the H-2D/H-2L region. Five class I genes map to the D/L region of BALB/c (H-2^d) mice. Two of these genes encode the serologically detectable H-2D^d and H-2L^d antigens. Three additional class I genes are found in the region between the proximal H-2D^d and distal H-2L^d genes. These genes, called D2^d, D3^d, and D4^d, are of unknown function. Only one class I gene has been identified in the H-2D region of B10 mice. The Q, T, and M regions contain a large number of class Ib genes, the functions of which are mostly unknown.

Genes within the human and mouse class II regions

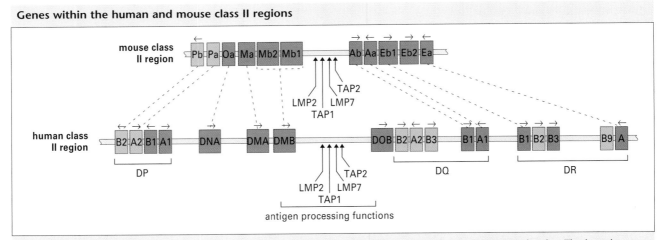

Fig. 5.18 The arrangement of the genes within the human and murine MHCs is shown. Homologous genes between the two species are indicated. Expressed genes are colored orange and pseudogenes are shown yellow. Mice of the b, s, f, and q haplotypes fail to express class II-E molecules. The b and s haplotypes fail to transcribe the Ea gene, but make normal cytoplasmic levels of Eb chain. Mice of f and q haplotypes fail to make both Ea and Eb chains.

ucts of the human MHC class II region, but additional genes have also been identified:

- the DR family comprises a single α gene (DRA) and up to nine β genes (DRB1–9), including pseudogenes and several different gene arrangements occur within the locus;
- the DQ and DP families each have one expressed gene for α and β chains and an additional pair of pseudogenes.

DR, DQ, and DP α chains associate in the cell primarily with β chains of their own loci. For example:

- the *DPA1* and *DPB1* gene products associate to generate the HLA-DP class II molecules detected using specific antibodies;
- similarly, *DQA1* and *DQB1* encode the HLA-DQ antigens.

The organization and length of the DRB region varies in different haplotypes (Fig. 5.19), with different numbers of β chains expressed.

The MHC class II region also contains genes that encode proteins involved in antigen presentation that are not expressed at the cell surface (see Chapter 7).

Mouse MHC class II genes are located in the H-2I region

The α and β chains of mouse MHC class II molecules are encoded by separate genes located in the I region of the H-2 complex (see Figs 5.5 and 5.18). The gene nomenclature indicates first the locus and then the type of chain it encodes:

- the Ab and Aa genes thus encode the β and α chains of the A molecule; and
- the Eb and Ea genes likewise encode the two chains of the E molecule (Fig. 5.5).

Several other class II b and a genes for which no gene product is known have been cloned:

- one of these – Pb – is a pseudogene;
- two others – Ob and Eb2 – may be functional.

The number of DRB loci varies with different haplotypes

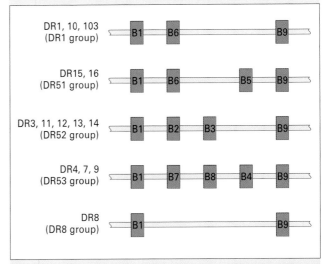

Fig. 5.19 The numbers of DRB loci varies between individuals. For example, a person who has a haplotype producing molecules of the type DR1 (see Appendix 1) has three loci for DRB (top line). Not all of these loci produce mRNA for DR β chains.

The Ob and Eb2 genes display a low level of polymorphism and are transcribed, but it is not known whether they are translated.

Different strains of mice vary in their expression of some of the MHC class II genes (see Fig. 5.18).

MHC polymorphism is concentrated in and around the peptide-binding cleft

A hallmark of the MHC is the extreme degree of polymorphism (structural variability) of the molecules encoded within it. The class Ib molecules are much less polymorphic than the classical class I and II molecules. A list of allelic variants of HLA class I and II molecules is given in Appendix 1.

Within a particular MHC class I or class II molecule, the structural polymorphisms are clustered in particular regions. The amino acid sequence variability in class I molecules is clustered in three main regions of the α_1 and α_2 domains. The α_3 domain appears to be much more conserved.

Q. Correlate the domains that show structural variability and structural conservation with the molecules that they interact with.

A. The α_1 and α_2 domains interact with the variable antigen peptides (see Fig. 5.7) and the TCR, while the α_3 domain interacts with the monomorphic CD8 molecule (see Fig. 5.15).

In MHC class II molecules, the extent of variability depends on the subregion and on the polypeptide chain. For example:

• most polymorphism occurs in DRβ and DQβ chains, whereas DPβ chains are slightly less polymorphic;
• DQα is polymorphic whereas DRα chains are virtually invariant, being represented by just two alleles.

In outbred populations in which individuals have two MHC haplotypes, hybrid class II molecules with one chain from each haplotype can be produced. This generates additional structural diversity in the expressed molecules.

Most of the polymorphic amino acids in MHC class I and class II molecules are clustered on top of the molecule around the peptide-binding site (see Fig. 5.7). Variation is therefore centered in the base of the antigen-binding groove or pointing in from the sides of the α helices. This polymorphism affects the ability of the different MHC molecules to bind antigenic peptides.

AN INDIVIDUAL'S MHC HAPLOTYPE AFFECTS SUSCEPTIBILITY TO DISEASE

Genetic variations in MHC molecules affect:
• the ability to make immune responses, including the level of antibody production;
• resistance or susceptibility to infectious diseases;
• resistance or susceptibility to autoimmune diseases and allergies.

Knowing this, we can start to answer the question why the MHC is so polymorphic. The immune system must handle many different pathogens. By having several different MHC molecules, an individual can present a diverse range of antigens and is therefore likely to be able to mount an effective immune response. There is therefore a selective advantage in having different MHC molecules.

Going beyond this, we know that different pathogens are prevalent in different areas of the world, so evolutionary pressures from pathogens will tend to select for different MHC molecules in different regions.

Q. The haplotype HLA-B53 is associated with protection against childhood malaria, a disease that is prevalent in equatorial regions. In which country would you expect to find the highest frequency of the HLA-B53 allele – China, Ghana, or South Africa?

A. The gene frequency is around 40% in Ghana and 1–2% in China and South Africa, which are outside the equatorial regions affected by malaria.

All nucleated cells of the body express MHC class I molecules

The function of MHC class I molecules is to present antigens that have entered the cell, such as viral peptides. Because any cell of the body may become infected with a virus or intracellular pathogen, all cells need to sample their internal molecules and present them at the cell surface to cytotoxic T cells.

By contrast, MHC class II molecules are used by APCs to present antigens to helper T cells. Consequently the distribution of class II molecules is much more limited (see Fig. 7.4).

MHC molecules are co-dominantly expressed

This means that, in one individual, all of the principal MHC gene loci are expressed from both the maternal and paternal chromosomes. As there are three MHC class I loci in humans (HLA-A, HLA-B, and HLA-C), each of which is highly polymorphic, most individuals will have genes for six different class I molecules, all of which will be present at the cell surface. Each MHC molecule will have:
• a slightly different shape; and
• present a different set of antigenic peptides.

A similar logic applies to MHC class II molecules. There are three principal class II loci in humans (HLA-DP, HLA-DQ, and HLA-DR), all of which are polymorphic. At first sight, it would appear that an APC could express six different class II molecules as well as its class I molecules. However, this is probably an underestimate. As noted above, hybrid class II molecules (using one polypeptide encoded by the maternal chromosome and one by the paternal chromosome) also occur.

The specificity of the TCR and MHC explains genetic restrictions in antigen presentation

Much of the original work on antigen presentation was carried out using strains of mice that had been inbred to the point where both maternal and paternal chromosomes were identical. Any offspring therefore inherited the same set of autosomes from each parent, and the offspring were genetically identical to their parents. Clearly the level of diversity in the MHC molecules was much less than in an outbred human population.

The artificial simplicity of the inbred mouse system, however, allowed immunologists to dissect how antigens were presented to T cells in a whole animal, when the molecular structures of the MHC molecules and the TCR were completely unknown.

The key experiment that demonstrated the importance of the MHC in antigen presentation revealed a phenomenon called **genetic restriction** (also known as **MHC restriction**). In essence, it was noted that cytotoxic T cells from a mouse infected with a virus are primed to kill cells of the same H-2 haplotype infected with that virus; they do not kill cells of a different haplotype infected with the same virus (Fig. 5.20).

These data, and similar experiments using APCs and helper T cells, showed that T cells that have been primed to recognize antigen presented on MHC molecules of one haplotype will normally respond again only when they see the same antigen on the same MHC molecule.

Q. Interpret these findings in relation to the way in which T cells recognize antigen.

A. The TCR interacts with residues from both the antigenic peptide and the associated MHC molecule. In other words, the T cell recognizes the specific combination of MHC molecule plus peptide.

Peter Doherty and Rolf Zinkernagel performed the key experiments delineating the phenomenon of MHC restriction of T cell responses in the mid 1970s and were awarded the Nobel Prize in Physiology or Medicine in 1996 for this work.

CD1 IS AN MHC CLASS 1-LIKE MOLECULE THAT PRESENTS LIPID ANTIGENS

CD1 molecules are structurally related to MHC class I molecules and are non-covalently bound to β_2-microglobulin.

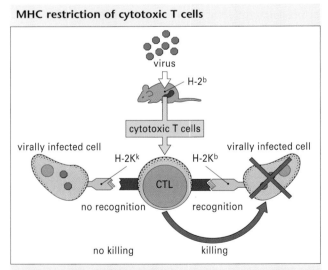

MHC restriction of cytotoxic T cells

Fig. 5.20 A mouse of the H-2^b haplotype is primed with virus and the cytotoxic T cells thus generated are isolated and tested for their ability to kill H-2^b and H-2^k cells infected with the same virus. The cytotoxic T cells kill H-2^b, but not H-2^k cells. In this instance, it is the H-2K class I gene product presenting the antigen to the T cells. The T cell is recognizing a specific structure produced by the association of a specific MHC molecule with a specific viral antigen.

The genes encoding CD1 molecules are located outside the MHC and are not polymorphic. In humans, they consist of five closely linked genes, of which four are expressed (Fig. 5.21), encoding proteins that fall into two separate groups:
- group 1 molecules in humans include CD1a, CD1b, and CD1c;
- CD1d proteins form the second group.

Murine CD1b has been crystallized and analyzed by X-ray crystallography. This shows that the molecule has a deep electrostatically neutral antigen-binding groove, which is highly hydrophobic and can accommodate lipid or glycolipid antigens (Fig. 5.22). One model for the binding places hydrophobic acyl groups of the lipids into the large hydrophobic pockets, leaving the more polar groups of the antigens such as phosphate and carbohydrate on the top, where they can interact with the TCR.

The binding requirements of the hydrophobic pockets on CD1 are fairly tolerant because they will accommodate acyl groups of different lengths, but the interactions with the TCR are much more specific – small changes in the structure of the carbohydrate moiety will destroy the ability to stimulate a T cell.

The antigens presented by the group I CD1 molecules and CD1d are different. For example, group I molecules present lipoarabinomannan, a component of the cell wall of mycobacteria (see Fig. 14.1), whereas CD1d cannot do this.

Another difference between CD1 and conventional MHC molecules is the way in which antigen is loaded into the antigen-binding groove:
- MHC class I molecules are loaded with antigenic peptides in the endoplasmic reticulum, and this requires transport of the peptides from the cytoplasm (see Chapter 7).
- group I CD1 molecules appear to be loaded in an acidic endosomal compartment because they do not bind to lipid antigens unless they are partially unfolded at low pH.

There is some debate about the physiological functions of the CD1 molecules in host defense:
- group I CD1 molecules present lipids from mycobacteria and *Haemophilus influenzae* and can stimulate both CD4$^+$ and CD8$^+$ cytotoxic T cells, and therefore appear to have a role in antimicrobial defense.

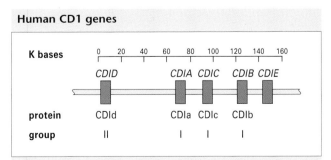

Human CD1 genes

Fig. 5.21 The genes of the human CD1 cluster extend over 160 kilobases on chromosome 1. A gene product for *CD1E* has not yet been identified.

Glycolipid antigens presented by CD1

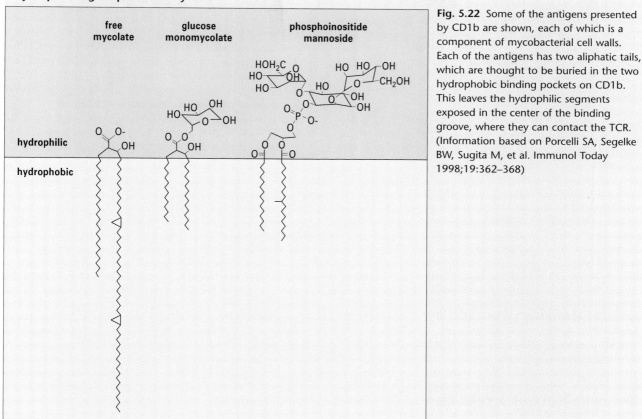

Fig. 5.22 Some of the antigens presented by CD1b are shown, each of which is a component of mycobacterial cell walls. Each of the antigens has two aliphatic tails, which are thought to be buried in the two hydrophobic binding pockets on CD1b. This leaves the hydrophilic segments exposed in the center of the binding groove, where they can contact the TCR. (Information based on Porcelli SA, Segelke BW, Sugita M, et al. Immunol Today 1998;19:362–368)

- most CD1d molecules appear to bind self antigens, though they also present lipids from parasites such as *Plasmodium falciparum* and *Trypanosoma brucei* (see Chapter 15) to T cells that use a restricted group of TCRs, indicating a role in defense against single-celled protozoal parasites.

FURTHER READING

Bentley GA, Mariuzza RA. The structure of the T cell antigen receptor. Annu Rev Immunol 1996;14:563–590.

Bjorkman PJ, Parham P. Structure, function and diversity of class I major histocompatibility complex molecules. Annu Rev Biochem 1990;59:253–288.

Bjorkman PJ, Saper MA, Samraoui B, et al. The structure of the human class I histocompatibility antigen HLA-A2. Nature 1987;329:506–512.

Bjorkman PJ, Samraoui B, Bennett WS, et al. The foreign antigen binding site and T-cell recognition regions of class I histocompatibility antigens. Nature 1987;329:512–516.

Bodmer JG, Marsh, SE, Albert ED, et al. Nomenclature for factors of the HLA system, 1994. Tissue Antigens 1994;44:1–18.

Brenner MB, MacLean J, Dialynas DP, et al. Identification of a putative second T-cell receptor. Nature 1986;322:145–149.

Brown JH, Jardetzky TS, Gorga JC, et al. Three-dimensional structure of the human class II histocompatibility antigen HLA-DR1. Nature 1993;364:33–39.

Burdin N, Kronenberg M. CD1-mediated immune responses to glycolipids. Curr Opin Immunol 1999;111:326–331.

Carosella ED, Dausett J, Kirzenbaum H. HLA-G revisited. Immunol Today 1996;17:407–409.

Chien Y-H, Jores R, Crowley MP. Recognition by γδ T cells. Annu Rev Immunol 1996;14:511–532.

Davis MM, Bjorkman PJ. T-cell antigen receptor genes and T-cell recognition. Nature 1988;334:395–402.

Davis MM, Boniface JJ, Reich Z, et al. Ligand recognition by αβ T cells. Annu Rev Immunol 1998;16:523–544.

Garcia KC, Degano M, Stanfield RL, et al. An αβ T cell receptor structure at 2.5Å and its orientation in the TCR–MHC. Complex Sci 1996;274:209–219.

Garcia KC, Teyton GL, Wilson IA. Structural basis of T cell recognition. Annu Rev Immunol 1999;17:369–398.

Garratt TPJ, Saper MA, Bjorkman PJ, et al. Specificity pockets for the side chains of peptide antigens in HLA-w68. Nature 1989;342:692–696.

Hass W, Pereira P, Tonegawa S. Gamma/delta cells. Annu Rev Immunol 1993;11:637–685.

Hayday AC. γδ cells: a right time and a right place for a conserved third way of protection. Annu Rev Immunol 2000;18:975–1026.

Hunkapiller T, Hood L. Diversity of the immunoglobulin gene superfamily. Adv Immunol 1989;44:1–63.

Lefranc M-P, Rabbitts TH. The human T-cell receptor γ (TRG) genes. Trends Biochem Sci 1989;14:214–218.

Leiden JM. Transcriptional regulation of T cell receptor genes. Annu Rev Immunol 1993;11:539–570.

Madden DR, Gorga JC, Strominger L, et al. The structure of

HLA-B27 reveals nonamer self-peptides bound in an extended conformation. Nature 1991;353:321–325.

Manning TC, Kranz DM. Binding energetics of T-cell receptors: correlation with immunological consequences. Immunol Today 1999;20:417–422.

Porcelli SA, Segelke BW, Sugita M, et al. The CD1 family of lipid antigen-presenting molecules. Immunol Today 1998;19:362–368.

Powis SH, Trowsdale J. Human major histocompatibility complex genes. Behring Inst Mitt 1994;94:17–25.

Raulet DH. How γδ T cells make a living. Curr Biol 1994;4:246–251.

Roth DB. Generating antigen receptor diversity. Lewin B, ed. www.ergito.com Immunology module of Virtual Text. 2005: Chapter 5.

Salter RD, Benjamin RJ, Wesley PK, et al. A binding site for the T-cell co-receptor CD8 on the α_3 domain of HLA-A2. Nature 1990;345:41–46.

San José E, Sahuquillo AG, Bragado R, Alarcón B. Assembly of the TCR/CD3 complex: CD3 epsilon/delta and CD3 epsilon/gamma dimers associate indistinctly with both TCR alpha and TCR beta chains. Evidence for a double TCR heterodimer model. Eur J Immunol 1998;28:12–21.

Sloan-Lancaster J, Allen PM. Altered peptide–ligand induced partial T cell activation: molecular mechanisms and role in T cell biology. Annu Rev Immunol 1996;14:1–27.

Stern LJ, Wiley DC. Antigenic peptide binding by class I and class II histocompatibility proteins. Structure 1994;2:245–251.

Stern LJ, Brown JH, Jardetzky TS, et al. Crystal structure of the human class II MHC protein HLA-DR1 complexed with an influenza virus peptide. Nature 1994;368:215–221.

Weiss A, Littman DR. Signal transduction by lymphocyte antigen receptor. Cell 1994;76:263–274.

Zeng ZH, Castaño LH, Segelke B, Stura EA, Peterson PA, Wilson IA. The crystal structure of mouse CD1: an MHC-like fold with a large hydrophobic binding groove. Science 1997;277:339–345.

Critical thinking: Somatic hypermutation (see p. 494 for explanation)

1 Can you think of reasons why TCRs do not undergo somatic hypermutation?

The specificity of T cells (see p. 494 for explanations)

SM/J mice of the haplotype H-2^v were immunized with the λ repressor protein, a molecule with 102 amino acid residues. After 1 week, T cells were isolated from the animals and set up in culture with APCs and antigen. The ability of APCs to activate the T cells was determined in a lymphocyte proliferation assay (see Method Box 7.2, p. 160).

It was found that when APCs from SM/J mice were used in the culture the T cells were activated, but that when APCs from Balb/c mice were used (H-2^d) they were not activated. APCs from F1 (SM/J•Balb/c) mice were able to activate the T cells just as well as the APCs from the parental SM/J strain.

2 Explain why the SM/J cells and the F1 cells can present antigen to the T cells, but the Balb/c cells cannot.

Using the primed T cells from the SM/J mouse and APCs from the same strain, the investigation continues, but peptides of the λ repressor protein are used instead of intact antigen. It is found that a peptide corresponding to residues 80–94 of the intact protein is able to stimulate the T cells, but that other peptides are much less effective or ineffective. The table below shows the sequences of some of these peptides and their ability to activate the T cells when included in the culture at a concentration of 10 μM.

peptide	amino acid sequence	T cell activation
12–36	QLEDARRLKAIYEKKKNELGLSQESV	–
80–102	SPSIAREIYEMYEAVSMQPSLRS	+++
73–88	ILKVSVEEFSPSIAREIY	–
80–94	SPSIAREIYEMYEAVS	++
84–98	AREIYEMYEAVSMQP	–

3 Explain why peptides 80–102 and 80–94 activate the T cells while the others do not.

In a final experiment the T cells are stimulated with a mutated variant of peptide 80–94 with aspartate (D) substituted for isoleucine (I) at position 87 (bold type). It is found that the mutated peptide is able to stimulate the T cells as well as the original peptide, even when present at lower concentrations (1 μM).

4 What term is used to describe this kind of mutated peptide? What would you predict about the binding affinity of this peptide within the TCR–MHC–peptide complex?

Modes of
Immune
Response

Mechanisms of Innate Immunity

CHAPTER

6

SUMMARY

- **Innate immune responses do not depend on immune recognition by lymphocytes,** but have co-evolved with and are functionally integrated with the adaptive elements of the immune system.

- **The body's responses to damage include inflammation, phagocytosis, and clearance of debris and pathogens, and remodeling and regeneration of tissues.** Inflammation is a response that brings leukocytes and plasma molecules to sites of infection or tissue damage.

- **The phased arrival of leukocytes in inflammation depends on chemokines and adhesion molecules expressed on the endothelium.** Adhesion molecules fall into families that are structurally related. They include the cell adhesion molecules (CAMs) of the immunoglobulin supergene family (which interact with leukocyte integrins), and the selectins (which interact with carbohydrate ligands).

- **Leukocyte migration to lymphoid tissues is also controlled by chemokines.** Chemokines are a large group of signaling molecules that initiate chemotaxis and/or cellular activation. Most chemokines act on more than one receptor, and most receptors respond to more than one chemokine.

- **Plasma enzyme systems modulate inflammation and tissue remodeling.** The kinin system and mediators from mast cells including histamine contribute to the enhanced blood supply and increased vascular permeability at sites of inflammation.

- **Pathogen-associated molecular patterns (PAMPs) are distinctive biological macromolecules that can be recognized by the innate immune system.** Innate antimicrobial defenses include molecules of the collectin, ficolin, and pentraxin families, which can act as opsonins, either directly or by activating the complement system. Macrophages also have surface lectins, which allow them to directly bind to pathogens. The Toll-like receptors recognize various PAMPs and cause macrophage activation. Their signaling systems and actions are closely related to those used by inflammatory cytokines TNFα and IL-1.

- **Microbicidal proteins are part of the innate immune system.** Many cell types synthesize and secrete antimicrobial proteins.

INNATE IMMUNE RESPONSES DO NOT DEPEND ON IMMUNE RECOGNITION BY LYMPHOCYTES

The immune system deals with pathogens by means of a great variety of different types of immune response, but these can be broadly divided into:
- adaptive responses; and
- innate immunity.

The adaptive immune responses depend on the recognition of antigen by lymphocytes, a cell type that has evolved relatively recently – lymphocytes are present in all vertebrates, but not invertebrates, though lymphocyte-like cells are present in closely related phyla, including the tunicates and echinoderms (Fig. 6.1).

Q. What are the two key characteristics of adaptive immune responses?

A. They display a high level of specificity for the particular pathogen, and the responses show long-lasting memory.

Electron micrographs of lymphocyte-like cells

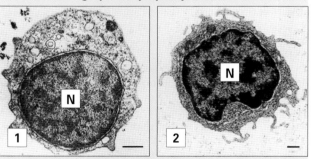

Fig. 6.1 **Electron micrographs of lymphocyte-like cells** from the tunicate *Ciona intestinalis* (**1**), and from a fish, the blenny, *Blennius pholis* (**2**). Note the similar morphology – both cells have a large nucleus and a thin rim of undifferentiated cytoplasm. Scale bar 0.5 μm. (Courtesy of Dr AF Rowley from Endeavour 1989:13;72–77. Copyright 1989 with permission from Elsevier)

Before the evolution of lymphocytes, and the emergence of specific antigen receptors – antibodies (see Chapter 3) and the T cell receptor (TCR, see Chapter 5) – we can infer that a number of different types of immune defense were already present in precursor organisms. Many of these systems have been retained in vertebrates and have continued to evolve alongside the adaptive immune system. Hence, in present-day mammals we see an integrated immune system in which different types of defense work in concert.

In reality it is quite artificial to try to segregate adaptive and innate immune responses. For example a macrophage:

- displays the very primitive immune defense of phagocytosis; but also
- expresses MHC molecules and acts as an antigen-presenting cell, a function that makes sense only in relation to the evolution of T cells.

We can identify some of the ancient innate immune defense systems because related systems are seen in distant phyla. For example, the family of **Toll-like receptors** (**TLRs**, see p. 143) present on mammalian macrophages and involved in phagocytosis were first identified in insects. We can therefore infer that the distant ancestor of mammals and insects had a receptor molecule of this type that probably recognized microbial components.

Q. Why would it be a mistake to think that the immune system seen in insects or worms was the precursor of the immune system seen in present-day vertebrates?

A. Both have been separately evolved for millions of years. The immune systems of worms and insects have developed to cope with the pathogens that they encounter in the context of their life cycles.

Having stated how the functional distinction between adaptive and immune systems is essentially artificial, this chapter outlines some of the immune defenses that do not depend on immune recognition by lymphocytes.

THE BODY'S RESPONSES TO DAMAGE INCLUDE INFLAMMATION

The body's response to tissue damage depends on:
- what has caused the damage;
- its location; and
- its severity.

In many cases damage can be caused by physical means, and does not involve infection or an adaptive immune response.

However, if an infection is present, the body's innate systems for limiting damage and repairing tissues work in concert with the adaptive immune responses. The overall process involves a number of overlapping stages, which typically take place over a number of days or weeks. These may include some or all of the following:
- stopping bleeding;
- acute inflammation;
- killing of pathogens, neutralizing toxins, limiting pathogen spread;
- phagocytosis of debris, pathogens, and dead cells;

- proliferation and mobilization of fibroblasts or other tissue cells to contain an infection and/or repair damage;
- removal or dissolution of blood clots and remodeling of the components of the extracellular matrix;
- regeneration of cells of the tissue and re-establishing normal structure and function.

Inflammation brings leukocytes and plasma molecules to sites of infection or tissue damage

Many immune responses lead to the complete elimination of a pathogen (sterile immunity), followed by resolution of the damage, disappearance of leukocytes from the tissue and full regeneration of tissue function – the response in such cases is referred to as **acute inflammation**.

Q. What three principal changes occur in the tissue during an acute inflammatory response?

A. An increased blood supply to the affected area, an increase in capillary permeability allowing larger serum molecules to enter the tissue, and an increase in leukocyte migration into the tissue (see Chapter 1).

In some cases an infection is not cleared completely. Most pathogenic organisms have developed systems to deflect the immune responses that would eliminate them. In this case the body often tries to contain the infection or minimize the damage it causes; nevertheless, the persistent antigenic stimulus and the cytotoxic effects of the pathogen itself lead to ongoing **chronic inflammation**.

The cells seen in acute and chronic inflammation are quite different, and reflect the phased arrival of different populations of leukocytes into a site of infection (Fig. 6.2). Consequently:
- sites of acute inflammation tend to have higher numbers of neutrophils and activated helper T cells; whereas
- sites of chronic inflammation have a higher proportion of macrophages, cytotoxic T cells, and even B cells.

The phased arrival of different populations of leukocytes at a site of inflammation is dependent on **chemokines** expressed on the endothelium (see below). These chemokines activate distinct leukocyte populations causing them to migrate into the tissue.

The cell types seen in sites of damage and the capacity of the tissue for repair and regeneration also depend greatly on the tissue involved. For example, in the brain the capacity for cell regeneration is very limited, so in chronic inflammatory diseases, such as multiple sclerosis, the area of damage often becomes occupied by scar tissue formed primarily by a specialized CNS cell type, the astrocyte.

The following sections explain the general principles of how inflammation develops, though the specific details depend on:
- the type of infection;
- the tissue; and
- the immune status of the individual.

The phased arrival of different populations of leukocytes into a site of infection

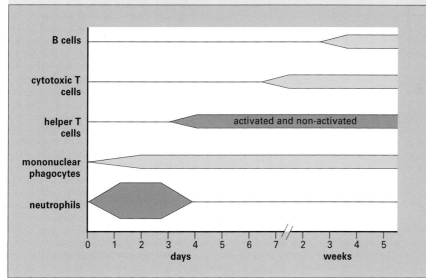

Fig. 6.2 Leukocytes enter sites of infection in phases. Sites of chronic inflammation have more macrophages and T cells.

Cytokines control the movement of leukocytes into tissues

Tissue damage leads to the release of a number of inflammatory cytokines, either from:
- patrolling leukocytes; or
- cells within the tissue, including resident mononuclear phagocytes.

The cytokine **tumor necrosis factor-α (TNFα)** is particularly important in this respect.

TNFα has many functions in the development of inflammation

TNFα is produced primarily by macrophages and other mononuclear phagocytes and has many functions in the development of inflammation and the activation of other leukocytes (Fig. 6.3).

Notably, TNFα induces the adhesion molecules and chemokines on the endothelium (which are required for the accumulation of leukocytes), and activates the microbicidal systems of phagocytes. In addition TNFα can induce **apoptosis** in susceptible cells.

TNFα and the related cytokines, the **lymphotoxins**, act on a family of receptors. One of the effects of these cytokines is to cause the activation of the transcription factor **NF-κB** (Fig. 6.4), which has been described as a master-switch of the immune system (see Fig. 9.21).

The signaling pathways that lead to NF-κB activation are evolutionarily very ancient, and are found in species as diverse as fruit flies, humans, and sea urchins.

IL-1 has wide-ranging functions that switch the body into a state to combat disease

Interleukin-1 (IL-1) is another important inflammatory cytokine. It is produced by many cell types in the body and shares some functions with TNFα, though both TNFα and IL-1 and their receptors are quite different.

For example, IL-1 induces adhesion molecules on endothelium that promote leukocyte migration.

IL-1 also has a number of distinct functions, of which the most important is the induction of fever. IL-1 acts directly on centers in the hypothalamus that control the body's temperature.

It is thought that the increase in temperature that accompanies inflammation in mammals gives the immune system a slight edge on the pathogens. A small increase in body temperature leads to much faster lymphocyte division, which means that the adaptive immune system (which relies on rapid expansion of pathogen-specific clones) can be mobilized more quickly.

IL-1 has an interesting variety of other constitutional effects. For example, it suppresses appetite and promotes one type of sleep. Another pro-inflammatory cytokine – interleukin-6 (IL-6), which is produced in the liver and by vascular endothelium in inflammation – also produces these constitutive symptoms, but this effect is due to the secondary induction of IL-1.

Taken together, we can see that in addition to its local effects in inflammation, IL-1 has wide-ranging functions that switch the body into a state to combat disease.

Interferons and NK cells delay viral spread

Viruses and many bacteria can replicate at an enormous rate and potentially have the capacity to overwhelm the individual before the adaptive immune system gets going – it takes several days to activate and expand clones of antigen-specific lymphocytes. During this time **interferons** (see Chapter 13, p. 247) and **NK cells** (see Chapter 10, p. 204) are particularly important in slowing the spread of infection:
- interferons act by inducing antiviral proteins, which limit the ability of a virus to replicate within a cell;
- NK cells have some capacity to recognize and kill virus-infected cells.

TNFα is a cytokine with many functions

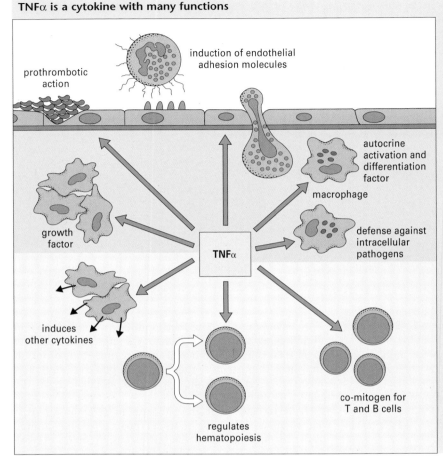

prothrombotic action

induction of endothelial adhesion molecules

autocrine activation and differentiation factor

macrophage

defense against intracellular pathogens

growth factor

TNFα

induces other cytokines

regulates hematopoiesis

co-mitogen for T and B cells

Fig. 6.3 TNFα has several functions in inflammation. It is prothrombotic and promotes leukocyte adhesion and migration (top). It has an important role in the regulation of macrophage activation and immune responses in tissues (center), and it also modulates hematopoiesis and lymphocyte development (bottom).

THE PHASED ARRIVAL OF LEUKOCYTES IN INFLAMMATION DEPENDS ON CHEMOKINES AND ADHESION MOLECULES

The mechanisms that control leukocyte migration into inflamed tissues have been carefully studied because of their biological and medical importance. These mechanisms are also applicable in principle to the cell movement that occurs between lymphoid tissues as the immune system develops and during normal life.

The routes that leukocytes take as they move around the body are determined by interactions between:
- circulating cells; and
- the endothelium of blood vessels.

Leukocyte migration is controlled by signaling molecules, which are expressed on the surface of the endothelium, and occurs principally in venules (Fig. 6.5). There are three reasons for this:
- the signaling molecules and adhesion molecules that control migration are selectively expressed in venules;
- the hemodynamic shear force in the venules is relatively low, and this allows time for leukocytes to receive signals from the endothelium and allows adhesion molecules on the two cell types to interact effectively;
- the endothelial surface charge is lower in venules (Fig. 6.6).

Although the patterns of leukocyte migration are complex, the basic mechanism appears to be universal. The initial interactions are set out in a three-step model (Fig. 6.7):
- leukocytes are slowed as they pass through a venule and roll on the surface of the endothelium before being halted – this is mediated primarily by adhesion molecules called **selectins** interacting with carbohydrates on glycoproteins;
- the slowed leukocytes now have the opportunity to respond to signaling molecules held at the endothelial surface – particularly important is the large group of cytokines called **chemokines,** which activate particular populations of leukocytes expressing the appropriate chemokine receptors;
- activation upregulates the affinity of the leukocytes' **integrins**, which now engage the cellular adhesion molecules on the endothelium to cause firm adhesion and initiate a program of migration.

Transendothelial migration is an active process involving both leukocytes and endothelial cells and occurs near the junctions between endothelial cells (Fig. 6.8).

There has been much controversy concerning whether leukocytes migrate through the junctions between endothelial cells or across the endothelium itself. In specialized tissues such as the brain and thymus, where the

Intracellular signaling pathways induced by TNFα

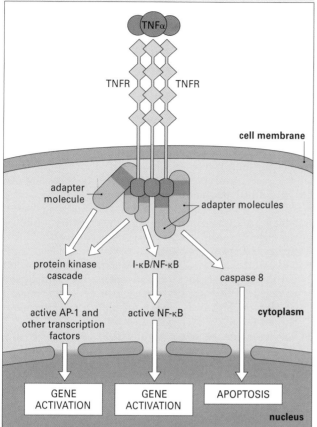

Fig. 6.4 TNFα induces the trimerization of the TNF receptor (TNFR) on the cell surface, which causes adapter molecules to be recruited to the receptor complex. One pathway leads to the activation of caspase 8 and apoptosis. Other pathways lead to the activation of transcription factors AP-1 and NF-κB, which activate many genes involved in adaptive and innate immune responses.

Leukocytes adhering to the wall of a venule

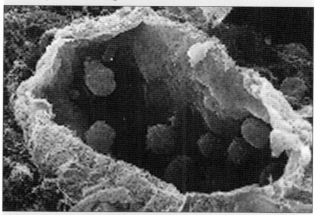

Fig. 6.5 Scanning electron micrograph showing leukocytes adhering to the wall of a venule in inflamed tissue. ×16 000. (Courtesy of Professor MJ Karnovsky)

Leukocyte migration across endothelium

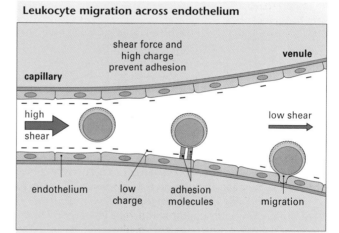

Fig. 6.6 Leukocytes circulating through a vascular bed may interact with venular endothelium via sets of surface adhesion molecules. In the venules, hemodynamic shear is low, surface charge on the endothelium is lower, and adhesion molecules are selectively expressed.

endothelium is connected by continuous tight junctions, it is clear that lymphocytes migrate across the endothelium in vacuoles and that the junctions do not break apart.

Migrating cells extend pseudopods down to the basement membrane and move beneath the endothelium using new sets of adhesion molecules. Enzymes are now released that digest the collagen and other components of the basement membrane, allowing cells to migrate into the tissue. Once there, the cells can respond to new sets of chemotactic stimuli, which allow them to position themselves appropriately in the tissue.

Leukocyte traffic into tissues is determined by where and when adhesion and signaling molecules are expressed

Intercellular adhesion molecules are membrane-bound proteins that allow one cell to interact with another. Often these molecules traverse the membrane and are linked to the cytoskeleton.

Q. Why is it important that cell adhesion molecules (CAMs) interact with the cytoskeleton?

A. By binding to the cytoskeleton the adhesion molecules allow a cell to gain traction on another cell or on the extracellular matrix, which allows the cell to move through tissues.

In many cases, a particular adhesion molecule can bind to more than one ligand, using different binding sites. Although the binding affinity of individual adhesion molecules to their ligands is usually low, clustering of the molecules in patches on the cell surface, means that the avidity of the interaction can be high.

131

Three-step model of leukocyte adhesion

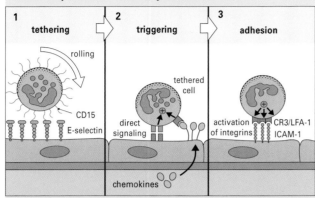

Fig. 6.7 The three-step model of leukocyte adhesion and activation is illustrated by a neutrophil, though different sets of adhesion molecules would be used by other leukocytes in different situations. **(1)** Tethering – the neutrophil is slowed in the circulation by interactions between E-selectin and carbohydrate groups on CD15, causing it to roll along the endothelial surface. **(2)** Triggering – the neutrophil can now receive signals from chemokines bound to the endothelial surface or by direct signaling from endothelial surface molecules. The longer a cell rolls along the endothelium, the longer it has to receive sufficient signal to trigger migration. **(3)** Adhesion – the triggering upregulates integrins (CR3 and LFA-1) so that they bind to ICAM-1 induced on the endothelium by inflammatory cytokines.

Lymphocyte migration

Fig. 6.8 Electron micrograph showing a lymphocyte adhering to brain endothelium close to the interendothelial cell junction in an animal with experimental allergic encephalomyelitis. Adhesion precedes transendothelial migration into inflammatory sites. (Courtesy of Dr C Hawkins)

Cells can modulate their interactions with other cell types by increasing the numbers of adhesion molecules on the surface or altering their affinity and avidity. They can alter the level of expression of adhesion molecules in two ways:
- many cells retain large intracellular stores of these molecules in vesicles, which can be directed to the cell surface within minutes following cellular activation;
- alternatively, new molecules can be synthesized and transported to the cell surface, a process that usually takes several hours.

Selectins bind to carbohydrates to slow the circulating leukocytes

The selectins include the molecules:
- E-selectin and P-selectin, which are expressed predominantly on endothelium and platelets; and
- L-selectin, which is expressed on some leukocytes (Fig. 6.9).

Selectins are transmembrane molecules with a number of extracellular domains homologous to those seen in complement control proteins (see Fig. 4.8). The extracellular region also has a domain related to the epidermal growth factor receptor and an N terminal domain that has lectin-like properties (i.e. it binds to carbohydrate residues), hence the name selectins.

The carbohydrate ligands for the selectins may be associated with several different proteins:
- at sites of inflammation, E-selectin and P-selectin, which are induced on activated endothelium, bind to the sialyl Lewis-X carbohydrate associated with CD15, present on many leukocytes;
- some of the selectin ligands are selectively expressed on particular populations of leukocytes, for example the molecule PSGL-1 (P-selectin glycoprotein ligand) present on TH1 cells binds to E- and P-selectin, but a variant found on TH2 cells does not.

When selectins bind to their ligands the circulating cells are slowed within the venules. Video pictures of cell migration show that the cells stagger along the endothelium. During this time the leukocytes have the opportunity of receiving migration signals from the endothelium. This is a process of signal integration – the

Selectins

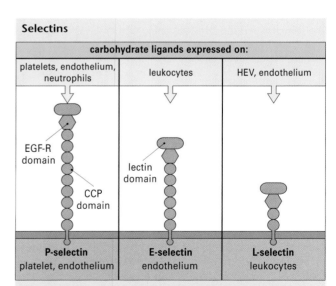

carbohydrate ligands expressed on:		
platelets, endothelium, neutrophils	leukocytes	HEV, endothelium
P-selectin platelet, endothelium	**E-selectin** endothelium	**L-selectin** leukocytes

Fig. 6.9 The structures of three selectins are shown. They have terminal lectin domains, which bind to carbohydrates on the cells listed. The EGF-R domain is homologous to a segment in the epidermal growth factor receptor. The CCP domains are homologous to domains found in complement control proteins, such as factor H, decay accelerating factor, and membrane cofactor protein (see Fig. 4.8).

more time the cell spends in the venule, the longer it has to receive sufficient signals to activate migration. If a leukocyte is not activated it detaches from the endothelium and returns to the venous circulation. A leukocyte may therefore circulate hundreds of times before it finds an appropriate place to migrate into the tissues.

Chemokines and other chemotactic molecules trigger the tethered leukocytes
Chemokines are small cytokines

The chemokines are a group of at least 40 small cytokines involved in cell migration, activation, and chemotaxis. They determine which cells will cross the endothelium and where they will move within the tissue. Most chemokines have two binding sites:

- one for their specific receptors; and
- a second for carbohydrate groups on proteoglycans (such as heparan sulfate), which allows them to attach to the luminal surface of endothelium (blood side), ready to trigger any tethered leukocytes (Fig. 6.10).

The chemokines may be produced by the endothelium itself. This depends on several factors including:

- the tissue;
- the presence of inflammatory cytokines; and
- hemodynamic forces.

In addition chemokines produced by cells in the tissues can be transported to the luminal side of the endothelium. Immune reactions or events occurring within the tissue can therefore induce the release of chemokines, which signal the inward migration of populations of leukocytes.

Q. **What advantage is there in having different types of inflammation occurring in different tissues?**

A. What constitutes an appropriate immune response depends on the pathogen, the amount of damage it is causing in a particular tissue, and the capacity of that tissue to repair and regenerate.

It is easiest to understand what chemokines do by considering their receptors

Chemokines fall into four different families, based on the spacing of conserved cysteine (C) residues. For example:

- α-chemokines have a CXC structure; and
- β-chemokines a CC structure.

All chemokines act via receptors that have seven transmembrane segments (**7tm receptors**) linked to GTP-binding proteins (**G-proteins**), which cause cell activation.

Most chemokines act on more than one receptor, and most receptors will respond to several chemokines. Because of this complexity, it is easiest to understand what chemokines do by considering their receptors:

- the receptors for the CXC chemokines are called CXCR1, CXCR2, and so on; while
- the receptors for the CC chemokines are called CCR1, CCR2, etc.

Until recently most chemokines had a descriptive name and acronym such as macrophage chemotactic protein-1 (MCP-1). The current nomenclature describes them according to their type, hence MCP-1 is CCL2, meaning that it is a **ligand** for the CC family of chemokine receptors (Fig. 6.11). A full list of chemokines is given in Appendix 4.

The chemokine receptors are selectively expressed on particular populations of leukocytes (see Fig. 6.11) and this determines which cells can respond to signals coming from the tissues.

The profile of chemokine receptors on a cell depends on its type and state of differentiation. For example:

- all T cells express CCR1;
- TH2 cells preferentially express CCR3; and
- TH1 cells preferentially express CCR5 and CXCR3.

After activation in lymph nodes, the levels of CXCR3 on a T cell increase, so that it becomes more responsive for the chemokines CXCL9, CXCL10, and CXCL11, which

Chemokines

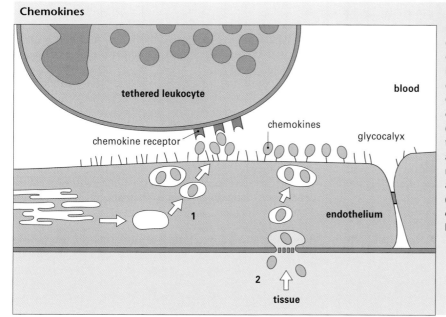

Fig. 6.10 Chemokines bind to glycosaminoglycans on endothelium via one binding site while a second site interacts with chemokine receptors expressed on the surface of the leukocyte. Chemokines may be synthesized by the endothelial cell and stored in vesicles (Weibel–Palade bodies) to be released to the luminal surface (blood side) following activation (1). Alternatively chemokines may be produced by cells in the tissues and transported across the endothelium (2). Cells in the tissue can therefore signal either directly or indirectly to circulating leukocytes.

Some chemokine receptors and their principal ligands

	TH1	MØ	TH2	eosinophil	basophil	neutrophil
	(CCR1)	CCR1		(CCR1)	CCR1	(CCR1)
	CCR2	CCR2	CCR2	CCR2	CCR2	
	CCR5 ●–● CCR5		CCR3 ●–● CCR3	●–● CCR3		CXCR1
	CXCR3					CXCR2
CCL3	+	+		+	+	+
CCL4	+	+				
CCL5	+	+	+	+	+	+
CCL2	+	+	+	+	+	
CCL7,8	+	+	+	+	+	+
CCL13	+	+	+	+	+	
CCL11			+	+	+	
CXCL8						+
CXCL1,2,3						+
CXCL9,10,11	+					

Fig. 6.11 Some of the chemokine receptors found on particular leukocytes and the chemokines they respond to are listed. The cells are grouped according the principal types of effector response. Note that TH1 cells and mononuclear phagocytes both express chemokine receptor CCR5, which allows them to respond to chemokine CCL3, while TH2 cells, eosinophils, and basophils express CCR3, which allows them to respond to CCL11. This allows selective recruitment of sets of leukocytes into areas with particular types of immune/inflammatory response. Both groups of cells express chemokine receptors CCR1 and CCR2, which allow responses to macrophage chemotactic proteins (CCL2, CCL7, CCL8, and CCL13). Neutrophils express chemokine receptors CXCR1 and CXCR2, which allow them to respond to CXCL8 (IL-8) and CXCL1 and CXCL2. Bracketed entries indicate that only a subset of cells express that receptor. Full details are given in Appendix 4.

activate that receptor. As a consequence, antigen-activated lymphocytes are more readily triggered to enter sites of inflammation where these chemokines are expressed.

Once a leukocyte has crossed the endothelium, it is capable of responding to a new set of chemokines, which direct its migration through the tissues.

Chemokines thus work in a hierarchical way, with a cell receiving successive signals for the next destination.

Other molecules are also chemotactic for neutrophils and macrophages

Several other molecules are chemotactic for neutrophils and macrophages, both of which have an f.Met-Leu-Phe (f.MLP) receptor. This receptor binds to peptides blocked at the N terminus by formylated methionine. Because prokaryotes (e.g. bacteria) initiate all protein translation with this amino acid, whereas eukaryotes do not, this provides a simple specific signal for the presence of bacteria, towards which phagocytes should move.

Neutrophils and macrophages also have receptors for:
- C5a, which is a fragment of a complement component generated at sites of inflammation following complement activation; and
- LTB4, which is generated at sites of inflammation following activation of a variety of cells, particularly macrophages and mast cells.

In addition, molecules generated by the blood clotting system, notably fibrin peptide B and thrombin, attract phagocytes, though many molecules such as these only act indirectly by inducing chemokines.

The first leukocytes to arrive at a site of inflammation, if activated, are able to release chemokines that attract others. For example:
- CXCL8 released by activated monocytes can induce neutrophil and basophil chemotaxis;
- similarly, macrophage activation leads to metabolism of arachidonic acid with release of LTB4.

Like chemokines, these other chemotactic molecules, including C5a and fMLP, act via 7tm receptors.

Q. The innate immune system has the capacity to recognize pathogen-associated molecular patterns (PAMPs). Which of the chemotactic molecules described above has a PAMP?

A. fMLP. It is the only molecule that comes from bacteria; all other chemotactic molecules are produced by cells of the body.

Integrins on the leukocytes bind to CAMs on the endothelium

Activation of leukocytes via their chemokine receptors initiates the next stage of migration.

Leukocytes and many other cells in the body interact with other cells and components of the extracellular matrix using a group of molecules called integrins.

In the third step of leukocyte adhesion (see Fig. 6.7), the leukocytes develop a firm adhesion to the endothelium using their surface integrins. Cell activation promotes this step in three ways:
- it can cause integrins to be released from intracellular stores;
- it can cause clustering of integrins on the cell surface into high-avidity patches;
- most importantly, the cell activation induced by the chemokines causes the integrins to become associated with the cytoskeleton and can switch them into a high-affinity form (Fig. 6.12) – this type of signaling is called inside-out signaling because activation inside the cell causes a change in the affinity of the extracellular portion of the integrin.

Normally the binding affinity of integrins for the CAMs on the endothelium is relatively weak, but when sufficient interactions take place, the cells adhere firmly.

Many of the CAMs on the endothelium have immunoglobulin-like domains (i.e. they belong to the immunoglobulin superfamily).

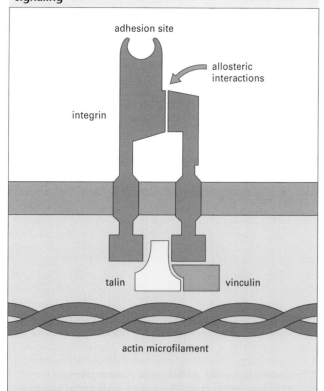

The affinity of integrins is controlled by inside-out signaling

Fig. 6.12 Activation of the cell causes a change in the position of the two chains of the integrin, which become linked to the cytoskeleton via the adapter molecules vinculin and talin. The association produces an allosteric change in the extracellular portion of the molecule, causing the binding site to open and allowing the integrin to attach to its ligand.

Some of the CAMs are constitutively expressed, while others are specifically induced on particular endothelia or at sites of inflammation.

Integrins and CAMs are very important groups of molecules

INTEGRINS COMPRISE A MAJOR GROUP OF ADHESION MOLECULES – Integrins are present on many cells, including leukocytes. Each member of this large family of molecules consists of two non-covalently bound polypeptides (α and β), both of which traverse the membrane.

Integrins fall into three major families depending on which β chain they have, because any β chain can associate with several α chains. Broadly speaking:
- the β_1-integrins are involved in binding of cells to extracellular matrix;
- the β_2-integrins are involved in leukocyte adhesion to endothelium or to other immune cells; and
- the β_3-integrins (cytoadhesins) are involved in the interactions of platelets and neutrophils at inflammatory sites or sites of vascular damage.

However, there are several exceptions to this rule, and some α chains can associate with more than one β chain (Fig. 6.13).

The ability of integrins to bind to their ligands depends on divalent cations. For example, LFA-1 ($\alpha_L\beta_2$-integrin) has a Mg^{2+} ion coordinated at the center of a binding site, which accommodates an aspartate residue from the ligand. Activation of the integrin causes the binding site to open, allowing access for the aspartate side chain.

Many of the integrins can bind to more than one ligand. For example:
- LFA-1 present on most lymphocytes binds to both intercellular CAM-1 (ICAM-1) and ICAM-2, which are expressed on endothelium;
- VLA-4 ($\alpha_4\beta_1$-integrin) binds to vascular CAM-1 (VCAM-1) expressed on endothelium, or to fibronectin (an extracellular matrix component).

ENDOTHELIAL CAMS INCLUDE ICAM-1, ICAM-2, VCAM-1, AND MAdCAM-1 – The CAMs on the endothelium that interact with integrins are all members of the immunoglobulin supergene family. They include ICAM-1 and ICAM-2, VCAM-1, and mucosal addressin CAM (MAdCAM-1) (Fig. 6.14). All members of this family are expressed or inducible on vascular endothelium:
- ICAM-1 and VCAM-1 are both induced by inflammatory cytokines;
- ICAM-2 is constitutively expressed at low levels on some endothelia and is downregulated by inflammatory cytokines.

Integrins

integrin		ligands	expression
VLA-1	$\alpha_1\beta_1$	?	T cells, fibroblasts
VLA-2	$\alpha_2\beta_1$	collagen	activated T cells, platelets
VLA-3	$\alpha_3\beta_1$	laminin, collagen, fibronectin	kidney, thyroid
VLA-4	$\alpha_4\beta_1$	VCAM-1, fibronectin	lymphocytes, some phagocytes
VLA-5	$\alpha_5\beta_1$	fibronectin	some leukocytes, platelets
VLA-6	$\alpha_6\beta_1$	laminin	widely distributed
LPAM-1	$\alpha_4\beta_7$	MAdCAM-1 (VCAM-1)	some T cells
	$\alpha_E\beta_7$	E-cadherin	intraepithelial T cells
LFA-1	$\alpha_L\beta_2$	ICAM-1, ICAM-2 (ICAM-3)	most leukocytes
CR3	$\alpha_M\beta_2$	C3b, C4b, ICAM-1	mononuclear phagocytes, neutrophils
CR4	$\alpha_X\beta_2$	C3b, C4b, ICAM-1 ?	macrophages
leukointegrin	$\alpha_D\beta_2$	ICAM-3, VCAM-1	macrophages

Fig. 6.13 The table gives the properties of some of the major integrins involved in leukocyte binding to endothelium or extracellular matrix.

Endothelial cell adhesion molecules

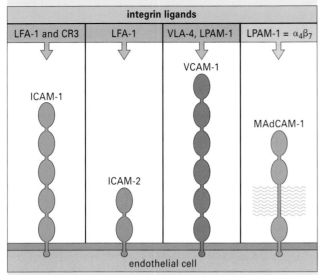

Fig. 6.14 The molecules ICAM-1, ICAM-2, VCAM-1, and MAdCAM-1 are illustrated diagrammatically with their immunoglobulin-like domains. Their integrin ligands (see Fig. 6.13) are listed above. MAdCAM-1 also has a heavily glycosylated segment, which binds L-selectin.

Mucosal addressin cell adhesion molecule of endothelium

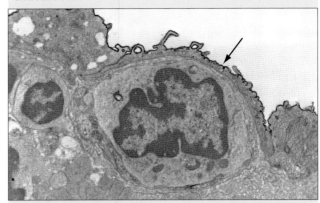

Fig. 6.15 The immunoelectron micrograph has been stained to show MAdCAM-1 as a dark border (arrow) on the luminal surface of endothelium. In this instance the molecule is expressed on brain endothelium in chronic relapsing experimental allergic encephalomyelitis induced by immunization of Biozzi AB/H mice with myelin basic protein. (Reproduced from Immunology, O'Neill JK, Butter C 1991;72:520–525. Copyright 1991 with permission from Blackwell Publishing)

The two N terminal domains of ICAM-1 are homologous to those of ICAM-2 and both molecules interact with LFA-1. (There are additional ligands for LFA-1, ICAM-3, and ICAM-4, which are expressed on lymphocytes.)

MAdCAM-1 is a composite molecule that includes:
*   two immunoglobulin-like domains that interact with an integrin; and
*   a glycosylated segment that can interact with selectins.

MAdCAM-1 was first identified on mucosal lymph node endothelium, but can also be induced at sites of chronic inflammation (Fig. 6.15)

Leukocyte migration in inflammation is controlled by both leukocytes and endothelium

Although the mechanisms described above are applicable to all leukocyte migration, the following discussion concerns just inflammation. Several factors account for the pattern of leukocyte accumulation, including:
*   the state of activation of the lymphocytes or phagocytes – the expression of adhesion molecules and their functional affinity vary depending on the type of cell and whether it has been activated by antigen, cytokines, or cellular interactions;
*   the types of adhesion molecule expressed by the vascular endothelium, which is related to its anatomical site and whether it has been activated by cytokines;
*   the particular chemotactic molecules and cytokines present – receptors vary between leukocyte populations so that particular chemotactic agents act selectively on some cells only.

Chemokines and adhesion molecules determine which leukocytes migrate where

Different sets of adhesion molecules and chemotactic agents are used by each type of cell.

E-selectin and P-selectin slow circulating leukocytes

When tissue is damaged, cells, including mononuclear phagocytes, release inflammatory cytokines such as TNFα or IL-1, which induce synthesis and expression of E-selectin.

In vitro, cells transfected with the gene for E-selectin bind neutrophils strongly, and this suggests that the slowing of neutrophils by E-selectin is a critical first step in neutrophil migration.

P-selectin acts similarly to E-selectin, but is held ready-made in the Weibel–Palade bodies of endothelium and released to the cell surface if the endothelium becomes activated or damaged. Both E-selectin and P-selectin can slow circulating platelets or leukocytes.

Different chemokines cause different types of leukocyte to accumulate

In the second step of migration, neutrophils are triggered by chemokines such as CXCL8 synthesized by cells in the tissue, or by the endothelium itself. CXCL8 acts on two different chemokine receptors – CXCR1 and CXCR2 (see Fig. 6.11) – to initiate neutrophil migration.

In some tissues different sets of chemokines cause the local accumulation of other groups of leukocytes. For example:
*   in the bronchi of individuals with asthma, CCL11 (eotaxin) is released, which causes the accumulation of eosinophils – CCL11 acts on CCR3, which is also

present on TH2 cells and basophils, so by releasing one chemokine, the tissue can signal to three different kinds of cell to migrate into the tissue and this particular set of cells is characteristic of the cellular infiltrates in asthma;

• in sites of chronic inflammation, the chemokines CXCL10 and CCL2 are released by endothelium in response to interferon-γ (IFNγ) and TNFα – CXCL10 acts on activated TH1 cells (via CXCR3), while CCL2 acts on macrophages (via CCR5); consequently macrophages and TH1 cells tend to accumulate at sites of chronic inflammation.

Q. In what type of inflammatory reaction would you expect to see the production of CXCL10 and the accumulation of activated macrophages?

A. In chronic inflammatory reactions.

Some endothelial adhesion molecules are induced by cytokines

Some endothelial adhesion molecules are induced at sites of inflammation by cytokines, particularly ICAM-1 and VCAM-1 (Fig. 6.16). Their level of expression is also tissue-specific. For example:

• ICAM-1 is expressed at higher levels on brain endothelium than VCAM-1;
• ICAM-I and VCAM-1 are equally expressed in skin endothelium.

By contrast ICAM-2 is not induced by inflammatory cytokines, and it has been suggested that ICAM-2 determines the basal level of binding of leukocytes to different types of endothelium, while ICAM-1 and VCAM-1 mediate migration into sites of inflammation.

ICAM-1 and ICAM-2 both interact with LFA-1 ($\alpha_L\beta_2$-integrin, see Fig. 6.13), which is present on most leukocytes, whereas VCAM-1 interacts with VLA-4 ($\alpha_4\beta_1$-integrin). Both of these integrins are upregulated on

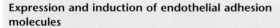

Expression and induction of endothelial adhesion molecules

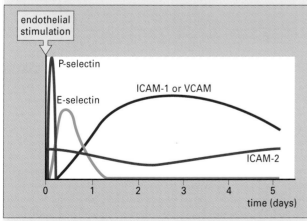

endothelial stimulation

P-selectin

ICAM-1 or VCAM

E-selectin

ICAM-2

0 1 2 3 4 5
time (days)

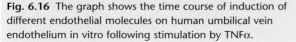

Fig. 6.16 The graph shows the time course of induction of different endothelial molecules on human umbilical vein endothelium in vitro following stimulation by TNFα.

activated lymphocytes, so the process of cell activation induces both:

• the chemokine receptors that allow activated lymphocytes to respond to inflammatory cytokines; and
• the integrins that allow activated lymphocytes to migrate.

CR3 is an important integrin expressed on monocytes

Another important integrin is CR3 ($\alpha_M\beta_2$-integrin, see Fig. 6.13), which is expressed on monocytes. Its function in phagocyte accumulation has been pinpointed by studies in vivo using antibodies to CR3, which inhibit phagocyte migration.

It is notable that a group of patients who have leukocyte adhesion deficiency (LAD) syndrome and suffer from severe infections due to poor phagocyte accumulation, are deficient in all β_2-integrins (LFA-1, CR3, etc., see Fig. 6.13).

CR3 recognizes a site on ICAM-1 separate from that recognized by LFA-1.

Lymphocyte binding to endothelium can be modulated using antibodies to adhesion molecules or inactive analogs of chemokines, and this holds out prospects for therapy of diseases where immunopathological inflammation occurs.

VLA molecules allow interaction with extracellular matrix and belong to the β_1-integrin group

Once leukocytes have crossed the endothelium and entered the tissues, they interact with the proteins of the extracellular matrix (collagen, laminin, fibronectin, etc.), as well as the tissue cells.

As lymphocytes leave the blood vessel they lose some of their surface molecules (e.g. L-selectin), which are no longer required. The functional phenotype changes from that of a circulating cell to one adapted to move through tissues.

Many of the molecules that allow interaction with extracellular matrix belong to the β_1-integrin group, and are known as very late antigens (VLAs), so-called because they were first identified on the T cell surface at a late stage after T cell activation. The whole group of β_1-integrins are now referred to as VLA molecules, though most of them are not just expressed on lymphocytes. This group includes:

• receptors for collagen (VLA-2 and VLA-3);
• receptors for laminin (VLA-3 and VLA-6); and
• receptors for fibronectin (VLA-3, VLA-4, and VLA-5).

The fact that some of these molecules appear late after lymphocyte activation suggests that cells go through a program of differentiation, and that the ability to interact with extracellular matrix is one of the last functions to develop.

LEUKOCYTE MIGRATION TO LYMPHOID TISSUES IS ALSO CONTROLLED BY CHEMOKINES

Migration of leukocytes into lymphoid tissues is also controlled by chemokines and adhesion molecules on the endothelium.

Up to 25% of lymphocytes that enter a lymph node via the blood may be diverted across the HEV. In contrast, only a tiny proportion of those circulating through other tissues will cross the regular venular endothelium at each transit. HEVs are therefore particularly important in controlling lymphocyte recirculation. Normally they are only present in the secondary lymphoid tissues, but they may be induced at sites of chronic inflammation.

In addition to their peculiar shape, HEV cells express distinct sets of heavily glycosylated sulfated adhesion molecules, which bind to circulating T cells and direct them to the lymphoid tissue.

The HEVs in different lymphoid tissues have different sets of adhesion molecules. In particular, there are separate molecules controlling migration to:
- Peyer's patches;
- mucosal lymph nodes; and
- other lymph nodes.

These molecules were previously called vascular addressins, and their expression on different HEVs accounts for the way in which lymphocytes relocalize to their own lymphoid tissue.

Naive lymphocytes express L-selectin, which contributes to their attachment to carbohydrate ligands on HEVs in mucosal and peripheral lymph nodes. Once they have stopped on the HEV, migrating lymphocytes may use the integrin $\alpha_4\beta_7$ (LPAM-1, see Fig. 6.13) to bind to MAdCAM on the HEV of mucosal lymph nodes or Peyer's patches.

Because the expression of $\alpha_4\beta_7$ allows migration to mucosal lymphoid tissue, whereas $\alpha_4\beta_1$ allows attachment to VCAM-1 on activated endothelium or fibronectin in tissues, expression of one or other of these molecules can alternately be used by naive lymphocytes migrating to lymphoid tissue or activated T cells to inflammatory sites.

Chemokines are important in controlling cell traffic to lymphoid tissues

Chemokines are also important in controlling cell traffic to lymphoid tissues. Naive T cells:
- express chemokine receptors CCR7 and CXCR4, which allow them to respond to chemokines expressed in lymphoid tissues;
- also respond to chemokines CCL18 and CCL19 produced by dendritic cells, which is thought to direct them to the appropriate T cell areas of the lymph node where dendritic cells can present antigen to them.

Once T cells have been activated they lose CXCR4 and CCR7, but gain new chemokine receptors (see Fig. 6.11), which allow them to respond to different chemokines (e.g. those produced at sites of inflammation).

Naive B cells also express:
- CCR7 and CXCR4, involved in migration to secondary lymphoid tissues;

- CXCR5, a receptor for CXCL13, which appears to be required for localization to lymphoid follicles within the lymph nodes.

Cells moving into lymphoid tissue therefore respond sequentially to signals on the endothelium and signals from the different areas within the tissue (Fig. 6.17).

PLASMA ENZYME SYSTEMS MODULATE INFLAMMATION AND TISSUE REMODELING

The change in vascular permeability is another important component of inflammation. However, whereas cell migration occurs across venules, serum exudation occurs primarily across capillaries where blood pressure is higher and the vessel wall is thinnest. This event is controlled in two ways:
- blood supply to the area increases;
- there is an increase in capillary permeability caused by retraction of the endothelial cells and possibly also by increased vesicular transport across the endothelium – this permits larger molecules to traverse the endothelium than would ordinarily be capable of doing so, and so allows antibody and molecules of the plasma enzyme systems to reach the inflammatory site.

Chemokines and cell migration into lymphoid tissue

Fig. 6.17 Cell migration occurs in stages. Naive T cells express CCR7, which allows them to respond to CCL21 expressed by secondary lymphoid tissues (1). Once the cells have migrated across the endothelium, the same receptor can respond to signals from CCL19 produced by dendritic cells (2), which promotes interactions with the T cells in the paracortex (T cell area) of the lymph node. B cells also express CCR7 and use similar mechanisms to migrate into the lymphoid tissues (1). However, they also express CXCR5, which allows them to respond to CXCL13, a chemokine produced in lymphoid follicles (2) – B cells are therefore directed to the B cell areas of the node. Mice lacking CXCR5 do not develop normal lymphoid follicles.

The four major plasma enzyme systems that have an important role in hemostasis and control of inflammation are the:
- clotting system;
- fibrinolytic (plasmin) system;
- kinin system; and
- complement system (see Chapter 4).

The kinin system generates powerful vasoactive mediators

The kinin system generates the mediators bradykinin and lysyl-bradykinin (kallidin).

Bradykinin is a very powerful vasoactive nonapeptide that causes:
- venular dilation;
- increased vascular permeability; and
- smooth muscle contraction.

Bradykinin is generated following the activation of Hageman factor (XII) of the blood clotting system, whereas tissue kallikrein is generated following activation of the plasmin system or by enzymes released from damaged tissues (Fig. 6.18).

The plasmin system has an important role in tissue remodeling and regeneration

The plasmin system can be activated by a soluble or a tissue-derived plasminogen activator, which leads to the enzymatic conversion of plasminogen into plasmin. Plasmin itself:
- was originally identified by its ability to dissolve fibrin;
- has several other activities, in particular it activates some metalloproteases – enzymes that are required for the breakdown and remodeling of collagen (Fig. 6.19);

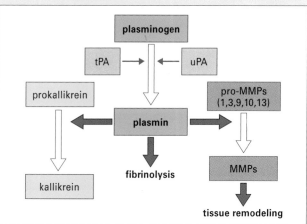

The plasmin system

Fig. 6.19 Plasmin is generated by the enzymatic activity of plasminogen activators. (MMP, matrix metalloproteinase; tPA, tissue plasminogen activator; uPA, urokinase plasminogen activator)

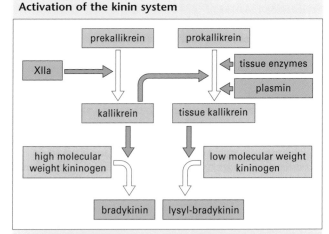

Activation of the kinin system

Fig. 6.18 Activated Hageman factor (XIIa) acts on prekallikrein to generate kallikrein, which in turn releases bradykinin from high molecular weight kininogen (HMWK). Prekallikrein and HMWK circulate together in a complex. Various enzymes activate prokallikrein to tissue kallikrein, which releases lysyl-bradykinin from low molecular weight kininogen. Bradykinin and lysyl-bradykinin are both extremely powerful vasodilators.

- additionally can promote angiogenesis (the formation of new blood vessels) by causing the release of cytokines that induce proliferation and migration of endothelial cells.

Auxiliary cells are also sources of inflammatory mediators

Auxiliary cells, including mast cells, basophils, and platelets, are also very important in the initiation and development of acute inflammation. They act as sources of the vasoactive mediators histamine and 5-hydroxytryptamine (serotonin), which produce vasodilation and increased vascular permeability.

Mast cells, basophils, and platelets release a variety of mediators

Many of the proinflammatory effects of C3a and C5a result from their ability to trigger mast cell granule release, because they can be blocked by antihistamines.

Mast cells and basophils are also:
- a route by which the adaptive immune system can trigger inflammation – IgE sensitizes these cells by binding to their IgE receptors and the cells can then be activated by antigen;
- an important source of slow-reacting inflammatory mediators, including the leukotrienes and prostaglandins, which contribute to a delayed component of acute inflammation and are synthesized and act some hours after mediators like histamine, which are pre-formed and released immediately following mast cell activation (see Chapter 23).

Fig. 6.20 lists the principal mediators of acute inflammation, and the interaction of the immune system with complement and other inflammatory systems is shown in Fig. 6.21.

Inflammatory mediators

mediator	main source	actions
histamine	mast cells, basophils	increased vascular permeability, smooth muscle contraction, chemokinesis
5-hydroxytryptamine (5HT – serotonin)	platelets, mast cells (rodent)	increased vascular permeability, smooth muscle contraction
platelet activating factor (PAF)	basophils, neutrophils, macrophages	mediator release from platelets, increased vascular permeability, smooth muscle contraction, neutrophil activation
IL-8 (CXCL8)	mast cells, endothelium, monocytes and lymphocytes	polymorph and monocyte localization
C3a	complement C3	mast cell degranulation, smooth muscle contraction
C5a	complement C5	mast cell degranulation, neutrophil and macrophage chemotaxis, neutrophil activation, smooth muscle contraction, increased capillary permeability
bradykinin	kinin system (kininogen)	vasodilation, smooth muscle contraction, increased capillary permeability, pain
fibrinopeptides and fibrin breakdown products	clotting system	increased vascular permeability, neutrophil and macrophage chemotaxis
prostaglandin E_2 (PGE$_2$)	cyclo-oxygenase pathway, mast cells	vasodilation, potentiates increased vascular permeability produced by histamine and bradykinin
leukotriene B_4 (LTB$_4$)	lipoxygenase pathway, mast cells	neutrophil chemotaxis, synergizes with PGE$_2$ in increasing vascular permeability
leukotriene D_4 (LTD$_4$)	lipoxygenase pathway	smooth muscle contraction, increasing vascular permeability

Fig. 6.20 The major inflammatory mediators that control blood supply and vascular permeability or modulate cell movement.

Platelets may be activated by:
- immune complexes; or
- platelet activating factor (PAF) from neutrophils, basophils, and macrophages.

Activated platelets release mediators. This is thought to be important in type II and type III hypersensitivity reactions (see Chapter 24).

Lymphocytes and monocytes release mediators that control the accumulation and activation of other cells

Once lymphocytes and monocytes have arrived at a site of infection or inflammation, they can also release mediators, which control the later accumulation and activation of other cells. For example:
- activated macrophages release the chemokine CCL3 (MIP-1α) and the leukotriene LTB$_4$, both of which are chemotactic and encourage further monocyte migration;
- lymphocytes can modulate later lymphocyte traffic by the release of chemokines and inflammatory cytokines, particularly IFNγ.

Q. What determines whether an immune response is acute or chronic?

A. Ultimately the outcome of an acute inflammatory response is related to the fate of the antigen. If the initiating antigen or pathogen persists, then leukocyte accumulation continues and a chronic inflammatory reaction develops. If the antigen is cleared then no further leukocyte activation occurs and the inflammation resolves.

In recurrent inflammatory reactions and in chronic inflammation the patterns of cell migration are different from those seen in an acute response.

We now know that the patterns of inflammatory cytokines and chemokines vary over the time course of an inflammatory reaction and this can be related to the successive waves of migration of different types of leukocyte into the inflamed tissue.

Chronic inflammation is characteristic of sites of persistent infection (see Chapter 9) or in autoimmune reactions where the antigen cannot ultimately be eradicated (see Chapter 20).

PAMPs ARE DISTINCTIVE BIOLOGICAL MACROMOLECULES THAT CAN BE RECOGNIZED BY THE INNATE IMMUNE SYSTEM

The molecules in this section are divided into families according to structure. Some of each family are also **acute phase proteins** (i.e. they are present in the blood and their levels increase during infection).

The immune system in acute inflammation

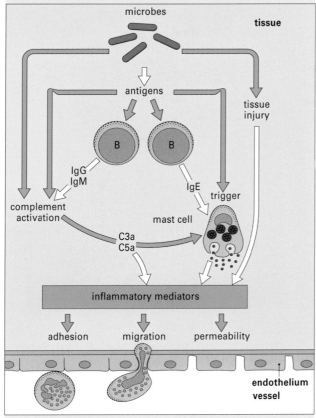

Fig. 6.21 The adaptive immune system modulates inflammatory processes via the complement system. Antigens (e.g. from microorganisms) stimulate B cells to produce antibodies including IgE, which binds to mast cells, while IgG and IgM activate complement. Complement can also be activated directly via the alternative pathway (see Fig. 4.7). When triggered by antigen, sensitized mast cells release their granule-associated mediators and eicosanoids (products of arachidonic acid metabolism, including prostaglandins and leukotrienes). In association with complement (which can also trigger mast cells via C3a and C5a), the mediators induce local inflammation, facilitating the arrival of leukocytes and more plasma enzyme system molecules.

Once phagocytes have entered the tissues, they bind, internalize, and destroy pathogens. Many pathogens have distinctive biological macromolecules on their surface, which can be recognized by elements of the innate immune system. These distinctive molecular structures are called **pathogen-associated molecular patterns (PAMPs)**.

In many cases, the innate recognition mechanisms allow phagocytes to bind and internalize the pathogens and this is often associated with activation of the phagocytes, which enhances their microbicidal activity.

The binding of the pathogen to the phagocyte can be direct or indirect:

- direct recognition involves the surface receptors on the phagocyte directly recognizing surface molecules on the pathogen;

- indirect recognition involves the deposition of serum-derived molecules onto the pathogen surface and their subsequent binding to receptors on the phagocyte (i.e. the process of opsonization) (Fig. 6.22)

Q. Give an example of an innate immune recognition system that allows macrophages to recognize and phagocytose bacteria.
A. Complement C3b can become deposited on bacteria following activation of either the lectin pathway or the alternative pathway (see Fig. 4.4). The deposited C3b acts as an opsonin and is recognized by the receptors CR1, CR3, and CR4 on macrophages (see Fig. 4.12).

Collectins and ficolins opsonize pathogens and inhibit invasiveness

The **mannan-binding lectin (MBL)** activates the lectin pathway and is one member of a group of serum proteins that recognize carbohydrates and act as opsonins (see Fig. 4.4). Each member of the group has subunits formed of a triple-helical collagenous tail and a lectin head (Fig. 6.23). A number of subunits may be linked together in the complete molecule and the overall structure of these molecules is similar to that of C1q (see Fig. 4.5), though C1q is not itself a lectin. Most of these molecules are produced by the liver and circulate in the blood, but the **surfactant proteins** are produced by lung epithelium.

MBL and the surfactant proteins are acute phase proteins

The synthesis of acute phase proteins is greatly increased in response to infection. Some acute phase proteins such as MBL increase 2–3-fold following infection, but others, for example C-reactive protein (CRP, see below), may increase several 100-fold.

By binding to the surface of bacteria or viruses the acute phase proteins can inhibit their ability to invade the tissues. For example surfactant protein-A (SP-A) binds to the glycosylated hemagglutin molecule on the surface of influenza virus and reduces the ability of the virus to infect cells.

In addition binding of collectins and ficolins can directly opsonize pathogens for uptake by phagocytes, though the receptors on the cells that bind to these molecules are not well defined.

Because some collectins and ficolins promote activation of the complement alternative pathway, their opsonizing activity may ultimately be mediated by the interaction of C3b with complement receptors.

The pentraxins CRP and SAP also opsonize bacteria

Two further acute phase proteins, **CRP** and **serum amyloid-P (SAP)**, both produced by the liver, are important opsonins. These molecules belong to a family called **pentraxins**, which have a characteristic protein fold.

CRP is a pentameric protein that binds to phosphorylcholine present on, for example, pneumococci and promotes their phagocytosis by binding to C1q

The binding of pathogen to the macrophage can be direct or indirect

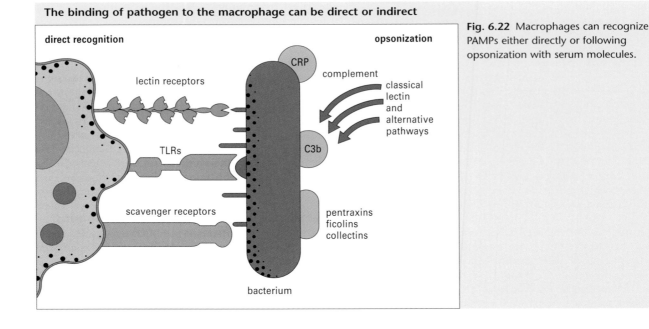

Fig. 6.22 Macrophages can recognize PAMPs either directly or following opsonization with serum molecules.

Structure of collectins and ficolins

Fig. 6.23 Collectins and ficolins are oligomers of triple-helical molecules with C-type lectin domains. They recognize a variety of microbial PAMPs.

and activating the complement classical pathway (see Fig. 4.4).

Because of its rapid synthesis in response to IL-6, CRP levels are often used clinically as a marker of infection or inflammation.

SAP also binds to bacteria and has a long evolutionary history (a homolog is present in horseshoe crabs), though its importance in host protection is still debated.

Other members of the pentraxin family are produced in different tissues and appear to have important roles in recognizing and clearing apoptotic cells.

Phagocytes have receptors that recognize pathogens directly

Even in the absence of opsonins, phagocytes have a number of receptors that allow them to recognize PAMPs. These include:

- scavenger receptors;
- carbohydrate receptors; and
- Toll-like receptors (TLRs).

Scavenger receptors and carbohydrate receptors (lectins) allow phagocytes to bind directly to microbes. Important examples include:

- the mannose receptor (CD206) on mononuclear phagocytes, which binds to mannan present in bacterial cell walls; and
- the dendritic cell receptors dectin-1 (which binds β1,3-glycan found in fungal cell walls) and dectin-2.

Each of these receptors has a C-type lectin domain, related to that found in the collectins and ficolins (see Fig. 6.23).

The scavenger receptors fall into two classes, members of which bind to lipopolysaccharide and lipoteichoic acid characteristic of Gram-negative bacteria. They are important, not just for recognition of pathogens, but also for clearing cell debris and apoptotic cells. The functions of these receptors in phagocytosis are described more fully in Chapter 9.

Q. Why do bacteria not just mutate their PAMPs so that they cannot be recognized by the innate immune system – after all, protein antigens of pathogens often mutate?

A. This is a difficult question because it requires deep insight into the evolutionary history of microbes, but many of the PAMPs are so fundamental to the structure of the bacterial or fungal cell walls that it is difficult to see how they could be altered without destroying the integrity of the microbe.

Toll-like receptors activate phagocytes and inflammatory reactions

The transmembrane protein Toll was first identified in the fruit fly *Drosophila* as a molecule required during embryogenesis. It was also noted that mutants lacking Toll were highly susceptible to infections with fungi and Gram-positive bacteria, suggesting that the molecule might be involved in immune defense. Subsequently a series of Toll-like receptors (TLRs) was identified in mammals that had very similar intracellular portions to the receptor in the flies.

The intracellular signaling pathways activated by the TLRs and the receptor for IL-1 are very similar and lead to activation of the transcription factor NK-κB (see Chapter 9).

The family of TLRs includes more than ten different receptors, many of which are capable of recognizing different microbial components (Fig. 6.24).

All of the TLRs are present on phagocytic cells, and some are also expressed on dendritic cells, mast cells, and B cells. Indeed, most tissues of the body express at least one TLR.

Q. TLR5 is present on the basal surface of epithelia in the gut, but not on the apical surface. What consequence might this have for immune reactions in the gut?

A. Bacteria within the gut would not stimulate the cell, whereas any microbes that have invaded the epithelial layer may do so. This may explain why non-pathogenic commensal bacteria in the gut do not elicit an inflammatory reaction, whereas pathogenic bacteria that have invaded the tissue do.

Expression of many of the TLRs is increased by inflammatory cytokines (e.g. TNFα, IFNγ) and elevated expression is seen in conditions such as inflammatory bowel disease.

The functional importance of the TLRs has been demonstrated in knockout mouse strains lacking individual receptors. Depending on the TLR involved, such animals fail to secrete inflammatory cytokines in response to pathogens and the microbicidal activity of phagocytes is not stimulated. These results show that the TLRs are primarily important in activating phagocytes in addition to any role they may have in endocytosis.

The TLRs make an important link between the innate and adaptive immune systems because their activation leads to the expression of co-stimulatory molecules on the phagocytes, which convert them into effective antigen-presenting cells.

The binding of microbial components to the TLRs effectively acts as a danger signal to increase the microbicidal activity of the phagocytes and allows them to activate T cells.

MICROBICIDAL PROTEINS ARE PART OF THE INNATE IMMUNE SYSTEM

Once a microbe has been endocytosed, it becomes subject to a number of microbicidal mechanisms.

In *Drosophila* fruit flies infection causes the release of various microbicidal proteins from the fat-body into the hemolymph.

In mammals, related proteins belonging to the **defensin** and **cathelicidin** families limit microbial spread by disrupting their outer membranes. For example the outer membrane of Gram-negative bacteria contains a higher level of negatively charged phospholipids than the mammalian plasma membrane. The positively charged defensins therefore preferentially insert into the bacterial membrane, particularly in conditions of low salt concentration.

Defensins constitute one of the major killing mechanisms of neutrophils and eosinophils. However, individual defensins are also produced by several cell types in tissues, particularly at epithelial surfaces in the lung, gut, and bladder. Some of these microbicidal peptides also cause mast cell degranulation with chemokine release and/or have direct chemotactic activity. They can therefore attract leukocytes to sites of infection.

The importance of these ancient antimicrobial defenses has been illustrated in gene-knockout animals, which often show increased susceptibility to particular types of

The Toll-like receptors

Toll-like receptor	ligand	pathogen
TLR1	lipopeptides	Gram-negative bacteria mycobacteria
TLR2	lipoteichoic acid lipoarabinomannan zymosan	Gram-positive bacteria mycobacteria fungi
TLR3	dsRNA	viruses
TLR4	lipopolysaccharide	Gram-negative bacteria
TLR5	flagellin	bacteria
TLR6	di-acyl lipopeptides	mycobacteria
TLR9	CpG-DNA	bacteria

Fig. 6.24 The Toll-like receptors recognize a variety of PAMPs. Gene duplication of the TLR precursor and divergence of function has led to a family of molecules capable of recognizing different types of pathogen.

infection. There is, however, little information on naturally occurring deficiencies of these molecules in humans. The functions of the microbicidal proteins are described in more detail in Chapter 9.

FURTHER READING

Akira S. Mammalian Toll-like receptors. Curr Opin Immunol 2003;15:5–11.

Binnerts ME, van Kooyk Y. How LFA-1 binds to different ligands. Immunol Today 1999;20:234–239.

Holmskov U, Thiel S, Jensenius JC. Collectins and ficolins: humoral lectins of innate immune defense. Annu Rev Immunol 2003;21;547–578.

Hynes RO. Integrins: bidirectional allosteric signalling machines. Cell 2002;110:673–678.

Lindhout E, Vissers JLM, Figdor CG, Adema GJ. Chemokines and lymphocyte migration. The Immunologist 1999;7:147–152.

Rossi D, Zlotnik A. The biology of chemokines and their receptors. Annu Rev Immunol 2000;18:217–242.

Springer TA. Traffic signals for lymphocyte recirculation and leukocyte emigration: the multistep paradigm. Cell 1994;76:301–314.

Underhill M, Ozinsky A. Phagocytosis of microbes: complexity in action. Annu Rev Immunol 2002;20:825–852.

Yang D, Biragyn A, Hoover DM, et al. Multiple roles of antimicrobial defensins. Cathelicidins and eosinophil-derived neurotoxin in host defense. Annu Rev Immunol 2004;22:181–216.

Critical thinking: The role of adhesion molecules in T cell migration (see p. 494 for explanations)

An experiment has been carried out to determine which CAMs mediate the migration of antigen-activated T cells across brain endothelium using a monolayer of endothelium overlaid with lymphocytes in vitro. The endothelium is either unstimulated or has been stimulated for 24 hours before the experiment with IL-1. In some cases the co-cultures were treated with blocking antibodies to different adhesion molecules. The results shown in the table below indicate the percentage of T cells that migrate across the endothelium in a 2-hour period.

blocking antibody	percentage of T cells migrating in 2 hours	
	unstimulated endothelium	IL-1-stimulated endothelium
none	18	48
anti-ICAM-1	3	16
anti-VCAM-1	19	28
anti-$\alpha_L\beta_2$-integrin (LFA-1)	2	14
anti-$\alpha_4\beta_1$-integrin (VLA-4)	17	32

1 Why does treatment of the endothelium with IL-1 cause an increase in the percentage of migrating cells in the absence of any blocking antibody?

2 Why does it require 24 hours of treatment with IL-1 to enhance the migration (1 hour of treatment does not produce this effect)?

3 Which adhesion molecules are important in mediating T cell migration across unstimulated endothelium?

4 Which adhesion molecules are important in mediating T cell migration across IL-1-activated endothelium?

Antigen Presentation

SUMMARY

- **T cells recognize peptide fragments that have been processed and become bound to major histocompatibility complex (MHC) class I or II molecules.** These MHC–antigen complexes are presented at the cell surface.

- **MHC class I molecules associate with endogenously synthesized peptides, binding to peptides produced by degradation of the cells' internal molecules.** This type of antigen processing is carried out by proteasomes (which cleave the proteins) and transporters (which take the fragments to the endoplasmic reticulum [ER]).

- **MHC class II molecules bind to peptides produced following the breakdown of proteins that the cell has endocytosed.** The peptides produced by degradation of these external antigens are loaded onto MHC class II molecules in a specialized endosomal compartment called MIIC.

- **Cross-presentation allows APCs to acquire antigens from infected cells.** A specialized pathway allows the acquisition of antigens from infected cells by APCs. This pathway, called cross-presentation, allows the display of exogenous antigens by MHC class I molecules.

- **Co-stimulatory molecules are essential for T cell activation.** Molecules such as B7 (CD80/86) on the APC bind to CD28 on the T cell to cause activation. Antigens presented without co-stimulation usually induce T cell anergy. Intercellular adhesion molecules also contribute to the interaction between a T cell and an antigen-presenting cell (APC). Interactions between intercellular cell adhesion molecule-1 (ICAM-1) and leukocyte functional antigen-1 (LFA-1) and between CD2 and its ligands extend the interaction between T cells and APCs.

- **CD4 binds to MHC class II and CD8 to MHC class I molecules.** These interactions increase the affinity of T cell binding to the appropriate MHC–antigen complex and bring kinases to the TCR complex.

- **The highly ordered area of contact between the T cell and APC is an immunological synapse.**

- **T cell activation induces enzyme cascades, leading to the production of interleukin-2 (IL-2) and the high-affinity IL-2 receptor on the T cell.** IL-2 is required to drive T cell division.

- **Antigen presentation affects the subsequent course of an immune response.** The immune system responds to clues that an infection has taken place before responding strongly to antigens.

T CELLS RECOGNIZE PEPTIDE FRAGMENTS BOUND TO MHC MOLECULES

Antigens recognized by T cells are degraded or processed in some way so that the determinant recognized by the T cell receptor (TCR) is only a small fragment of the original antigen.

Antigen processing refers to the degradation of antigen into peptide fragments, which become bound to major histocompatibility complex (MHC) class I or class II molecules (see Chapter 5). These are the critical fragments involved in triggering T cells. TCRs are sensitive to the sequences of amino acids in the MHC molecule peptide-binding groove rather than the conformational determinants recognized by antibodies.

Antigen presentation plays a central role in initiating and maintaining an appropriate immune response to antigen. The process is tightly controlled at several levels as follows:

- different types of antigen-presenting cell (APC) are brought into play depending on the situation, dendritic cells (DCs) being crucial for initiating responses;
- a complex series of molecular interactions takes place to ensure that small fragments of antigens are recognized in a highly specific manner by T cells;
- another level of control is exerted by **co-stimulatory molecules** on APCs, resulting in T cell activation only when appropriate, such as in an infection;
- adhesion molecules on the interacting cells also contribute to the stable binding of the cells, which promotes effective antigen presentation;
- signals from the cell surface are then transmitted by a series of signal transduction pathways that regulate gene expression in the nucleus;

- in the final stages the actions of cytokines on the lymphocytes drive cell division.

The four stages of antigen presentation are outlined in Fig. 7.1.

Different types of APC are involved depending on the situation
Interaction with APCs is essential for T cell activation

The interaction between T cells and the heterogeneous group of cells collectively termed APCs is the most extensively studied example of cell interaction in the immune system. It is the first such interaction to occur after antigen challenge and its outcome largely dictates the subsequent course of events:

- if a sufficient number of CD4+ helper T (TH) cells are triggered, then the activation of B cells or the development of cell-mediated immunity follows;
- if TH cells are not triggered, a form of immunological tolerance can develop, so that no other immunological events follow.

Several cell types can act as APCs

A wide spectrum of cells can present antigen, depending on how and where the antigen is first dealt with by cells of the immune system. In a lymphoid organ, the three main types of APC are:

- DCs;
- macrophages; and
- B cells (Fig. 7.2).

Activation of naive T cells on first encounter with antigen on the surface of an APC is called **priming**, to distinguish it from the responses of effector T cells to antigen on the surface of their target cells and the responses of primed memory T cells.

Summary of the key intercellular signals in T cell activation

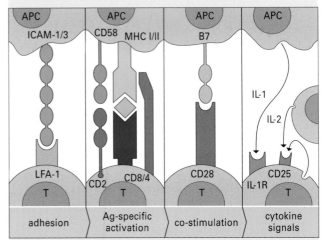

Fig. 7.1 Adhesion – association of APCs and T cells first involves non-specific, reversible binding through adhesion molecules, such as LFA-1 with ICAM-1 or ICAM-3. Antigen-specific recognition – recognition of the peptide antigen in the MHC molecule by the TCR, which provides the specificity of the interaction, results in prolonged cell–cell contact. Co-stimulation – a second signal (co-stimulation) is necessary for the T cell to respond efficiently, otherwise tolerance may result. Cytokine signals – activation results in upregulation of cytokines and their receptors, which boosts the activating signals and helps to decide the cell's fate.

Localization of antigen-presenting cells (APCs) in lymph nodes

area	antigen-presenting cells	antigen	persistence of antigen
subcapsular (marginal) sinus	marginal zone macrophages	polysaccharides Ficoll (T_{ind})	+ + + +
follicles and B cell areas	follicular dendritic cells	immune complexes that fix complement	+ + +
medulla	classic macrophages	most antigens	+
T cell areas	interdigitating dendritic cells	most antigens	+ +

Fig. 7.2 A lymph node represented schematically showing afferent and efferent lymphatics, follicles, the outer cortical B cell area, and the paracortical T cell area. Different APCs predominate in these areas and selectively take up different types of antigen, which then persist on the surface of the cells for variable periods. Polysaccharides are preferentially taken up by marginal zone macrophages and may persist for months or years, whereas antigens on recirculating macrophages in the medulla may last for only a few days or weeks. Note that recirculating 'veiled' cells (Langerhans' cells), which originally come from the skin, change their morphology to become interdigitating dendritic cells within the lymph node. Both these cells and the follicular dendritic cells have long processes, which are in intimate contact with lymphocytes.

Rapid Reference Box 7

CD2 – Receptor for CD58 and CD48, expressed by T cells.

CD11a – LFA-1 expressed by T, B, and NK cells, monocyte/macrophages, and granulocytes.

CD28 – binds CD80 and CD86, expressed by subpopulations of T cells and activated B cells.

CD40 – binds CD154, co-stimulatory, expressed by B cells, monocyte/macrophages, and FDCs.

CD45 – leukocyte common antigen expressed by populations of T, B, and NK cells, and monocyte/macrophages.

CD54 – ICAM-1 expressed by T, B, and NK cells, monocyte/macrophages, granulocytes, platelets, DCs, and other cells.

CD58 – a ligand for CD2.

CD80 – B7-1, expressed by subpopulations of activated B and T cells and monocyte/macrophages, and binds CD28 and CD152.

CD86 – B7-2, expressed by activated B cells and monocyte/macrophages, and binds CD28 and CD152.

CD152 – CTLA-4, binds CD80 and CD86, a downregulatory signaling molecule that competes with CD28 for ligation of B7 on APCs, expressed by a subpopulation of activated T cells.

CD154 – CD40 ligand (CD40L).

(APC, antigen-presenting cell; CR, complement receptor; DC, dendritic cell; FDC, follicular dendritic cell; ICAM-1, intercellular adhesion molecule-1; LCA, leukocyte common antigen; LFA, lymphocyte functional antigen)

Q. A number of bacterial components enhance the expression of MHC molecules and co-stimulatory molecules on macrophages. What effect would you expect this to have on the immune response? Would it be advantageous for the individual?

A. In the presence of infection, the action of the microbial components would enhance the ability of macrophages to present antigen to T cells. This would generally be advantageous because it would allow the immune system to respond more effectively to the infection. However, in some circumstances it might be disadvantageous because microbial components would also enhance unwanted immune responses such as autoimmune reactions.

B cells can:

- bind to a specific antigen through surface IgM or IgD;
- internalize it; and
- then degrade it into peptides, which associate with MHC class II molecules.

If antigen concentrations are very low, B cells with high-affinity antigen receptors (IgM or IgD) are the most effective APC because other APCs simply cannot capture enough antigen. Therefore, for secondary responses, when the number of antigen-specific B cells is high, B cells may be a major type of APC.

B cells do not normally express co-stimulatory molecules such as B7, but these can be induced by bacterial constituents.

The properties and functions of some APCs are summarized in Figs 7.3 and 7.4.

DCs ARE CRUCIAL FOR INITIATING RESPONSES – DCs, which are found in abundance in the T cell areas of lymph nodes and spleen, are the most effective cells for the initial activation of naive T cells. They pick up antigens in peripheral tissues, then migrate to lymph nodes, where they express high levels of adhesion and co-stimulatory molecules, as well as MHC class II molecules, which interact with the TCR and CD4 on TH cells.

Once they have migrated, DCs stop synthesizing MHC class II molecules, but maintain high levels of stable expression of MHC class II molecules containing peptides from antigens derived from the tissue where the DCs originated.

Interdigitating DCs are believed to be the major APCs involved in primary immune responses because they induce T cell proliferation more effectively than any other APC.

Remarkably, DCs are able to present internalized antigens to T cells via MHC class I as well as class II molecules, in a phenomenon called **cross-presentation**. This results in activation of cytotoxic T lymphocytes (CTLs), which are then available for killing of infected cells.

Macrophages and B cells express appropriate co-stimulatory molecules for activation of naive T cells only upon infection. Macrophages:

- ingest microbes and particulate antigens;
- digest them in phagolysosomes; and
- present fragments at the cell surface on MHC molecules.

A series of molecular interactions ensures highly specific antigen recognition by T cells
Antigens are processed before they are presented to T cells

Antigen processing involves degrading the antigen into peptide fragments. The vast majority of epitopes recognized by T cells are fragments from a peptide chain (see Chapter 5).

Only a minority of peptide fragments from a protein antigen are able to bind to a particular MHC molecule. Furthermore, different MHC molecules bind different sets of peptides (see Chapter 5). For example, studies using a viral antigen that is recognized by mouse strains of several different haplotypes (that is, having different MHC molecules) showed that TH cells from each haplotype recognized a distinct peptide from that antigen (Fig. 7.5). This depended largely on whether the strain possessed an MHC class II molecule that could bind to the particular peptide.

Q. The APCs of BALB/c mice present peptide 10–26 of the λ-repressor, whereas APCs of the C57BL/6 mouse present peptide 70–86 (see Fig. 7.5). Which of these peptides would be presented by APCs of an F1 mouse derived from a cross of these two strains?

A. Because MHC molecules are co-dominantly expressed, the APCs in the F1 strain will express both types of APC, and will therefore be able to present both peptides.

Antigen presentation

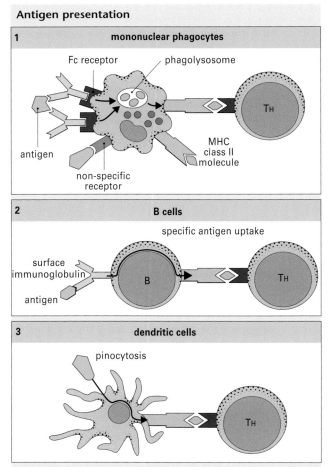

Fig. 7.3 Mononuclear phagocytes (**1**), B cells (**2**), and DCs (**3**) can all present antigen to MHC class II restricted TH cells. Macrophages take up bacteria or particulate antigen via non-specific receptors or as immune complexes, process it, and return fragments to the cell surface in association with MHC class II molecules. Activated B cells can take up antigen via their surface immunoglobulin and present it to T cells associated with their MHC class II molecules. DCs constitutively express MHC class II molecules and take up antigen by macropinocytosis.

Antigen-presenting cells

	phago-cytosis	type	location	class II expression
phagocytes (monocyte/ macrophage lineage)	+	monocytes macrophages marginal zone macrophages Kupffer cells microglia	blood tissue spleen and lymph node liver brain	(+) → + + + inducible
non-phagocytic constitutive APCs	–	Langerhans' cells	skin	+ + constitutive
		interdigitating DCs (IDCs)	lymphoid tissue	
		follicular dendritic cells	lymphoid tissue	–
lymphocytes	–	B cells and T cells	lymphoid tissues and at sites of immune reactions	– → + + inducible
facultative APCs	+	astrocytes	brain	inducible
	–	follicular cells	thyroid	inducible
	–	endothelium fibroblasts other types in appropriate tissue	vascular and lymphoid tissue connective tissue	– → + + inducible

Fig. 7.4 Many APCs are unable to phagocytose antigen, but can take it up in other ways, such as by pinocytosis. Endothelial cells (not normally considered to be APCs) that have been induced to express MHC class II molecules by interferon-γ (IFNγ) are also capable of acting as APCs, as are some epithelial cells. Another example is the thyroid follicular cell, which acts as an APC in the pathogenesis of Graves' autoimmune thyroiditis.

T cell antigenic peptides in the λ repressor protein

strain	haplotype	antigenic peptide position
BALB/c	d	>96%
C57BL/6	b	>92%
B10.BR	k	20% 50% 30%
B10	s	50% 50%
SM/J	v	100%

% = % of hybridomas recognizing both the protein and the peptide

Fig. 7.5 Diversity of antigenic peptides in relation to MHC class II molecules. Mice were immunized with λ repressor protein. T cell hybridomas generated from mouse cells were tested against a panel of overlapping peptides, which spanned the entire protein. Positions of antigenic peptides are shown in dark blue. One peptide was always immunodominant, though more than one peptide was antigenic in some mouse strains. Usually only a few peptides from a protein are stimulators. (Adapted from data of Roy S, Scherer MT, Briner TJ, et al. Science 1989;244:572–575)

Originally researchers carrying out these experiments would have to use particular antigenic peptides or whole molecules presented by APCs of the appropriate type. Now it is possible to use synthetic MHC–peptide combinations (Method Box 7.1).

METHOD BOX 7.1
Tetramers

Tetrameric complexes of MHC molecules may be used to identify clones of T cells specific to presentation of a particular peptide in a particular MHC molecule. These are usually tetramers of MHC class I molecules, though MHC class II tetramers are being developed.

The tetramer assay allows the detection of antigen-specific cytotoxic T lymphocytes (CTLs) in ex-vivo cell preparations without the need for in-vitro expansion.

The basis of this technique is to directly stain antigen-specific T cells with the MHC molecule–peptide complex that they recognize via their T cell receptors (TCRs).

Because the affinity of single TCR molecules for the MHC molecule–peptide is low, direct staining is not possible because of rapid dissociation. The formation of an MHC tetramer with four copies of the MHC molecule–peptide complex results in a very enhanced avidity for the TCR.

MHC molecules of the appropriate allotype are fused to a peptide (bsp), which acts as a substrate for biotinylation. MHC-bsp and β_2-microglobulin are expressed in *Escherichia coli* mixed with the specific CTL epitopic peptide under folding conditions, and the MHC molecule–peptide complexes thus formed are purified. The complexes are biotinylated and mixed at a ratio of 4:1 with fluorescence-labeled streptavidin to produce the tetramers (Fig. 1). The binding of these labeled tetramers by antigen-specific CTLs can then be analyzed by the fluorescence-activated cell sorter (FACS, see Method Box 2.1, p. 32).

A class I MHC tetramer

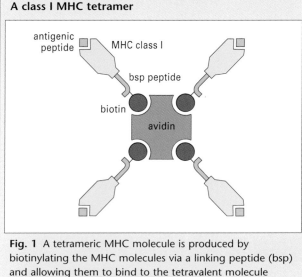

Fig. 1 A tetrameric MHC molecule is produced by biotinylating the MHC molecules via a linking peptide (bsp) and allowing them to bind to the tetravalent molecule avidin – a natural receptor for biotin.

Antigens are partially degraded into peptides before binding to MHC molecules

The processing of antigens to generate peptides that can bind to MHC class II molecules occurs in intracellular organelles (Fig. 7.6). Phagosomes containing endocytosed proteins fuse with lysosomes where a number of proteases are involved in breaking down the proteins to smaller fragments. The proteases include:

- cathepsins B and D;
- an acidic thiol reductase, γ-interferon-inducible lysosomal thiol reductase (GILT), which acts on disulfide-bonded proteins.

Alkaline agents such as chloroquine or ammonium chloride diminish the activity of proteases in the phagolysosomes and therefore interfere with antigen processing.

In laboratory studies, the requirement for internal degradation of antigen by APCs can be circumvented by the use of synthetic peptides. This ability to use synthesized peptides of known sequences has enabled researchers to readily identify epitopes recognized by T cells with different specificities.

The relative importance of different amino acids within a defined epitope can also be investigated by amino acid replacements at different sites. Comparison of the effects of amino acid substitution on MHC molecule binding and T cell reactivity has enabled conclusions to be drawn as to:

- which amino acid residues contact the MHC molecule; and
- which amino acid residues contact the TCR

MHC CLASS I MOLECULES ASSOCIATE WITH ENDOGENOUS PEPTIDES

MHC class I-restricted T cells (CTLs) recognize endogenous antigens synthesized within the target cell, whereas

Antigen processing

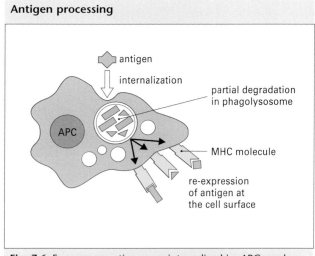

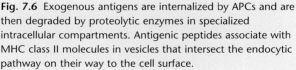

Fig. 7.6 Exogenous antigens are internalized by APCs and are then degraded by proteolytic enzymes in specialized intracellular compartments. Antigenic peptides associate with MHC class II molecules in vesicles that intersect the endocytic pathway on their way to the cell surface.

class II-restricted T cells (TH) recognize exogenous antigen.

Manipulation of the location of a protein can determine whether it elicits an MHC class I- or class II-restricted response. For example:

- influenza virus hemagglutinin (HA), a glycoprotein associated with the membrane of an infected host cell, normally elicits only a weak CTL response, but influenza virus HA can be generated in the cytoplasm by deleting that part of its sequence that encodes the N terminal signal peptide (required for translation across the membrane of the endoplasmic reticulum [ER]) and, when this is done, there is a strong CTL response to HA;

- the introduction of ovalbumin into the cytoplasm of a target cell (using an osmotic shock technique) generates CTLs recognizing ovalbumin, whereas the addition of exogenous ovalbumin generates an exclusively TH cell response.

Proteasomes are cytoplasmic organelles that degrade cytoplasmic proteins

Although the assembly of MHC class I molecules occurs in the ER of the cell, peptides destined to be presented by MHC class I molecules are generated from cytosolic proteins. The initial step in this process involves an organelle called the proteasome – a complex of 14–17 different subunits, which form a barrel-like structure (Fig. 7.7).

Proteasomes provide the major proteolytic activity of the cytosol. They have a range of different endopeptidase activities and they degrade denatured or ubiquitinated proteins to peptides of about 5–15 amino acids (ubiquitin is a protein that tags other proteins for degradation).

Two genes, *LMP2* and *LMP7*, located in the class II region of the MHC (Fig. 7.8), encode proteasome components that subtly modify the range of peptides produced by proteasomes. The expression of these genes is induced by interferon-γ (IFNγ), and the protein products:

- displace constitutive subunits of the proteasome. LMP2 and LMP7 along with a third inducible proteasome component encoded on a different chromosome;

Generation of immunoproteasomes by replacement of active subunits

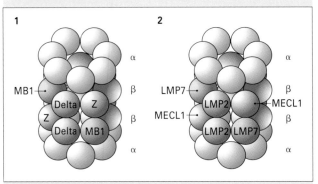

Fig. 7.7 The 20S proteasome, shown in cartoon form, is composed of four stacked disks, two identical outer disks of α subunits, and two similar inner disks comprised of β subunits. Each disk has seven different subunits. Peptides enter into the body of the proteasome for cleavage into peptides. Only three of the β subunits are active. In normal proteasomes, these are called MB1, delta, and Z (**1**). Interferon-γ treatment of cells results in replacement of these three subunits by the two MHC-encoded proteins, LMP2 and LMP7, as well as a third inducible protein, MECL1 (**2**). These subunits are shown adjacent to each other here, whereas they are actually in separate parts of the β ring and some would be hidden at the back of the structure shown.

- influence processing of peptides by creating peptide fragments suitable for binding MHC class I molecules from pathogens such as viruses, in addition to self proteins.

Additional subunits associate with the ends of core (20S) proteasomes and may influence antigen processing. These include interferon-inducible PA28 molecules as well as a complex of proteins that result in a larger 26S particle.

Proteasomes may not be the only proteases involved in producing peptides for presentation by MHC class I molecules. There is evidence for the involvement of enzymes, such as the giant tripeptidyl aminopeptidase II (TPPII) complex.

MHC genes involved in antigen processing and presentation

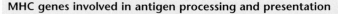
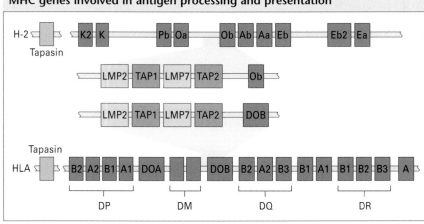

Fig. 7.8 Genes encoding the two subunits of the peptide transporter (TAP) and two components (LMP) of the multisubunit proteasome (see Fig. 7.7) are located in the murine and human class II regions. The Tapasin gene is located just centromeric (left) of the MHC.

Ribosomes are error prone during the course of rapid synthesis of viral proteins and there is evidence that defective ribosomal products (also known as DRiPs) are a direct source of peptides for MHC class I molecules.

Q. What advantage might there be in presenting DriPs on MHC class I molecules rather than fragments of mature viral peptides?

A. DriP-derived peptides will be generated earlier in infection than fragments produced by the degradation of mature viral proteins. This allows the CTLs to recognize virus-infected cells more quickly.

How do the peptides produced by proteasomes traverse the ER?

The products of two genes, *TAP1* and *TAP2*, that map adjacent to *LMP2* and *LMP7* in the MHC (see Fig. 7.8), function as a heterodimeric transporter that translocates peptides into the lumen of the ER. TAP is a member of the large ATP-binding cassette (ABC) family of transporters localized in the ER membrane. Microsomes from cells lacking TAP1 or TAP2 could not take up peptide in

experiments in vitro. Using a similar system it was shown that the most efficient transport occurred with peptide substrates of 8–15 amino acids. Although this size is close to the length preference of MHC class I molecule binding sites, it suggests that some additional trimming may be required by enzymes in the lumen of the ER. These include an ER amino peptidase, ERAP, and enzymes such as the TPPII complex may also contribute to trimming the N termini of peptides for class I binding.

Recent evidence has suggested that some of the components of the processing pathway are physically associated in the ER (Fig. 7.9). For example:

- newly synthesized MHC class I molecule–β_2-microglobulin complexes are associated with TAP in the ER;
- another MHC-encoded protein, called **tapasin**, forms a bridge between the MHC class I molecule and TAP, until peptide is associated with the class I molecule; dissociation occurs upon transport to the cis-Golgi.

Peptide loading involves other proteins such as calnexin, calreticulin, and ERp57. These chaperones promote and guide the assembly of stable MHC class I molecule–β_2-microglobulin–peptide complexes.

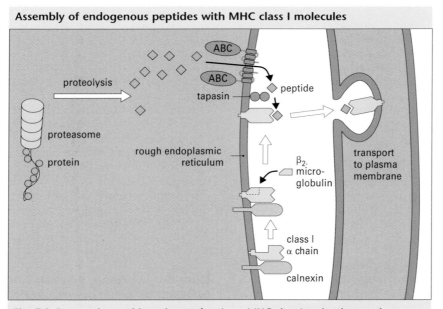

Fig. 7.9 Proposed assembly pathway of antigen–MHC class I molecule complex. Cytoplasmic antigens are processed by proteasomes (see Fig. 7.7). Peptides are transported by two members of the 'ABC' superfamily of transporters, also encoded within the MHC (TAP1 and TAP2). Antigenic peptides associate with class I heavy chains (see Fig. 5.6) and β_2-microglobulin in the ER. Molecular chaperones, such as calnexin and calreticulin, associate with partially assembled class I complexes. The class I molecule waiting to be loaded with peptide is engaged in a complex of proteins. The complex includes calreticulin, a lectin-like chaperone that binds to a sugar residue on the class I molecule. ERp57, a thiol oxido-reductase non-covalently associates with calreticulin and is disulfide bonded to tapasin. The immunoglobulin superfamily molecule tapasin forms a bridge between TAP and the MHC class I molecule, and may also act as a peptide 'editor'. An intact loading complex is essential for efficient MHC class I association with peptide. The fully assembled class I molecules are transported to the cell surface.

MHC class I molecule complexes lacking peptide are unstable, ensuring that only functionally useful complexes are available for interaction with TCRs.

A number of class I-like molecules can present very limited sets of antigens

In addition to the standard MHC class I molecules (class Ia), a number of class I-like molecules (class Ib), encoded in the MHC or elsewhere on the genome, can present very limited sets of antigens.

HLA-E–signal peptide complex interacts with the NKG2A inhibitory receptor on NK cells

HLA-E molecules bind a restricted set of peptides consisting of hydrophobic leader sequence peptides from class Ia molecules. Intriguingly, though these leader sequences are generated by signal peptidase within the ER, HLA-E is dependent on TAP transporters. By binding and presenting sequences from class Ia molecules HLA-E signals the fact that MHC class Ia expression has not been downregulated (e.g. by a virus).

The HLA-E–signal peptide complex interacts with the NKG2A inhibitory receptor on NK cells (see Fig. 10.4). A cell that expresses HLA-E is therefore not killed by NK cells.

Q. Why would conventional HLA-A, HLA-B, or HLA-C molecules be less well suited to the presentation of signal peptide to receptors on NK cells than HLA-E?
A. The conventional MHC molecules have evolved as highly diverse molecules that present the great range of microbial polypeptides to the diverse repertoire of T cell receptors. In contrast HLA-E molecules have a single function – to present well-defined signal peptides to a monomorphic receptor.

CD1 molecules present lipids and glycolipids

CD1 molecules, encoded on chromosome 1, present lipids and glycolipids. Humans have five *CD1* genes and mice have two. CD1b presents the bacterial lipid mycolic acid to T cells with αβ TCRs. Other CD1 molecules are recognized by γδ T cells.

The location of antigen-processing genes in the MHC may not be fortuitous

The finding of a cassette of antigen-processing genes such as the LMPs and TAPs in the class II region of the MHC is striking.

There is some evidence, especially from studies in rats, that particular alleles of *TAP* are genetically linked with alleles of class I genes that are most suited to receive the kind of peptides preferentially transported by the products of that *TAP* allele (Fig. 7.10).

The rat data suggest that localization of some antigen-processing genes in the MHC provides a selective advantage. In fact, the clustering of antigen processing and presenting genes in the MHC of most vertebrate species may not be fortuitous. It may help to coordinate co-evolution of some molecules as well as facilitating exchange of sequences between loci.

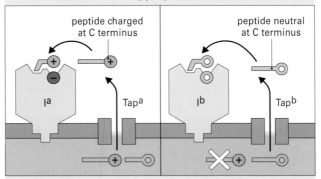

In rats, *TAP* genes are polymorphic and different alleles are linked in *cis* to the appropriate class I allele

Fig. 7.10 Different MHC class I molecules in rats can accommodate peptides (blue bars) with either a positive charge at the C terminus (+) or a neutral amino acid (o). Similarly, TAP molecules (orange) come in two forms, which differ in the types of peptide they preferentially transport into the ER. Most rat strains have the appropriate *TAP* allele on the same haplotype as the class I gene that it serves best.

MHC CLASS II MOLECULES ARE LOADED WITH EXOGENOUS PEPTIDES

MHC class II molecule α and β chains (see Chapter 5) are found in the ER complexed to a polypeptide called the invariant chain (Ii). This protein is encoded outside the MHC. The αβ–Ii complex is transported through the Golgi complex to an acidic endosomal or lysosomal compartment called MIIC. These MIIC vesicles appear to be specialized for the transport and loading of MHC class II molecules. They have characteristics of both endosomes and lysosomes and have an onion-skin appearance under the electron microscope, comprising multiple membrane structures. The αβ complex spends 1–3 hours in this compartment before reaching the cell surface. The Ii chain is cleaved to small fragments, one of which, termed CLIP (class II-associated invariant peptide), is located in the groove of the class II molecule until replaced by peptides destined for presentation (Figs 7.11 and 7.12).

How do antigenic peptides derived from exogenous proteins meet MHC molecules in the appropriate compartment?

The answer to this question lies in the intracellular traffic routes of MHC molecules. After synthesis in the ER both types of MHC molecule are transported through the Golgi compartment, class I in association with antigenic peptide and class II bound to invariant chain Ii. Class II molecules segregate from class I molecules in the trans-Golgi network. They then join the endosomal/lysosomal MIIC compartment en route to the plasma membrane.

Exogenous antigen can also enter APCs via an endocytic route (either receptor mediated or fluid phase, see Fig. 7.11) where in some cells, such as DCs, it can load onto:
- MHC class II molecules in MIIC vesicles; and

Proposed routes of intracellular trafficking of MHC molecules involved in antigen presentation

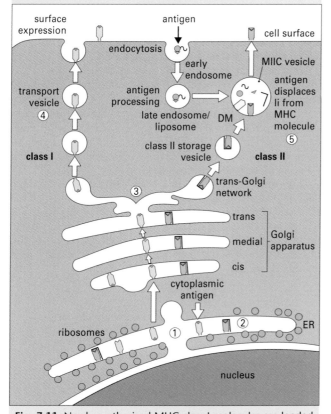

Fig. 7.11 Newly synthesized MHC class I molecules are loaded with peptide (**1**). MHC class II molecules associate with Ii in the ER (**2**). Ii prevents loading with peptide and contains sequences that enable the MHC class II molecule to exit from the rough endoplasmic reticulum (RER). MHC class I and class II molecules segregate after transit through the Golgi (**3**). Class I molecules go directly to the cell surface (**4**). Class II molecules enter an acidic compartment called MIIC, where they are loaded with peptide derived from exogenous antigen, and the CLIP peptide that occupies the binding groove dissociates (**5**).

MHC class II molecule processing compartment

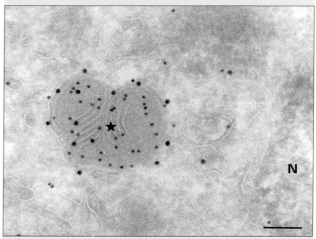

Fig. 7.12 Electron micrograph of ultrathin cryosections from B cells showing a multilaminar MIIC vesicle. The bar represents 100 nm. MHC class II molecules are revealed by antibodies coupled to 10 nm gold particles and HLA-DM by large gold particles (15 nm). (Courtesy of Dr Monique Kleijmeer)

- MHC class I molecules in the ER, in a TAP-dependent manner.

The exchange of CLIP for other peptides is orchestrated by a class II-related molecule called HLA-DM (Fig. 7.13). This glycoprotein consists of an α chain and a β chain, both of which are encoded in the class II region of the MHC (see Fig. 7.8).

HLA-DM acts by stabilizing empty MHC class II molecules so that when CLIP is released other peptides get a chance to associate. The DM molecule itself has a closed groove and it is not capable of binding peptide.

In cell lines lacking *DMA* and *DMB* genes, class II molecules are unstable and the cells no longer process and present proteins. Their class II molecules end up at the cell surface occupied by CLIP fragments of the invariant chain (Fig. 7.14).

HLA-DM acts like a catalyst to influence binding of peptides in exchange for CLIP

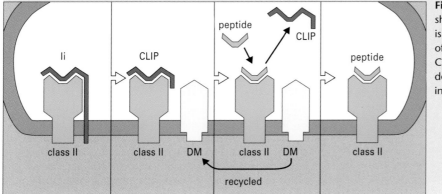

Fig. 7.13 An MHC class II molecule is shown loaded with the Ii chain. The Ii chain is cleaved to the CLIP fragment. Association of the complex with HLA-DM then allows CLIP to be exchanged for other peptides derived from endocytosed proteins present in MIIC vesicles.

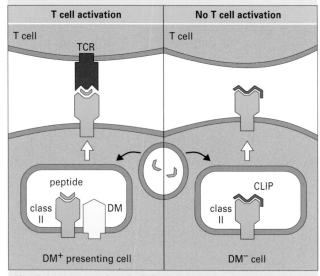

Absence of HLA-DM leads to failure of MHC class II molecules to bind appropriate peptides

T cell activation	No T cell activation
T cell	T cell
TCR	
peptide	CLIP
class II DM	class II
DM⁺ presenting cell	DM⁻ cell

Fig. 7.14 In normal APCs (left) peptides are loaded onto class II molecules, as shown in Fig. 7.13. In the absence of HLA-DM (right), the CLIP fragment is not removed, and the blocked MHC molecule is unable to activate T cells.

A further MHC-encoded molecule, HLA-DO (see Fig. 7.8), which associates with DM, is also involved in peptide loading. Like conventional MHC class II molecules, HLA-DO is a heterodimer (see Chapter 5), consisting of the DOA (formerly DNA) and DOB chains. Similar genes and molecules to DM and DO are found in other species, for example in mouse they are encoded by the Ma, Mb, and Oa, Ob genes, respectively.

CROSS-PRESENTATION ALLOWS APCs TO ACQUIRE ANTIGENS FROM INFECTED CELLS

Cross-presentation occurs when exogenous peptides are presented by MHC class I molecules. The principle that endogenously synthesized proteins are the source of peptides for MHC class I molecules appears to be violated by the phenomenon of cross-presentation. There is a specialized pathway in which T cells recognize MHC class I molecule–peptide complexes formed from exogenous protein antigens endocytically acquired by DCs.

Q. What function could cross-presentation fulfil in defense against viral infections?
A. Presumably such a mechanism is required so that, even if a virus fails to infect an APC directly, a successful cytotoxic CD8 T cell-mediated immune response can be generated.

In this process of cross-presentation, APCs acquire remnants of virus-infected cells by phagocytosis and present them on MHC class I molecules. Internalized proteins appear to be transferred from the endocytic pathway into the cytosol where they are then subject to processing and transport by proteasomes and TAP, respectively, as for other peptides (Fig. 7.15).

CO-STIMULATORY MOLECULES ARE ESSENTIAL FOR T CELL ACTIVATION

The process of activating T cells generally takes place in the lymph node nearest to the infection. The TCR recognizes a specific peptide lodged in the peptide-binding groove of the MHC molecule. This interaction dictates immunological specificity because a peptide associated with an MHC molecule forms a unique structure to be recognized by the TCR. Other molecules have a complementary role in this interaction.

The initial encounter of T cells with APCs is by non-specific binding through adhesion molecules. This transient binding by adhesion molecules permits the T cell to encounter a large number of different MHC molecule–peptide combinations on different APCs. In the absence of a specific interaction, the APC and T cell rapidly dissociate.

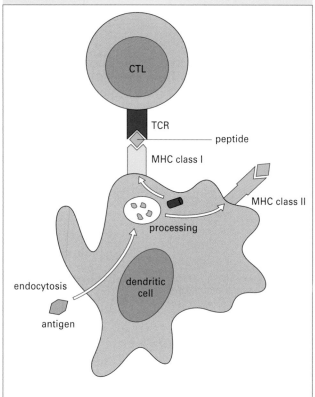

Cross-presentation when exogenous peptides are presented by MHC class I molecules

Fig. 7.15 DCs can present internalized antigen via both the MHC class I and class II pathways. This is atypical – external antigen is usually presented via the class II pathway. Peptides are transferred from the endosome to the cytosol where they are processed by the proteasome to enter the class I pathway.

Crucially, co-stimulatory molecules act together with the antigen-specific signals before the T cell is sanctioned for proliferation. Co-stimulatory and antigen-specific signals must be present simultaneously on the same cell.

Overall, antigen presentation through MHC class I or class II molecules can be split into four stages – adhesion, antigen-specific activation, co-stimulation, and cytokine signaling (see Fig. 7.1).

Multiple cell surface molecules interact during antigen presentation to T cells

Intercellular adhesion molecules (ICAMs), particularly ICAM-1 (CD54), interact with the integrin, lymphocyte functional antigen-1 (LFA-1 or CD11a/CD18), present on all immune cells.

If mouse cells are transfected with both human MHC and human ICAM-1, their capacity to act as human APCs is augmented.

When the T cell encounters the appropriate MHC molecule–peptide, which happens rarely except during an ongoing infection, a conformational change in LFA-1 on the T cell, signaled via the TCR, results in tighter binding to ICAM-1, which results in prolonged cell–cell contact. The joined cells can exist as a pair for long periods, allowing time for the T cell to proliferate and differentiate.

The specific MHC molecule–peptide–TCR interaction, though necessary, is not sufficient to fully activate the T cell. A second signal is required, otherwise the T cell will become unresponsive. This second signal, also referred to as co-stimulation, is of crucial importance.

Some co-stimulatory molecules that interact with ligands on the T cell's surface are shown in Fig. 7.16.

The most potent co-stimulatory molecules known are B7s, which are members of the immunoglobulin superfamily molecules; they include B7-1 (CD80) and B7-2 (CD86).

Several other B7-related molecules are beginning to emerge.

B7s exist as homodimers on the cell surface. These proteins are constitutively expressed on DCs, but can be upregulated on monocytes, B cells, and probably other APCs.

Upregulation of co-receptors is stimulated by inflammation and by interaction of microbial products with Toll-like receptors (TLRs, see Fig. 6.24) on the APC.

Co-receptors are the ligands for other immunoglobulin superfamily molecules – CD28 and its homolog CTLA-4 (CD152), which is expressed after T cell activation. CD28 is the main co-stimulatory ligand expressed on naive T cells. CD28 stimulation:

- has been shown to prolong and augment the production of IL-2 and other cytokines; and
- is probably important in preventing the induction of tolerance.

Although the CD28–B7 interaction is extremely important, CD28 knockout mice do respond to antigen, but require higher doses, so CD28 triggering is not obligatory, even for naive T cells. In CD28 knockout mice other co-stimulatory signals probably replace that delivered by CD28–B7.

CTLA-4, the alternative ligand for B7, is an inhibitory receptor limiting T cell activation, resulting in less IL-2 production. Thus CD28, constitutively expressed, initially interacts with B7, leading to T cell activation. Once this has peaked, the upregulation of CTLA-4 with its higher affinity limits the degree of activation because available B7 will interact with CTLA-4 (Fig. 7.17).

Q. What effect would you expect to see in mice that have the CTLA-4 gene knocked out?

A. They suffer from an aggressive lymphoproliferative disorder, because they do not inactivate dividing T cells efficiently (see Fig. 7.17).

Critical molecules involved in antigen presentation

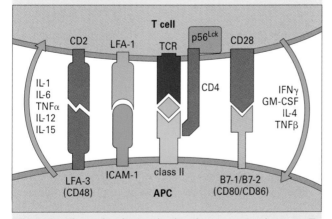

Fig. 7.16 The molecules involved in the interaction between T cells and APCs. The various cytokines and their direction of action are also shown. In humans LFA-3 (CD58) acts as a ligand for CD2, but in rodents CD48 performs this function.

Role of CTLA-4 in controlling T cell activation

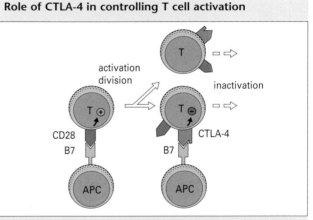

Fig. 7.17 Before activation, T cells express CD28, which ligates B7-1 and B7-2 on APCs (e.g. B cells). After activation, CTLA-4 is expressed, which is an alternative high-affinity ligand for B7. CTLA-4 ligates B7, so the T cells no longer receive an activation signal.

The CD2 molecule on T cells is also involved in T cell activation, in conjunction with the TCR. CD2 is a receptor for LFA-3 (CD58), which is widely distributed on cells and is present on all APCs. In rodents CD48 binds to CD2 and appears to be functionally equivalent to LFA-3 in humans. Both CD2 and LFA-3 are members of the immunoglobulin superfamily.

Co-stimulation via B7 is a necessary signal for T cell activation

Resting T cells cannot respond optimally without co-stimulation via B7, and if they recognize their antigen in a non-stimulating manner they become inactivated, producing a state of immunological tolerance (Fig. 7.18). This tolerance is specific, only affecting TH cells that respond to a particular antigen. Persistent tolerance without cell death is known as **clonal anergy**.

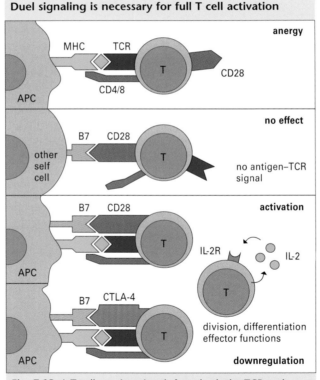

Duel signaling is necessary for full T cell activation

Fig. 7.18 A T cell requires signals from both the TCR and CD28 for activation. Anergy – in the absence of co-stimulatory molecules inactivation or anergy results. This situation would prevail to tolerize T cells not removed by central tolerance to self antigens expressed on peripheral tissues. No effect – in the absence of an antigen-specific signal (e.g. wrong peptide) there is no effect on the T cell. Activation – co-reception of both signals, from the surface of a professional APC, activates the T cell to produce IL-2 and its receptor (IL-2R). The cell divides and differentiates into an effector T cell, which no longer requires signal 2 for its effector function. Downregulation – at the termination of the immune response, CTLA-4 replaces CD28 and downregulates T cell function.

As discussed in Chapters 2 and 12, many T cells are made tolerant to self molecules during their development in the thymus. However, the process is not perfect and many autoreactive T cells are present in the circulation. These cells may still be tolerized outside the thymus because, although they are specific for self MHC–peptide, this is often first encountered on cells that lack the appropriate co-stimulatory signals.

CD4 AND CD8 BINDING TO MHC MOLECULES INCREASE T CELL BINDING AFFINITY

CD4 and CD8 co-receptors for MHC molecules increase the sensitivity of T cells to antigen-presenting molecules by about 100-fold. The two major subsets of T cells, TH and CTLs, express either CD4 or CD8, respectively.

CD4 and CD8 are only distantly related, but serve similar functions as co-receptors for MHC molecule–peptide–TCR interactions. In association with the MHC molecule–peptide–TCR complex:

- CD8 interacts with MHC class I molecules and consists of two chains with immunoglobulin-like domains on long stalks, coupled by a disulfide bridge;
- CD4 interacts with MHC class II molecules and consists of four immunoglobulin domains external to the cell, and its cytoplasmic tail has a docking site for the tyrosine kinase, Lck (see below);

CD8 co-receptor binds to conserved portions of the α_3 domains of class I molecules (see Fig. 5.6), leaving the portion enclosing peptide free to interact with the TCR. Like CD4, CD8 associates with Lck.

Both CD4 and CD8 co-receptors increase the sensitivity of T cells to antigen-presenting molecules by about 100-fold.

THE HIGHLY ORDERED AREA OF CONTACT BETWEEN A T CELL AND AN APC IS AN IMMUNOLOGICAL SYNAPSE

The junction between a T cell and an APC does not just consist of interacting molecules arranged randomly on the cell surfaces. There is a clustering of TCRs in a patch on the cell surface in an area of membrane with distinct properties, surrounded by a ring of adhesion molecules.

Immunological synapse formation is thought to be an active dynamic process that helps T cells to distinguish potential antigenic ligands.

Experiments show that initially TCR ligands are relegated to the outer ring of the nascent synapse. Subsequently, there is transport of the complexes to a central cluster, which is dependent, in an unknown way, on TCR–ligand interaction kinetics.

Productive T cell proliferation appears to depend on the formation of a stable central cluster of TCRs interacting with MHC molecules (Fig. 7.19). The final configuration of the synapse has MHC molecule–peptide–TCR interactions at the hub of the synapse ringed by ICAM-1–LFA-1 interactions (Fig. 7.20). Large

Diagram of an immunological synapse

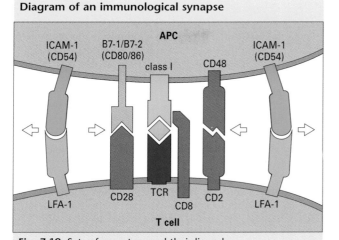

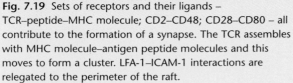

Fig. 7.19 Sets of receptors and their ligands – TCR–peptide–MHC molecule; CD2–CD48; CD28–CD80 – all contribute to the formation of a synapse. The TCR assembles with MHC molecule–antigen peptide molecules and this moves to form a cluster. LFA-1–ICAM-1 interactions are relegated to the perimeter of the raft.

Color-enhanced reconstruction of an immunological synapse

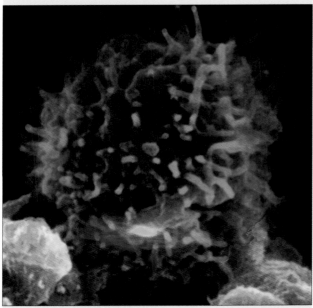

Fig. 7.20 A live-cell fluorescence image, showing the peripheral zone of adhesion molecules (red) surrounding the core containing TCRs (green), is superimposed on a scanning electron micrograph of a T cell (purple) interacting with a DC (dark green). (Courtesy of Dr Mike Dustin and Science)

CD45 molecules, also known as the leukocyte common antigen, are excluded to an outer ring. The precise arrangement of the immunological synapse is cell specific and may be different on T cells and other cells such as NK cells.

Although the interaction between CD4$^+$ T cells and APCs has been reasonably well studied, that between CD8$^+$ T cells and APCs is less well understood. CD4$^+$ cells help in the activation of most CD8$^+$ T cells. Because a single interdigitating DC (IDC) can bind many T cells, it has been proposed that activation takes place in a cluster of CD4$^+$ and CD8$^+$ T cells gathered on the surface of IDCs.

T CELL ACTIVATION LEADS TO PRODUCTION OF IL-2 AND HIGH-AFFINITY IL-2R

Receptors on the surface of T cells signal to the interior of the cell using signal transduction pathways that are common to many other cell types, including B cells. A key principle is the clustering of receptors upon ligand binding. This leads to activation of associated tyrosine kinases, which phosphorylate tyrosine residues in the cytoplasmic tails of the clustered receptors, followed by recruitment of additional kinases and signaling molecules, in cascades. The end-result of these complex pathways is the induction of gene synthesis by the activation of transcription factors (Fig. 7.21).

Activation is initiated by the actions of tyrosine kinases

TCR α and β chains are associated with the CD3γ, δ, and ε molecules, the ζ and η chains (see Fig. 5.3), and the enzyme Lck (p56^{lck}), which is attached to the intracellular portions of CD4 or CD8 (see Fig. 7.21). The label p56^{lck} signifies a lymphocyte-specific tyrosine kinase of 56 kDa.

Recognition of an antigen–MHC molecule complex by the TCR and ligation of co-stimulatory molecules initiates the signaling events.

The earliest events involve tyrosine kinases of the Src family, particularly Lck associated with CD4 and CD8, and Fyn, which phosphorylate target sequences found in the ζ chain (also present on Igα, Igβ, and FcγR, see Fig. 3.20), termed **immunoreceptor tyrosine-based activation motifs (ITAMs)**.

Phosphorylation of the ITAMs initiates a series of steps (see Fig. 7.21), that lead to the activation of transcription factors and their translocation to the nucleus. The transcription factors act on genes required for T cell activation, including the IL-2 and the **IL-2 receptor (IL-2R)** genes.

Q. What occurs when a cell generates both a cytokine and the receptor for that cytokine?

A. This allows autocrine stimulation, where the cell can activate itself as well as similar cells in the immediate vicinity.

Cell division occurs after IL-2 production and is secondary to ligation of the IL-2R.

Intracellular signaling in T cell activation

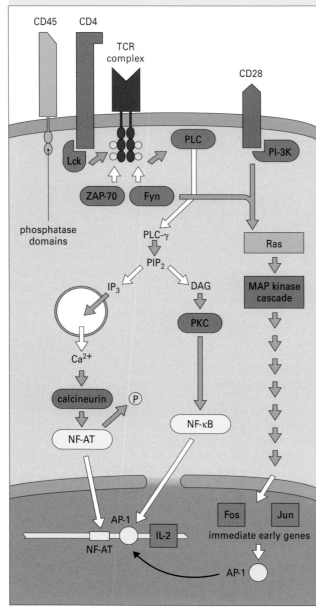

Fig. 7.21 T cell activation involves the transduction of signals from both the TCR and CD28. Clustering of surface receptors such as TCR, CD4, CD28, and CD45 results in activation of tyrosine kinases Fyn and Lck. CD4, which is associated with the TCR complex, binds to the kinase, Lck. Such kinases become activated by dephosphorylation, possibly by phosphatase domains on CD45 (leukocyte common antigen). Lck can now phosphorylate the ITAM domains on the γ chains of CD3 (see Figs 5.3 and 5.15), which allows them to associate with other kinases including Fyn and ZAP-70. Fyn activates phospholipase C (PLCγ), which leads to two pathways by the cleavage of phosphatidylinositol bisphosphate (PIP$_2$) into diacylglycerol (DAG) and inositol trisphosphate (IP$_3$). IP$_3$ releases Ca^{2+} from intracellular (ER) stores to activate calcium-dependent enzymes such as calcineurin. Calcineurin removes phosphate from the transcription factor NF-AT (nuclear factor of activation of T cells), which causes its translocation to the nucleus. DAG activates protein kinase C (PKC), which then activates the transcription factor NF-κB. Meanwhile, ZAP-70, Fyn, and PI-3 kinase (PI-3K) (associated with CD28) integrate signals via kinase cascades in the cytoplasm that activate specific transcription factors. Adapter proteins are used to link the various receptors to the common intracellular signaling components. GTP-binding proteins (G proteins) are involved in activating a set of protein kinases in the MAP kinase cascade. The transcription factors translocate to the nucleus to activate genes, including 'immediate early genes' Fos and Jun for cell division and the promoter AP-1, which acts with NF-AT on the IL-2 gene.

In summary, TCR stimulation results in activation of a variety of tyrosine kinases and downstream effectors that regulate cellular responses, resulting in the regulation of IL-2 gene expression, which is largely responsible for activating the T cell.

B cell activation and T cell activation follow similar patterns

In B cells, the function of CD3 is replaced by Igα and Igβ, which also carry ITAM motifs in their cytoplasmic tails. Cross-linking of surface immunoglobulin leads to activation of the Src family kinases, which in B cells are Fyn, but also Lyn and Blk. A series of analogous activation steps occurs in B cells (see Chapter 8).

An activating signal is integrated from both the antigen receptor and co-stimulatory molecules

It is still not clear exactly what is an effective antigenic signal. For a T cell, interaction at a single TCR is not sufficient, but exactly how many interactions are necessary may depend on other lymphocyte stimulatory signals and the type and activation state of the T cell being stimulated.

Murine T cell hybrids (derived from the fusion of a normal T cell with a tumor T cell) are known to be easily triggered. To stimulate a T cell hybrid:
- an effective APC, such as a macrophage, need carry no more than 60 MHC class II molecule–antigen fragment complexes;

- a weak APC, such as a class II-transfected fibroblast, needs 5000 such complexes.

Recent work has suggested that about 8000 TCR molecules need to interact with MHC molecule–peptide complexes and become activated, as judged by their loss from the T cell surface, for T cell clones to be triggered.

As TCR–MHC molecule interactions are of low affinity, one MHC molecule–peptide complex could activate multiple TCRs.

In the presence of a co-stimulatory signal such as CD28–B7 ligation (see Fig. 7.16), 1500 activated and internalized TCRs are sufficient for the activation of T cell clones.

As discussed above, interaction at the TCR or membrane immunoglobulin alone cannot mediate a positive activation signal for T or B cells. On the contrary it may induce a negative or tolerogenic signal.

Co-stimulatory molecules such as CD2 and CD11a/CD18 (LFA-1) (see Fig. 7.16) are not responsible only for binding – their cytoplasmic domains are also involved in signaling. For example, experimental deletion of the intracytoplasmic domain of CD2 interfered with activation, but left its adhesion function unaltered.

CD28 ligation appears to result in induction of IL-2 synthesis by a pathway distinct from that regulated by calcineurin.

As shown in Fig. 7.21, the induction of IL-2 gene expression requires integrated signals from the activation of PLC, Ras, and the calcium-dependent serine phosphatase calcineurin.

The IL-2 enhancer contains a binding site for a nuclear factor, **NF-AT (nuclear factor of activation of T cells)**, that is induced upon T cell activation. NF-AT is activated by calcineurin. It then translocates to the nucleus where it interacts with Fos and Jun to induce IL-2 gene expression.

IL-2 expression is dependent on the additional signals initiated upon ligation of CD28 by B7 (see Figs 7.19 and 7.21). How the signal from CD28 complements the TCR signal is not established, but it may act by stabilizing IL-2 mRNA as well as increasing transcription.

Ciclosporin, an immunosuppressive drug, causes inhibition of the phosphatase activity of calcineurin.

Rapamycin, another immunosuppressive agent, blocks signaling downstream of IL-2 activation.

Mitogens and superantigens can also activate T cells

T cells can also be activated by some mitogens. Most T cells are stimulated by:
- phytohemagglutinin (PHA), a lectin isolated from red kidney beans; or
- concanavalin-A, extracted from castor beans.

These molecules are able to bind to T cell surface molecules including the TCR complex and CD2, causing them to cluster on the cell surface, thereby mimicking the clustering caused by antigen presentation. Such mitogens, however, will activate the T cells regardless of their antigen specificity.

Another group of molecules that can activate T cells non-specifically are the **superantigens**. These are mostly of bacterial origin and include:

- staphylococcal enterotoxins (responsible for some types of acute food poisoning);
- toxic shock syndrome toxin (responsible for tampon sepsis-induced shock); and
- exfoliative dermatitis toxin.

Superantigens bind to MHC class II molecules on APCs and are recognized by TCRs, but not in the same way as an MHC molecule–peptide complex. Binding is to the Vβ chain of the TCR (see Fig. 5.2) alone. Depending on experimental conditions, the effects are the same as with antigen in that either activation or clonal anergy may occur (Fig. 7.22). A key point about superantigens is that they stimulate families of clones using common Vβ gene segments.

CTLA-4 expression downregulates T cells

The role of the B7 counter-receptor CTLA-4 (CD152) in downregulating T cell activation has been referred to above (see Fig. 7.17).

The negative signal generated by CTLA-4 may be propagated through the cytoplasmic tail of the molecule, which bears a motif known as an **ITIM (immunoreceptor tyrosine-based inhibitory motif)**, which has the characteristic sequence IxYxxL. ITIM motifs are thought to work by recruiting inhibitory phosphatases such as SHIP, which remove phosphate groups added by tyrosine kinases.

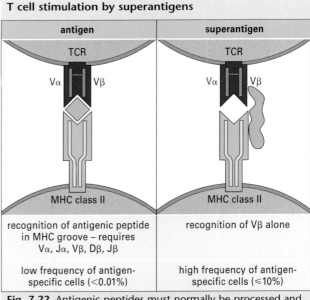

T cell stimulation by superantigens

antigen	superantigen
TCR	TCR
Vα Vβ	Vα Vβ
MHC class II	MHC class II
recognition of antigenic peptide in MHC groove – requires Vα, Jα, Vβ, Dβ, Jβ	recognition of Vβ alone
low frequency of antigen-specific cells (<0.01%)	high frequency of antigen-specific cells (≤10%)

Fig. 7.22 Antigenic peptides must normally be processed and presented on MHC molecules to trigger the TCR. However, superantigens, such as staphylococcal enterotoxins, are not processed, but bind directly to MHC class II molecules and Vβ of the TCR. Each superantigen activates a distinct set of Vβ-expressing T cells, depending on which Vβ gene segment the T cell is expressing.

Q. Which other receptors have ITIMs?

A. The inhibitory Fc receptor FcγRIIb expressed on B cells has ITIMs (see Fig. 3.20). Other inhibitory receptors with similar motifs include the killer inhibitory receptors (KIRs) expressed on NK cells as well as T cells (see Figs 10.3 and 10.5).

Interleukin-2 drives T cell division

Apart from the cell surface interactions, cytokines, acting locally, are required for promoting T cell division (see Fig. 7.18).

Triggering of the TCR along with co-receptors results in IL-2 synthesis by the T cell itself. In most CD4$^+$ cells and some CD8$^+$ T cells, there is a transient production of IL-2 for 1–2 days. During this time the interaction of IL-2 with the high-affinity IL-2R results in T cell division.

On resting T cells, the IL-2R is predominantly present as a low-affinity form consisting of two polypeptide chains, a β chain (p75) that binds IL-2 and a γ chain that signals to the cell. When the T cell is activated, it produces an α chain (p55 = CD25), which contributes to IL-2 binding and, together with the β and γ chains, forms the high-affinity receptor (Fig. 7.23).

The transient expression of the high-affinity IL-2R for about 1 week after stimulation of the T cell, together with the induction of CTLA-4, helps limit T cell division. In the absence of positive signals, the T cells will start to die by apoptosis.

An understanding of the requirements for T cell division has allowed researchers to generate long-lived T cell lines, which are used in many areas of immunological research (Method Box 7.2).

Other cytokines contribute to activation and division

Other cytokines may also contribute to T cell proliferation. For example, IL-1 and IL-6 induce the expression of IL-2R on resting T cells.

Q. Which cells generate IL-1 and IL-6?

A. Mononuclear phagocytes among others. Thus the production of these cytokines enhances their antigen-presenting function.

Additionally IL-4 and IL-15 may provide stimulatory signals through their own receptors.

IL-12 is also of major importance in T cell activation:
- helping to enhance IFNγ production; and
- directing naive T cells to develop into TH1 cells.

IL-15 made by APCs can also induce T cell proliferation and may be very important before IL-2 is produced.

ANTIGEN PRESENTATION AFFECTS THE COURSE OF AN IMMUNE RESPONSE

APCs may be activated rapidly in an immune response, for example by:
- the immunogenic entity itself, in the case of bacteria and some viruses; or
- the antigen in conjunction with the adjuvant component of a vaccine.

METHOD BOX 7.2
T cell lines

To test the response of lymphocytes to a specific antigen that is being presented, the lymphocyte stimulation test (Fig. 1) may be used. This test measures the response of the T cells to antigen as indicated by their entering the cell cycle and incorporating precursors of DNA synthesis.

The lymphocyte stimulation test

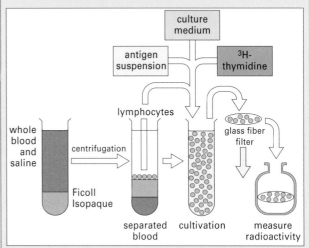

Fig. 1 In the lymphocyte stimulation test, whole blood in saline solution is first layered on Ficoll Isopaque (which has a density between, and therefore separates, white cells and red cells) and centrifuged (400 *g*). This separates the lymphocytes from the other cell and serum constituents. The cells are washed (to remove contaminants such as antigen) and then put into test tubes with a suspension of antigen and culture medium. Triticated thymidine (³H-thymidine) is added 16 hours before the cells are harvested. The cells are harvested on a glass-fiber filter disk and their radioactivity measured by placing the disk in a liquid scintillation counter. A high count indicates that the lymphocytes have undergone transformation and confirms their responsiveness to the antigen. This test can also be used for cells from lymphoid tissue.

Antigen presentation is not a unidirectional process. T cells, as they become activated:
- release cytokines such as IFNγ and granulocyte–macrophage colony stimulating factor (GM–CSF);
- express surface molecules such as CD40 ligand, which enhance antigen presentation.

When APCs are activated, they express more MHC class I and II molecules, Fc receptors, and co-stimulatory adhesion molecules, including B7-1 and B7-2, CD11a/b/c, ICAM-1, and ICAM-3. They also produce numerous cytokines (e.g. IL-1, IL-6, TNFα), enzymes, and other mediators.

Activation of lymphocytes leads to two partially competing processes:
- cell proliferation; and
- cell differentiation into effector cells.

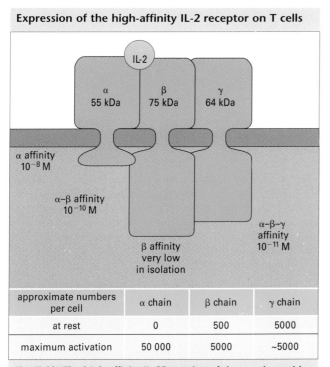

Expression of the high-affinity IL-2 receptor on T cells

IL-2

α
55 kDa

β
75 kDa

γ
64 kDa

α affinity
10^{-8} M

α–β affinity
10^{-10} M

α–β–γ
affinity
10^{-11} M

β affinity
very low
in isolation

approximate numbers per cell	α chain	β chain	γ chain
at rest	0	500	5000
maximum activation	50 000	5000	~5000

Fig. 7.23 The high-affinity IL-2R consists of three polypeptide chains, shown schematically. Resting T cells do not express the α chain, but after activation they may express up to 50 000 α chains per cell. Some of these associate with the β chain to form the high-affinity IL-2R.

Cells at the end stage of differentiation, such as plasma cells, may become so specialized that they lose surface molecules such as MHC class II, and are unable to respond to regulatory signals or to proliferate.

The fate of lymphocytes responding to antigen is varied:

- some can persist for a long time as memory cells – the life span of memory cells can be more than 40 years in humans, as judged by the chromosome abnormalities (e.g. cross-linking of DNA which would prevent mitosis) found in the blood cells of Hiroshima survivors;
- other lymphocytes have a short life span, which explains why moderate antigenic stimulation does not lead to lymphoid enlargement – this is nevertheless sufficient for generating effective cell-mediated and antibody responses.

Apoptosis is critically important for disposing of unwanted cells after an immune response.

The immune system responds to clues that an infection has taken place before responding strongly to antigens

In recent years it has become appreciated that APCs must respond appropriately to an infection, for example, but not to high levels of harmless substances that may fluctuate in the environment.

APC activation is generally a response to infection, or at least the presence of substances, such as constituents of bacterial cell walls, characteristic of infection. This requirement neatly explains the need for **adjuvants**, which are typically derived from bacterial components.

Adjuvants are generally necessary in vaccines to stimulate a robust immune response. The concept of immune activation only in response to infection (or adjuvant as a surrogate for infection), and not to other antigens, has been popularized as the **'danger' hypothesis**. This idea proposes that the immune system does not merely distinguish self from non-self, but responds to clues that an infection has taken place before responding strongly to antigens.

In other words, foreign substances may be innocuous or invisible to the immune system unless accompanied by danger signals, such as infection. These danger signals are provided by receptors for microbial products on APCs, such as the Toll-like receptors (TLRs, see Fig. 6.24).

FURTHER READING

Ackerman, AL, Cresswell P. Cellular mechanisms governing cross-presentation of exogenous antigens. Nat Immunol 2004;5:678–684.

Alberola IJ, Takaki S, Kerner JD, Perlmutter RM. Differential signaling by lymphocyte antigen receptors. Annu Rev Immunol 1997;15:125–154.

Bell D, Young JW, Banchereau J. Dendritic cells. Annu Rev Immunol 1999;17:255–305.

Boes M, Ploegh HL. Translating cell biology in vitro to immunity in vivo. Nature 2004;430:264–271.

Brocke P, Garbi N, Momburg F, Hammerling GJ. HLA-DM, HLA-DO and tapasin: functional similarities and differences. Curr Opin Immunol 2002;14:22–29.

Clements JL, Boerth NJ, Ran Lee J, Koretzky GA. Integration of T cell receptor-dependent signaling pathways by adapter proteins. Annu Rev Immunol 1999;17:89–108.

Germain RN, Stefanova I. The dynamics of T cell receptor signaling: complex orchestration and the key roles of tempo and cooperation. Annu Rev Immunol 1999;17:467–522.

Grakoui A, Bromley SK, Sumen C, et al. The immunological synapse: a molecular machine controlling T cell activation. Science 1999;285:221–227.

Healy JI, Goodnow CC. Positive versus negative signaling by lymphocyte antigen receptors. Annu Rev Immunol 1998;16:645–670.

Kloetzel PM. Generation of MHC class I antigens: functional interplay between proteasomes and TPPII. Nat Immunol 2004;5:661–669.

Lehner PJ, Cresswell P. Recent developments in MHC class I-mediated antigen presentation. Curr Opin Immunol 2004;16:82–89.

Lehner PJ, Trowsdale J. Antigen processing: coming out gracefully. Curr Biol 1998;8:R605–R608.

Mellman I, Turley SJ, Steinman RM. Antigen processing for amateurs and professionals. Trends Cell Biol 1998;8:231–237.

Nelson CA, Fremont DH. Structural principles of MHC class II antigen presentation. Rev Immunogenet 1999;1:47–59.

Pamer E, Cresswell P. Mechanisms of MHC class I-restricted antigen processing. Annu Rev Immunol 1998;16:323–358.

Parham P. Accessory molecules in the immune response. Immunol Rev 1996;153.

Parham P. Mechanisms of antigen-processing. Immunol Rev 1996;151.

Rodriguez A, Regnault A, Kleijmeer M, et al. Selective transport of internalized antigens to the cytosol for MHC class I presentation in dendritic cells. Nat Cell Biol 1999;1:362–368.

Terhorst C, Spits H, Staal F, Exley M. T lymphocyte signal transduction. In: Hames BD, Glover DM, eds. Molecular Immunology. Oxford: IRL Press; 1996.

Watts C, Powis S. Pathways of antigen processing and presentation. Rev Immunogenet 1999;1:60–74.

Critical thinking: Antigen processing and presentation (see p. 495 for explanations)

Two T cell clones have been produced from a mouse infected with influenza virus. One of the clones reacts to a virus peptide when it is presented on APCs that have the same MHC class I (H-2K) locus as the original mouse (i.e. the clone is MHC class I restricted). The other clone is MHC class II restricted. The two clones are stimulated in tissue culture using syngeneic macrophages as APCs. The macrophages have been either infected with live influenza virus or treated with inactivated virus. The patterns of reactivity of the two clones are shown in the table below. In the last two lines of the table the macrophages are pretreated with either emetine or chloroquine before they are infected with virus. Emetine is a protein synthesis inhibitor. Chloroquine inhibits the fusion of lysosomes with phagosomes.

antigen	APCs treated with	reactivity of clone	
		clone 1	clone 2
none	–	–	–
live virus	–	+	+
inactivated virus	–	–	+
live virus	emetine	–	+
live virus	chloroquine	+	–

1 Why are macrophages used as APCs in this experiment? Would you get the same results if you used infected fibroblasts?
2 Why does the live influenza virus stimulate both clones whereas the inactivated virus stimulates only the MHC class II-restricted clone?
3 Why does emetine prevent the macrophages from presenting antigen to the MHC class I-restricted T cells whereas chloroquine prevents them from presenting to MHC class II-restricted cells?
4 One of these clones expresses CD4 and the other CD8. Which way round is it?

Cell Cooperation in the Antibody Response

SUMMARY

- **The primary development of B cells is antigen-independent.** Pre-B cells recombine genes for immunoglobulin heavy and light chains to generate their surface receptor for antigen.

- **T-independent (TI) antigens activate B cells without requiring T cell help.** They can be divided into two groups. TI-1 antigens can act as polyclonal stimulators, while TI-2 antigens are polymers that activate by cross-linking the B cell receptor.

- **T-dependent (TD) antigens are taken up by B cells, processed, and presented to helper T (TH) cells.** T cells and B cells usually recognize different parts of an antigen.

- **B and T cell activation follow similar patterns.** B cell activation requires signals from the B cell receptor (BCR) and co-stimulation. CD40 is the most important co-stimulatory molecule on B cells. Ligation of B cell co-receptor complex can lower the threshold of antigen needed to trigger the B cell. Intracellular signaling pathways are analogous in B and T cells.

- **Cytokine secretion from CD4$^+$ T cells is important in B cell proliferation and differentiation.** Activated B cells proliferate and differentiate into antibody-forming cells (AFCs).

- **B cell affinity maturation takes place in the germinal centers.** Mutation of immunoglobulin genes followed by selection of high-affinity clones is the basis of affinity maturation.

- **B cells switch to another immunoglobulin class (class switching) by recombining heavy chain genes.** Differential splicing of long RNA transcripts is a second mechanism by which B cells can produce more than one type of antibody.

THE PRIMARY DEVELOPMENT OF B CELLS IS ANTIGEN INDEPENDENT

Over a lifetime, an individual may encounter a vast array of unique and different pathogens. To protect the individual, the immune system has evolved a complex system to be able to respond to any conceivable antigen that it encounters. One of the tactics our immune system uses to fight off these foreign antigens is the production of protective proteins, or antibodies.

Antibodies are produced by B cells, and are exceptional in their almost unlimited potential for diversity.

The development of an antibody response is the culmination of a series of cellular and molecular interactions occurring in an orderly sequence between a B cell and a variety of other cells of the immune system.

In this chapter, the principles of B cell development, activation, proliferation, and differentiation leading to the generation of antibody-producing plasma and memory cells are discussed in the context of immune cell cooperation. In addition, some of the critical molecules involved are described and the consequences of the interactions, including affinity maturation and class switching, are examined.

Within the bone marrow, a sequence of immunoglobulin rearrangements and phenotypic changes takes place during B cell ontogeny that leads to the production of the B cell receptor (BCR). This process is analogous to the generation of the T cell receptor (TCR) in thymic T cells (see Chapter 5).

The BCR complex includes the:
- membrane-bound immunoglobulin (mIg);
- Igα; and
- Igβ.

The molecular processes involved in immunoglobulin gene rearrangement are described in Chapter 3, and this section relates these events to B cell development.

The earliest stage of antigen-independent B cell development is the progenitor B (pro-B) cell (Fig. 8.1).

Pro-B cells are divided into early and late pro-B cell groups based on the expression of:
- terminal deoxynucleotidyltransferase (TdT), which is an intranuclear enzyme uniquely expressed during VH gene rearrangement (see Chapter 3); and
- a marker called B220, which identifies a particular variant of leukocyte common antigen (CD45R), a tyrosine phosphatase that appears to be important in regulating BCR signaling.

Early pro-B cells express TdT alone whereas late pro-B cells express B220 and have reduced TdT (intermediate pro-B cells express both markers).

B cell development

	stem cell	pro-B cell		pre-B cell		immature B cell	mature B cell	activated B cell	memory B cell	plasma cell
		early	late	large	small					
H chain gene rearrangement		DJ V-DJ VDJ								
L chain gene rearrangement					V-J VJ					
RAG-1,2/TdT		(bar)			(bar)					
surrogate L chain		(bar)								
immunoglobulin				μ chain	IgM	IgM	IgM & IgD	IgM	IgG/IgA/IgE	secreted Ig
Igα, Igβ		(bar extends across)								
CD34	(bar)									
c-kit	(bar)									
CD43		(bar)								
CD45R		(bar extends across)								
B220	(bar)									
MHC class II		(bar extends across)								
CD19		(bar extends across)								
CD20				(bar extends across)						
CD40		(bar extends across)								

Fig. 8.1 B cells differentiate from lymphoid stem cells into naive B cells and may then be driven by antigen to become memory cells or plasma cells. Upon antigen stimulation, the B cell proliferates and develops into a plasma cell or a memory cell after a phase of proliferation, activation, and blast transformation. During early B cell development, the heavy chain gene (IgH) undergoes a DJ recombination, followed by a VDJ recombination. The recombined heavy chain is initially expressed with a surrogate light chain and the Igα and Igβ chains (CD79) to produce the pre-B cell receptor. Later, light chain genes undergo a VJ recombination and surface IgM is produced as the B cell receptor (BCR). Pre-B cells express cytoplasmic μ chains only. The immature B cell has surface IgM, and the mature B cell other immunoglobulin isotypes. The diagram also shows the time of expression of a number of B cell markers.

B220 remains expressed on the surface throughout the remainder of B cell ontogeny.

Genes for immunoglobulin H and L chains are recombined to generate the surface receptor for antigen

Cells progressing through the pro-B cell stage rearrange their immunoglobulin heavy chain genes and express the **recombination-activating genes *RAG-1* and *RAG-2*** (see Chapter 3). As late pro-B cells pass into the pre-B cell stage, they downregulate TdT, RAG-1, and RAG-2 (see Fig. 8.1).

Pre-B cells can be divided into:
• mitotically active pre-B cells; and
• small non-dividing pre-B cells.
Both large and small pre-B cells express immunoglobulin μ heavy chains (see Chapter 3) in the cytoplasm (cμ) and the pre-B cell receptor complex on their surface (Fig. 8.2).

Large pre-B cells have successfully rearranged their immunoglobulin heavy chain genes. As these cells pass from the large pre-B cell group into the small pre-B cell group, they begin to rearrange their immunoglobulin light chain genes and express *RAG-1* and *RAG-2* again.

The final stage of B cell development is the immature B cell stage. Immature B cells have successfully rearranged their light chain genes and express surface IgM as their antigen receptor, at which time *RAG-1* and *RAG-2* gene expression is again turned off.

Q. What is the significance of the observation that RAG genes are expressed at two distinct times during B cell development?

A. The heavy and the light chain genes undergo rearrangements at different times and the RAGs are expressed at the times when recombination is taking place in either the heavy or the light chain gene loci.

Rapid Reference Box 8

activation-induced cytidine deaminase (AID) – an enzyme expressed in activated B cells that causes somatic mutation.

affinity maturation – the increase in average antibody affinity frequently seen during a secondary immune response.

B cell coreceptor complex – a complex of three cell surface molecules, including CD19, CD81, and the complement receptor CD21, which enhances the sensitivity of the B cell to activation by low quantities of antigen.

CD40 – a critical co-stimulatory receptor on B cells that is ligated by CD40L (= CD154) on helper T cells.

class switching – the process by which an individual B cell can link immunoglobulin heavy chain C genes to its recombined VDJ gene to produce a different class of antibody with the same specificity; this process is also reflected in the overall class switch seen during the maturation of an immune response.

iccosomes – immune complexes in the form of small inclusion bodies found on follicular dendritic cells.

interleukin-4 (IL-4) – previously called B cell growth factor, a key cytokine for B cell division and differentiation.

receptor editing – a process in which the genes for the B cell antigen receptor (antibody) undergo a secondary process of recombination, which allows production of non-self reactive antibodies.

somatic mutation – a process during B cell maturation affecting the antibody gene region, that permits refinement of antibody specificity.

T-dependent and T-independent antigens – describe the requirements of B cells in producing secreted antibody in response to antigenic stimulation; T-independent antigens can induce antibody production by B cells without T cell help.

The pre-B cell receptor

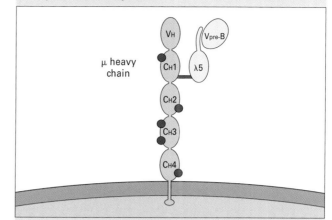

Fig. 8.2 The surrogate BCR complex is composed of a μ heavy chain and V_{pre-B} and λ5 proteins (surrogate light chains). The receptor has a role in early differentiation and development of B cells. The unit shown here associates with the signaling molecules Igα and Igβ.

they undergo activation, proliferation, and differentiation, leading to the generation of plasma cells and memory B cells.

The immune response to most antigens depends on both T cells and B cells recognizing the antigen in a linked fashion. This type of antigen is called a **T-dependent (TD) antigen**.

A small number of antigens, however, can activate B cells without MHC class II-restricted T cell help and are referred to as **T-independent (TI) antigens** (Fig. 8.3).

T-independent antigens

antigen	polymeric	polyclonal activation	resistance to degradation
lipopolysaccharide (LPS)	+	+ + +	+
Ficoll	+ + +	–	+ + +
dextran	+ +	+	+ +
levan	+ +	+	+ +
poly-D amino acids	+ + +	–	+ + +
polymeric bacterial flagellin	+ +	+ +	+

Fig. 8.3 The major common properties of some of the main TI antigens are listed. TI antigens induce the production of cytokines interleukin-1 (IL-1), tumor necrosis factor-α (TNFα), and IL-6 by macrophages. (Note that both poly-L amino acids and monomeric bacterial flagellin are TD antigens, demonstrating the role of antigen structure in determining TI properties.)

As immature B cells develop further into mature B cells, they begin to express both IgM and IgD on their surface. These mature B cells are then free to exit the bone marrow and migrate into the periphery.

Other phenotypic markers can also help to identify particular populations of pro-B, pre-B, or immature B cells (see Fig. 8.1).

In addition, a number of growth and differentiation factors are required to drive the B cells through the early stages of development. Receptors for these factors are expressed at various stages of B cell differentiation:

• IL-4, IL-3, and low molecular weight B cell growth factor (L-BCGF) are important in initiating the process of B cell differentiation;

• other factors are active in the later stages.

TI ANTIGENS DO NOT REQUIRE T CELL HELP TO ACTIVATE B CELLS

Naive mature B cells are free to exit the bone marrow and migrate into the periphery. If these cells do not encounter antigen, they die within a few weeks by apoptosis. If, however, these mature B cells encounter specific antigen,

Importantly, many TI antigens are particularly resistant to degradation. TI antigens can be divided into two groups (TI-1 and TI-2) based on the manner in which they activate B cells:

- TI-1 antigens are predominantly bacterial cell wall components – the prototypical TI-1 antigen is lipopolysaccharide (LPS), a component of the cell wall of Gram-negative bacteria;
- TI-2 antigens are predominantly large polysaccharide molecules with repeating antigenic determinants (e.g. Ficoll, dextran, polymeric bacterial flagellin, and poliomyelitis virus).

Q. What common characteristic can you see in many of the TI antigens, and how are such antigens recognized by the immune system?

A. Many TI antigens have **pathogen-associated molecular patterns (PAMPs)** recognized by **Toll-like receptors** (e.g. TLR4 recognizes LPS and TLR5 recognizes flagellin, see Fig. 6.24). They therefore have an intrinsic ability to activate the immune system irrespective of their ability to bind to the specific antigen receptor on individual B cell clones.

Many TI-1 antigens possess the ability in high concentrations to activate B cell clones that are specific for other antigens – a phenomenon known as polyclonal B cell activation. However, in lower concentrations they only activate B cells specific for themselves. TI-1 antigens do not require a second signal.

TI-2 antigens, on the other hand, are thought to activate B cells by clustering and cross-linking immunoglobulin molecules on the B cell surface, leading to prolonged and persistent signaling. TI-2 antigens require residual non-cognate T cell help, such as cytokines.

Several signal transduction molecules are necessary for mediating TI antigen responses in B cells. These include:

- CD19;
- HS1 protein;
- Lyn;
- IL-5Rα;
- receptors for TNFα and lymphotoxin α.

TI antigens induce poor memory

Primary antibody responses to TI antigens in vitro are generally slightly weaker than those to TD antigens. They peak fractionally earlier and both generate mainly IgM.

The secondary responses to TD and TI antigens differ greatly:

- the secondary response to TI antigens resembles the primary response; whereas
- the secondary response to TD antigens is far stronger and has a large IgG component (Fig. 8.4).

It seems, therefore, that TI antigens do not usually induce the maturation of a response leading to **class switching** or to an increase in antibody affinity, as seen with TD antigens. This is most likely due to a lack of co-stimulation mediated via CD40 (see below) and a lack of key cytokines released by T cells (IL-2, IL-4, IL-5).

Memory induction to TI antigens is also relatively poor.

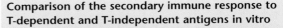
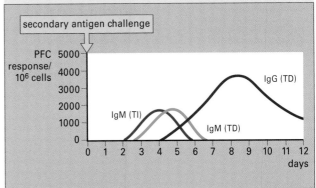

Comparison of the secondary immune response to T-dependent and T-independent antigens in vitro

Fig. 8.4 The secondary response to TD antigens is stronger and induces a greater number of IgG-producing cells, as measured in a plaque-forming cell (PFC) assay (see Method Box 8.1).

A number of assays for measuring antibody production by B cells are outlined in Method Box 8.1.

There are potential survival advantages if the immune response to bacteria does not depend on complex cell interactions because it could be more rapid.

Many bacterial antigens bypass T cell help because they are very effective inducers of cytokine production by macrophages – they induce IL-1, IL-6, and TNFα from macrophages. Some such antigens directly stimulate B cells.

TI antigens tend to activate the CD5⁺ subset of B cells

TI antigens predominantly activate the B-1 subset of B cells found mainly in the peritoneum. These B-1 cells can be identified by their expression of CD5, which is induced upon binding of TI antigens. In contrast to conventional B cells, B-1 cells have the ability to replenish themselves.

TD ANTIGENS REQUIRE T CELL HELP TO ACTIVATE B CELLS
T cells and B cells recognize different parts of antigens

In the late 1960s and early 1970s, studies by Mitchison and others, using chemically modified proteins, led to significant advances in understanding of the different functions of T cells and B cells.

To induce an optimal secondary antibody response to a small chemical group or **hapten** (which is immunogenic only if bound to a protein carrier), it was found that the experimental animal must be immunized and then challenged using the same hapten–carrier conjugate – not just the same hapten. This was referred to as the **carrier effect**.

METHOD BOX 8.1
Measuring antibody production – the PFC assay and ELISPOT

Various methods have been developed for assaying antibody production. Two such methods are the plaque-forming cell (PFC) assay and the enzyme-linked immunospot assay (ELISPOT).

Antibody-forming cells (AFCs) are measured by means of a quantitative PFC assay (Fig. 1), originally developed by Niels Jerne in the 1960s. B cells (e.g. spleen cells) are plated in agar with sheep red blood cells sensitized by binding the specific antigen to their surface. Antibody produced by any B cell will coat the red blood cells. Following the addition of complement, these coated cells may be lyzed, causing the appearance of a zone of lyzed cells (plaque) in the agar. The panel on the right in Fig. 1 shows the appearance of such a plaque, with a B cell in the center, under the microscope. The plaques are then counted to give a quantitative measure of the number of PFCs.

Another way of detecting antibody-producing cells is by means of an enzyme-linked immunospot assay (ELISPOT, Method Box 2.1, Fig. 3). An ELISPOT assay starts out by coating a plastic well with antigen and adding a known quantity of B cells. The antigen coated onto the plastic will then capture any antibody in the vicinity of the activated B cell that is producing the antibody. After a period of time, the B cells are removed, and the specific antibody can be detected by adding an enzyme-labeled anti-immunoglobulin plus chromogen. Development of the label in this assay results in a spot surrounding the active B cell. Counting each spot and knowing the quantity of B cells originally added to the well allows one to enumerate the frequency of B cells producing the specific antibody. Method Box 2.1, Fig. 3 shows the method of detecting antibodies and the appearance of the spots on the developed plates. In addition to analyzing specific antibody-secreting B cells, the ELISPOT assay has been adapted to measure the frequency of cytokine-secreting T cells and various other cell types (right panel). With the improvement in ELISPOT assay plate design and in ELISPOT detection equipment, antibody- or cytokine-secreting cells can now be detected at the single cell level.

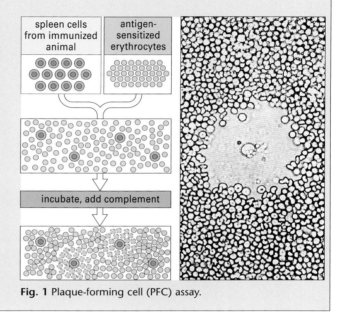

Fig. 1 Plaque-forming cell (PFC) assay.

By manipulating the cell populations in these experiments, it was shown that:
- helper T cells (TH) cells are responsible for recognizing the carrier; whereas
- the B cells recognize hapten.

These experiments were later reinforced by details of how:
- B cells use antibody to recognize epitopes; while
- T cells recognize processed antigen fragments.

One consequence of this system is that an individual B cell can receive help from T cells specific for different antigenic peptides provided that the B cell can present those determinants to each T cell.

In an immune response in vivo, it is believed that the interactions between T and B cells that drive B cell division and differentiation involve T cells that have already been stimulated by contact with the antigen on other antigen-presenting cells (APCs), for example dendritic cells.

This has led to the basic scheme for cell interactions in the antibody response set out in Fig. 8.5. It is proposed that antigen entering the body is processed by cells that present the antigen in a highly immunogenic form to the TH and B cells. The T cells recognize determinants on the antigen that are distinct from those recognized by the B cells, which differentiate and divide into antibody-forming cells (AFCs). Therefore two processes are required to activate a B cell:
- antigen interacting with B cell immunoglobulin receptors – this involves 'native' antigen;
- stimulating signal(s) from TH cells that respond to processed antigen bound to MHC class II molecules.

B AND T CELL ACTIVATION FOLLOW SIMILAR PATTERNS

In B cells the signaling function of CD3 in T cells is carried out by a heterodimer of Igα and Igβ. Two molecules of the Igα–Igβ heterodimer associate with surface immunoglobulin to form the BCR. The cytoplasmic tails of Igα and Igβ carry **immunoreceptor tyrosine activation motifs (ITAMs)**.

Cross-linking of surface immunoglobulin leads to activation of the Src family kinases, which in B cells are Fyn, but also Lyn, and Blk. Syk is analogous to ZAP-70 in T cells, and binds to the phosphorylated ITAMs of Igα and Igβ (Fig. 8.6). This leads to activation of a kinase cascade and translocation of nuclear transcription factors

Cell cooperation in the antibody response

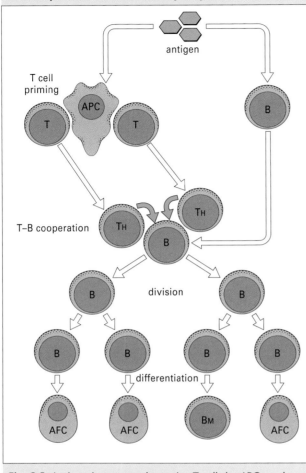

Fig. 8.5 Antigen is presented to naive T cells by APCs such as dendritic cells. B cells also take up antigen and present it to the T cells, receiving signals from the T cells to divide and differentiate into antibody-forming cells (AFCs) and memory B cells (BM).

Intracellular signaling in B cell activation

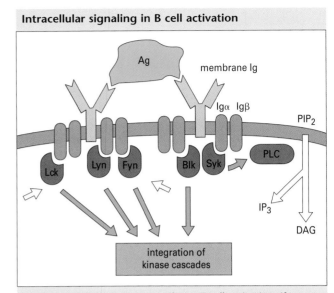

Fig. 8.6 B cell activation is similar to T cell activation. If membrane immunoglobulin becomes cross-linked (e.g. by a TI antigen), tyrosine kinases, including Lck, Lyn, Fyn, and Blk, become activated. They phosphorylate the ITAM domains in the Igα and Igβ chains of the receptor complex. These can then bind another kinase, Syk, which activates phospholipase C. This acts on membrane phosphatidylinositol bisphosphate (PIP$_2$) to generate inositol trisphosphate (IP$_3$) and diacyl glycerol (DAG), which activates protein kinase C. Signals from the other kinases are transduced to activate nuclear transcription factors.

Q. If an animal was depleted of complement C3 during the primary immune response, what effect do you think this would have on the development of the secondary antibody response?

A. Lack of C3 means that immune complexes containing C3b and C3d do not form. Therefore they cannot bind to follicular dendritic cells (FDCs) via CR2 or engage with B cells via the B cell co-receptor complex (see Fig. 8.7); consequently B cell activation and the development of the secondary immune response is greatly impaired. (These experiments have been done by depleting mice of C3 using cobra venom factor.)

analogous to the process that occurs in T cells (see Fig. 7.21).

B cell activation is also markedly augmented by the 'co-receptor complex' comprising three proteins:
- CD21 (complement receptor-2, CR2);
- CD19; and
- CD81 (target of antiproliferative antibody, TAPA-1) (Fig. 8.7).

Follicular dendritic cells are known to retain antigen on their surface for prolonged periods of time as immune complexes (**iccosomes**). The antigen in such complexes can bind to:
- CD21 (via the complement fragment C3d); and
- surface immunoglobulin on the B cells.

Phosphorylation of the cytoplasmic tail of CD19 can then occur, leading to binding and activation of Lyn. It is likely that these kinases enhance the activation signal through the phospholipase C and phosphatidylinositol 3-kinase pathways, particularly when antigen concentration is low.

Direct interaction of B cells and T cells involves co-stimulatory molecules

Antigen-specific T cell populations can be obtained by growing and cloning T cells with antigens, APCs, and IL-2. It is therefore possible to visualize directly B cell and T cell clusters interacting in vitro:
- the T cells become polarized, with the TCRs concentrated on the B cell side;
- the B cells also become polarized and express most of their MHC class II molecules and intercellular adhesion molecule-1 (ICAM-1) in proximity to the T cells.

B cell co-receptor complex

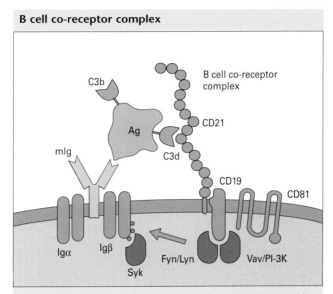

Fig. 8.7 The B cell co-receptor complex consists of CD21 (the complement receptor type 2), CD19, and CD81 (a molecule with four transmembrane segments). Antigen with covalently bound C3b or C3d can cross-link the membrane immunoglobulin to CD21 of the co-receptor complex. This greatly reduces the cell's requirement for antigen to activate it. CD19 can associate with tyrosine kinases including Lyn, Fyn, Vav, and PI-3 kinase (PI-3K). Compare this with CD28 on the T cell (see Fig. 7.21). Receptor cross-linking causes phosphorylation of the Igα and Igβ chains of the antigen–receptor complex and recruitment and activation of Syk.

The interactions in these clusters strongly suggest an intense exchange of information, which leads to two important events in the B cell life cycle:

• induction of proliferation; and
• differentiation into AFCs.

The initial interaction between a naive B cell and a **cognate antigen** via the BCR in the presence of cytokines or other growth stimuli induces activation and proliferation of the B cell. This then leads to processing of the TD antigen and presentation to T cells (see Chapter 7).

The interaction between B and T cells is a two-way process in which:

• B cells present antigen to T cells; and
• receive signals from the T cells for division and differentiation (Fig. 8.8).

The central antigen-specific interaction is that between the MHC class II molecule–antigen complex and the TCR. This interaction is augmented by interactions between pairs of adhesion molecules and co-stimulatory molecules.

Q. Which co-stimulatory molecules, present on B cells and other APCs, promote T cell proliferation? What mechanisms are involved?

A. B7-1 (CD80) and B7-2 (CD86) act on antigen-activated T cells by ligating CD28, leading to expression of the high-affinity IL-2 receptor (see Fig. 7.16).

Cell surface molecules involved in the interaction between B and TH cells

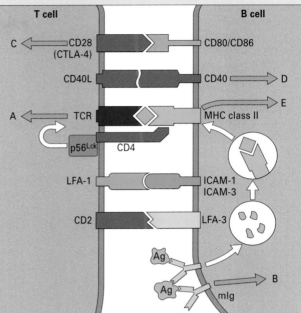

Fig. 8.8 Membrane immunoglobulin (mIg) takes up antigen (Ag) into an intracellular compartment where it is degraded and peptides can combine with MHC class II molecules. Other arrows show the discrete signal transduction events that have been established. A and B are the antigen receptor signal transduction events involving tyrosine phosphorylation and phosphoinositide breakdown. The antigen receptors also regulate LFA-1 affinity for ICAM-1 and ICAM-3, possibly through the signal transduction events. In the T cell, CD28 also sends a unique signal to the T cell (C). In the later phases of the response CTLA-4 can supplant CD28 to cause downregulation (see Fig. 7.18). In the B cell, stimulation via CD40 is the most potent activating signal (D). In addition, MHC class II molecules appear to induce distinct signaling events (E). Not shown is the exchange of soluble interleukins and binding to the corresponding receptors on the other cell. (Adapted from DeFranco A. Nature 1991;351:603–605)

The interaction between B and T cells is a two-way event as follows:

• CD40, a member of the TNF receptor family, delivers a strong activating signal to B cells, more potent even than signals transmitted via surface immunoglobulin;
• upon activation, T cells transiently express a ligand, termed CD40L (a member of the TNF family), which interacts with CD40;
• CD40–CD40L interaction helps to drive B cells into cell cycle;
• transduction of signals through CD40 induces upregulation of CD80/CD86 and therefore helps to provide further co-stimulatory signals to the responding T cells.

Signaling through CD40 is also essential for germinal center development and antibody responses to TD antigens.

Q. Some individuals have a mutation that produces a non-functional variant of CD40L. In its homozygous form, what effect would you expect this mutation to have on serum antibody levels?

A. The mutation produces hyper-IgM syndrome, with high serum IgM and low IgG, IgA, and IgE levels, due to lack of germinal centers and failure of the B cells to switch isotype.

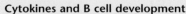

CYTOKINE SECRETION FROM CD4⁺ T CELLS CONTROLS B CELL PROLIFERATION AND DIFFERENTIATION

The cytokine milieu is critical for determining the outcome of an immune response following B cell–T cell interaction. Recent work has shown that CD4⁺ T cells in both mouse and human can be divided into different subsets, depending on their cytokine profile (Fig. 8.9):

- TH1 cells – CD4⁺ T cells that produce IL-2 and interferon-γ (IFNγ), but not IL-4, are designated TH1 and are chiefly responsible for delayed-type hypersensitivity responses, but can also help B cells produce IgG2a (mouse), but not much IgG1 or IgE;
- TH2 cells – CD4⁺ T cells that produce IL-4, IL-5, IL-10, and IL-13, but not IL-2 or IFNγ, are designated TH2 and are very efficient helper cells for production of antibody, especially IgG1 and IgE;
- TH0 cells – many CD4⁺ T cells, especially in humans, have cytokine profiles intermediate between TH1 cells and TH2 cells, and are known as 'TH0' cells. These cells are capable of producing both the TH1 cytokine IFNγ and the TH2 cytokine IL-4. However, classic TH1 and TH2 cells have been well documented in humans, especially in diseased tissues.

During B cell–T cell interaction, T cells can secrete a number of cytokines that have a powerful effect on B cells (see Fig. 8.9). IL-2, for example, is an inducer of proliferation for B cells.

The specific cytokines produced by TH2 cells also affect B cells. These cytokines include IL-4, IL-5, IL-6, IL-10, and IL-13:

- IL-4 (previously known as B cell activating or differentiation factor-1) acts on B cells to induce activation and differentiation, and acts on T cells as a growth factor and promotes differentiation of TH2 cells, thus reinforcing the antibody response – excess IL-4 plays a part in allergic disease, causing production of IgE;
- IL-5 in humans is chiefly a growth and activation factor for eosinophils and is responsible for the eosinophilia of parasitic disease (in the mouse it also acts on B cells to induce growth and differentiation);
- IL-6 is produced by many cells including T cells, macrophages, B cells, fibroblasts, and endothelial cells, and acts on most cells, but is particularly important in inducing B cells to differentiate into AFCs – IL-6 is considered to be an important growth factor for multiple myeloma, a malignancy of plasma cells;
- IL-10 acts as a growth and differentiation factor for B cells in addition to modulating cytokine production by TH1 cells;
- IL-13, which shares a receptor component and signaling pathways with IL-4, acts on B cells to produce IgE.

Other cytokines such as IL-7, originally isolated from a stromal cell line as a factor supporting pre-B cell growth, have been shown to be indispensable for B cell development.

Q. Give three different ways in which IL-4 can reinforce the TH2-type immune response.

A. It promotes differentiation of TH0 cells into TH2 cells. It acts on B cells to promote their division, differentiation, and antibody synthesis. It also acts on endothelium and tissue cells to promote the synthesis of chemokines that selectively attract TH2 cells.

Cytokines and B cell development

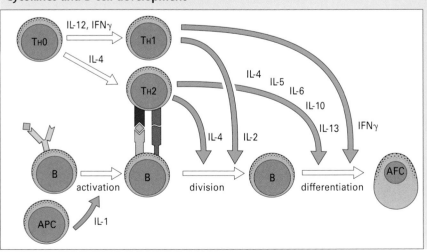

Fig. 8.9 B cell development is influenced by cytokines from T cells and APCs, and by direct interactions with TH2 cells. IL-4 is most important in promoting division, and and a variety of cytokines including IL-4, IL-5, IL-6, IL-10, and IFNγ influence development into antibody-forming cells (AFCs), and affect the isotype of antibody that will be produced.

Cytokines can also influence antibody affinity. Antibody affinity to most TD antigens increases during an immune response, and a similar effect can be produced by certain immunization protocols. For example, high-affinity antibody subpopulations are potentiated after immunization with antigen and IFNγ (Fig. 8.10).

A number of adjuvants are capable of enhancing levels of antibody, but few have this characteristic of also potentiating affinity. As affinity markedly influences the biological effectiveness of antibodies, IFNγ may be an important adjuvant for use in vaccines.

Q. Why do adjuvants not generally enhance antibody affinity, though they do enhance antibody titers? – think of when and how adjuvants act.

A. Most adjuvants act as depots for antigen or have components that promote antigen presentation to T cells. They do not act directly on B cells.

In addition to the effects of cytokines on B cell proliferation and differentiation, cytokines are capable of influencing the class switch from IgM to other immunoglobulin classes (see below).

Cytokine influence on antibody affinity

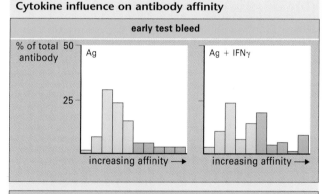

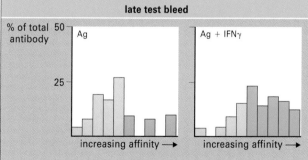

Fig. 8.10 Mice were immunized either with antigen alone (Ag) or with antigen plus 30 000 units of IFNγ (Ag + IFNγ). The affinity of the antibodies was measured either early or late after immunization. Mice receiving IFNγ showed more high-affinity antibody (darker bars) in both the early and late bleeds than mice that received antigen alone. (Adapted from Holland GP, Holland N, Steward MW. Clin Exp Immunol 1990;82:221–226)

Cytokine receptors aid in B cell growth and differentiation

Receptors for the many growth and differentiation factors required to drive the B cells through their early stages of development are expressed at various stages of B cell differentiation. Receptors for IL-7, IL-3, and low molecular weight B cell growth factor are important in the initial stages of B cell differentiation whereas other receptors are more important in the later stages (Fig. 8.11).

B cell–T cell interaction may either activate or inactivate (anergize)

The above description of B cell–T-cell interaction suggests that the only possible outcome is activation of the B cell. However, this is not the case.

APC–T cell interaction may yield two diametrically opposing results, namely activation or inactivation (**clonal anergy**, see Fig. 7.18).

In the same way, B cells frequently become anergic. This is an important process because affinity maturation of B cells (see below) during the immune response as a result of rapid mutation in the genes encoding the antibody variable regions could easily result in high-affinity autoantibodies.

Clonal anergy and other forms of tolerance in the periphery are important for silencing these potentially damaging clones. However, the molecular details of this process are still unclear. Moreover, the respective roles of IgM and IgD, the two cell surface receptors for antigen on B cells, are also not understood in terms of activation or inactivation. Both IgM and IgD appear to be capable of transmitting signals for both functions.

Following activation, antigen-specific B cells can follow either of two separate developmental pathways:
• the first pathway involves proliferation and differentiation into AFCs in the lymph nodes or in the periarteriolar lymphoid sheath of the spleen – these AFCs function to rapidly clear antigen, but the great majority of these cells die via apoptosis within 2 weeks, so it is unlikely that these AFCs are responsible for long-term antibody production;
• in the second pathway some members of the expanded B cell population migrate into adjacent follicles to form germinal centers before differentiating into memory B cells.

The mechanism that determines which path a B cell takes is unknown. However, it is likely that the decision can be influenced by the nature of the naive B cells initially recruited into the response, the affinity and specificity of the BCR, the type of antigen driving the response, and the levels of T cell help.

Q. Which type of APC is specifically located in the germinal center?

A. FDCs (see Fig. 7.2), and these turn out to be very important in driving B cell development.

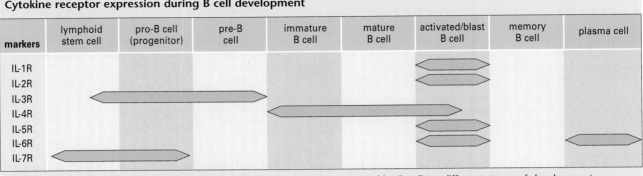

Cytokine receptor expression during B cell development

markers	lymphoid stem cell	pro-B cell (progenitor)	pre-B cell	immature B cell	mature B cell	activated/blast B cell	memory B cell	plasma cell
IL-1R						◇		
IL-2R						◇		
IL-3R	◁———————————▷							
IL-4R				◁————————————————————▷				
IL-5R						◇		
IL-6R						◇		◇
IL-7R	◁————————▷							

Fig. 8.11 The whole life history of B cells from stem cell to mature plasma cell is regulated by cytokines present in their environment. Receptors for these cytokines are selectively expressed by B cells at different stages of development. Many of these receptors now have CD nomenclature (see Appendix 2).

B CELL AFFINITY MATURATION TAKES PLACE IN THE GERMINAL CENTERS

The germinal center is important in that it provides a microenvironment whereby B cells can undergo developmental events that ultimately result in an affinity-matured, long-lived memory B cell compartment of the immune system (Fig. 8.12). These developmental events come about due to complex interactions between B cells, CD4⁺ helper T cells, and FDCs. These events include:

- clonal proliferation;
- antibody variable region somatic hypermutation;
- receptor editing;
- isotype switch recombination;
- affinity maturation; and
- positive selection.

The germinal center initially contains only dividing centroblasts. Shortly thereafter, the germinal center polarizes itself into a dark zone containing centroblasts and a light zone containing non-dividing (resting) centrocytes (Figs 8.13 and 8.14). Centroblasts proliferate rapidly in the dark zone and downregulate the expression of their surface immunoglobulin. **Somatic hypermutation** then occurs to diversify the rearranged variable region genes (see Chapter 3, p. 83). Somatic hypermutation allows a single B cell to give rise to a clone that contains variants with different affinities for the antigen.

B cell development in germinal centers

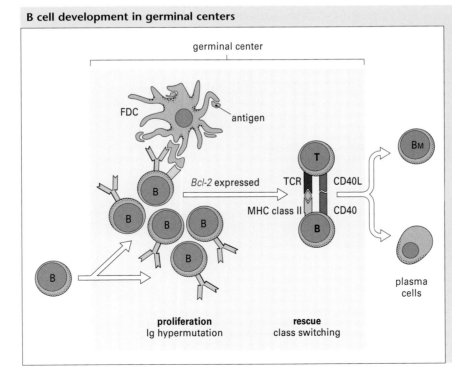

Fig. 8.12 A B cell enters a germinal center and undergoes rapid proliferation and hypermutation of its immunoglobulin genes. Antigen is presented by the follicular dendritic cell (FDC), but only B cells with high-affinity receptors will compete effectively for this antigen. B cells that do have a higher-affinity immunoglobulin express *Bcl-2* and are rescued from apoptosis by interaction with T cells (i.e. the B cell presenting antigen to the T cell). Interaction with T cells promotes class switching. The class switch that takes place depends on the T cells present, which partly relates to the particular secondary lymphoid tissue and the type of current immune response (TH1 versus TH2). B cells leave the germinal center to become either plasma cells or B memory cells (BM).

Schematic organization of the germinal center

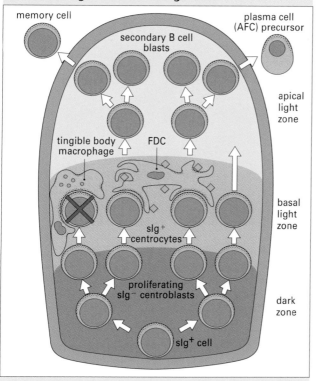

Fig. 8.13 The functions of the germinal center are clonal proliferation, somatic hypermutation of immunoglobulin receptors, receptor editing, isotype class switching, affinity maturation, and selection by antigen. In this model, the germinal center is composed of three major zones – a dark zone, a basal light zone, and an apical light zone. These zones are predominantly occupied by centroblasts, centrocytes, and secondary blasts, respectively. Primary B cell blasts carrying surface immunoglobulin receptors (sIg⁺) enter the follicle and leave as memory B cells or AFCs. Antigen-presenting follicular dendritic cells (FDCs) are mainly found in the two deeper zones, and cell death by apoptosis occurs primarily in the basal light zone where tingible body macrophages are also located. Blue squares are iccosomes on the FDC. (Adapted from Roitt IM. Essential Immunology, 7th edn. Oxford: Blackwell Scientific, 1991. Copyright 1991 with permission from Blackwell Publishing)

Isotype switch recombination (see below) occurs following somatic hypermutation and requires cell cycling. Receptor editing of immunoglobulin light chain genes also occurs in centroblasts.

Following these developmental changes, the centroblasts migrate to the FDC light zone of the germinal center and give rise to centrocytes, which then re-express surface immunoglobulin BCR. In the light zone, centrocytes encounter antigen bound to the FDCs and antigen-specific T$_H$2 cells. FDCs and T cells interact with centrocytes through:

- surface molecules such as the BCR, CD40, CD80 (B7-1), CD86 (B7-2), LFA-1, VLA-4, CD54 (ICAM-1), and CD106 (VCAM-1); and

Zoning of the germinal center of a lymph node

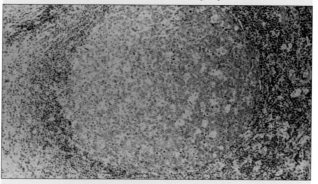

Fig. 8.14 This Giemsa-stained section (× 40) shows the light part (left) and the more actively proliferating dark part (right). There is a well-developed mantle of small resting lymphocytes, which have less cytoplasm and therefore appear more densely packed. (Courtesy of Dr K McLennan)

- cytokines such as IL-2, IL-4, IL-5, IL-6, IL-10, IL-13, and lymphotoxin-α.

After the centrocytes have stopped dividing, they are selected according to their ability to bind antigen. Those with high-affinity receptors for foreign antigen are positively selected whereas those without adequate affinity undergo Fas-dependent apoptosis (see Chapter 10).

Self-reactive B cells generated by somatic mutation are deleted

Centrocytes that respond to soluble antigen or do not receive T cell help are negatively selected and undergo **Fas-independent apoptosis**. In this way, selection provides a mechanism for elimination of self-reactive antibodies that may be generated during somatic hypermutation.

Positively selected centrocytes can re-enter the dark zone for successive rounds of expansion, diversification, and selection.

Somatic hypermutation and selection improve the average affinity of the germinal center B cell population for presented antigen.

Following these B cell developmental stages, the centrocytes exit the germinal center and lose their susceptibility to apoptosis by:
- reducing Fas; and
- increasing the expression of Bcl-2.

Three possible outcomes are associated with exit from the germinal center:
- antibody-secreting bone marrow homing effector B cells;
- marginal zone memory B cells;
- recirculating memory B cells.

The factors that regulate the decision to exit the germinal center are poorly understood.

In-vivo antibody responses show isotype switching, affinity maturation, and memory

The earliest studies on antibody responses followed the development of specific antibodies in animals immunized

with TD or TI antigens. With our improved knowledge of B cell development and maturation, it is now possible to understand the features of immune responses in vivo in terms of the underlying cellular events. Features of antibody responses in vivo include:
• the enhanced secondary response;
• isotype switching;
• affinity maturation;
• the development of memory.

However, some of these events can be understood only by viewing the B cell population as a whole, rather than as a collection of individual cells. The elements of the antibody response in vivo are detailed as follows.

Following primary antigenic challenge, there is an initial lag phase when no antibody can be detected. This is followed by phases in which the antibody titer increases logarithmically to a plateau and then declines. The decline occurs because the antibodies are either:
• naturally catabolized; or
• bind to the antigen and are cleared from the circulation (Fig. 8.15).

An examination of the responses following primary and secondary antigenic challenge shows that the responses differ in the following four major respects (Fig. 8.16):
• time course – the secondary response has a shorter lag phase and an extended plateau and decline;
• antibody titer – the plateau levels of antibody are much greater in the secondary response, typically 10-fold or more than plateau levels in the primary response;
• antibody class – IgM antibodies form a major proportion of the primary response, whereas the secondary response consists almost entirely of IgG, with very little IgM;

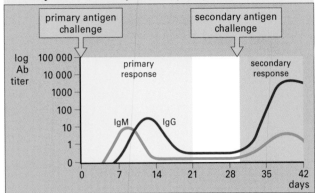

Primary and secondary antibody responses

Fig. 8.16 In comparison with the antibody response after primary antigenic challenge, the antibody level after secondary antigenic challenge in a typical immune response appears more quickly, persists for a longer period of time, attains a higher titer, and consists predominantly of IgG antibodies.

• antibody affinity – the affinity of the antibodies in the secondary response is usually much higher; this is referred to as 'affinity maturation'.

The functions of the different antibody classes are detailed in Chapter 3.

Affinity maturation of B cells depends on cell selection

The antibodies produced in a primary response to a TD antigen generally have a low average affinity. However, during the course of the response, the average affinity of the antibodies increases or 'matures'. As antigen becomes limiting, the clones with the higher affinity have a selective advantage. This process is called **affinity maturation**.

The degree of affinity maturation is inversely related to the dose of antigen administered. High antigen doses produce poor maturation compared with low antigen doses (Fig. 8.17). It is thought that:
• in the presence of low antigen concentrations only B cells with high-affinity receptors bind sufficient antigen and are triggered to divide and differentiate;
• in the presence of high antigen concentrations, there is sufficient antigen to bind and trigger both high- and low-affinity B cells.

Although individual B cells do not usually change their overall specificity, the affinity of the antibody produced by a clone may be altered.

Affinity maturation is achieved through two processes

Affinity maturation is achieved through two processes:
• somatic mutation of the variable (V), diversity (D), and joining (J) gene segments encoding the variable regions of antibodies (see Chapter 3);

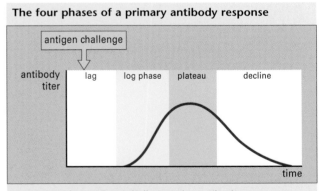

The four phases of a primary antibody response

Fig. 8.15 After antigen challenge, the antibody response proceeds in four phases – a lag phase when no antibody is detected; a log phase when the antibody titer increases logarithmically; a plateau phase during which the antibody titer stabilizes; and a decline phase during which the antibody is cleared or catabolized. In a primary immune response, IgM initially predominates, followed by IgG. The actual time course and titers reached depend on the nature of the antigenic challenge and the nature of the host.

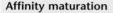

Affinity maturation

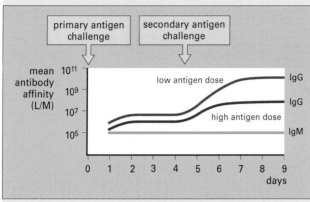

Fig. 8.17 The average affinity of the IgM and IgG antibody responses after primary and secondary challenge with a TD antigen is shown. The affinity of the IgM response is constant throughout. The affinity maturation of the IgG response depends on the dose of the secondary antigen. Low antigen doses produce higher-affinity immunoglobulin than high antigen doses because the high-affinity clones compete effectively for the limiting amount of antigen.

- antigen-driven selection and expansion of mutant clones expressing higher-affinity antibodies.

The mechanism by which affinity maturation occurs is thought to involve B cell progeny binding to antigen on FDCs in order to proliferate and differentiate further. It is thought that unprocessed antigen in immune complexes is captured by FDCs via their Fc and complement receptors (see Fig. 2.18) and held there. As B cells encounter the antigen, there is competition for space on the surface of the FDC, leading to selection. When a cell with higher affinity arises, it will stay there longer and presumably be given a stronger signal. B cells with higher affinity will therefore have a selective advantage.

An alternative theory is that B cells with higher-affinity receptors compete more effectively to bind and internalize antigen and therefore have a greater potential of presenting antigen to T cells, and receiving T cell help.

Somatic hypermutation and receptor editing lead to changes in the BCR

Somatic hypermutation is a common event in AFCs during TD responses and is important in the generation of high-affinity antibodies.

Somatic hypermutation introduces point mutations at a very high rate into the variable regions of the rearranged heavy and light chain genes (see Fig. 3.32). This results in mutated immunoglobulin molecules on the surface of the B cell. Mutants that bind antigen with higher affinity than the original surface immunoglobulin provide the raw material for the selection processes mentioned above.

The mechanism by which somatic hypermutation occurs involves an enzyme called **activation-induced cytidine deaminase (AID)**, which converts cytidine bases in DNA into uracil. The enzyme is specifically expressed in active B cells and is induced by IL-4 and ligation of CD40. Animals lacking this enzyme have deficient somatic hypermutation and class switch recombination (see below).

The abnormal uracil bases produced in the DNA are processed by a number of DNA repair systems, which fix the mutation in the immunoglobulin gene sequence.

AID appears to be targeted to the actively transcribing DNA genes by association with RNA polymerase, though it acts preferentially on the non-transcribing strand. The mechanism that preferentially targets AID to immunoglobulin genes is still uncertain, but it may involve secondary structures in the displaced (non-coding) DNA, or additional proteins expressed in B cells that are associated with the immunoglobulin V region gene.

Receptor editing is another mechanism by which diversity can be introduced into B cells during affinity maturation. Secondary V(D)J recombination can occur in immature B cells whose antigen receptors bind self antigen. The resulting immunoglobulin rearrangement converts these cells into non-self-reactive cells. In this way, specificity for foreign antigens can be improved and self-reactivity avoided.

B CELLS SWITCH IMMUNOGLOBULIN CLASS BY RECOMBINING HEAVY CHAIN GENES

B cells produce antibodies of five major classes – IgM, IgD, IgG, IgA, and IgE. In humans, there are also four subclasses of IgG and two of IgA (see Chapter 3). Each terminally differentiated plasma cell is derived from a specific B cell and produces antibodies of just one class or subclass.

All classes of immunoglobulin use the same set of variable region genes.

The first B cells to appear during development carry surface IgM as their antigen receptor. Upon activation, other classes of immunoglobulin are seen, each associated with different effector functions.

When a mature AFC switches antibody class, all that changes is the constant region of the heavy chain. The expressed V(D)J region and light chain do not change. Antigen specificity is therefore retained.

This has been shown by the analysis of double myelomas, in which two monoclonal antibodies are present in the serum at the same time:
- IgM and IgG antibodies from a patient with multiple myeloma have been found to have identical light chains and VH regions – only the constant regions are switched, from μ to γ;
- similarly, IgM and IgD are often found on the surface of a lymphocyte at the same time.

Again, although the classes are different, the antigen-binding specificities are identical.

The constant region genes encoding the different heavy chains (CH) are responsible for the generation of antibody classes and subclasses. These genes are clustered at the 3′ end of the immunoglobulin heavy chain (IGH) locus, downstream of the J segment genes.

Constant region genes of mouse

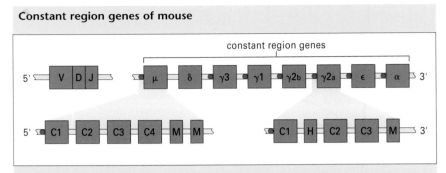

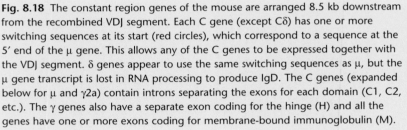

Fig. 8.18 The constant region genes of the mouse are arranged 8.5 kb downstream from the recombined VDJ segment. Each C gene (except Cδ) has one or more switching sequences at its start (red circles), which correspond to a sequence at the 5' end of the μ gene. This allows any of the C genes to be expressed together with the VDJ segment. δ genes appear to use the same switching sequences as μ, but the μ gene transcript is lost in RNA processing to produce IgD. The C genes (expanded below for μ and γ2a) contain introns separating the exons for each domain (C1, C2, etc.). The γ genes also have a separate exon coding for the hinge (H) and all the genes have one or more exons coding for membrane-bound immunoglobulin (M).

The arrangement of the constant genes in mouse and humans is shown in Figs 8.18 and 8.19. Upstream of the μ genes is a switch sequence (S), which is repeated upstream to each of the other constant region genes except δ. These sequences are important in the recombination events that occur during class switching, as explained below.

Class switching occurs during maturation and proliferation

Most class switching occurs during proliferation. However, it can also take place before encounter with exogenous antigen during early clonal expansion and maturation of the B cells (Fig. 8.20). This is known

because some of the progeny of immature B cells synthesize antibodies of other immunoglobulin classes, including IgG and IgA.

Further B cell differentiation results in synthesis of surface IgD, an antibody class found almost exclusively on B cell membranes.

Different classes of surface immunoglobulin on the same B cell have the same antigen specificity, that is, they express the same V region genes, though later additional diversity within a single clone may be generated by somatic mutation after class switching.

Evidence that some class switching occurs independently of antigen comes from experiments with vertebrates

Constant region genes and class switching in humans

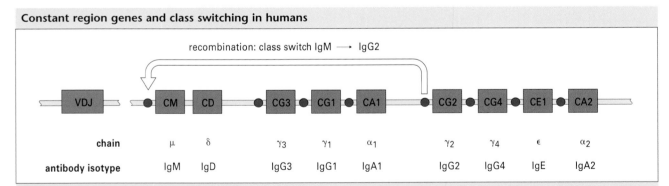

Fig. 8.19 The human immunoglobulin heavy chain gene locus (IGH) is shown. Initially, B cells transcribe a VDJ gene and a μ heavy chain that is spliced to produce mRNA for IgM. Under the influence of T cells and cytokines, class switching may occur, illustrated here as a switch from IgM to IgG2. Each heavy chain gene except CD (which encodes IgD) is preceded

by a switch region. When class switching occurs, recombination between these regions takes place, with the loss of the intervening C genes – in this case CM, CD, CG3, CG1, and CA1. (Note that pseudogenes have been omitted from this diagram.)

B cell differentiation – class diversity

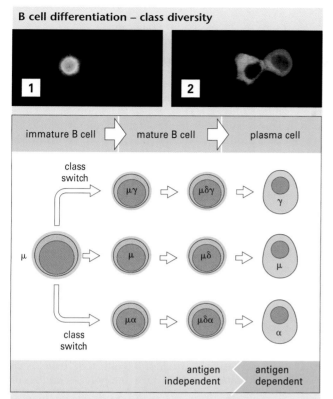

Fig. 8.20 Immature B cells produce IgM only, but mature B cells can express more than one cell surface antibody because mRNA and cell surface immunoglobulin remain after a class switch. IgD is also expressed during clonal maturation. Maturation can occur in the absence of antigen, but the development into plasma cells (which have little surface immunoglobulin, but much cytoplasmic immunoglobulin) requires antigen and (usually) T cell help. The photographs show B cells stained for surface IgM (green – 1) and plasma cells stained for cytoplasmic IgM and IgG (green and red – 2). IgM is stained with fluorescent anti-μ chain and IgG with rhodaminated anti-γ chain.

raised in gnotobiotic (virtually sterile) environments where exposure to exogenous antigens is severely restricted.

Class switching is achieved by gene recombination

B cells switch from IgM to the other classes or subclasses by an intrachromosomal deletion process in which the intervening genetic material between highly repetitive switch regions 5′ to each C_H gene is excised as a circle (Fig. 8.21).

Switching involves cytokine-dependent transcription of DNA in the region of the new constant region, reflecting changes in the chromatin in that region. This occurs before recombination of the 5′ switch regions that precede the genes for each of the heavy chain isotype constant region domains.

Class switching may also be achieved by differential splicing of mRNA

Class switching is important in the maturation of the immune response and may be accompanied or preceded by somatic mutation.

Initially, a complete section of DNA that includes the recombined VDJ region and the δ and μ constant regions is transcribed. Two mRNA molecules may then be produced by differential splicing, each with the same VDJ segment, but having either μ or δ constant regions.

It is suggested that much larger stretches of DNA are sometimes also transcribed together, with differential splicing giving other immunoglobulin classes sharing V_H regions (Fig. 8.22). This has been observed in cells simultaneously producing IgM and IgE.

Production of membrane and secreted immunoglobulin results from differential transcription of the H chain region

Membrane-bound immunoglobulin (BCR) is identical to secreted immunoglobulin (antibody) except for an extra stretch of amino acids at the C terminus of each heavy chain.

Class switching by gene recombination

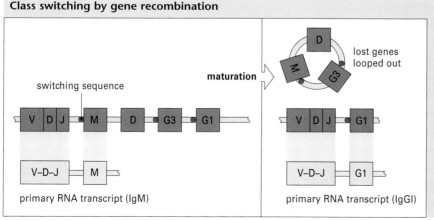

primary RNA transcript (IgM)

primary RNA transcript (IgGl)

Fig. 8.21 Initially the VDJ region is transcribed together with the M gene for the IgM heavy chain (left). After removal of introns during processing, mRNA for secreted IgM is produced. During B cell maturation, class switch recombination occurs between the Sμ (the switch region of the μ heavy chain gene) recombination region and a downstream switch region (G1 in this example). The intervening region (containing genes for IgM, IgD, and IgG3 in this instance) is looped out and then cut, with deletion of the intervening regions and joining of the two switch regions.

Isotype switching by differential RNA splicing

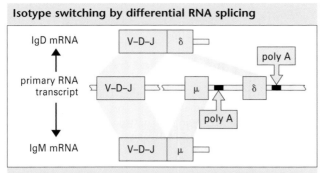

Fig. 8.22 Single B cells produce more than one antibody isotype from a single long primary RNA transcript. A transcript containing μ and δ is shown here. Polyadenylation can occur at different sites, leading to different forms of splicing, producing mRNA for IgD (top) or IgM (bottom). Even within this region, there are additional polyadenylation sites that determine whether the translated immunoglobulin is the secreted or membrane-bound form.

Membrane immunoglobulins are therefore slightly larger than their secreted counterparts. Their additional amino acids traverse the cell membrane and anchor the molecule in the lipid bilayer. In membrane IgM, for example, a section of hydrophobic (lipophilic) amino acids is sandwiched between hydrophilic amino acids, which lie on either side of the membrane (Fig. 8.23).

Membrane immunoglobulins:
- exist only as the basic four-chain unit;
- do not polymerize further; and
- are associated with molecules involved in signal transduction (e.g. Igα and Igβ).

Production of the two forms of immunoglobulin (membrane and secreted) occurs by differential transcription of the germline C region (Fig. 8.24). It is thought that the poly A sequence is important in determining which RNA transcript is produced, but exactly how this is controlled is uncertain.

Immunoglobulin class expression is influenced by cytokines and antigenic stimulus

During a TD immune response, there is a progressive change in the predominant immunoglobulin class of the specific antibody produced, usually to IgG. This class switch is not seen in TI responses, in which the predominant immunoglobulin usually remains IgM.

There is now considerable evidence for the involvement of T cells and their cytokines in the de-novo isotype switching:
- in mice, T cells in mucosal sites have been shown to stimulate IgA production;
- IL-4 preferentially switches B cells that have been either polyclonally activated (by lipopolysaccharide) or specifically activated by antigen to the IgG1 or IgE isotype, with concomitant suppression of other isotypes, and in a similar system IL-5 induces a 5–10-fold increase in IgA production with no change in other isotypes;

Membrane and secreted IgM

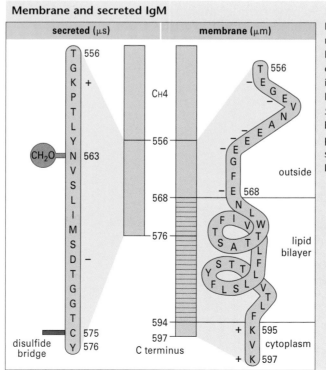

Fig. 8.23 C terminal amino acid sequences for both secreted and membrane-bound IgM are identical up to residue 556. Secreted IgM has 20 further residues. Residue 563 (asparagine) has a carbohydrate unit attached to it, while residue 575 is a cysteine involved in the formation of interchain disulfide bonds. Membrane IgM has 41 residues beyond 556. A stretch of 26 residues between 568 and 595 contains hydrophobic amino acids sandwiched between sequences containing charged residues. This hydrophobic portion may traverse the cell membrane as two turns of a helix. A short, positively charged, section lies inside the cytoplasm. Mouse IgM is shown in this example.

Production of membrane and secreted IgM

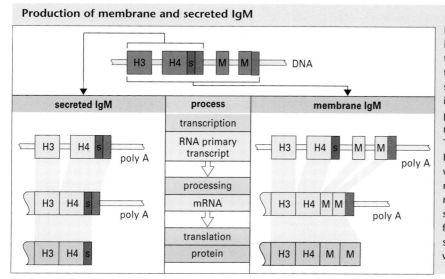

Fig. 8.24 Part of the DNA coding for IgM is shown diagrammatically. The exons for the μ3 and μ4 domains (H3 and H4) and the transmembrane and cytoplasmic segment of membrane IgM (M) are indicated. The 3′ untranslated sequence is present at the end of the H4 and second membrane segments (S = stop codons). The DNA can be transcribed in two ways. If transcription stops after S, the transcript with a poly A tail is processed to produce mRNA for secreted IgM. If transcription runs through to include the membrane segments, processing removes the codons for the terminal amino acids and the stop signal of H4, so translation yields a protein with a different C terminus.

Isotype regulation by mouse T cell cytokines

TH	cytokines	immunoglobulin isotypes					
		IgG1	IgE	IgA	IgG3	IgG2b	IgG2a
TH2	IL-4	↑	↑	↓	↓	↓	↓
	IL-5	=	=	↑	=	=	=
TH1	IFNγ	↓	↓	↓	↓	↓	↑

Fig. 8.25 The effects of IFNγ (product of TH1 cells) and IL-4 and IL-5 (products of TH2 cells), which result in an increase (↑), a decrease (↓), or no change (=) in the frequency of isotype-specific B cells after stimulation with the polyclonal activator lipopolysaccharide (LPS) in vitro.

- IFNγ enhances IgG2a responses in mice, but suppresses all other isotypes (Fig. 8.25).

It is interesting that IL-4 and IFNγ, which act as reciprocal regulatory cytokines for the expression of antibody isotypes, are derived from different TH subsets. In addition, IL-12 and IL-18 stimulation of mouse T cells can induce the production of IFNγ. These cells can therefore act as immunoregulatory cells by differentially inducing IgG2a expression, while inhibiting IgG1, IgE, and IgG2b expression. Transforming growth factor-β (TGFβ) induces the switch to IgA or IgG2b. In humans, the situation is somewhat different:

- IL-4 induces the expression of IgG4 and IgE; and
- TGFβ induces the expression of IgA alone.

FURTHER READING

Hardy RR, Hayakawa K. B cell development pathways. Annu Rev Immunol 2001;19:595–621.

Henderson A, Calamé K. Transcriptional regulation during B cell development. Annu Rev Immunol 1998;16:163–200.

Lane P. Development of B cell memory and effector function. Curr Opin Immunol 1996;8:331–336.

Lipsky PE, Attrep JF, Grammer AC, et al. Analysis of CD40–CD40 ligand interactions in the regulation of human B cell function. Ann NY Acad Sci 1997;815:372–383.

Liu Y-J, de Bouteiller O, Fugier-Vivier I. Mechanisms of selection and differentiation in germinal centers. Curr Opin Immunol 1997;9:256–262.

McHeyzer-Williams LJ, McHeyzer-Williams MG. Antigen-specific memory B cell development. Annu Rev Immunol 2005;23:487–513.

Osmond DG, Rolink A, Melchers F. Murine B lymphopoiesis: towards a unified model. Immunol Today 1998;19:65–68.

Przylepa J, Himes C, Kelsoe G. Lymphocyte development and selection in germinal centers. Curr Top Microbiol Immunol 1998;229:85–104.

Smith KG, Fearon DT. Receptor modulators of B cell receptor signaling – CD19/CD22. Curr Top Microbiol Immunol 2000;245:195–212.

Snapper CM, Mond JJ. A model for induction of T cell-independent humoral immunity in response to polysaccharide antigens. J Immunol 1996;157:2229–2233.

Stavnezer J. Antibody class switching. Adv Immunol 1996;61:79–146.

Tarlington D. Germinal centers: form and function. Curr Opin Immunol 1998;10:245–251.

Critical thinking: Development of the antibody response (see p. 495 for explanations)

A project is under way to develop a vaccine against mouse hepatitis virus, a pathogen of mice that may become a serious problem in colonies of mice. The vaccine consists of capsid protein of the virus, which is injected subcutaneously as a depot in alum on day 0. At days 5 and 14, the group of six mice is bled and the serum is tested for the presence of antibodies against the viral capsid protein. Separate assays are done for each of the immunoglobulin classes, IgM, IgG, and IgA. The amounts, expressed in mg/ml of antibody are shown in the figure.

When the data are analyzed it appears that two of the animals have high titers of antibody, particularly of IgG and IgA, at both days 5 and 14.

1   Why do the titers of IgG antibodies increase more rapidly between days 5 and 14 than the titers of IgM antibodies, in all animals?

2   Propose an explanation for the high titers of IgG antibodies in the two animals indicated at day 5. Can this explanation also account for the relatively high levels of IgA antibodies also seen in these mice?

The spleens from mice taken at day 14 are used to produce B cells making monoclonal antibodies against the viral protein (see Method Box 3.1). Of the clones produced, 15 produce IgG, three produce IgM, and none produces IgA.

3   Why do you suppose there are no IgA-producing clones, despite the good IgA response?

4   You want a high-affinity antibody for use in an assay. Which of the clones you have produced are likely to be of higher affinity?

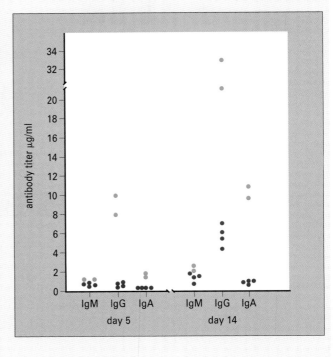

Mononuclear Phagocytes in Immune Defense

SUMMARY

- **Macrophages, myeloid dendritic cells, and osteoclasts all differentiate from circulating blood monocytes.**

- **Resident macrophages are widely distributed throughout the body.** Phenotypically distinct populations are present in each organ and within the different zones of spleen and lymph nodes.

- **Resident and recruited macrophages respond to injury and immune stimuli.** TH1 cytokines such as IFNγ enhance inflammation and antimicrobial activity. TH2 cytokines induce an alternate activation with efficient antigen presentation to B cells. TGFβ, corticosteroids, and IL-10 can induce an anti-inflammatory phenotype.

- **Resident macrophages clear apoptotic cells using scavenger receptors and the vitronectin receptor.** Endocytosis by this pathway does not activate the macrophage killing mechanisms.

- **Macrophages internalize pathogens using a variety of specific and opsonic receptors.** These include the LPS receptor and Toll-like receptors, the β-glucan receptor, the mannose receptor (MR), the Fc receptors, and complement receptors CR1, CR3, and CR4.

- **Activated macrophages secrete cytokines, enzymes, complement system molecules, and procoagulant.** Resting macrophages have only a limited killing activity.

- **Activated macrophages produce reactive oxygen and nitrogen intermediates which are highly toxic for endocytosed bacteria and fungi.** Recently recruited cells are most effective at antimicrobial killing.

- **Macrophages can initiate, promote, prevent, suppress, and terminate immune responses.**

MACROPHAGES DIFFERENTIATE FROM CIRCULATING BLOOD MONOCYTES

Mononuclear phagocytes comprise a family of cells that share common hematopoietic precursors and are distributed via the blood stream as monocytes to all tissues of the body, including secondary lymphoid organs, even in the absence of an overt inflammatory stimulus.

Within tissues the mononuclear phagocytes undergo maturation, adapt to their local microenvironment, and differentiate into various cell types:
- macrophages;
- myeloid-derived dendritic cells; and
- osteoclasts.

These various cell types perform specific housekeeping, trophic, and immunologic functions (Fig. 9.1).

The macrophages for the most part become and remain highly efficient phagocytes and play an important role in pathogen recognition and clearance during infection, as well as removal of senescent and dying cells and immune complexes (Fig. 9.2).

In response to particulate and other potential antigenic stimuli:
- the dendritic cells are uniquely efficient inducers of primary immune responses by naive T cells; whereas

- macrophages produce a range of secretory products that affect the migration and activation of other immune cells.

Macrophages are actively endocytic and degrade antigens, but can present peptides to already primed T cells in secondary responses after MHC and other accessory molecules have been induced by cytokines such as IFNγ derived from TH1 cells and NK cells. Once recruited and activated by such interactions, the macrophage plays a major role in the effector limb of cell-mediated immunity to intracellular pathogens such as mycobacteria, often within focal accumulations of cells known as granulomas.

Macrophages are extremely heterogeneous in their gene expression and cellular activities, with beneficial as well as destructive roles in tissue homeostasis and host defense.

Through their varied plasma membrane receptor repertoire and secretory responses, macrophages interact with other leukocytes as well as non-hematopoietic cells in all tissues, so regulating both innate and acquired immunity.

Although the concept of the mononuclear phagocyte system is central to our understanding of immunity, this is but one role in a wider context of physiologic and pathologic contributions to tissue maintenance, response to injury, and repair.

Differentiation of monocytes

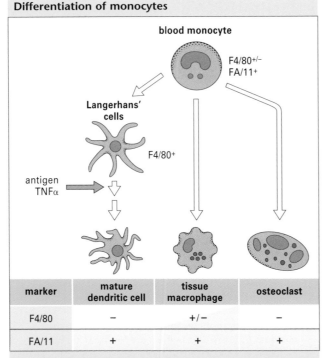

marker	mature dendritic cell	tissue macrophage	osteoclast
F4/80	–	+/–	–
FA/11	+	+	+

Fig. 9.1 Circulating monocytes give rise to myeloid dendritic cells (distinct from plasmacytoid dendritic cells, which are thought to originate from distinct precursors), tissue macrophages, and osteoclasts. F4/80 and FA/11 (macrosialin, the murine homolog of CD68) are differentiation antigens of mouse macrophages and closely related cells.

Rapid Reference Box 9

chemokines – a large group of cytokines falling into four separate families. The main families are the CC group and the CXC group. They include interleukin-8 (CXCL8), monocyte chemotactic protein-1 (MCP-1, CCL2), RANTES, (CCL5) macrophage inflammatory protein-1α (MIP-1α, CCL3) interferon-inducible protein 10 (IP-10, CCL10), and many others. They act on seven-transmembrane pass receptors and have a variety of chemotactic and cell-activating properties, acting on selected populations of target cells (see Appendix 4).

CSFs (colony stimulating factors) – a group of cytokines that control the differentiation of hematopoietic stem cells.

cytokines – a generic term for soluble molecules that mediate interactions between cells (see Appendix 3).

IFNs (interferons) – a group of molecules involved in signaling between cells of the immune system and in protection against viral infections.

IL-1–IL-27 (interleukins) – a group of molecules involved in signaling between cells of the immune system.

LTs (leukotrienes) – a collection of metabolites of arachidonic acid that have powerful pharmacological effects.

LPS (lipopolysaccharide) – a product of some Gram-negative bacterial cell walls that can act as a B cell mitogen.

PGs (prostaglandins) – pharmacologically active derivatives of arachidonic acid. Different prostaglandins are capable of modulating cell mobility and immune responses.

TGFs (transforming growth factors) – a group of cytokines identified by their ability to promote fibroblast growth; they are also generally immunosuppressive.

RESIDENT MACROPHAGES ARE WIDELY DISTRIBUTED THROUGHOUT THE BODY

Some of the key features of resident macrophage populations in tissues are shown in Fig. 9.3. The cells vary in their life span, morphology, and phenotype, for example the microglial cells in the brain appear quite unlike mononuclear phagocytes in other tissues (Fig. 9.4).

Resident cells have usually ceased to proliferate, but retain the ability to express a range of mRNA and proteins, often as relatively long-lived cells, with low turnover, unlike neutrophils.

Plasma membrane differentiation markers such as the F4/80 antigen have proved useful in defining the distribution of mature macrophages in many (but not all)

Role of macrophages and dendritic cells in immune defense

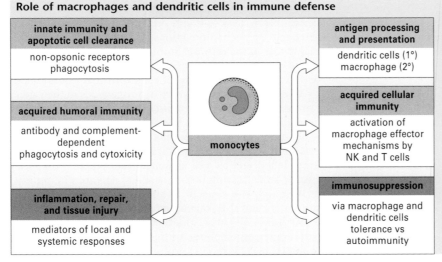

Fig. 9.2 Both macrophages and dendritic cells play important roles in innate immune responses, inflammation, and tissue remodeling, as well as in specific immune responses.

Resident tissue macrophage populations

organ	name/site	functions/properties
bone marrow	stromal macrophage	interacts with hematopoietic cells, removes erythroid nuclei
liver	Kupffer cells	clearance of cells and complexes from the blood
spleen	red pulp macrophages white pulp tingible body macrophages marginal zone macrophages	clearance of senescent blood cells phagocytosis of apoptotic B cells interface between circulation and immune system
lymph node	subcapsular sinus macrophages medullary macrophages	interface with afferent lymph interface with efferent lymph
thymus	thymic macrophage	clearance of apoptotic cells
gut	lamina propria	endocytosis
lung	alveolar macrophage	clearance of particulates and infectious agents
brain	microglia in neuropil choroid plexus	interacts with neurons interface with cerebrospinal fluid
skin	Langerhans' cells	antigen capture
reproductive tract	ovary, testis	clearance of dying cells
endocrine organs	adrenal, thyroid, pancreas, etc.	metabolic homeostasis
bone	osteoclasts	bone remodeling

Fig. 9.3 Resident tissue macrophage populations.

Microglia in mouse brain stained for F4/80

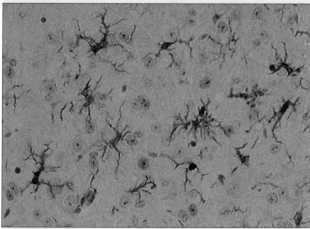

Fig. 9.4 Microglia are widely distributed in non-overlapping fields and show a dendritic morphology. (Courtesy of Dr Payam Rezaie)

murine tissues. In humans, the CD68 antigen, an intracellular vacuolar marker, is widely expressed; the murine homolog (macrosialin) is a pan-macrophage marker, also present in many myeloid dendritic cells and osteoclasts, unlike F4/80.

It is possible to reconstruct a constitutive migration pathway in which monocytes become endothelial-like and line vascular sinusoids, as in the liver (Kupffer cells, see Fig. 2.3), or penetrate between endothelial cells. They underlie endothelia or epithelia, which can also be penetrated by, for example, Langerhans' cells (F4/80+ precursors of dendritic cells), or enter the interstitial space or serosal cavities (Fig. 9.5).

Although macrophages are often regarded as sessile cells compared with freely migratory dendritic cells, they readily migrate to draining lymph nodes after an inflammatory stimulus and become arrested there. They are therefore absent from efferent lymph and do not, as a rule, re-enter the circulation.

Q. Why is there no advantage for the immune system in the recirculation of macrophages, whereas recirculation of lymphocytes is a central element in immune defense?
A. Macrophages do not develop an immunological memory, and do not undergo the selective clonal expansion of antigen-stimulated lymphocytes that occurs in lymphoid tissues. Therefore there is no advantage in having macrophages return to the circulation from lymphoid tissues.

Mature macrophages are themselves part of the stromal microenvironment in bone marrow. They associate with developing hematopoietic cells to perform poorly defined non-phagocytic trophic functions, as well as removing effete cells and erythroid nuclei.

Secondary lymphoid organs contain several distinct types of macrophage and related cells, which are still poorly understood. Fig. 9.6 illustrates the complexity of

Differentiation and distribution of macrophages

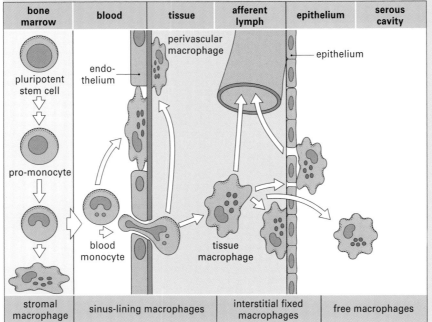

Fig. 9.5 Blood monocytes are derived from bone marrow in the adult host and enter tissues initially as sinus-lining or extravascular mature cells. Interstitial or intraepithelial adherent macrophages and serosal macrophages can enter afferent lymphatics. Monocyte-derived dendritic cells can arise from tissue macrophages by reverse migration across endothelium. Stromal macrophages in bone marrow may also derive from the circulating monocyte population.

macrophage-like cells in rodent spleen (red and white pulp, marginal zone) and normal lymph nodes (subcapsular sinus, medulla).

Differentiation antigens such as sialoadhesin, a lectin-like receptor for sialylated glycoconjugates, are particularly strongly present on marginal metallophils (inner marginal zone) and on subcapsular sinus macrophages. These cells are present at the interface between:

- blood (spleen);
- afferent lymph (lymph nodes); and
- organized lymphoid structures.

They play a role in the capture of organisms, particulates, polysaccharides, and soluble antigens, as well as of circulating host cells or migrating dendritic cells, which have their own characteristic distribution in T and B cell-dependent areas.

The molecular mechanisms of constitutive macrophage distribution and induced migration are beginning to be defined, and involve cellular adhesion molecules, cytokines, and growth factors, as well as chemokines and chemokine receptors, as summarized in Fig. 9.7.

Macrophage colony stimulating factor (M-CSF or CSF-1) is a major growth, differentiation, and survival factor selective for macrophages, whereas granulocyte–macrophage colony stimulating factor (GM-CSF) regulates myeloid cell production and function.

Chemokines are produced by a range of hematopoietic and tissue cells, including macrophages themselves, and act on various leukocyte subpopulations depending principally on their chemokine receptor profile.

RESIDENT AND RECRUITED MACROPHAGES RESPOND TO INJURY AND IMMUNE STIMULI

Inflammatory stimuli (e.g. local infection) enhance the recruitment of monocytes (and often other myeloid cells) from blood, and ultimately from bone marrow stores.

Monocytes adhere to activated endothelium through a series of well-described interactions involving selectins, β_2 integrins, and CD31, as well as chemotactic molecules acting on their transmembrane G protein-coupled receptors (Fig. 9.8, see also Chapter 6). When ligands bind to these receptors it causes the recruitment of intracellular proteins to the area of membrane activation of integrins and polarization of the cells (Fig. 9.9).

Diapedesis results in local tissue interactions and accumulation of macrophages with enhanced turnover and an altered phenotype (e.g. the upregulation of endocytic receptors and production of proinflammatory mediators).

Phagocytosis by recently recruited monocytes profoundly alters their differentiation into:

- migratory dendritic cells; or
- more sessile macrophages.

Recent studies have confirmed the potential of monocytes to differentiate into either of these cell types in vivo, as they do in cell culture.

It is convenient to distinguish the macrophages 'elicited' by a non-specific inflammatory stimulus from 'immunologically activated' macrophages. The latter cells:

- respond to IFNγ by acquiring enhanced antimicrobial properties; and

Macrophages in secondary lymphoid tissues

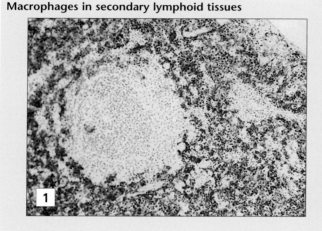

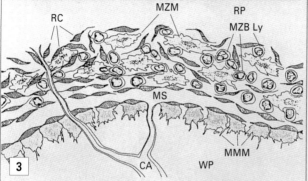

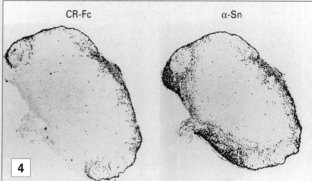

Fig. 9.6 Heterogeneity of macrophages in secondary lymphoid organs of mouse. (**1**) Red pulp of spleen stained for F4/80. Macrophages stain strongly positive. (Courtesy of Dr DA Hume) (**2**) Mouse spleen stained with antibody to sialoadhesin. The marginal metallophils of spleen are strongly sialoadhesin positive. (Courtesy of Dr PR Crocker) (**3**) The marginal zone contains inner metallophilic and outer zones. In the diagram of the marginal zone of the spleen, the central arteriole (CA) branches into small capillaries, which either pass through the marginal zone and end in the red pulp (RP) or open into the marginal sinus (MS). The marginal zone is composed of reticular cells (RCs). Within this reticular framework, the large marginal zone macrophages (MZMs), dendritic cells, and marginal zone B cells (MZBs) are localized. The marginal metallophilic macrophages (MMM) are situated at the inner border of the marginal sinus and the white pulp (WP) (Courtesy of Dr G Kraal) (**4**) Lymph node contains subcapsular sinus macrophages, which are sialoadhesin positive and bind CR-Fc, a chimeric probe of the mannose receptor cysteine-rich domain, and human Fc (left); medullary macrophages express only sialoadhesin (right). (Courtesy of Dr L Martinez-Pomares)

- express enhanced MHC class II molecules, whereas other genes (e.g. the mannose receptor) are downregulated.

Q. What will be the functional effect of the changes in cell surface molecules described above?

A. The increase in MHC class II molecules will enhance the ability to present antigen to CD4$^+$ T cells, while the reduction in the MR may mean a reduced ability to take up some microbes by non-immune mechanisms.

Cytokines produced by NK cells, lymphocytes, and various antigen-presenting cells (APCs) influence the pattern of gene expression by macrophages. Work in vitro, and some studies in vivo, especially with cytokine/receptor knockout mouse strains, have made it possible to classify macrophages differing in their functional state (Fig. 9.10).

The initial and further interactions with endocytic and phagocytic stimuli give rise to further heterogeneity in phenotype. It should be emphasized that, although the evidence for individual molecules as mediators of activation is good, we have little insight into the complex interactions that pertain in vivo.

Fig. 9.11 illustrates a mycobacterium-induced granuloma, rich in macrophages. Cytokines, for example TNFα, and receptors such as CR3 play an important role in granuloma formation.

Environmental influences on macrophages

stimulus	example/receptors	response
growth factors	M-CSF, GM-CSF	growth, differentiation, survival
cytokines	IFNγ TNFα IL-4, IL-13 IL-10	activation activation alternate activation deactivation
chemokines	CCL2 (macrophage chemotactic protein-1, MCP-1)	migration
extracellular matrix	fibronectin / β_1-integrin	adhesion, phagocytosis
peptides	vasoactive peptide (VIP)	modulation of various functions
eicosanoids	prostaglandin E_2 (PGE_2) leukotriene B_4 (LTB_4)	modulation of various functions
cellular interactions: endothelium T cells	fibronectin / β_1- integrin accessory molecules (CD80, CD86)	recruitment antigen presentation
microbial interactions	LPS (CD14)	secretion, activation
proteases	neutral proteinases (e.g. plasmin)	adhesion, secretion

M-CSF, macrophage colony stimulating factor; GM-CSF, granulocyte—macrophage colony stimulating factor; IFNγ, interferon-γ; IL, interleukin; LPS, lipopolysaccharide; TNFα, tumor necrosis factor-α

Fig. 9.7 Some of the mediators that act on macrophages.

Macrophage 7tm G protein-coupled receptors for chemotactic stimuli

receptors	ligands	sources
fMLP	fMet-Leu peptides	prokaryote protein synthesis
C5a receptor	complement C5a	lytic activation
LTB_4 receptor	leukotriene B_4	mast cells, macrophages
PAF receptor	platelet-activating factor	platelets, neutrophils, macrophages
CCR1, CCR2, CCR5	chemokines CCL2, 3, 4, 5, 7, 8	leukocytes, tissue cells
CXCR1, CXCR2	CXCL8 (IL-8)	endothelium, lymphocytes
CXCR3	CXCL9, 10, 11	endothelium, tissue cells
CX3CR1	CX3CL1 (fractalkine)	endothelium, epithelium, neurons, smooth muscle cells

7tm, seven-transmembrane segments; CCL, CC chemokine ligand; CXCL, CXC chemokine ligand; CCR, CC chemokine receptor; CXCR, CXC chemokine receptor; fMLP, f.Met-Leu-Phe; PAF, platelet-activating factor

Fig. 9.8 Macrophages express a variety of receptors for chemotactic agents. Fractalkine (CX3CL1) is unique as a transmembrane ligand – its receptor, CX3CR1, and CCR2 may be differentially expressed by monocytes, giving rise to inflammatory and resident macrophages.

Intracellular signaling via chemotactic agents such as f-met-leu-phe (fMLP)

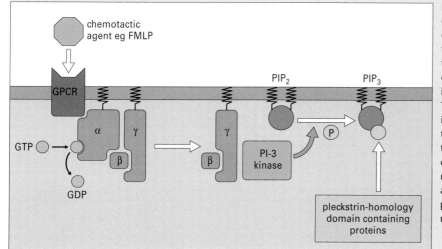

Fig. 9.9 fMLP binds to its receptor and causes guanosine triphosphate (GTP) to displace guanosine diphosphate (GDP) on the heterotrimeric G protein. This causes the β and γ chains to dissociate from the α chain and they in turn recruit phosphatidyl inositol (PI)-3 kinase to the membrane. The kinase phosphorylates phosphatidyl inositol diphosphate (PIP_2) to the triphosphate PIP_3. A number of proteins that have pleckstrin homology (PH) domains are then recruited to the membrane at this point, causing focal adhesion, activation of integrins, and polarization of the cell, in preparation for migration.

Activation of macrophages

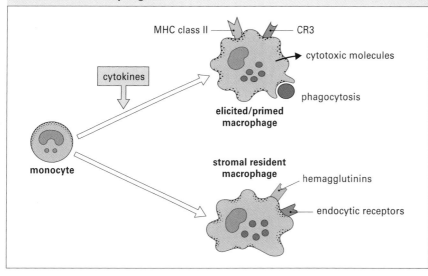

Fig. 9.10 Elicited and immunologically primed macrophages differ from resident macrophages. Monocyte recruitment is enhanced and yields macrophages with proinflammatory and cytotoxic properties. Activation by cytokines enhances expression of MHC class II molecules and the complement receptor CR3. Phagocytosis and the production of proinflammatory mediators and cytotoxic products are increased. By contrast, resident macrophages (e.g. in bone marrow) lack inflammatory functions, but participate in trophic reactions (e.g. with developing hematopoietic cells) as well as performing endocytosis. Microbial stimuli can act directly on resident macrophages to induce distinct surface and secretory properties.

Immunologically activated macrophages express the capacity to produce antimicrobial products including lysozyme and reactive oxygen and nitrogen species (see below). However, characteristic morphologic features such as epithelioid cell and giant cell formation, hallmarks of mycobacterial granulomas, remain mysterious in origin.

Cytokines modulate the phenotype of macrophages

A further level of heterogeneity derives from the distinct effects of TH1- and TH2-type cytokines on monocyte/macrophage differentiation (Fig. 9.12).

In-vitro studies with macrophages treated with different cytokines have indicated that there is a spectrum of gene expression induced by different cytokines (Fig. 9.13):

- IFNγ characteristically enhances proinflammatory and antimicrobial activities ('immune activation');
- IL-10 efficiently counteracts proinflammatory and antimicrobial activities ('deactivation');
- IL-4 and IL-13 exert distinctive effects on MHC class II and MR expression, which we have termed 'alternative activation', rather than focusing on the modest inhibition of proinflammatory products.

Broadly speaking:

- 'activated' macrophages mediate cellular immunity;
- 'alternatively activated' macrophages may promote humoral immunity, including repair processes.

It is well established that macrophages and myeloid dendritic cells produce IL-12 and IL-18, which enhance the production of IFNγ by NK cells and T cells. There is, as yet, no comparable IL-4/IL-13-inducing activity that can be ascribed to the APCs, though subsets of dendritic cells have been implicated in TH2 differentiation, which has also been postulated to constitute a 'default' pathway.

A granulomatous reaction in pulmonary tuberculosis

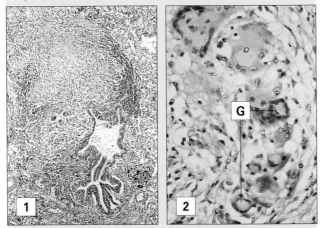

Fig. 9.11 The central area of caseous necrosis in which much of the cellular structure is destroyed is characteristic of tuberculosis in the lung. Apart from this necrosis, the histology is typical of chronic T cell-dependent 'tuberculoid' granulomas. The lesion is surrounded by a ring of epithelioid cells and mononuclear cells. Multinucleate giant cells, believed to be derived from the fusion of epithelioid cells, are also present (left, × 170). Giant cells (G) are illustrated at a higher magnification (right). Hematoxylin and eosin stain. (Courtesy of Dr G Boyd)

The links between innate and acquired immune responses are therefore understood only in part.

MACROPHAGES CLEAR APOPTOTIC CELLS USING SCAVENGER RECEPTORS AND THE VITRONECTIN RECEPTOR

Macrophages express a very wide range of plasma membrane receptors, which underlie their interactions with:

- other cells;
- extracellular ligands derived from plasma;
- extracellular matrix; and
- microorganisms.

It is useful to distinguish:

- opsonic receptors (e.g. for antibody and complement); from
- 'non-opsonic' receptors.

The processes of phagocytosis mediated by opsonic receptors are shown in Fig. 9.14. Whereas neutrophils express similar opsonic receptors, they lack most of the opsonin-independent receptors for phagocytosis.

Q. What groups of receptors do not require opsonins for their actions?

A. The Toll-like receptors, lectin receptors, and scavenger receptors, which recognize pathogen-associated molecular patterns (PAMPs) (see Fig. 6.24).

Modulation of macrophage activation

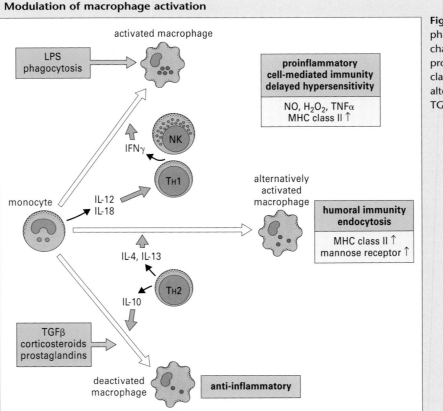

Fig. 9.12 Signals from microbial products, phagocytosis, and cytokines result in changes to the surface and secretory properties of macrophages, which can be classified as activated, deactivated, or alternatively activated. (NO, nitric oxide; TGFβ, transforming growth factor-β)

Regulation of macrophage phenotype

	TH1 type	TH2 types		significance
	IFNγ	IL-4/IL-13	IL-10	
MHC class II molecule (Ia)	++	+	–	immune cell interactions
respiratory burst NO	++ ++	(–) (–)	– –	cell-mediated immunity tissue injury (e.g. tuberculosis)
TNFα IL-1 IL-6	++	(–)	–	proinflammatory
mannosyl receptor	–	++	0	phagocytosis/endocytosis (e.g. antigens)
growth	–	+	0	local growth of MØ in immune lesions
fusion	0	++	0	giant cell formation–granulomas (e.g. tuberculosis)
growth factor secretion	–	++	+	healing of lesions

Fig. 9.13 TH1 and TH2 cytokines act on macrophages to induce distinctive functions, which can be described as 'activation' (TH1-type), 'alternative activation', or deactivation (TH2-type). (+, increase; -, decrease; 0, no effect)

Phagocytosis mediated by opsonic receptors

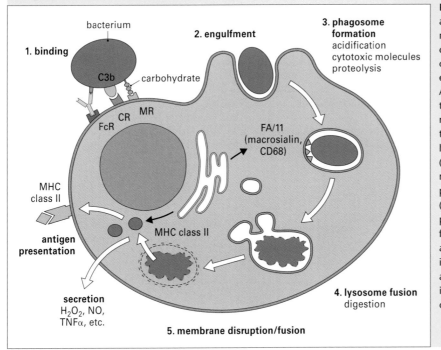

Fig. 9.14 (1) Pathogens, such as bacteria, are taken up by binding to opsonic receptors including the Fc receptor, complement receptors, and receptors for carbohydrate (MR). (2) The particle is engulfed and the phagosome forms (3). Acidification of the phagosome follows as toxic molecules (reactive oxygen and nitrogen intermediates) are pumped into the phagosome. The marker FA/11 is located in the phagosome membrane. (4) Lysosomes fuse with the phagosome, releasing proteolytic enzymes into the phagolysosome, which digest the bacteria. (5) On completion the membrane of the phagolysosome is disrupted. Antigenic fragments may become diverted to the acidic endosome compartment for interaction with MHC class II molecules and antigen presentation. The process induces secretion of toxic molecules and cytokines.

However, pattern recognition clearly extends to endogenous, host-derived molecules (self, which may be modified), though there may be intriguing differences in the outcome of these receptor–ligand interactions regarding cytokine responses and the inflammatory consequences.

In particular, macrophage receptors play a dual role in clearance of both macromolecules and apoptotic cells, which differs from their role in uptake of microbial invaders or foreign antigens:

- in the first case there is no or even a suppressed inflammatory response;
- in the second, the immune system may need to be alerted.

The roles of cell type, receptor profile, signal pathway, and mediator release in these dual responses are all under investigation.

Q. In what ways can macrophages alert lymphocytes that microbial antigens are present?
A. They can express co-stimulatory molecules and inflammatory cytokines, which are induced following for example ligation of Toll-like receptors by microbial products (see Chapters 6 and 7).

To maintain appropriate numbers of all cell types in development and normal tissue homeostasis, as well as during immune, inflammatory, and other pathologic responses, cells die naturally by:
• programmed death (apoptosis); or
• necrosis, the latter releasing potentially injurious products.

Cellular and biochemical pathways resulting in apoptosis are conserved in evolution; apoptotic cells are rapidly and efficiently cleared by macrophages (e.g. in thymus; Fig. 9.15), though they can also be engulfed by non-professional phagocytes.

The receptors implicated in apoptotic cell recognition show considerable redundancy and include a range of scavenger receptors (e.g. SR-AI; Fig. 9.16), vitronectin receptor, an ATP-transporter, and CD14 (see below). Thrombospondin and C1q can act as opsonins.

The ligands expressed by apoptotic cells are not well defined. Recently a conserved, widely distributed receptor has been postulated for phosphatidylserine, a phospholipid displayed on the outer leaflet of apoptotic cells.

Ligation of the vitronectin receptor results in production of anti-inflammatory products (e.g. PGE$_2$ and TGFβ), which can overcome proinflammatory responses induced by potent stimuli such as LPS. Indeed, intracellular pathogens can induce and exploit this downregulation, which is presumably a host protective reaction, to promote their own survival.

Inefficient clearance of apoptotic cells may also contribute to autoimmune disorders such as systemic lupus erythematosus (see Chapter 20), and may explain their association with genetic deficiencies of complement components.

Macrophages are more efficient than mature dendritic cells in the capture and digestion of apoptotic cells. Macrophages and dendritic cells may express different receptor profiles, but other differences could also contribute to a different fate for ingested dying cells.

Phagocytosis of apoptotic thymocyte by thymic macrophage

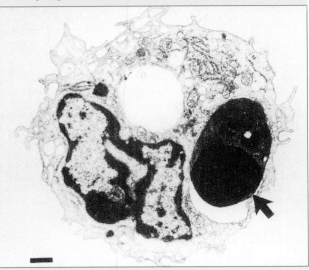

Fig. 9.15 Thymic macrophages phagocytose the large numbers of thymocytes that die during T cell development. The arrow indicates the nucleus of a phagocytosed thymocyte.

Class A and related scavenger receptors

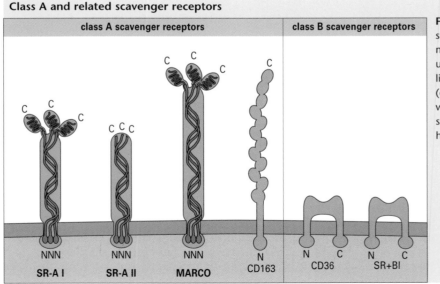

Fig. 9.16 Selected scavenger receptors are shown. Scavenger receptors of macrophages are responsible for the uptake of apoptotic cells, modified lipoproteins, and other polyanionic ligands (e.g. LPS and lipoteichoic acids [LTA]), as well as selected bacteria such as *Neisseria* spp. CD163 is involved in endocytosis of hemoglobin–haptoglobin complexes.

Clearance of dead cells

	apoptotic cells	necrotic cells
receptors	scavenger receptors phosphatidyl serine receptors	Fc receptors complement receptors
cytokines	TGFβ1	TNFα, IL-1β, IL-8

Fig. 9.17 Receptors involved in the uptake of apoptotic and necrotic cells, and the cytokines released following uptake.

Q. Give examples in the immune system where macrophages phagocytose apoptotic cells.
A. Thymocytes that fail the processes of positive and negative selection die by apoptosis and are phagocytosed by thymic macrophages (see Chapter 2). B cells that die within lymphoid follicles are taken up by tingible body macrophages (see Chapter 8).

The recognition mechanisms of normally senescent hematopoietic cells (e.g. erythrocytes, platelets) and of necrotic cells are still obscure.

Fig. 9.17 compares the differential recognition and cytokine production following the uptake of apoptotic and necrotic cells.

MACROPHAGES INTERNALIZE PATHOGENS USING A VARIETY OF SPECIFIC AND OPSONIC RECEPTORS
The mannose receptor is the best studied lectin-like receptor

Although macrophages can express a range of lectins specific for various sugar ligands, the MR is the best studied and may play a unique role in tissue homeostasis as well as host defense (Fig. 9.18). Endogenous ligands include lysosomal hydrolases and myeloperoxidase, and a range of pro- and eukaryotic organisms express mannose-rich structures, which may serve as ligands.

An N terminal cysteine-rich domain of the MR is a distinct lectin for sulfated glycoconjugates highly

Lectin receptors

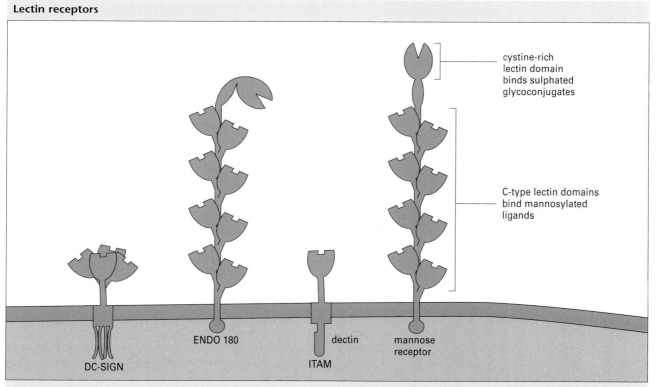

cystine-rich
lectin domain
binds sulphated
glycoconjugates

C-type lectin domains
bind mannosylated
ligands

ENDO 180

DC-SIGN

dectin

ITAM

mannose
receptor

Fig. 9.18 The mannose receptor contains eight C-type lectin domains involved in binding to mannosylated carbohydrates and related glycoconjugates. It is related to a more broadly expressed endocytic receptor, ENDO 180. A distinct lectin domain located in the distal (C terminal) segment binds sulfated glycoconjugates. The β-glucan receptor (dectin-1) contains a single lectin domain and an intracellular immunoreceptor tyrosine-based activation motif (ITAM). DC-SIGN (another mannose-binding C-type lectin) has four associated lectin domains.

expressed in secondary lymphoid organs (marginal metallophils, subcapsular sinus macrophages, and follicular dendritic cells).

A novel antigen transport pathway has been postulated by which cell-associated or soluble MRs could deliver antigen to B and/or T cells, modulating their immune response.

The cysteine-rich domain also contributes to the clearance of hormones such as lutropin, which contains similar sulfated structures.

DC-SIGN, another mannose-binding C-type lectin, can be expressed on selected macrophages. It has been implicated in interactions between APCs and T cells and in microbial recognition (see Fig. 9.18).

Dectin-1 is a β-glucan receptor with a single lectin-like domain and an intracellular ITAM, responsible for the uptake of fungi and intracellular signaling (Fig. 9.19, see Fig. 9.18).

CD14 interacts with Toll-like receptors to initiate signal transduction

Monocytes and to a lesser extent tissue macrophages express a glycosyl phosphatidylinositol (GPI)-anchored molecule – CD14 – implicated in the cellular response to bacterial LPS. A plasma LPS-binding protein enhances LPS responses markedly; genetic ablation of CD14 in mice renders them highly resistant to septic shock, mainly mediated by TNFα release into the circulation. Toll-like receptors (TLRs, see Fig. 6.24) play a major role in LPS signaling in macrophages.

Zymosan particles phagocytosed by a macrophage

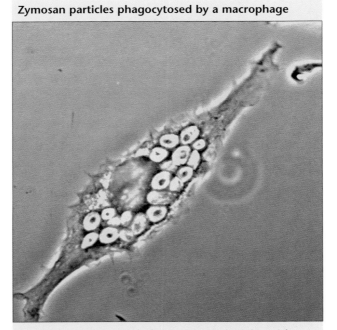

Fig. 9.19 The micrograph shows zymosan (yeast) particles phagocytosed by a macrophage, a process dependent on dectin-1. Truncation of the receptor cytoplasmic tail prevents phagocytosis.

Activation of macrophages by lipopolysaccharide and IL-1

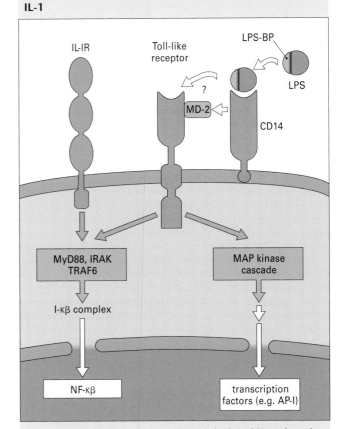

Fig. 9.20 LPS binds leukocyte CD14 (which is GPI-anchored to the membrane) through LPS binding protein (LPS-BP) and interacts with transmembrane TLRs by interaction with MD-2 to initiate signal transduction. Signaling pathways of the receptor share elements with the IL-1R pathway (e.g. IRAK – IL-1R-associated kinase). Cell activation proceeds via both the mitogen-activated protein (MAP) kinase pathways and the induction of NF-κB. (IL-1R, IL-1 receptor)

The signaling pathway for IL-1 and TLR shows many similarities (Fig. 9.20), resulting in nuclear factor kappa B (NF-κB) activation. Details of the NF-κB signaling pathway, which is activated following clustering of the TLRs, are shown in Fig. 9.21.

A distinct pathway leads to the induction of type 1 interferon (IFN) genes (*IFNα*, *IFNβ*), which can then act on type 1 interferon receptors in an autocrine pathway that induces many other genes (Fig. 9.22).

Q. What can you infer about the role of IFNs in immune defense against pathogens from their intracellular signaling pathways?
A. IFNs are involved in both antibacterial and antiviral defenses because they can activate many genes involved in inflammation.

Other receptors involved in LPS clearance, such as SR-A (see Fig. 9.16), may serve to downregulate responses induced via the CD14 pathway (see Fig. 9.20) and

The nuclear factor kappa B activation pathway

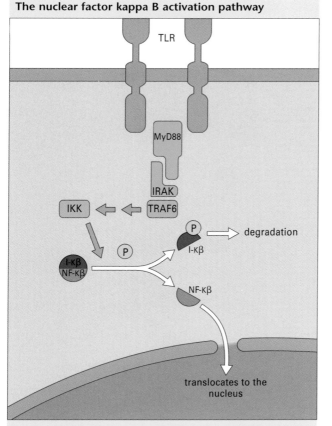

Fig. 9.21 Activation of NF-κB can be induced by ligation of a number of cell surface receptors including the Toll-like receptors (TLRs) illustrated. Apart from MyD88, a small number of other adapters transmit signals from the TLRs to cause NF-κB activation. An intracellular signaling cascade leads to the activation of inhibitor of kappa B kinase (IKK). NF-κB is normally retained in the cytosol by interaction with an inhibitor (I-κB). Phosphorylation of I-κB by IKK leads to dissociation and degradation of the inhibitor and NF-κB translocates to the nucleus to act as a transcription factor that activates a set of genes involved in inflammatory reactions.

therefore limit the systemic release of TNFα and resultant septic shock.

Monocytes and macrophages express a range of complement receptors

Monocytes and macrophages express a range of hetero-dimeric receptors for C3 cleavage products (CR1, CR3, CR4) and interact with other components of the classical, alternative, or lectin-induced pathways of complement activation (see Fig. 4.12).

CR3 contributes to myelomonocytic cell recruitment by adhesion to induced endothelial ligands, including intercellular adhesion mlecule-1 (ICAM-1), as shown in human and murine genetic deficiency syndromes.

CR3 is a promiscuous receptor, with ligands other than iC3b, including fibrinogen. Its role in regulated phago-

cytosis has been well studied, and the mechanism of CR3-mediated ingestion differs strikingly from that mediated by Fc receptors (see below). Inflammatory and secretory responses also differ after complement and antibody-dependent uptake.

Complement receptors:
- contribute to apoptotic cell clearance as well as to host defense to infection; but also
- serve as a 'safe' entry receptor for organisms such as mycobacteria by direct interaction with microbial ligands or after opsonization.

Fc receptor-mediated uptake proceeds by a zipper-like process

Fc receptors are opsonic receptors for a variety of immunoglobulin subclasses, especially IgG. The receptors are themselves immunoglobulin superfamily members, with two or three domains (see Fig. 3.20).

Fc receptors contain immunoreceptor tyrosine-based activation motifs (ITAMs) or immunoreceptor tyrosine-based inhibitory motifs (ITIMs), which, by interaction with other membrane molecules (e.g. γ chain) and cyto-plasmic kinases (e.g. Syk) and/or phosphatases, regulate complex signaling pathways.

Apart from activation of effector responses (phago-cytosis, endocytosis, antibody-dependent cytotoxicity), different Fc receptors can also downregulate inflammatory cascades and may provide a link between innate and adaptive immunity.

The mechanism for ingestion of antibody-coated particles is distinct from that mediated by CR3 (Fig. 9.23). Fc receptor-mediated uptake proceeds by a zipper-like process where sequential attachment between receptors and ligands guides pseudopod flow around the circumference of the particle. CR3 contact sites are discontinuous for complement-coated particles which 'sink' into the macrophage cytoplasm. Small GTPases play distinct roles in actin cytoskeleton engagement by each receptor-mediated process.

Macrophages express several receptors with ITIMs

Recent studies have discovered several new receptors with ITIMs expressed on macrophages, which deactivate their effector functions (e.g. signal regulatory proteins [SIRPs]) or resemble NK inhibitory receptors in their ability to ligate MHC class I molecules (see Chapter 10).

Transmembrane glycoproteins such as DAP-12 promote the surface expression of C-type lectins analogous to NK cell receptors. These may play an important regulatory function in monocytes and macrophages, for example in deactivation of cellular cytotoxicity.

Macrophages express a range of G protein-coupled receptors

Macrophages express a range of G protein-coupled receptors in addition to multispan receptors for chemokines. The F4/80 antigen (see Fig. 9.1) contains:
- a seven-transmembrane spanning portion homologous to a family of peptide receptors (e.g. vasoactive intestinal peptide, VIP); and

Activation of the *IFNβ* gene by Toll-like receptors

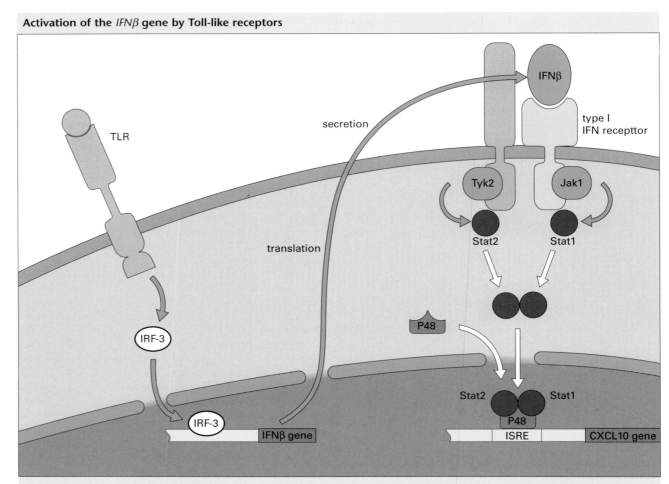

Fig. 9.22 TLRs can activate the *IFNβ* gene via a pathway that is independent of MyD88, but involves activation of the transcription factor interferon regulatory factor-3 (IRF-3). Released IFNβ acts on type 1 IFN receptors causing the aggregation of the two subunits of the receptor. This leads to activation and phosphorylation of two Jak kinases, Jak1 and Tyk2. These two transcription factors form a complex with a DNA-binding protein, P48. The complex moves to the nucleus and induces transcription of genes bearing an IFN-specific response element (ISRE), such as the chemokine CXCL10.

- a large extracellular domain consisting of multiple epidermal growth factor (EGF) domains.

The F4/80 molecule has been implicated in the induction of peripheral tolerance.

Non-opsonic phagocytosis can lead to intracellular infection

In the absence of opsonins, macrophages use multiple receptors to recognize and engulf a range of microorganisms, parasites, and viruses directly. These include:

- CR3;
- SR-As;
- MR;
- the β-glucan receptor; and
- CD14.

SR-As use selected polyanionic ligands including LPS (Gram-negative) and lipoteichoic acid (Gram-positive) for bacterial recognition.

MR ligands are found on mycobacteria, HIV gp120, *Pneumocystis carinii*, *Klebsiella* spp., as well as yeasts (*Candida albicans*).

CR3 ligands include phosphatidylinositol mannoside (PIM), and a direct saccharide binding site on CR3 has been implicated in opsonin-independent recognition.

Different receptors often collaborate (e.g. CR3 and MR in the uptake of *Leishmania* promastigotes).

Non-opsonic uptake or invasion results in a range of survival strategies by intracellular pathogens enabling them to:

- avoid phagosome maturation;
- inhibit fusion with lysosomes and acidification (mycobacteria); or conversely
- promote invasion by rapid recruitment of lysosomes (*C. albicans*, *Trypanosoma cruzi*).

Legionella pneumophila induces a coiling phagocytosis, and recruits various intracellular organelles (endoplasmic

Zipper model of phagocytosis

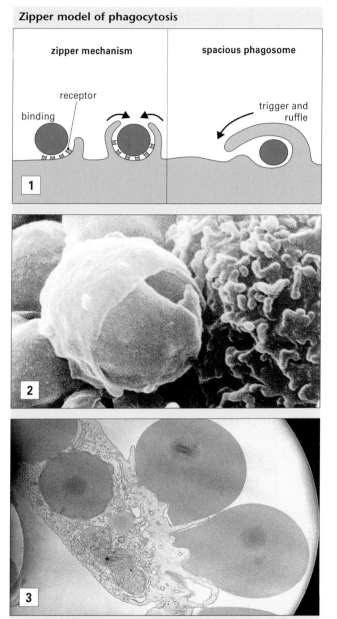

Fig. 9.23 (1) During phagocytosis, receptor–ligand interactions guide the extension of tightly apposed pseudopods around the particle's total circumference until a fusion of the plasma membrane occurs at the tip. This is known as the zipper mechanism. Alternative 'trigger' mechanisms, in which spacious phagosomes result from flipping over of ruffles back onto the plasma membrane, have also been described. The cytoskeleton of phagocytes plays a key role in engulfment, during which there is extensive remodeling of actin filaments. Some microorganisms and intracellular parasites induce novel mechanisms to recruit cell membranes during entry into phagocytes. (2 and 3) Electron micrographs of ingestion of antibody (IgG)-coated sheep erythrocytes by peritoneal macrophage by the zipper mechanism. (Scanning electron micrograph (2), courtesy of Dr GG MacPherson. Transmission electron micrograph (3), courtesy of Dr SC Silverstein)

reticulum, mitochondria), whereas salmonellae induce the formation of spacious phagosomes.

Once within vacuoles:

- the organism can replicate in secondary lysosomes (*Leishmania* spp.); or
- escape into the cytosol by membrane dissolution (*Listeria monocytogenes*).

IFNγ can overcome many of these evasion strategies, resulting in killing or stasis of the organisms by mechanisms described below.

Opsonization by antibody and/or complement can alter the fate of the organism by extracellular lysis or by targeting it to lysosomes.

Some organisms induce apoptosis in macrophages (e.g. *Salmonella* spp.); others spread between cells by fusion (e.g. HIV) or by intercellular infection (e.g. *Listeria* spp.).

The ability of macrophages to present processed peptide antigens derived from intracellular pathogens to T cells is poorly defined. It is possible that they collaborate with dendritic cells by releasing breakdown products, so activating naive T cells. Once MHC class II molecules are induced by IFNγ, exogenous antigens are presented by the MHC class II pathway (see Fig. 7.11). Endogenous antigens are presented by the MHC class I pathway (see Fig. 7.9), so infected macrophages can become targets for CD8+ cytotoxic T cells.

Q. How are lipid antigens such as mycolic acids of mycobacteria presented to T cells?

A. CD1 molecules present these antigens, which are inducible on selected macrophage populations.

Macrophages contain intracellular receptors for pathogens

Recently a number of intracellular proteins have been discovered in macrophages and other cells, that are able to sense microbial wall degradation products. These proteins contain leucine-rich repeats, pyrin, caspase-associated recruitment domains (CARD), and **nucleotide oligomerization domains (NOD)**. Ligation induces expression of proinflammatory cytokines (e.g. IL-1).

As illustrated for NOD-1 (Fig. 9.24), signal transduction involves the formation of protein–protein complexes that are involved in IL-1 processing (**inflammasomes**). Mutations in the pyrin domain have been implicated in rare hyperinflammatory syndromes such as familial Mediterranean fever. IL-1 receptor antagonists can be remarkably effective as therapy in related conditions.

The *NOD-2* gene is frequently mutated in people with Crohn's disease, a chronic granulomatous inflammatory bowel disease (Fig. 9.25). It is expressed by monocytes and macrophages and recognizes cytosolic muramyl dipeptides, resulting from the degradation of both Gram-negative and Gram-positive organisms.

NOD-2 deficiency leads to increased susceptibility to bacterial infection via the oral route, and may be required for expression of antimicrobial peptides. Other genes have also been implicated in susceptibility to inflammatory bowel disease.

NOD-1 signal transduction

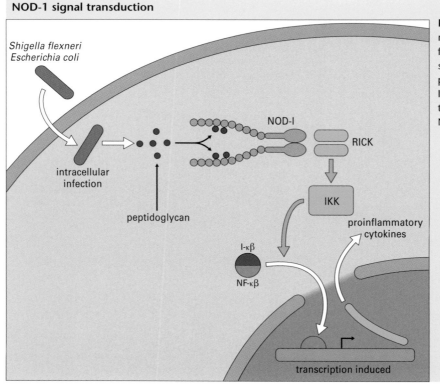

Fig. 9.24 NOD-1 is an intracellular pattern recognition molecule. Peptidoglycan from, for example, *Shigella flexneri* and some strains of *Escherichia coli* binds to the protein. A domain (RICK) then activates IKK (see Fig. 9.21) leading to the transcription of proteins dependent on NF-κB.

Crohn's disease

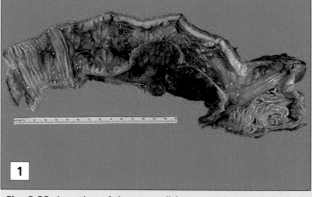

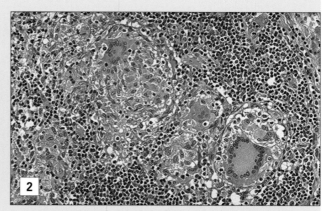

Fig. 9.25 A section of the gut wall from a patient with Crohn's disease, showing the intense inflammation of the tissue (**1**). The histological section shows a granulomatous reaction with lymphocyte and macrophage infiltration and the formation of giant cells (**2**).

ACTIVATED MACROPHAGES SECRETE A VARIETY OF MOLECULES

Following encounters with microorganisms and antigens, resident macrophages are able to enhance their transcription and translation of a wide range of gene products, including secreted molecules, which often act locally close to the cell surface.

Secretory products include:
- eicosanoids;
- cytokines;
- complement proteins; and
- enzymes, especially lysozyme (Fig. 9.26).

After priming by IFNγ, macrophages triggered by surface-acting stimuli such as LPS release increased levels of various products, which promote an inflammatory reaction, recruit other cells, regulate their activities, and induce adhesion.

Macrophages also release inhibitory molecules (e.g. TGFβ, PGE₂, IL-10), which suppress inflammatory and immune responses, including T cell proliferation.

Secretory products of macrophages

category	example	function
low molecular weight metabolites	reactive oxygen intermediates reactive nitrogen intermediates eicosanoids – prostaglandins, leukotrienes platelet-activating factor (PAF)	killing, inflammation killing, inflammation regulation of inflammation clotting
cytokines	IL-1β, TNFα, IL-6 IFNα/IFNβ IL-10 IL-12, IL-18 TGFβ CCL2, CCL3, CCL4, CCL5, CXCL8	local and systemic inflammation antiviral, innate immunity, immunomodulation deactivation of MØ, B cell activation IFNγ production by NK and T cells repair, modulation, inflammation chemokines
adhesion molecules	fibronectin thrombospondin	opsonization, matrix adhesion, phagocytosis of apoptotic cells
complement	C3, all others	local opsonization
procoagulant	tissue factor	clotting cascade
enzymes	lysozyme urokinase (plasminogen activator) collagenase elastase	Gram-positive bacterial lysis fibrinolysis matrix catabolism matrix catabolism

Fig. 9.26 Macrophages produce a wide range of secreted molecules.

IFNγ, IL-1, and TNFα are potent regulators of leukocyte and other cellular activities.

Q. Describe four roles of IFNγ in the development of the immune response, each modulating a different group of cells.
A. IFNγ induces MHC molecules and co-stimulatory molecules on APCs, and induces adhesion molecules and chemokines on endothelium. It also activates macrophage microbicidal activity, modulates class switching by B cells, and regulates the balance between Tн1 and Tн2 populations of T cells.

IL-6 and IL-1 act as circulating mediators of the acute phase response. Distant targets of these macrophage-derived cytokines include thermoregulatory centers in the central nervous system, muscle and fat stores, and the neuroendocrine system.

Cytotoxic products and powerful neutral proteinases such as elastase, collagenase, and urokinase (generating plasmin) (Fig. 9.27) are able to induce tissue injury and contribute to destructive chronic inflammation in joints and lung.

Monocyte-derived procoagulant/tissue factor can also induce vascular occlusion and tissue damage.

Macrophages themselves express receptors for cytokines, as well as producing molecules that are cleaved by metalloproteinases and shed into the circulation. By contrast, soluble receptors and receptor antagonists (eg. IL-1Ra, soluble TNFR) are potential inhibitors of receptor–ligand interactions.

mRNA microarray methods to analyze gene expression generate complex profiles of selective induction and inhi-bition of large numbers of genes, some highly restricted to macrophages, others shared with different cell types. Patterns of macrophage mRNA and protein expression now provide insights into intrinsic and extrinsic regulation of macrophage differentiation and activation.

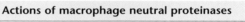

Actions of macrophage neutral proteinases

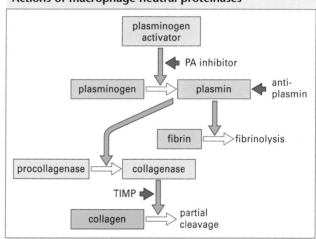

Fig. 9.27 Macrophage-derived neutral proteinases interact with plasma and tissue enzymes and their inhibitors (which can also be generated by macrophages) to regulate fibrinolysis and matrix catabolism. (PA, plasminogen activator; TIMP, tissue inhibitor of matrix metalloproteinase)

Resting macrophages have limited antimicrobial killing activity

Following phagocytosis, pathogens are subjected to a variety of killing mechanisms, which are generally more diverse and more effective in activated macrophages.

Following lysosome fusion, there is a transient rise in the pH of the phagolysosome, followed by a fall in pH, which occurs within 10–15 minutes. The acidification of the phagolysosome may, by itself, contribute to the killing of some organisms, but the additional killing mechanisms, described below, may be more effective at specific pH values. For example:

- the production of reactive oxygen intermediates (ROIs) in activated macrophages occurs immediately after internalization;
- cationic proteins are most active during the early alkaline phase; and
- many digestive lysosomal enzymes are more active in the later acidic phase (Fig. 9.28).

Lysozyme acts directly on the bacterial cell wall proteoglycans

The resident macrophage has a relatively limited killing capacity, which may be sufficient to restrict growth of many, if not most, organisms, including viruses. Lysozyme acts directly on the bacterial cell wall proteoglycans, present especially in the exposed cell wall of Gram-positive bacteria (Fig. 9.29).

The cell walls of Gram-negative bacteria may also become exposed to lysozyme if they have been damaged by complement membrane attack complexes.

Lysozyme is constitutively produced by macrophages.

Defensins also contribute to macrophage antibacterial activities

A group of highly cationic proteins and polypeptides called defensins also contribute to macrophage antibacterial activities.

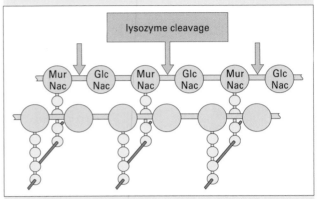

Action of lysozyme on the cell wall of *Staphylococcus aureus*

Fig. 9.29 The structure of the cell wall of Gram-positive bacteria such as *Staphylococcus aureus* includes a backbone of N-acetylglucosamine (GlcNac) alternating with N-acetylmuramic acid (MurNac) cross-linked by amino acid side chains (yellow) and bridges of five glycine residues (orange). Lysozyme splits the molecules at the places indicated.

The defensins:

- are small peptides (30–33 amino acids) found in some macrophages of many species and specifically in human neutrophils, where they comprise up to 50% of the granule proteins;
- form ion-permeable channels in lipid bilayers and probably act before acidification of the phagolysosome;
- are able to kill a range of pathogens, including bacteria (*S. aureus*, *Pseudomonas aeruginosa*, *E. coli*), fungi (*Cryptococcus neoformans*), and enveloped viruses (herpes simplex).

Q. What other molecule can generate ion-permeable channels in lipid bilayers?
A. The final component of the lytic complement pathway, C9 (see Chapter 4).

In resident macrophages, endocytosis, lysosome delivery and fusion, and acidification favor destruction of phagocytosed pathogens, but may facilitate escape of an organism from vacuole to cytosol.

The **N-ramp multispanning glycoprotein** found in macrophage phagosomes contributes to cellular and ultimately host resistance or susceptibility to a range of intracellular pathogens (mycobacteria, *Leishmania* spp., *Salmonella* spp.) by influencing iron transport into or possibly out of the vacuole.

ACTIVATED MACROPHAGES PRODUCE REACTIVE OXYGEN AND NITROGEN INTERMEDIATES

Elicited (i.e. recruited by a non-immune inflammatory stimulus) and immunologically activated macrophages produce higher levels of lysozyme than resting macrophages,

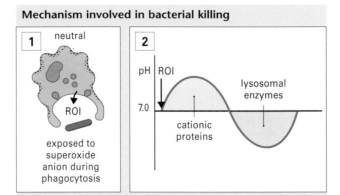

Mechanism involved in bacterial killing

Fig. 9.28 During phagocytosis there is immediate exposure to reactive oxygen intermediates (ROIs) (**1**). This leads to a transient increase in pH, when cationic proteins may be most effective (**2**). Subsequently the pH falls as H⁺ ions are pumped into the phagolysosome and neutral proteinases and lysosomal enzymes with low pH optima become effective. Lactoferrin acts by chelating free iron and can do so at alkaline or acidic pH.

Oxygen-dependent microbicidal activity

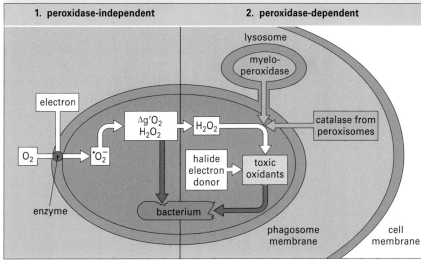

Fig. 9.30 (1) An enzyme (NADPH oxidase, see p. 307) in the phagosome membrane reduces oxygen to the superoxide anion ($^\bullet O_2^-$). This can give rise to hydroxyl radicals ($^\bullet OH$), singlet oxygen ($\Delta g' O_2$), and hydrogen peroxide (H_2O_2), all of which are potentially toxic. Lysosome fusion is not required for these parts of the pathway, and the reaction takes place spontaneously following formation of the phagosome. (2) If lysosome fusion occurs, myeloperoxidase (or, under some circumstances, catalase from peroxisomes) acts on peroxides in the presence of halides (preferably iodide). Then additional toxic oxidants, such as hypohalite (HIO, HClO), are generated.

as well as proinflammatory cytokines, chemokines, growth factors, and proteases.

One major difference between resting and activated macrophages is the ability to generate hydrogen peroxide (H_2O_2), and other metabolites generated by the respiratory burst (Fig. 9.30). The phagocyte oxidase (Phox) membrane and cytosolic proteins found in neutrophils and activated macrophages assemble to form an NADPH oxidase complex, which contains a novel cytochrome.

In the presence of myeloperoxidase, released by myelomonocytic cells, the Klebanoff reaction generates even higher levels of reactive oxygen metabolites. Patients with chronic granulomatous disease lack essential oxidase components and suffer from repeated infections.

Macrophages in mouse as well as human can be activated by IFNγ to express high levels of **inducible nitric oxide synthase (i-NOS)**, which catalyzes the production of nitric oxide (NO) from arginine (Fig. 9.31). Release of NO by macrophages affects neighboring vessels and leukocytes, and contributes to the killing of intracellular pathogens such as *Leishmania* spp. either directly or by production of peroxynitrites.

Failure of macrophage activation in AIDS contributes to opportunistic pathogen infections and persistence of HIV, as well as reactivation of latent tuberculosis (e.g. by anti-TNFα therapy).

Rare inborn errors in humans for IL-12 and IFN receptors have confirmed experimental gene ablation studies in the mouse, which render the host susceptible to infection by intracellular bacteria.

Recently recruited cells are particularly effective in microbial killing

Macrophages vary considerably in their antimicrobial activity. Monocytes produce more reactive oxygen metabolites and myeloperoxidase than differentiated tissue macrophages.

It is the recently recruited and further activated cell that is primarily responsible for host defense. In-situ

The nitric oxide pathway

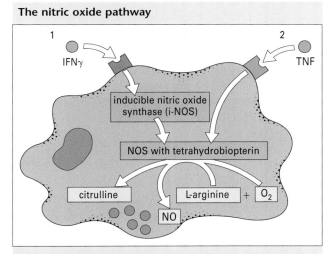

Fig. 9.31 The inducible nitric oxide synthase (i-NOS) combines oxygen with guanidino nitrogen of L-arginine to give nitric oxide (NO), which is toxic for bacteria and tumor cells. Toxicity may be increased by interactions with products of the oxygen reduction pathway, leading to the formation of peroxynitrites. Tetrahydrobiopterin is needed as a cofactor. In murine macrophages IFNγ activates the pathway (1), which is then optimally triggered by TNF (2). Triggering release of NO from human macrophages is more complex and usually involves cross-linking of membrane CD23. Human macrophages can sometimes express i-NOS but they contain little tetrahydrobiopterin, and maximal NO release may require interaction with other cell types.

analysis shows that granuloma macrophages are the major source of newly produced proteins such as lysozyme, TNFα, and IL-1. The latter cytokines are more tightly regulated than lysozyme, and further exposure to microbial components such as LPS is needed to induce the majority of macrophages to express these mediators.

Role of activated macrophages in immunopathology

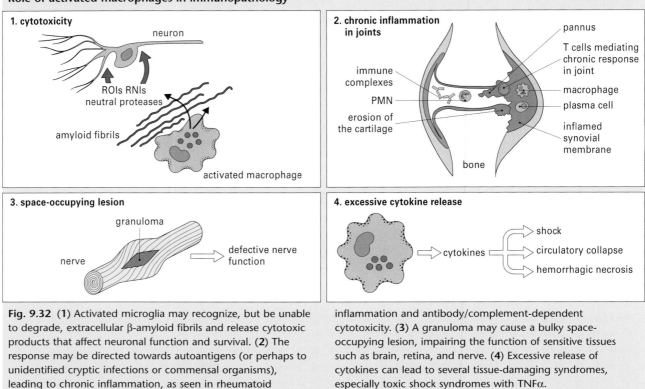

Fig. 9.32 **(1)** Activated microglia may recognize, but be unable to degrade, extracellular β-amyloid fibrils and release cytotoxic products that affect neuronal function and survival. **(2)** The response may be directed towards autoantigens (or perhaps to unidentified cryptic infections or commensal organisms), leading to chronic inflammation, as seen in rheumatoid arthritis. Non-internalizable immune complexes may perpetuate inflammation and antibody/complement-dependent cytotoxicity. **(3)** A granuloma may cause a bulky space-occupying lesion, impairing the function of sensitive tissues such as brain, retina, and nerve. **(4)** Excessive release of cytokines can lead to several tissue-damaging syndromes, especially toxic shock syndromes with TNFα.

Once effector mechanisms are activated, local surface reactions also influence the release of potentially injurious macrophage molecules. If ligands are presented on a non-internalizable surface ('frustrated phagocytosis'), secretory products can be released into the extracellular environment.

Activated macrophages contribute considerably to tissue damage in autoimmune and chronic inflammatory diseases in joints, lung, and the nervous system (Fig. 9.32).

MACROPHAGES INITIATE, PROMOTE, PREVENT, SUPPRESS, AND TERMINATE IMMUNE RESPONSES

The macrophage is able to initiate, promote, prevent, suppress, or terminate an immune response. Its actions may seem antigen non-specific, though antigen dependent.

Apart from a major role in host defense, macrophages:
- are participants in autoimmunity (failure to prevent immunity) and peripheral tolerance;
- may contribute to T cell downregulation in placenta (a macrophage-rich organ) and at immunologically privileged sites such as the anterior chamber of the eye;
- can nurse or kill neighboring cells and partners, and we need to learn more about how they discriminate friend from foe, and danger from safety.

The host is not viable without macrophages, which perform vital functions within and beyond the immune system.

FURTHER READING
Reviews

Aderem A, Underhill DM. Mechanisms of phagocytosis in macrophages. Annu Rev Immunol 1999;17:593–623.

Akira S, Takeda K. Toll-like receptor signaling. Nat Rev Immunol 2004;4:499–511.

Brown GD, Gordon S. Fungal β-glucans and mammalian immunity. Immunity 2003;19:311–315.

Desjardins M. ER-mediated phagocytosis: a new membrane for new functions. Nat Rev Immunol 2003;3:280–291.

Ezekowitz RAB, Hoffmann JA, eds. Innate immunity. New Jersey: Humana Press; 2003.

Geijtenbeek TBH, Engering A, Van Kooyk Y. DC-SIGN, a C-type lectin on dendritic cells that unveils many aspects of dendritic cell biology. J Leuk Biol 2002;71:921–931.

Girardin SE, Philpott DJ. The role of peptidoglycan recognition in innate immunity. Eur J Immunol 2004;34:1777–1782.

Gordon S. Macrophages and the immune response In: Paul W, ed. Fundamental immunology, 5th ed. Philadelphia: Lippincott Raven; 2003:481–495.

Gordon S. Alternative activation of macrophages. Nat Rev Immunol 2003;3:23–35.

Gordon S. Pattern recognition receptors: doubling up for the innate immune response. Cell 111:927–930.

Hull KM, Shoham N, Chae JJ, et al. The expanding spectrum of systemic autoinflammatory disorders and their rheumatic manifestations. Curr Opin Rheumatol 2003;15:61–69.

Kaufmann SHE, Medzhitov R, Gordon S, eds. The innate immune response to infection. Washington, DC: ASM Press; 2004.

Kuijpers TW, Roos D. Neutrophils: the power within. In: Kaufmann SHE, Medzhitov R, Gordon S, eds. The innate immune response to infection. Washington, DC: ASM Press; 2004:47–70.

Luster AD. Chemokines linking innate and adaptive immunity. Curr Opin Immunol 2002;14:129–135.

O'Neill LAJ. TLRs: Professor Mechnikov, sit on your hat. Trends Immunol 2004;25:687–693.

Peiser L, Mukhopadhyay S, Gordon S. Scavenger receptors in innate immunity. Curr Opin Immunol 2002;14:123–128.

Portnoy DA, Auerbuch V, Glomski IJ. The cell biology of *Listeria monocytogenes* infection. J Cell Biol 2002;158:409–414.

Puel A, Picard C, Cheng-Lung K, et al. Inherited disorders of NF-kappaB-mediated immunity in man. Curr Opin Immunol 2004;16:34–41.

Rabinovitch M. Professional and non-professional phagocytes: an introduction. Trends Cell Biol 1995;5:85–87.

Randolph GJ. Dendritic cell migration to lymph nodes: cytokines, chemokines and lipid mediators. Semin Immunol 2001;13:267–274.

Russell DG. *Mycobacterium tuberculosis*: here today and here tomorrow. Nat Rev Mol Cell Biol 2001;2:569–577.

Savill J, Dransfield I, Gregory C, Haslett C. A blast from the past: clearance of apoptotic cells regulates immune responses. Nat Rev Immunol 2002;2:965–975.

Taylor PR, Martinez-Pomares L, Stacey M, et al. Macrophage receptors and immune recognition. Annu Rev Immunol 2005;23:901–944.

Tschopp J, Martinon F, Burns K. NALPs: a novel protein family involved in inflammation. Nat Rev Mol Cell Biol 4:95–104.

Selected papers

Brown GD, Herre J, Williams DL, et al. Dectin-1 mediates the biological effects of β-glucans. J Exp Med 2003;197:1119–1124.

Dalton DK, Pitts-Meek S, Keshav S, et al. Multiple defects of immune cell function in mice with disrupted interferonγ genes. Science 1993;259:1739–1742.

Geissmann F, Jung S, Littman DR. Blood monocytes consist of two principal subsets with distinct migratory properties. Immunity 2003;19:71–82.

Kindler Y, Sappino AP, Grau GE, et al. The inducing role of TNF in the development of bactericidal granulomas during BCG infection. Cell 1981;56:731–740.

Lin H-H, Faunce DE, Stacey M, et al. The macrophage F4/80 receptor is required for the induction of antigen-specific efferent regulatory T cells in peripheral tolerance. J Exp Med 2005;201:1615–1625.

Medzhitov R, Preston-Hurlburt P, Janeway CA Jr. A human homologue of the *Drosophila* Toll protein signals activation of adaptive immunity. Nature 1997;388:394–397.

Poltorak A, He X, Smirnova I, et al. Defective LPS signaling in C3H/HeJ and C57 Bl/10 ScCr mice: mutations in the *TLR4* gene. Science 1998;282:2085–2088.

Critical thinking: The role of macrophages in toxic shock syndrome (see p. 495 for explanations)

In an experimental model of septic shock, mice are infected systemically with bacille Calmette–Guérin (BCG), a non-lethal vaccine strain of mycobacteria. After 12 days, the mice are challenged intraperitoneally with graded doses of lipopolysaccharide (LPS). Blood samples are taken at 2 hours and the clinical condition of the mice is monitored for up to 24 hours. Experiments are terminated earlier if mice show severe signs of distress.

1 What cytokines would you measure in the 2-hour serum sample?

2 What clinical signs would be indicative of incipient septic shock?

3 What mechanisms contribute to septic shock?

4 What outcome would you expect if the following knockout mouse strains were used instead of wild-type controls: CD14, scavenger receptor class A (SR-A), IFNγ?

5 Interpret your results.

6 Suggest further experiments.

7 What is the clinical significance of this experiment?

The distinction between inflammatory responses and house-keeping of apoptotic cells (see p. 495 for explanations)

Mouse peritoneal macrophages are fed a meal of apoptotic cells in culture, and then challenged with an intracellular pathogen, *Trypanosoma cruzi*. Subsequent single cell analysis of parasite survival shows that *T. cruzi* growth is enhanced by prior uptake of apoptotic cells, but not of necrotic cells or control particles.

8 How would you investigate the macrophage surface receptors responsible for apoptotic cell uptake?

9 Suggest a possible mechanism by which apoptotic cell uptake promotes *T. cruzi* survival.

10 How would you investigate this experimental model?

11 What is the possible in vivo and clinical significance of this observation?

The role of macrophages in TH1 and TH2 responses (see p. 496 for explanations)

Isolated mouse peritoneal macrophages are treated for 2 days with selected cytokines (IFNγ, IL-4, IL-13, IL-10) in culture and a range of assays for cell activation is employed. It is found that IFNγ enhances the respiratory burst (after LPS challenge), MHC class II expression, and proinflammatory cytokine production, but downregulates mannose receptor (MR)-mediated endocytosis. IL-10 is an efficient antagonist of the above effects. IL-4 and IL-13 are weak antagonists of respiratory burst and proinflammatory cytokine production and markedly induce MHC class II molecules and MR activity.

12 Interpret the significance and possible functional relevance of these results in relation to concepts of TH1/TH2 differentiation.

13 What further work could be done to investigate the possibility that macrophage activation could by analogy be classified as M1/M2?

14 How would you investigate the role of macrophages and dendritic cells as possible inducers of CD4$^+$ T cell subset differentiation?

Cell-mediated Cytotoxicity

CHAPTER 10

SUMMARY

- **Cell-mediated cytotoxicity is an essential defense against intracellular pathogens, including viruses, some bacteria, and parasites.** CTLs recognize antigen presented on MHC molecules. Most CTLs are CD8+ and recognize antigenic peptides presented on MHC class I molecules. NK cells react against cells that do not express MHC class I molecules. They can interact with these cells using a variety of receptors.

- **NK cells express a variety of receptors.** The lectin-like receptor CD94 interacts with HLA-E. KIRs (killer immunoglobulin-like receptors) are members of the immunoglobulin superfamily – those with short tails are activating, and those with long tails are inhibitory. Immunoglobulin-like transcripts (ILTs) have a wider cell distribution than other NK cell receptors.

- **Interactions with NK receptors determine NK cell action.** NK cells use several different receptors to positively identify their targets, and intracellular signaling pathways coordinate inhibitory and activating signals.

- **Cytotoxicity is effected by direct cellular interactions, cytokines, and granule exocytosis.** Fas ligand and TNF can signal apoptosis to the target cell. Granules containing perforin and granzymes contribute to target cell damage. Ligation of Fas or the type 1 TNF receptor on the target cell leads to the activation of caspases, which are the ultimate mediators of apoptosis in the target.

- **Macrophages, neutrophils, and eosinophils are non-lymphoid cytotoxic effectors.** Macrophages damage targets using their non-specific toxic effector systems or via cytokines. Eosinophils mediate cytotoxicity by exocytosis of their granules.

CELL-MEDIATED CYTOTOXICITY IS AN ESSENTIAL IMMUNE DEFENSE MECHANISM

Cytotoxicity describes the ways in which leukocytes recognize and destroy other cells.

Cell-mediated cytotoxicity is an essential defense against:
- intracellular pathogens, including viruses;
- some bacteria;
- some parasites.

Tumor cells, eukaryotic pathogens, and even cells of the body may also become the target of cytotoxic cells.

Cytotoxicity is also important in the destruction of allogeneic tissue grafts.

Several types of cell have cytotoxic activity including:
- cytotoxic T lymphocytes (CTLs);
- natural killer (NK) cells; and sometimes
- myeloid cells.

The mechanisms of recognition and killing used by the lymphoid cells are quite distinct from those of the myeloid cells, and will be considered first.

CTLs recognize antigen presented on MHC molecules and NK cells react against cells that do not express MHC class I

CTLs and NK cells recognize their targets in different ways (Fig. 10.1):

Recognition of target cells by cytotoxic T lymphocytes (CTLs) and NK cells

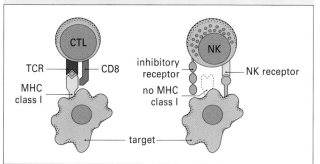

Fig. 10.1 CTLs recognize processed antigen presented on the target cell by MHC molecules using their T cell receptor (TCR). Most CTLs are CD8+ and recognize antigen presented by MHC class I molecules, but a minority are CD4+ and recognize antigen presented by MHC class II molecules. In contrast, NK cells have receptors that recognize MHC class I on the target and signal inhibition of cytotoxicity. They use a number of different receptors (NK receptors) to identify their targets positively, including CD2, CD69, or antibody bound to their Fc receptor (CD16).

Rapid Reference Box 10

ADCC (antibody-dependent cell-mediated cytotoxicity) – a cytotoxic reaction in which Fc receptor-bearing cells recognize target cells via specific antibodies.

Caspases – a group of enzymes that initiate and act as effectors of apoptosis.

CD94 – lectin-like receptor that recognizes MHC class I peptides presented by HLA-E molecules.

CD95 – Fas, a molecule expressed on a variety of cells that acts as a target for ligation by CD95L on cytotoxic cells.

Granzymes – granule associated enzymes that are released by cytotoxic cells and which induce apoptosis in target cells.

HLA-E molecules – class Ib molecules encoded within the MHC which present leader peptides of MHC class I molecules for recognition by CD94/NKG2 receptors on NK cells.

HLA-G molecules – class Ib molecules encoded within the MHC which are expressed on cells of the placenta and inhibit NK cell-mediated cytotoxicity.

ITAMs and ITIMs (immunoreceptor tyrosine activation/inhibitory motifs) – these are target sequences for phosphorylation by kinases involved in cell activation or inhibition.

KIRs (killer immunoglublin-like receptors) – a group of molecules present on NK cells that, when ligated can activate or inhibit cytotoxicity.

Lymphotoxins – a group of cytokines that act on TNF/LT receptors and which may induce apoptosis in target cells.

Perforin –a molecule contained in the granules of cytotoxic cells which is related to complement C9, and when released can form pores in the plasma membrane of a target cell.

TNFα – a cytokine encoded within the MHC, that may induce apoptosis in target cells.

- CTLs recognize specific antigens (e.g. viral peptides on infected cells) presented by MHC molecules – most CTLs cells are CD8⁺ and recognize antigen presented on MHC class I molecule, though some CD4⁺ cells are cytotoxic and recognize antigen presented on MHC class II molecules;
- NK cells recognize cells that fail to express MHC class I molecules and also use a variety of receptors to recognize their targets positively (e.g. they can bind to antibody already attached to antigen on a target cell using their Fc receptors (CD16) – a process known as **antibody-dependent cell-mediated cytotoxicity [ADCC]**).

The most important role of CTLs is the elimination of cells infected with virus (see Chapter 13).

Nearly all nucleated cells express MHC class I molecules and if they become infected can therefore present antigen to CD8⁺ CTLs (see Chapters 5 and 7).

Cellular molecules that have been partly degraded by proteasomes are transported to the endoplasmic reticulum to become associated with MHC class I molecules and are then transported to the cell surface.

Q. How does a virus-infected cell know which molecules are viral antigens and should therefore be presented to CTLs?
A. It does not. Each cell samples its own molecules and presents them for review by CD8⁺ CTLs. Both the cell's own molecules and those of intracellular pathogens will be presented in this way. It is the T cells that can distinguish self molecules from non-self antigens, not the infected cell.

Additional interactions may be required to stabilize the bond between the CTL and the target (Fig. 10.2), and can even help trigger the killing event. For example, by adding antibodies against CD3 or CD2 on the CTL in vitro, it is possible to trigger the killing of target cells that are bound to the CTL. It is probable that binding of physiological ligands to these molecules (CD3 and CD2) can also trigger CTLs in this way.

CTLs and NK cells are complementary in the immune defense against virally infected cells

Several viruses (particularly herpes viruses) have evolved mechanisms to avoid recognition by CTLs. They reduce the expression of MHC molecules or even produce proteins that pick MHC molecules out of the endoplasmic reticulum to reduce the likelihood that processed viral peptides will be presented at the cell surface.

Because NK cells specifically recognize cells that have lost their MHC class I molecules, we can see that CTLs and NK cells act in a complementary way to protect the body. In effect:

- the NK cells check that cells of the body are carrying their identity card (MHC class I);
- the CTL checks the specific identity (antigen specificity) on the card.

Experiments involving the micromanipulation of individual cells have shown that a single CTL can sequentially kill several target cells. To do this CTLs must be:

- resistant to their own killing mechanisms; and
- able to detach effectively from dying target cells.

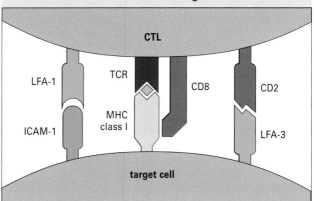

Interactions between CTLs and target cells

Fig. 10.2 Some of the ligands involved in the interaction between CTLs and their targets. (ICAM-1, intercellular adhesion molecule-1; TCR, T cell receptor; LFA-3, leukocyte functional antigen-1)

Cytokine-activated killer (LAK) cells are related to NK cells

Immunologists have experimented with several potential treatments for cancer. One approach has been to activate the patient's own lymphocytes in vitro with interleukin-2 (IL-2), and then to reinfuse them. These cells, which are initially derived from blood or spleen, are called **cytokine-activated killer cells** or, originally, **lymphokine-activated killers** (**LAKs**). They:

- show enhanced MHC non-restricted cytotoxicity; and
- appear to be largely derived from precursor cells that are indistinguishable from NK cells.

Therefore LAK cells probably do not represent a separate lineage, but rather a consequence of activation. This type of cell is undergoing trials for the treatment of cancer in humans.

NK CELLS EXPRESS A VARIETY OF RECEPTORS

NK cells are mostly derived from large granular lympho-cytes (LGLs), which comprise about 5% of human periph-eral blood lymphocytes. The majority of NK cells are:

- CD3$^-$, CD16$^+$, CD56$^+$, CD94$^+$ (see Appendix 2); and
- do not contain productive rearrangements of the TCR genes.

Initial experiments on the specificity of NK cells showed that MHC class I expression protected cells from NK cell-mediated cytotoxicity and that particular allotypes of HLA-C were dominant genes for producing resistance.

This led to a search for receptors on NK cells that could inhibit cytotoxicity and that might be expressed in a variety of different forms capable of:

- reacting with MHC class I; and
- signaling the presence of MHC class I molecules to the NK cell.

Two major types of molecule were identified and termed **killer inhibitory receptors** (**KIRs**):

- one group of molecules was identified as type 2 membrane glycoproteins (C terminus outside) with a C-type lectin domain (Ca^{2+}-dependent);
- the other group of molecules were members of the immunoglobulin superfamily.

Subsequently it was realized that, although some members of each group did indeed act as killer inhibitory receptors, others could actually activate the killer cell. So it was not correct to call all members of both groups 'inhibitory receptors'. It was therefore proposed that the term '**KIR**' now meaning '**killer immunoglobulin-like receptor**', should be used for just the second group of molecules.

The lectin-like receptor CD94 interacts with HLA-E

The lectin-like receptor **CD94** is a characteristic marker of human NK cells, but is also found on a subset of CTLs. It covalently assembles with different members of another group of type 2 membrane molecules called **NKG2**, and the dimers are expressed at the cell membrane (Fig. 10.3).

There are at least six members of the NKG2 family (NKG2A–NKG2F). The dimer of CD94–NKG2A is

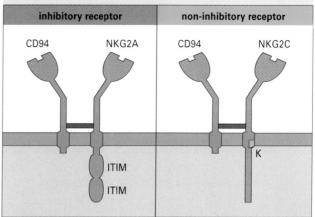

Lectin-like receptors of NK cells

Fig. 10.3 The inhibitory receptors consist of CD94 disulfide-bonded (red) to peptides from the *NKG2* locus, such as NKG2A, which have intracellular domains carrying ITIM motifs (immunoreceptor tyrosine inhibitory motif). Non-inhibitory receptors (such as CD94/NKG2C) lack the ITIMs, but have a charged lysine residue (K) in the transmembrane segment that allows them to interact with signal transducing molecules.

an inhibitory receptor that blocks NK cell-mediated cytotoxicity. By contrast CD94–NKG2C is an activating receptor (see Fig. 10.3). Although these two NKG2 molecules are very similar, they differ in their intracellular segments, and this determines whether the receptor is inhibitory or activating.

In vivo, the role of the inhibitory version is clear, but that of the activating variant is not. Possibly, it may act as one of the receptors by which NK cells carrying CD94–NKG2C actively engage their targets.

CD94 is distantly related to the mouse molecule Ly-49, which is present in the NK cell gene complex (NKC). Indeed, it was partly this homology of CD94 to mouse NK cell receptors that alerted researchers to the possibility that CD94 was an NK cell receptor in humans.

The ligand for both CD94–NKG2A and CD94–NKG2C is the **HLA-E** molecule.

HLA-E molecules present peptides from other MHC class I molecules

The *HLA-E* gene locus encodes an **MHC class I-like molecule**. These are sometimes called **class Ib molecules** to distinguish them from the classical MHC molecules that present antigen to CTLs.

The extraordinary function of HLA-E is to present peptides from other MHC class I molecules. The leader peptides from other MHC molecules are transported to the endoplasmic reticulum and are required to stabilize functional HLA-E molecules (Fig. 10.4). Cells lacking classical MHC class I molecules do not express HLA-E at the cell surface. Hence an inhibitory signal is not passed to the NK cell.

In effect HLA-E is a sensitive mechanism for monitoring whether viruses or tumors have downregulated MHC class I molecule expression in a cell.

HLA-E presents peptides of other MHC class I molecules

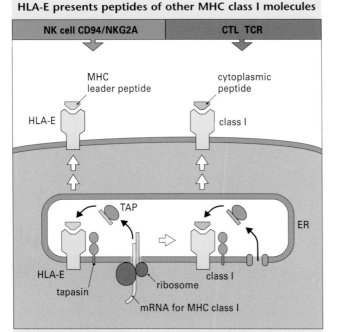

Fig. 10.4 Leader peptides from MHC class I molecules are loaded onto HLA-E molecules in the endoplasmic reticulum, a process that requires TAP transporters and tapasin to assemble functional HLA-E molecules. These are presented at the cell surface for review by the CD94 series of receptors on NK cells (left). The MHC class I molecules meanwhile present antigenic peptides from cytoplasmic proteins that have been transported into the endoplasmic reticulum. These complexes are presented to the TCR on CD8+ CTLs.

Q. Unlike the MHC molecules themselves, their leader peptides are very similar, regardless of the haplotype of the molecules. From this observation, what can you infer about immune recognition, mediated by NK cells?

A. The combination of HLA-E plus leader peptide is similar regardless of the haplotype, therefore the CD94–NKG2 receptor does not need to be highly polymorphic to recognize MHC molecules of different haplotypes. Compare this with antigen presentation by HLA-A and -B and immune recognition by the TCR.

Although CD94 has a lectin domain, the recognition of the HLA-E–peptide occurs via interaction with residues from the peptide and the α1 and α2 domains of the MHC molecule. The lectin domain could, however, reinforce this interaction by binding to carbohydrate associated with the MHC molecule.

KIRs are members of the immunoglobulin superfamily

The second group of NK cell receptors are members of the immunoglobulin superfamily. They fall into two subsets, having either two or three immunoglobulin domains (Fig. 10.5).

Killer immunoglobulin-like receptors

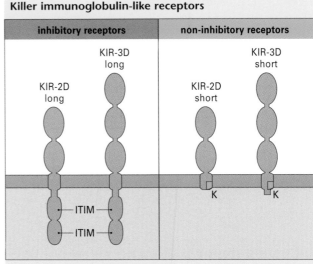

Fig. 10.5 KIRs consist of either two or three extracellular immunoglobulin superfamily domains. The inhibitory forms are longer and have intracellular ITIMs (immunoreceptor tyrosine inhibitory motifs), whereas the non-inhibitory forms have the charged residue in the membrane comparable to the non-inhibitory forms of CD94–NKG2 (see Fig. 10.3).

Thirteen groups of KIRs have been identified encoded in a gene cluster on chromosome 19q13.4. The molecules are highly diverse:

• the two-domain members (KIR-2D) are defined as CD158;
• the three-domain members are KIR-3D.

The nomenclature also indicates whether the variant has a short or long cytoplasmic tail (e.g. KIR-2DL1 for a two-domain variant with a long cytoplasmic tail).

KIRs with short tails are activating, and those with long tails are inhibitory

Two of the two-domain members have been shown to bind to allelic variants of HLA-C, and these isoforms have inhibitory cytoplasmic domains (see below). The specificity of these receptors can:

• partly explain why particular HLA-C allotypes inhibited some NK cells;
• explain why these allotypes produce dominant resistance – if a cell expresses a particular HLA-C allotype, then that is sufficient to inhibit an NK cell that has engaged it.

Interestingly the expression of KIRs varies on individual NK cells. Not all cells express all KIRs, though the total population of NK cells does express all of the KIR genes present in that individual.

Other isoforms of the KIRs have activating domains. These generally engage HLA molecules with a lower affinity than the inhibitory forms, and, like the activating forms of CD40–NKG2, their physiological functions are uncertain.

Immunoglobulin-like transcripts (ILTs) have a wider cell distribution than other NK cell receptors

A third group of receptors is clustered in the same region as the KIRs and have either two or four immunoglobulin-like domains. These receptors, called **immunoglobulin-like transcripts (ILTs)**, have a wider cellular distribution than the other NK cell receptors. Some of these interact with a broad spectrum of MHC molecules, and others with none at all – their functions are therefore still uncertain.

INTERACTIONS WITH NK RECEPTORS DETERMINE NK CELL ACTION
HLA-G inhibits NK cell action against the placenta

An intriguing recent discovery is that the HLA-G molecule, which is expressed only on placental trophoblasts, is a dominant NK cell inhibitor that confers resistance to all types of NK cell (HLA-G is another MHC class Ib molecule). Trophoblast cells are derived from the fetus and invade the maternal circulation as the placenta is established.

Q. What can you say about trophoblast cells with regard to their susceptibility to damage by CTLs?

A. The fetal cells contain paternal MHC genes so are allogeneic in the mother, and one might therefore expect them to be susceptible to destruction by CTLs.

Q. Because trophoblasts are not destroyed by maternal CTLs, what can you predict about their expression of MHC molecules, and what is the consequence of this?

A. *HLA-A* and *HLA-B* genes are downregulated on trophoblasts, and consequently one would expect the cells to become susceptible to damage by NK cells (*HLA-C* is still expressed.) In practice, therefore, *HLA-G* expression is required to protect the placenta from attack by NK cells.

There is some debate as to which of the inhibitory receptors recognize HLA-G. One ligand for HLA-G is ILT-2. The leader peptide of HLA-G can also be presented in complex with HLA-E to CD94. It is possible that HLA-G can also be directly recognized by a KIR (KIR-2DL4).

NK cells use several different receptors to positively identify their targets

NK cells may engage their targets using a variety of receptors, including CD2, CD16, and CD69, and receptors related to those that inhibit cytotoxicity.

The Fc receptor (CD16) binds antibody bound to target cells and mediates ADCC (Fig. 10.6). Historically this was referred to as killer (K) cell activity, but this function may also be performed by several other cell types with Fc receptors, including T cells.

Myeloid cells expressing Fc receptors can also show antibody-dependent cytotoxicity, but probably use different killing mechanisms to those of T cells and NK cells.

K cell activity

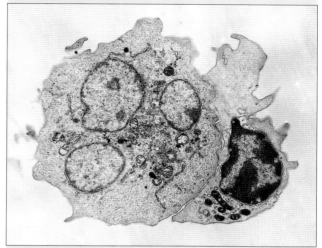

Fig. 10.6 Electron micrograph of a large granular lymphocyte (right) engaging a target cell sensitized with antibody (left). × 2500. (Courtesy of Dr P Penfold)

Potential targets for ADCC include:
* viral antigens on cell surfaces;
* MHC molecules; and
* some epitopes present on tumors.

Therefore monocytes and (according to some controversial reports) polymorphs may also be active against antibody-coated tumor targets. Some myeloid cells (monocytes and eosinophils) are certainly important effectors of damage to antibody-coated schistosomulae (see Chapter 15).

Intracellular signaling pathways coordinate inhibitory and activating signals

The next question is how does an NK cell decide between cytotoxic action or inaction. This decision is thought to depend on the coordination of intracellular signaling pathways, and may involve the balance between activating and inhibitory signals.

Both the lectin-like receptor and the KIRs occur as inhibitory or activating molecules. The key difference is the presence of **immunoreceptor tyrosine inhibitory motifs (ITIMs)**:
* If ITIM motifs become phosphorylated, they can recruit phosphatases, which downregulate the activity of the NK cell (Fig. 10.7).
* In contrast, other KIRs that lack the ITIMs can associate with a molecule (DAP12) which is related to the ζ chain of the TCR complex. DAP12 has **immunoreceptor tyrosine activation motifs (ITAMs)**, which allow it to phosphorylate and recruit tyrosine kinases including ZAP-70 (see Figs 10.7 and 7.21), which lead to cell activation.

At present, it is not known how the balance of activation and inhibition is resolved. In particular it is uncertain how a ligand such as HLA-C will act when it can bind to both inhibitory and activating receptors on the same cell.

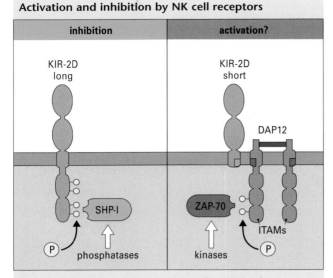

Fig. 10.7 Following phosphorylation of its ITIMs, the inhibitory receptors of NK cells can bind to phosphatases, including SHP-1 and SHP-2, which inhibit killing. The non-inhibitory forms of the receptor associate with a dimeric molecule DAP12, via the complementary charged residues in their membranes. DAP12 has immunoreceptor tyrosine activation motifs (ITAMs). When phosphorylated this recruits kinases of the Syk family or ZAP-70 (see Chapter 7). Whether this leads to NK cell activation or whether it modulates the inhibitory signals is not known.

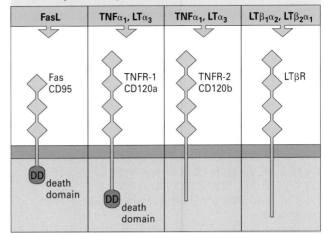

Fig. 10.8 The molecule Fas (CD95), the two TNF receptors, and the lymphotoxin receptor are illustrated. The extracellular domains are similar to those found in the NGF (nerve growth factor) receptor. Both Fas and TNFR-1 have death domains, which are involved in the recruitment of caspases. The ligands for these receptors are indicated at the top. Lymphotoxin-α can form homotrimers or heterotrimers with lymphotoxin-β. Up to 25 other members of these families have been identified by database searching.

CYTOTOXICITY IS EFFECTED BY DIRECT CELLULAR INTERACTIONS, CYTOKINES, AND GRANULE EXOCYTOSIS

CTLs and NK cells use a variety of different mechanisms to kill their targets. These include:

- direct cell–cell signaling via surface molecules; and
- indirect signaling via cytokines.

In addition, CTLs and large granular lymphocytes (NK cells) have granules that contain proteins that damage target cells if they are released directly against the target cell plasma membrane.

Exactly which combination of these three mechanisms is used depends on the CTL involved.

Cytotoxicity may be signaled via Fas or a TNF receptor on a target cell

CTLs signal to their targets using members of the **tumor necrosis factor (TNF)** receptor group of molecules, which include:

- Fas (CD95); and
- the TNF receptors (Fig. 10.8).

Both CD4 and CD8 T cells can initiate cell death via expression of Fas ligand, a member of the TNF family (Fig. 10.9). Fas ligand recognizes the widely expressed cell surface protein Fas. Cross-linking leads to trimerization of Fas and recruitment of FADD to the death domain in the cytoplasmic tail of Fas. FADD recruits caspase 8 or 10, leading to Ca^{2+}-dependent apoptosis.

Activated caspase 8 can cleave and activate other caspases, in addition to its own direct actions in the pathways of apoptosis.

Other members of the TNF receptor family with death domains in their cytoplasmic tails, such as TNFR-1, can also trigger caspase-dependent cell death upon engagement with their ligand by a similar mechanism.

This ability to induce cell death is dependent on the presence of the death domain in the cytoplasmic tail. TNF receptor members lacking the death domain do not mediate caspase-dependent cell death.

Granules of CTLs contain perforin and granzymes

Activated CTL and NK cells contain numerous cytoplasmic granules termed **lytic granules**. Upon recognition of a target cell, these granules polarize to the site of contact, an area referred to as the 'immunological synapse', releasing their contents into a small cleft between the two cells (Fig. 10.10).

The lytic granules contain the pore-forming protein, **perforin**, as well as a series of granule-associated enzymes, **granzymes**, all of which are secreted upon recognition of a target.

Perforin is a monomeric pore-forming protein

Although NK cells and CTLs use different mechanisms to recognize their targets, the lytic mechanisms used to destroy the targets are the same. The key protein is perforin, a monomeric pore-forming protein that is

Mechanisms of cell killing

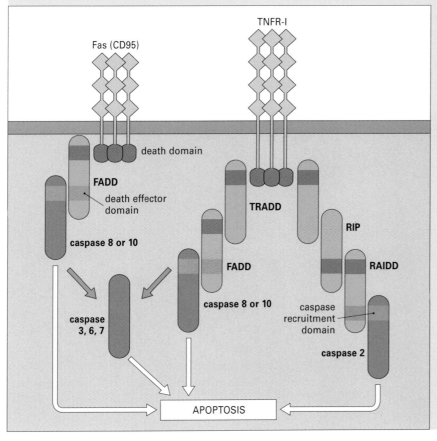

Fig. 10.9 Ligation of CD95 or TNFR-1 causes trimerization of the receptors. Death domains in the cytoplasmic portion of CD95 bind to the adapter protein FADD (MORT1), which recruits caspase 8 or 10. TNFR-1 can activate either caspase 8 or 10, via TRADD and FADD, or caspase 2 via RIP and RAIDD. Caspase 8 can further activate other caspases, and these in concert lead to apoptosis of the target cell.

related both structurally and functionally to the complement component C9 (see Chapter 4).

Q. What function does C9 perform?

A. It polymerizes to form channels across membranes as the final step in the lytic pathway.

Perforin is inactive when located within the granules, but undergoes a conformational activation, which depends on the concentration of Ca^{2+} ions (Fig. 10.11).

Like C9, perforin is able to form homopolymers, inserting into the membrane to form a circular pore of approximately 16 nm in diameter.

Unlike C9, perforin possesses a domain that can bind phospholipid membranes directly in the presence of Ca^{2+} ions.

Perforin-deficient mice show greatly reduced cytotoxicity. The fact that some cytotoxicity remains demonstrates that other mechanisms contribute to CTL and NK cell-mediated death. Some of this residual killing is likely to come from the Fas ligand and TNF pathways.

Granzymes cleave substrates in the target cell, leading to the rapid initiation of apoptosis

Also contained within the lytic granules are the **granzymes**, which are a series of serine proteases that

require perforin to enter the cytoplasm of the target cell (Fig. 10.12). Once in the cytoplasm, granzymes can cleave a number of substrates, leading to the rapid initiation of apoptosis:

- Granzyme B cleaves a number of pro-caspases, leading to the activation of caspases 10, 3, and 7, so triggering apoptosis of the target cell. Granzyme B-deficient mice show delayed but not ablated cytotoxicity, revealing the role of other pathways.
- Another mechanism is provided by granzyme A, which triggers apoptosis via a caspase-independent pathway. Granzyme A acts on one of its substrates, SET (an endoplasmic reticulum-associated protein complex), activating a DNAse, which nicks the DNA and leads to nuclear breakdown.
- Granzyme C also contributes to apoptosis via a caspase-independent pathway, though the details of this pathway are not yet known.

Eleven granzymes have been identified in the mouse and five in humans, though the functions of all of these are not yet known. The large number of granzymes is likely to provide multiple pathways to trigger apoptosis, ensuring that cell death ensues.

In summary, recognition of a target leads to rapid polarization of the lytic granules to the immunological synapse. The contents of the granules are released,

Intracellular reorganizations during effector–target cell interaction

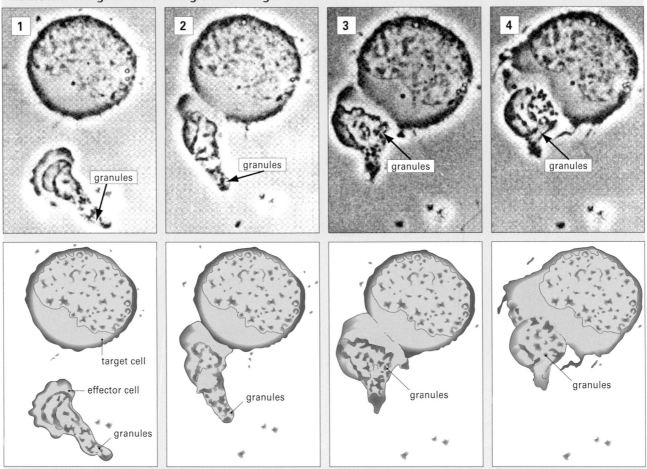

Fig. 10.10 Early events in the interaction of CTLs with specific targets were studied with high-resolution cinematographic techniques. The figure shows four frames (together with interpretative drawings), taken at different times, of a CTL interacting with its target. The location of the granules within the effector cell is indicated in each case. Before contact with the target (**1**), the effector has granules located in a uropod at the rear, and is seen to move randomly by extending pseudopods from the organelle-free, broad, leading edge of the cell. Within 2 minutes of contacting the target (**2**), the CTL has begun to round up and initiate granule reorientation (**3**). After 10 minutes (**4**), the granules occupy a position in the zone of contact with the target, where they appear to be in the process of emptying their contents into the intercellular space between the two cells. (Courtesy of Dr VH Engelhard)

including the pore-forming protein perforin, which allows granzymes to enter the cytoplasm of the target cell and rapidly trigger apoptosis.

CTL and NK cells kill targets without killing themselves

Although CTLs can be killed by other CTLs they do not destroy themselves when they kill another target. A number of mechanisms contribute to this:

- Both perforin and granzymes are synthesized as inactive precursors that need to be activated by removal of a small pro-piece.
- Activation takes place only after perforin and granzymes have been released from the granules, where the pH, Ca^{2+} levels, and the presence of proteoglycans

that bind both perforin and granzymes are thought to keep both perforin and granzymes inactive.

Nevertheless the CTL is still resistant to its own perforin as it releases the granule contents into the immunological synapse. Some recent work has shown that a membrane-bound form of cathepsin B contributes to the CTL resistance to lysis because it lines the granule membranes and cleaves perforin on the CTL side of the synapse.

Additional mechanisms render CTLs more resistant to lysis, for example CTLs express:

- cFLIP, a protein that inhibits the cleavage of caspase 8 and prevents apoptosis triggering via the caspase 8 pathway;
- the serpin, protease inhibitor 8 (PI-8), which can prevent the action of granzyme B.

Perforin undergoes a conformational activation

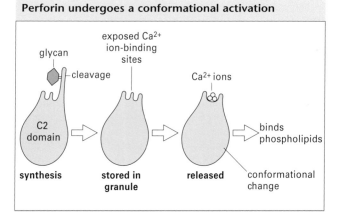

Fig. 10.11 Perforin is synthesized with a tailpiece of 20 amino acid residues with a large glycan residue attached. In this form it is inactive. Cleavage of the tailpiece within the granules allows Ca^{2+} ions to access a site associated with the C2 domain of the molecule, but the molecule is thought to be maintained in an inactive state by low Ca^{2+} concentrations in the granules. Following secretion the increased Ca^{2+} concentration permits a conformational change, which exposes a phospholipid-binding site, allowing the perforin to bind to the target membrane as a precursor to polymerization.

Diseases resulting from a loss of lytic granule proteins

A number of genetic diseases have been identified that result from loss of function of several different effector proteins involved in CTL-mediated killing. Strikingly, these give rise to very different clinical syndromes.

Mutations that cause loss of perforin expression or function give rise to **familial hemophagocytic lympho-histiocytosis**, a disease characterized by massive infil-tration of organs with activated macrophages engulfing lymphocytes.

Q. What effect would you expect lack of perforin to have in affected individuals?
A. CTLs are unable to kill virally infected cells, and it is thought that the associated macrophage infiltration is a consequence of the inability to regulate the response to viral infections.

Loss of Fas ligand expression gives rise to **autoimmune lymphoproliferative syndrome type 2 (ALPS2)**, which results in aberrant lymphoproliferation in affected patients. The gld mouse model also lacks Fas ligand and has a similar pathology. The symptomatology of ALPS2 is very similar to that caused by mutations that result in loss of Fas (ALPS1).

Mutations that prevent activation of granzymes have now been identified. Cathepsin C is required to activate granzymes by proteolytic cleavage. Patients lacking cathepsin C present with **Papillon–Lefèvre syndrome**. This rare condition appears in young children and is characterized by severe inflammation around the teeth and dry scaly skin, which may become infected. Only a small number of the patients show increased susceptibility to infections and, interestingly, do not appear to have an increased susceptibility to viral infections.

MACROPHAGES, NEUTROPHILS, AND EOSINOPHILS ARE NON-LYMPHOID CYTOTOXIC EFFECTORS
Macrophages can damage targets using their non-specific toxic effector systems or via cytokines

A number of non-lymphoid cells may be cytotoxic to other cells or invading microorganisms, such as bacteria or parasites. Cytotoxicity may be triggered specifically to a

Granule-associated killing mechanisms

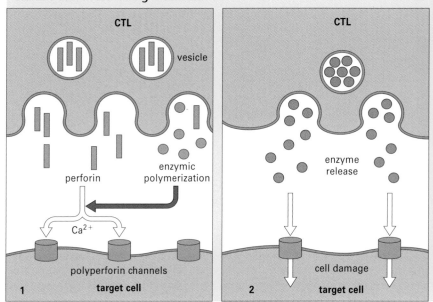

Fig. 10.12 The CTL degranulates, releasing perforin and various enzymes (granzymes) into the immediate vicinity of the target cell membrane. In the presence of Ca^{2+}, perforin binds to the target cell membrane and forms polyperforin channels (**1**). Enzymes that activate the apoptosis pathways, degradative enzymes, and other toxic substances released from the cytotoxic cell may pass through the channels in the target cell membrane and cause cell damage or killing (**2**).

target by ADCC or may involve a range of non-specific toxic mediators. For example, macrophages and neutrophils both express FcγRI and FcγRII which allows them to engage tumors by ADCC.

In general macrophages and neutrophils aim to destroy pathogens by internalizing them and subjecting them to toxic molecules and enzymes within the phagolysosome. These include:
- the production of reactive oxygen intermediates, toxic oxidants, and nitric oxide (Fig. 10.13, see Chapter 9); as well as
- the secreted molecules such as neutrophil defensins, lysosomal enzymes, and cytostatic proteins.

If the phagocyte fails to internalize its target, then these mediators may be released into the extracellular environment and contribute to localized cell damage. This action is referred to as '**frustrated phagocytosis**' and occurs when the target is engaged by surface receptors, but is too large to phagocytose. The actions of the mediators produced by the phagocyte damage the target rather than induce apoptosis. For this reason, the cytotoxic action of phagocytes tends to produce necrosis and inflammation.

Additionally, activated macrophages secrete TNF, which can induce apoptosis in a similar way to NK cells and CTLs. Macrophages can therefore induce necrosis, apoptosis, or a combination of both, depending on the state of activation of the macrophages and the target involved.

Eosinophils mediate cytotoxicity by exocytosis of their granules

Mature eosinophils are characterized by their granules, which have a crystalloid core that binds the dye eosin. Generally, eosinophils are only weakly phagocytic – they ingest some bacteria following activation, but are less efficient than neutrophils at intracellular killing.

The major function of eosinophils appears to be the secretion of various toxic granule constituents following activation. They are therefore effective for the extra-cellular killing of microorganisms, particularly large parasites such as schistosomes (see Chapter 15).

The components of the eosinophil granule include the following:
- Major basic protein (MBP) – not to be confused with myelin basic protein of oligodendrocytes. MBP is the major component of eosinophil granules, forming the crystalloid core, and has been shown to damage, and sometimes kill, parasites, but also damages host tissue cells.
- Eosinophil peroxidase (EPO) – a highly cationic heterodimeric 71–77-kDa hemoprotein that is distinct from the myeloperoxidase of neutrophils and macrophages. In the presence of H_2O_2, also produced by eosinophils, EPO will oxidize a variety of substrates, including halide ions to produce hypohalite, and this may represent the eosinophil's most potent killing mechanism for some parasites.
- Eosinophil cationic protein (ECP) – an eosinophil-specific toxin that is very potent at killing many parasites, particularly the schistosomulae of *Schistosoma mansoni*. The molecule is a ribonuclease, which, because of its high charge, binds avidly to negatively charged surfaces and it is possible that it forms membrane channels, which allow other mediators access to the target organism.

Other molecules produced by eosinophils are lysophospholipase and eosinophil-derived neurotoxin (EDN), which is also a ribonuclease but with strong neurotoxic activity.

Degranulation of eosinophils can be triggered in a number of ways:
- binding to IgG-coated parasites via surface FcγRII triggers the release of some mediators including ECP, but not EPO;
- in contrast triggering via FcεRII leads to the release of EPO, but not ECP.

Parasite killing may involve contact-dependent degranulation or may simply require deposition of toxins within the local tissue.

Degranulation may also be triggered directly in vitro by several cytokines, including:
- interleukin-3 (IL-3);
- IL-5;
- granulocyte–macrophage colony stimulating factor (GM-CSF);
- TNF;
- interferon-β (IFNβ); and
- platelet-activating factor (PAF).

These mediators also enhance ADCC-mediated degranulation.

Eosinophils are prominent in the inflammatory lesion of a number of diseases, particularly atopic disorders of the gut, skin, and respiratory tract, where they are often closely associated with fibrotic reactions. Examples are atopic eczema, asthma, and inflammatory bowel disease.

Although eosinophils may play some regulatory role in these conditions, such as inactivating histamine, their toxic products and cytotoxic mechanisms are a major cause of the tissue damage. For example, in asthma, eosinophil

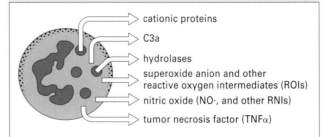

Mechanisms that may contribute to the cytotoxicity of myeloid cells

- cationic proteins
- C3a
- hydrolases
- superoxide anion and other reactive oxygen intermediates (ROIs)
- nitric oxide (NO·, and other RNIs)
- tumor necrosis factor (TNFα)

Fig. 10.13 Reactive oxygen intermediates (ROIs) and reactive nitrogen intermediates (RNIs), cationic proteins, hydrolytic enzymes, and complement proteins released from myeloid cells may damage the target cell in addition to cytokine-mediated attack.

granule proteins are detectable in the blood and lungs following asthmatic attacks. MBP can kill some pneumocytes and tracheal epithelial cells while EPO kills type II pneumocytes. MBP can also induce mast cells to secrete histamine, so exacerbating allergic inflammation.

FURTHER READING

Berke G. The binding and lysis of target cells by cytotoxic lymphocytes. Annu Rev Immunol 1994;12:735.

Bleackle RC, Lobe CG, Duggan B, et al. The isolation of a family of serine protease genes expressed in activated cytotoxic T lymphocytes. Immunol Rev 1988;103:5.

Kagi D, Ledermann B, Burki K, et al. Cytotoxicity mediated by T cells and natural killer cells is greatly impaired in perforin-deficient mice. Nature 1994;369:31–37.

Lanier LL. NK cell recognition. Annu Rev Immunol 2005;23:225–274.

Lee N, Llano M, Carreto M, et al. HLA-E is a major ligand for the natural killer inhibitory receptor CD94/NKG2A. Proc Natl Acad Sci 1998;95:5199–204.

López-Botet M, Bellón T. Natural killer cell activation and inhibition by receptors for MHC class I. Curr Opin Immunol 1999;11:301–307.

Navarro F, Llano M, Bellón T, et al. The ILT2 (LIR-1) and CD94NKG2A cell receptors respectively recognise HLA-G1 and HLA-E molecules on coexpressed targets. Eur J Immunol 1999;29:277–283.

Rathmell JC, Thompson CB. The central effectors of cell death in the immune system. Annu Rev Immunol 1999;17:781–828.

Wallach D, Varfolomeev EE, Malanin NL, et al. Tumor necrosis factor receptors and Fas signalling mechanisms. Annu Rev Immunol 1999;17:331–368.

Watanabe-Fukunga R, Brannan CI, Copeland NG, et al. Lymphoproliferation disorder in mice explained by defects in Fas antigen that mediates apoptosis. Nature 1992;356:314.

Yanelli JR, Sullivan JA, Mandell GL, Engelhard VH. Reorientation and fusion of cytotoxic T cell granules after interaction with target cells as determined by high resolution cinematography. J Immunol 1986;136:377.

Yokoyama WM, Kim S, French AR. The dynamic life of natural killer cells. Annu Rev Immunol 2004;22:405–430.

Critical thinking: Mechanisms of cytotoxicity (see p. 496 for explanations)

Lymphocytes from a normal individual were stimulated in vitro by co-culture with irradiated T lymphoma cells. (Irradiation of these stimulator cells prevents them from dividing in the co-culture.) After 7 days the lymphocytes were harvested and fractionated to obtain a population of cytotoxic cells (CD8+) and a population of NK cells (CD94+, CD16+). These effector cells were set up in a cytotoxicity assay with the tumor cells as targets. The tumor cells were labeled to detect both DNA fragmentation and cell lysis. The results shown in the table were obtained in these assays.

treatment	lysis (%)	DNA fragmentation (%)
no effector cells	4	1
CD8+ CTLs	82	80
NK cells	12	11
anti-tumor cell antibody	5	1
NK cells + anti-tumor cell antibody	28	28
purified perforin	95	2

1 Why do CTLs lyze the targets and induce DNA fragmentation? What are these cells recognizing on the tumor cell surface?

2 Why might the NK cells cause some damage to the tumor? Why does the presence of antibody to the tumor enhance the cytotoxic capacity of the NK cells?

3 Explain the result with purified perforin.

Regulation of the Immune Response

CHAPTER 11

SUMMARY

- **Many factors govern the outcome of any immune response.** These include the antigen itself, its dose and route of administration, and the genetic background of the individual responding to antigenic challenge. A variety of control mechanisms serve to restore the immune system to a resting state when the response to a given antigen is no longer required.

- **The APC may affect the immune response** through its ability to provide co-stimulation to T cells. Different types of APC promote different modes of immune response.

- **Immunoglobulins can influence the immune response,** positively as an anti-idiotype or through immune complex formation. They may also negatively influence immune responses by reducing antigenic challenge or by feedback inhibition of B cells.

- **T cells regulate the immune response.** Cytokine production by T cells influences the type of immune response elicited by antigen. CD4$^+$ T cells can deviate immune responses to TH1- or TH2-type responses. Regulatory T cells may belong to the CD4 or CD8 subpopulations. They can inhibit responses by the production of suppressive cytokines such as IL-10 and TGFβ.

- **Senescence of cells is regulated by telomere erosion.** Upregulation of telomerase by cells during an immune response compensates for telomere shortening caused by cell division.

- **Selective migration of lymphocyte subsets to different sites can modulate the local type of immune response** because TH1 cells and TH2 cells respond to different sets of chemokines.

- **The neuroendocrine system influences immune responses.** Corticosteroids in particular downregulate TH1 responses and macrophage activation.

- **Genetic factors influence the immune system and include both MHC-linked and non-MHC-linked genes.** They affect the level of immune response and susceptibility to infection.

MANY FACTORS GOVERN THE OUTCOME OF ANY IMMUNE RESPONSE

The immune response, like all biological systems, is subject to a variety of control mechanisms. These mechanisms restore the immune system to a resting state when responsiveness to a given antigen is no longer required.

An effective immune response is an outcome of the interplay between antigen and a network of immunologically competent cells.

The nature of the immune response, both qualitatively and quantitatively, is determined by many factors, including:
- the form and route of administration of the antigen;
- the antigen-presenting cell (APC);
- the genetic background of the individual; and
- any history of previous exposure to the antigen in question or to a cross-reacting antigen.

Specific antibodies may also modulate the immune response to an antigen.

T cells and B cells are triggered by antigen after effective engagement of their antigen-specific receptors together with appropriate co-stimulation. In the case of the T cell, this engagement is not with antigen itself, but with processed antigenic peptide bound to MHC class I or class II molecules on APCs (see Chapter 7).

The nature of an antigen, the dose, and the route of administration have all been shown to have a profound influence on the outcome of an immune response. An effective immune response removes antigen from the system.

Repeated antigen exposure is required to maintain T and B cell proliferation, and during an effective immune response there is often a dramatic expansion of specifically reactive effector cells.

At the end of an immune response reduced antigen exposure results in a reduced expression of IL-2 and its receptor leading to **apoptosis** (or programmed cell death, see Chapter 10) of the antigen-specific T cells. The majority of antigen-specific cells therefore die at the end of an immune response leaving a minor population of long-lived T and B cells to survive and give rise to the memory population.

Q. What process leads to the inactivation of T cells and loss of the IL-2 receptor?
A. Ligation of CTLA-4, the alternative receptor for the co-stimulatory molecule B7 (see Fig. 7.18).

Different antigens elicit different kinds of immune response

Intracellular organisms such as some bacteria, parasites, or viruses induce a cell-mediated immune response. Cell-mediated immune responses are also induced by agents such as silica.

In contrast extracellular organisms and soluble antigens induce a humoral response, with the polysaccharide capsule antigens of bacteria generally inducing IgM responses.

In some situations, antigens (e.g. those of intracellular microorganisms) may not be cleared effectively leading to a sustained immune response. This has pathological consequences for autoimmunity and hypersensitivity (see Chapters 20 and 23–26).

Large doses of antigen can induce tolerance

Very large doses of antigen often result in specific T and sometimes B cell tolerance.

Administration of antigen to neonatal mice often results in tolerance to the antigen. It was speculated that this might be the result of immaturity of the immune system. However, more recent studies have shown that neonatal mice can develop efficient immune responses (Fig. 11.1) and that non-responsiveness may in some cases be attributable, not to the immaturity of T cells, but to immune deviation. In this case a non-protective TH2-type cytokine response would dominate a protective TH1-type cytokine response.

T-independent polysaccharide antigens have been shown to generate tolerance in B cells after administration in high doses. Tolerance and its underlying mechanisms are discussed in Chapter 19.

Effect of antigen dose on the outcome of the immune response to murine leukemia virus

virus (pfu)	antiviral cytotoxicity	TH1 response (IFNγ)	TH2 response (IL-4)
0.3	+++		
1000	+		
		80 60 40 20 0 20 40 60 80	

Fig. 11.1 Newborn mice were infected with either 0.3 or 1000 plaque-forming units (pfu) of virus and the CTL response against virally infected targets was assessed together with the production of interferon-γ (IFNγ – a helper T cell type 1 [TH1] cytokine) or interleukin-4 (IL-4 – a TH2 cytokine) in response to viral challenge. Mice infected with a low dose of virus make a TH1-type response and are protected. The results are presented as arbitrary units.

Antigen route of administration can determine whether an immune response occurs

The route of administration of antigen has been shown to influence the immune response:
- antigens administered subcutaneously or intradermally evoke an active immune response; whereas
- antigens given intravenously, orally, or as an aerosol may cause tolerance or an immune deviation from one type of CD4+ T cell response to another.

For example, rodents that have been fed ovalbumin or myelin basic protein (MBP) do not respond effectively to a subsequent challenge with the corresponding antigen. Moreover, in the case of MBP, the animals are protected from the development of the autoimmune disease experimental allergic encephalomyelitis (EAE).

Q. Considering the type of immune responses generated in mucosal tissues why might oral administration of antigen deviate the immune response, and in what way?
A. Mucosal tissues have high levels of antibody-producing B cells. Consequently antigens that first encounter the immune system at these sites may be presented by B cells, which tend to induce TH2-type responses.

This phenomenon may have some therapeutic value in allergy. Recent studies have shown that oral administration of a T cell epitope of the Der p1 allergen of house dust mite (*Dermatophagoides pteronyssimus*) could tolerize to the whole antigen. The potential mechanisms of such tolerance induction include anergy, immune deviation, and the generation of regulatory T cells that act through the production of cytokines such as TGFβ and IL-10.

Similar observations have been made when antigen is given as an aerosol. Studies in mice have shown that aerosol administration of an encephalitogenic peptide inhibits the development of experimental allergic encephalomyelitis (EAE) that would normally be induced by a conventional (subcutaneous) administration of the peptide (Fig. 11.2). This may also have therapeutic implications because the inhibition of the response is not limited to the antigen administered as an aerosol, but also includes other antigens capable of inducing EAE, such as proteolipid protein.

A clear example of how different routes of administration affect the outcome of the immune response is provided by studies of infection with lymphocytic choriomeningitis virus (LCMV). Mice primed subcutaneously with peptide in incomplete Freund's adjuvant develop immunity to LCMV. However, if the same peptide is repeatedly injected intraperitoneally the animal becomes tolerized and cannot clear the virus (Fig. 11.3).

THE APC MAY AFFECT THE IMMUNE RESPONSE

The nature of the APC initially presenting the antigen may determine whether immune responsiveness or tolerance ensues.

Effective activation of T cells requires the expression of co-stimulatory molecules on the surface of the APC. Therefore presentation by dendritic cells or activated

Aerosol administration of antigen modifies the immune response

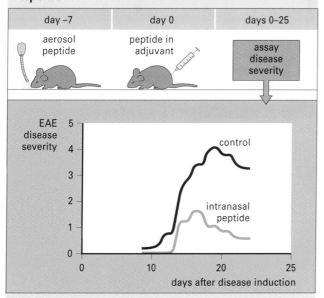

Fig. 11.2 Mice were treated with a single aerosol dose of either 100 µg peptide (residues 1–11 of MBP) or just the carrier. Seven days later the same peptide, this time in adjuvant, was administered subcutaneously. The subsequent development of experimental allergic encephalomyelitis (EAE) was significantly modified in pretreated animals.

Peptide-induced inactivation of LCMV-specific T cells

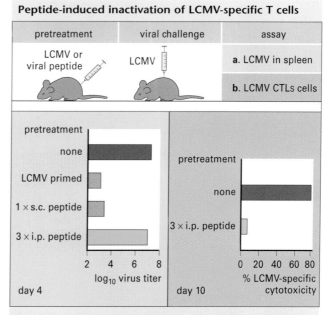

Fig. 11.3 Mice were either primed with LCMV or injected with 100 mg LCMV peptide. The peptide was given either subcutaneously (s.c.) or three times intraperitoneally (i.p.) with incomplete Freund's adjuvant. The animals were later infected with LCMV (day 0). The titer of virus in the spleen was measured on day 4. Animals that had been pretreated with subcutaneous peptide or with LCMV developed neutralizing antibody and protective immunity against the virus; animals pretreated with peptide i.p. did not develop immunity. Cytotoxic T lymphocyte (CTL) activity was assessed in the mice on day 10. Mice that had received no pretreatment demonstrated CTLs specific for the LCMV peptide. Mice pretreated with peptide i.p. failed to show such activity.

macrophages that express high levels of MHC class II molecules in addition to co-stimulatory molecules results in highly effective T cell activation (see Fig. 7.18).

Furthermore, the interaction of CD40L on activated T cells with CD40 on dendritic cells is important for the high-level production of IL-12 necessary for the generation of an effective TH1 response.

If antigen is presented to T cells by a 'non-professional' APC that is unable to provide co-stimulation, unresponsiveness or immune deviation results. For example, when naive T cells are exposed to antigen by resting B cells they fail to respond and become tolerized. Recent experimental observations illustrate this point.

Neonatal animals are more susceptible to tolerance induction. Therefore mice administered MBP in incomplete Freund's adjuvant during the neonatal period are resistant to the induction of EAE. This is due to the development of a dominant TH2 response (see Fig. 11.1). The prior TH2 response to MBP prevents the development of the TH1 pathological response, which mediates EAE.

Adjuvants may facilitate immune responses by inducing the expression of high levels of MHC and co-stimulatory molecules on APCs. Furthermore, their ability to activate Langerhans' cells leads to the migration of these skin dendritic cells to the local draining lymph nodes where effective T cell activation can occur.

The importance of dendritic cells in initiating a cytotoxic T lymphocyte (CTL) response is illustrated by experiments showing that newborn female mice injected with male spleen cells fail to develop a CTL response to the male antigen, H-Y. However if male dendritic cells are injected into female newborn mice, a good H-Y-specific CTL response develops.

IMMUNOGLOBULINS CAN INFLUENCE THE IMMUNE RESPONSE

Antibody has been shown to exert feedback control on the immune response.

Passive administration of IgM antibody together with an antigen specifically enhances the immune response to that antigen, whereas IgG antibody suppresses the response. This was originally shown with polyclonal antibodies, but has since been confirmed using monoclonal antibodies (Fig. 11.4).

The ability of passively administered antibody to enhance or suppress the immune response has certain clinical consequences and applications:

• certain vaccines (e.g. mumps and measles) are not generally given to infants before 1 year of age because levels of maternally derived IgG remain high for at least

Feedback control by antibody

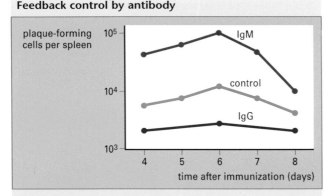

Fig. 11.4 Mice received either a monoclonal IgM anti-SRBC (sheep red blood cells), IgG anti-SRBC, or medium alone (control). Two hours later all groups were immunized with SRBC. The antibody response measured over the following 8 days was enhanced by IgM and suppressed by IgG.

Antibody-dependent B cell suppression

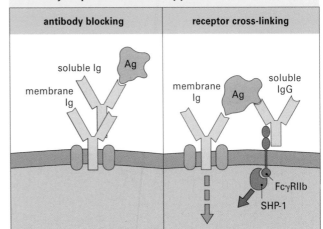

Fig. 11.5 Antibody blocking – high doses of soluble immunoglobulin (Ig) block the interaction between an antigenic determinant (epitope) and membrane immunoglobulin on B cells. The B cell is then effectively unable to recognize the antigen. This receptor-blocking mechanism also prevents B cell priming, but only antibodies that bind to the same epitope to which the B cell's receptors bind can do this. Receptor cross-linking – low doses of antibody allow cross-linking by antigen of a B cell's Fc receptors and its antigen receptors. The FcγRIIb receptor associates with a tyrosine phosphatase (SHP-1), which interferes with cell activation by tyrosine kinases associated with the antigen receptor. This allows B cell priming, but inhibits antibody synthesis. Antibodies against different epitopes on the antigen can all act by this mechanism.

6 months after birth and the presence of such passively acquired IgG at the time of vaccination would result in the development of an inadequate immune response in the baby;

- in cases of Rhesus (Rh) incompatibility, the administration of anti-RhD antibody to Rh⁻ mothers prevents primary sensitization by fetally derived Rh⁺ blood cells, presumably by removing the foreign antigen (fetal erythrocytes) from the maternal circulation (see Chapters 24 and 25).

The mechanisms by which antibody modulates the immune response are not completely defined. In the case of IgM-enhancing plaque-forming cells, there are thought to be two possible interpretations:

- IgM-containing immune complexes are taken up by Fc or C3 receptors on APCs and are processed more efficiently than antigen alone;
- IgM-containing immune complexes stimulate an **anti-idiotypic response** to the IgM, which amplifies the immune response.

IgG antibody can suppress specific IgG synthesis

For IgG-mediated suppression there are also various ways in which the antibody is known to act.

Passively administered antibody binds antigen in competition with B cells (antibody blocking)

The impact of the IgG in antibody blocking (Fig. 11.5) in this case is highly dependent on the concentration of the antibody, and on its affinity for the antigen compared with the affinity of the B cell receptors. Only high-affinity B cells compete successfully for the antigen. This mechanism is independent of the Fc portion of the antibody.

Immunoglobulin can inhibit B cell differentiation by cross-linking (receptor cross-linking)

IgG antibody is also known to have an effect that is Fc dependent. Immunoglobulin can inhibit B cell differen-

tiation by cross-linking the antigen receptor with the Fc receptor (FcγRIIb) on the same cell (see Fig. 11.5). In this case, the antibodies may recognize different epitopes.

Increasing average antibody affinity

Doses of IgG that are insufficient to inhibit the production of antibodies completely have the effect of increasing the average antibody affinity because only those B cells with high-affinity receptors can successfully compete with the passively acquired antibody for antigen. For this reason, antibody feedback is believed to be an important factor driving the process of **affinity maturation** (Fig. 11.6).

Immune complexes may enhance or suppress immune responses

One of the ways in which antibody (either IgM or IgG) might act to modulate the immune response involves an Fc-dependent mechanism and immune complex formation with antigen.

Immune complexes can inhibit or augment the immune response (Fig. 11.7). By activating complement, immune complexes may become localized via interactions with CR2 on follicular dendritic cells (FDCs). This could facilitate the immune response by maintaining a source of antigen.

Antibody feedback on affinity maturation

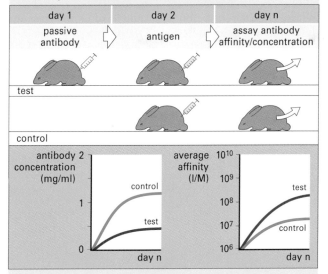

Fig. 11.6 The effect of passive antibody on the affinity and concentration of secreted antibody. One of two rabbits was injected with antibody (passive antibody) on day 1. Both rabbits were immunized with antigen on day 2 and the affinity and concentration of antibody raised to this antigen were assayed at a later time (day n). The antibody assay results show that passive antibody reduces the concentration, but increases the affinity of antibody produced.

Q. How does the presence of antigen on FDCs facilitate the immune response?

A. The antigen is available for uptake by B cells and presentation to T cells within the follicle, a process required for **class switching** and affinity maturation (see Fig. 8.12).

CR2 is also expressed on B cells and, as co-ligation of CR2 with membrane IgM has been shown to activate B cells, immune complex interaction with CR2 of the B cell–co-receptor complex and membrane Ig might lead to an enhanced specific immune response.

The immune response of patients with malignant tumors is often depressed, and it has been postulated that this is the result of the presence of circulating immune complexes composed of antibody and tumor cell antigens.

Idiotypic interactions may enhance or suppress antibody responses

Individual T cell receptors (TCRs) and immunoglobulins are immunogenic by virtue of unique sequences within their variable regions known as **idiotypes**. Antibodies formed against these antigen-binding sites are called **anti-idiotypic antibodies**, and are capable of influencing the outcome of an immune response.

Idiotypic determinants may be:
• encoded in the germline V region genes; or
• generated by the process of recombination and mutation involved in producing functional V region elements (see Chapter 5).

Regulatory effects of immune complexes

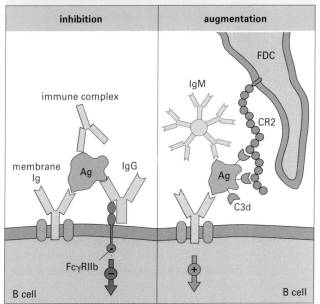

Fig. 11.7 Immune complexes can act either to inhibit or to augment an immune response. Inhibition – when the Fc receptor of the B cell is cross-linked to its antigen receptor by an antigen–antibody complex, a signal is delivered to the B cell, inhibiting it from entering the antibody production phase. Passive IgG may have this effect. Augmentation – antibody encourages presentation of antigen to B cells when it is present on an APC, bound via Fc receptors or, in this case, complement receptors (CR2) on a follicular dendritic cell (FDC). Passive IgM may have this effect.

Immunogenic epitopes in or around the binding site are termed **idiotopes** (Fig. 11.8).

Jerne proposed that an immune network existed within the body that interacted by means of idiotype recognition. According to this proposition, when an antibody response is induced by antigen, this antibody will in turn evoke an anti-idiotypic response to itself. This hypothesis is conceptually interesting, but the role of such an idiotype network in controlling a normal immune response remains unclear.

There is good evidence that anti-idiotypes can affect the representation of recognized idiotypes in an immune response. For example, when strain C57Bl/6 mice are challenged with the hapten nitrophenyl (NP), they produce antibodies that are largely restricted to a few defined idiotypes. The anti-idiotype 146 can enhance or suppress the production of idiotype 146 when the mice are subsequently challenged with NP on a carrier protein. The observed effect depends on the amount of anti-idiotype given and is idiotype specific; the overall level of anti-NP antibody is hardly affected. Most importantly, the amounts of anti-idiotype used are within the normal physiological range for particular idiotype-bearing antibodies, which suggests that idiotypic regulation may occur in vivo.

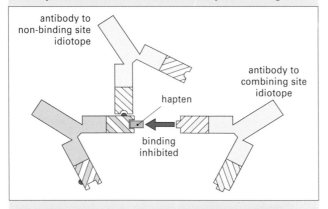

Idiotopes associated with the antibody-combining site

antibody to
non-binding site
idiotope

antibody to
combining site
idiotope

hapten

binding
inhibited

Fig. 11.8 An anti-idiotype serum may contain antibodies directed to various sites on the immunoglobulin molecule. The sites associated with the combining site are site-associated idiotopes. Binding to these can be inhibited by hapten. Antibodies to non-binding site idiotopes (non-site associated) are not inhibited by hapten.

T CELLS REGULATE THE IMMUNE RESPONSE

Cytokines are part of an extracellular signaling network that controls every function of the innate and adaptive immune system and have:

- numerous effects on cell phenotypes; and
- the ability to regulate the type of immune response generated and its extent.

Differentiation into CD4⁺ TH subsets is an important step in selecting effector functions

A single TH cell precursor is able to differentiate into either a TH1 or a TH2 phenotype. The TH1/TH2 decision is crucial to the effective immunity and it is likely that many factors contribute to that decision. Factors that may influence the differentiation of TH cells include:

- the sites of antigen presentation;
- co-stimulatory molecules involved in cognate cellular interactions;
- peptide density and binding affinity – high MHC class II peptide density favors TH1, low densities favor TH2;
- APCs and the cytokines they produce;
- the cytokine profile and balance of cytokines evoked by antigen;
- activity of co-stimulatory molecules and hormones present in the local environment;
- host genetic background.

The cytokine balance is one of the major stimuli.

IL-12 is a potent initial stimulus for IFNγ production by T cells and natural killer (NK) cells and therefore regulates TH1 differentiation.

IFNα, a cytokine produced early during viral infection, induces IL-12 and can also switch cells from a TH2 to a TH1 profile.

By contrast, early production of IL-4 favors the generation of TH2 cells.

If polarizing signals are not present, CD4⁺ TH0 cells have a less differentiated cytokine profile and represent a heterogeneous population with individual clones that can differentiate along the TH1 or TH2 pathway.

Cytokines from TH1 cells inhibit the actions of TH2 cells and vice versa. Thus, cross-regulation of TH subsets has been demonstrated whereby IFNγ secreted by TH1 cells can inhibit the responsiveness of TH2 cells (Fig. 11.9) whereas IL-10 produced by TH2 cells downregulates B7 and IL-12 expression by APCs, which in turn inhibits TH1 activation.

The TH1/TH2 balance is modulated not only by the level of expression of IL-12, but also by expression of the IL-12 receptor (IL-12R). The high-affinity IL-12R is composed of two chains, β1 and β2, with both chains being expressed only in TH1 cells. Both TH1 and TH2 cells express the β1 chain, but expression of the β2 chain is induced by IFNγ and inhibited by IL-4 (Fig. 11.10).

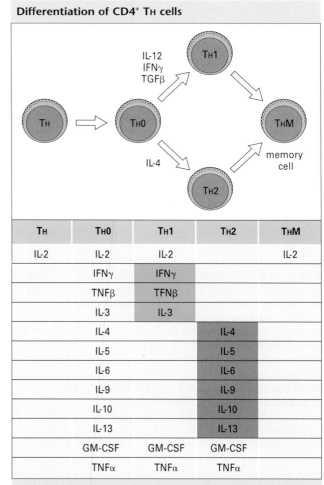

Differentiation of CD4⁺ TH cells

TH	TH0	TH1	TH2	THM
IL-2	IL-2	IL-2		IL-2
	IFNγ	IFNγ		
	TNFβ	TFNβ		
	IL-3	IL-3		
	IL-4		IL-4	
	IL-5		IL-5	
	IL-6		IL-6	
	IL-9		IL-9	
	IL-10		IL-10	
	IL-13		IL-13	
	GM-CSF	GM-CSF	GM-CSF	
	TNFα	TNFα	TNFα	

Fig. 11.9 The diagram illustrates the differentiation of murine TH cells. IL-12, IFNγ, and transforming growth factor-β (TGFβ) favor differentiation of TH1 cells, and IL-4 favors differentiation of TH2 cells. (GM-CSF, granulocyte–macrophage colony stimulating factor; TNF, tumor necrosis factor)

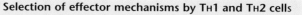

Regulation of the TH1 response by IL-12

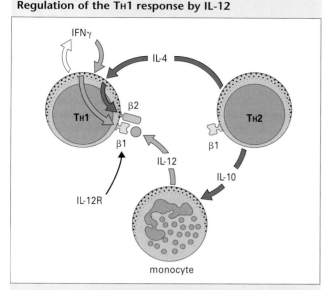

Fig. 11.10 The high-affinity IL-12R consisting of the β1 and β2 chains is expressed only on TH1 cells. IL-12 released by mononuclear phagocytes promotes the development and activation of TH1 cells, but IL-12 production is inhibited by IL-10 released by TH2 cells. IFNγ from TH1 cells promotes production of the β1 chain and therefore production of the high-affinity IL-12R. However, this is inhibited by IL-4.

Selection of effector mechanisms by TH1 and TH2 cells

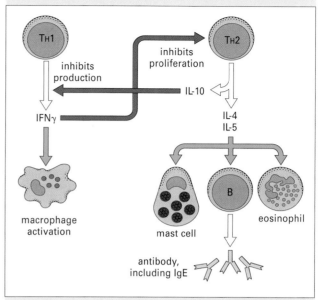

Fig. 11.11 The cytokine patterns of TH1 and TH2 cells drive different effector pathways. TH1 cells activate macrophages and are involved in antiviral and inflammatory responses. TH2 cells are involved in humoral responses and allergy.

An immune response therefore tends to settle into a TH1 or TH2 type of response.

Immune responses are not always strongly polarized in this way and the phenomenon works more closely in mice than humans.

TH1 and TH2 cells are best considered as extremes on a scale, but TH1 and TH2 responses do play different protective roles and may contribute to immunopathology.

Q. Apart from the cross-regulation by cytokines described above, in what other ways can a TH1-type or TH2-type immune response reinforce itself?

A. The chemokines induced by TH1 and TH2 cells tend to induce the accumulation of the same sets of lymphocytes and their associated effector cells (see Chapter 6).

TH cell subsets determine the type of immune response

It is clear that:
- local patterns of cytokine and hormone expression help to select lymphocyte effector mechanism; and
- the polarized responses of CD4⁺ TH cells seem to be based on their profile of cytokine secretion (Fig. 11.11).

Q. In what way do cytokines that are normally associated with TH1 responses (IFNγ, IL-2) affect B cell differentiation?

A. IL-2 promotes B cell division. IFNγ promotes affinity maturation and class switching to IgG2a (see Chapter 8, Figs 8.9 and 8.10) which acts as an opsonin and fixes complement.

TH1 cytokines including IFNγ, TNFβ, and IL-2 (see Fig. 11.9) also promote:
- macrophage activation;
- antibody-dependent cell-mediated cytotoxicity; and
- delayed-type hypersensitivity.

TH2 clones are typified by production of IL-4 and IL-5, with IL-6, IL-9, IL-10, and IL-13 also commonly produced (see Fig. 11.9). These cells provide optimal help for humoral immune responses biased towards:
- IgG1 and IgE isotype switching;
- mucosal immunity;
- stimulation of mast cell and eosinophil growth and differentiation; and
- IgA synthesis.

Therefore, in essence, TH1 cells are associated with cell-mediated inflammatory reactions and TH2 cells are associated with strong antibody and allergic responses.

CD8⁺ T cells can be divided into subsets on the basis of cytokine expression

Many CD8⁺ CTLs make a spectrum of cytokines similar to TH1 cells and are termed CTL1 cells. CD8⁺ cells that make TH2-associated cytokines are associated with regulatory functions. The differentiation of these cells may be affected by the CD4⁺ cell cytokine profile, with CTLs commonly associated with TH1 responses and less commonly found when TH2 cells are present. Thus:
- IFNγ and IL-12 may encourage CTL1 generation; and
- IL-4 may encourage CTL2 generation.

However, both CTL1 and CTL2 cells can be cytotoxic and kill mainly by a Ca²⁺/perforin-dependent mechanism (see Figs 10.11 and 10.12).

CD4⁺ Tregs can be derived in two ways

Although T cells modulate the immune response in a positive sense by providing T cell help, which may favor either cell-mediated (TH1) or humoral (TH2) immunity as discussed above, T cells are also capable of down-regulating immune responses, and both CD4⁺ and CD8⁺ T cell subsets can induce this inhibition.

A naturally occurring population of CD4⁺CD25⁺ regulatory T cells (Tregs) is generated in the thymus. Additionally, CD4⁺ Tregs can be induced from non-regulatory T cells in the periphery. These induced Tregs are a heterogeneous population of cells with a regulatory function.

Although Tregs do not prevent initial T cell activation, they inhibit a sustained response and prevent chronic and potentially damaging immunopathology.

The generation and mechanisms of suppression by the different CD4⁺ Treg populations vary, but:

- both populations are anergic (non-responsive) in vitro;
- neither have characteristics of TH1 or TH2 CD4⁺ cells; and
- they both inhibit cellular responses.

The characteristics of both cell types are compared in Fig. 11.12.

CD4⁺CD25⁺ Tregs are naturally occurring

The immunosuppressive functions of CD4⁺ cells were initially observed by adoptively transferring T cells depleted of CD25⁺ cells into immunodeficient mice. This resulted in multiorgan autoimmunity suggesting that CD25⁺ cells play an important role in preventing self-reactivity. When the CD25⁺ T cells were replaced, autoimmune disease was prevented.

CD4⁺CD25⁺ Tregs constitute 5–10% of peripheral CD4⁺ cells in both mice and humans. The presence of these cells in cord blood suggests that they have a thymic origin. In support of this notion, CD4⁺CD8⁻CD25⁺ cells from the thymus can suppress T cell proliferation, suggesting that they are a naturally occurring, distinct lineage of cells.

Q. What function does CD25 serve on developing thymocytes and on activated T cells?

A. It is part of the IL-2R (see Chapter 7 and Fig. 7.23), which is required for cell proliferation.

Naturally occurring CD4⁺CD25⁺ Tregs are educated in the thymus during the negative selection phase and then exit the thymus as a regulatory population.

Comparison of CD4⁺CD25⁺ Tregs with naive and activated CD4⁺ T cells shows that regulatory cells selectively express **Foxp3**, a member of the forkhead/winged helix transcription factors (Fig. 11.13) essential for the development and function of CD4⁺CD25⁺ Tregs. Mutations in the *Foxp3* gene cause immune dysregulation, polyendocrinopathy enteropathy, X-linked syndrome (IPEX). Individuals with this disease have increased autoimmune and inflammatory diseases.

The importance of Foxp3 in the development of CD4⁺CD25⁺ Tregs was underlined following transduction of Foxp3 into naive T cells (which do not express Foxp3). This increased expression of CD25 and induced suppressor function.

The study of CD4⁺CD25⁺ Tregs has been difficult because of problems in separating these cells from activated T cells, which also express CD25.

Comparison of CD4⁺ regulatory T cells

CD4⁺ CD25⁺ Treg	Tr1/TH3
differences	
generated in the thymus	generated in the periphery
express Foxp3	variable expression of Foxp3
CD25 high, CD45R low	CD45R0 high, CD45RB low variable CD25 expression
cell contact dependent	cell contact independent
require IL-2 for suppression	IL-2-independent suppression
similarities	
triggered by specific antigen	triggered by specific antigen
secrete IL-10/TGFβ	secrete IL-10/TGFβ
unresponsive to anti-CD3 in vitro	unresponsive to anti-CD3 in vitro

Fig. 11.12 This table outlines the similarities and differences in generation and function of the subsets of naturally occurring thymic and peripherally induced CD4⁺ regulatory T cells.

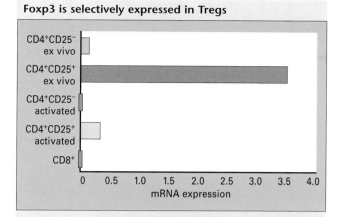

Fig 11.13 Cell populations were collected and real-time polymerase chain reaction (PCR) was performed to assess levels of Foxp3. Foxp3 mRNA is expressed selectively in CD4+CD25+ cells ex vivo. It was expressed at low levels in activated CD4+CD25+ cells and was not present in CD25− cells or CD8+ cells. (Adapted from Fontenot JD, Gavin MA, Rudensky AY. Nat Immunol 2003;4:330–336)

The expression of a number of cell surface molecules on CD4+CD25+ Tregs has been examined and include:
- CTLA-4;
- CD45RB (which is weakly expressed on CD4+CD25+ cells); and
- GITR (glucocorticoid-induced TNF-related receptor).

However, none of these cell surface molecules exclusively identifies the naturally occurring Treg cell population, and CTLA-4, for example, is expressed in both activated T cells and Tregs.

Thymic-derived CD4+CD25+ Tregs work in a cell contact-dependent manner

Naturally occurring CD4+CD25+ Tregs respond to numerous environmental stimuli.

IL-2 is required for suppression, suggesting that CD25 (the IL-2Rα chain, see Fig. 7.23) has a functional role in these cells.

CD4+CD25+ Treg-induced suppression in vitro is cell contact dependent. It is thought that the GITR might be involved in this interaction, but the exact nature is not known.

Induced CD4+ regulatory T cells can be generated following exposure to antigen

In addition to naturally occurring CD4+CD25+ Tregs, which are generated in the thymus, some populations of CD4+ regulatory T cells can be induced to develop in the periphery. Thymectomized mice are able to generate regulatory cells, therefore there must be a thymic-independent induction of these cells in the periphery. For example they arise:
- following allograft transplantation; and
- after oral administration of antigen.

CD4+ regulatory T cells can also be generated from antigen-experienced cells in the presence of certain cytokines. Upon stimulation with IL-10, antigen-experienced cells can differentiate into **Tr1 cells** – these cells do not express CD25 or Foxp3 and they mediate suppression through the secretion of IL-10.

Alternatively, if induced CD4+ regulatory T cells are generated in the presence of TGFβ, they express Foxp3 and upregulate expression of CD25. These induced regulatory cells mediate suppression via production of TGFβ (Fig. 11.14).

Although induced CD4+CD25+ Tregs have an overlapping phenotype with thymus-derived CD4+CD25+ Tregs, they are a different population of cells and have different mechanisms for inducing suppression.

The role of CD4+ Tregs in infections is not clear

Although CD4+ Tregs play a vital role in the prevention of autoimmune diseases (see Chapter 20), their role in infections is less clear.

CD4+ Tregs have a protective role against immune-mediated pathology and their ability to suppress both TH1 and TH2 responses is important in reducing inflammation. For example, lesions in the eye in stromal keratitis are less severe in the presence of CD4+CD25+ Tregs.

CD4+ Tregs can also suppress virus-specific responses. Many pathogens induce high levels of IL-10 and TGFβ, which promote the induction of CD4+CD25+ Tregs. In chronic viral infections, including HIV, cytomegalovirus

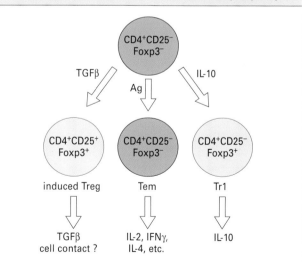

Fig 11.14 CD4+CD25− cells in the periphery can be stimulated to become suppressive. If TGFβ is present cells upregulate Foxp3 and CD25. In the presence of IL-10 cells become suppressive, but they do not express Foxp3 or CD25. Induced Tregs suppress via cytokine-dependent mechanisms. In the presence of antigen and co-stimulation, effector T cells are generated. (Tem, T effector memory cells)

(CMV), and herpes simplex virus (HSV) infections, increased numbers of Tregs are responsible for decreased antigen-specific responses by CD4$^+$ and CD8$^+$ T cells. This can lead to disease development.

CD8$^+$ T cells negatively regulate secondary immune responses

CD8$^+$ cells can be induced to become suppressive.

CD8$^+$ Tregs are generated in vitro by stimulating highly differentiated CD8$^+$ cells with antigen and IL-10. Like CD4$^+$CD25$^+$ cells, CD8$^+$ Tregs express the forkhead protein Foxp3.

Many CD8$^+$ Tregs work in a cell contact-dependent manner. They cause the downregulation of co-stimulatory molecules on dendritic cells and endothelial cells. This induces tolerance because upon the interaction with the TCR and peptide there is insufficient co-stimulation to generate a functional immune response.

In mice the MHC class Ib molecule, Qa-1, is crucial for suppression. Mice lacking Qa-1 are unable to suppress responses. However when Qa-1 is replaced into these cells their ability to suppress immune responses is restored (Fig. 11.15).

CD8$^+$ Tregs:
- need to be primed by CD4$^+$ cells during a primary response; they then suppress secondary immune responses;
- can downregulate both TH1 and TH2 responses and also control CD4$^+$ responses to superantigen;
- can suppress immune responses through the secretion of cytokines including IFNγ, IL-6, and IL-10.

NK cells produce immunoregulatory cytokines and chemokines

NK cells make cytokines and chemokines and therefore play an important role in the innate immune response to infections and tumors.

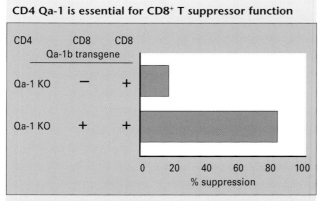

CD4 Qa-1 is essential for CD8$^+$ T suppressor function

Fig. 11.15 Qa-1 knockout (KO) mice were generated. Qa-1 KO CD4$^+$ cells were mixed with CD8$^+$ cells and the level of suppression was assessed. CD8$^+$ cells could not suppress CD4 cells lacking Qa-1 expression. Insertion of the Qa-1b allele into CD4$^+$ cells resulted in effective suppression of responses. (Adapted from Hu D, Ikizawa K, Lu L, et al. Nat Immunol 2004;5:516–523)

The production of immunoregulatory cytokines and chemokines at early stages in the immune response influences the characteristics of the subsequent adaptive immune response and can therefore influence the outcome of the immune response.

NK cells play a key role in the early immune response to intracellular pathogens, largely through their production of IFNγ, which activates macrophages and facilitates differentiation of TH1 cells.

NK cell activity itself is induced by a variety of cytokines including:
- IFNα/β;
- IL-15;
- IL-18; and
- IL-12.

NK cells in turn are negatively regulated by cytokines such as IL-10 and TGFβ.

Q. Which cells will tend to promote the development of NK cells?

A. The TH1 population and macrophages through the production of IL-12, IL-15, and IL-18, whereas the TH2 population will tend to inhibit their development through the production of IL-10.

NK T cells produce cytokines when their TCR engages glycolipids in association with CD1d (see Chapter 10). It has been suggested that these cells play an immunoregulatory role in the control of autoimmunity, parasite infection, and tumor cell growth.

Recent experiments suggest that NK T cells secreting IFNγ are able to induce NK cell activation, increasing both NK proliferation and cytotoxicity. They are capable of making both TH1-type (IFNγ) and TH2-type (IL-4) cytokines depending on the cytokines present in the microenvironment when they are activated (Fig. 11.16).

The presence of IL-7, for example, has been shown to elicit IL-4 production in NK T cells and therefore to promote a TH2 response. This ability to make IL-4, particularly in the thymus, has been associated with the prevention of autoimmunity. For example, non-obese diabetic (NOD) mice have a deficit in NK T cells, and injection of NK T cells into these mice prevents the spontaneous development of autoimmune diabetes.

Deficiencies of NK T cells have also been reported in human autoimmune diseases including:
- rheumatoid arthritis;
- psoriasis;
- ulcerative colitis; and
- multiple sclerosis.

SENESCENCE OF CELLS IS REGULATED BY TELOMERE EROSION

Cells age by the process of cellular senescence, causing growth arrest and limiting their proliferative life span. This influences the extent of the immune response. The mechanisms that control cell senescence are an important part of immune regulation.

NK T cells produce both TH1- and TH2-type cytokines

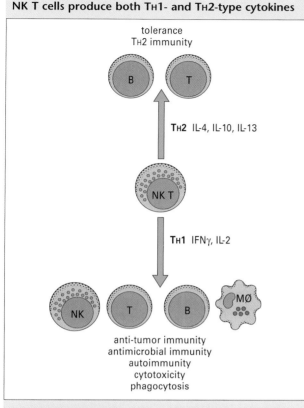

Fig. 11.16 NK T cells exert effects on many cell types. They can produce TH1 cytokines and TH2 cytokines and are involved in all aspects of the immune response.

Telomeres visualized by confocal microscopy

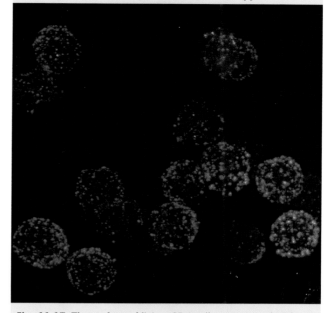

Fig. 11.17 The surface of living CD4 cells was stained with a red anti-CD4 antibody and then treated to destroy subcellular membranes, following which the telomeres were hybridized with a blue probe specific for the telomere sequences and visualized by confocal microscopy. Telomeres cap the ends of eukaryotic chromosomes and are repeating GGGTTA sequences at the ends of chromosomes with up to 2000 copies per cell. They protect chromosome stability and integrity, and are a mechanism for replicating DNA ends. (Courtesy of Dr J Skok and Dr JM Fletcher)

Telomeres are repeats of the DNA sequence GGGTTA and protein located at the end of chromosomes (Fig. 11.17).

Telomeres provide stabilization to chromosomes and protect the chromosomal ends from damage; they are also important in regulating the replicative capacity of cells.

During every cell division telomeres shorten by 50–100 base pairs because DNA polymerase cannot replicate the ends of chromosomes. The mechanism of telomere shortening prevents uncontrolled cell proliferation, which could lead to cancer.

When telomeres become too short the chromosome becomes unstable and DNA damage can occur. To prevent damaged cells being replicated, cells with unstable chromosomes:

• die by **apoptosis**; or
• enter cell cycle arrest, also known as **cellular senescence**.

Studies on T cells in elderly individuals show that they have significantly shorter telomeres than young individuals (Fig. 11.18).

In addition individuals with some premature ageing syndromes have short telomeres, are more susceptible to infections, and usually have a low life expectancy.

The decrease in telomere length with age is reflected in the increased exposure to antigens that elderly people have encountered. Memory T cells have shorter telomeres than naive T cells because they can have undergone many cell divisions (see Fig. 11.18). However, recent studies have shown that the extent of telomere erosion is dependent on which antigens are encountered. For example, CMV-specific cells have shorter telomeres than those of other antigen-specific cells, including EBV and VZV. Too much telomere erosion leads to senescence (i.e. effective loss of cells through cell cycle arrest) and this may cause the loss of specific populations of cells during ageing.

Cellular senescence can be delayed by maintaining telomere length; this occurs through the action of the enzyme **telomerase**. Telomerase contains an RNA template for the telomeric sequence GGGTTA. The enzyme is a reverse transcriptase that adds multiple telomere sequences to the 3′ end of replicated DNA and prevents telomere shortening (Fig. 11.19).

T cells can upregulate the expression of telomerase in certain situations, including during antigen stimulation. This prevents telomere loss during clonal expansion of antigen-specific cells and ensures that cells entering the memory pool retain their function. However, after repeated stimulation the ability to upregulate telomerase

Telomere erosion in ageing and antigen-specific memory

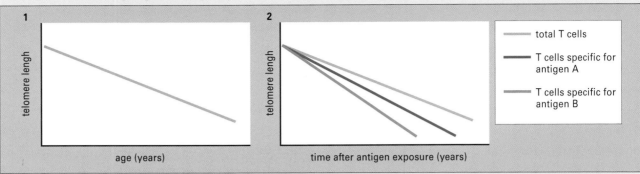

Fig. 11.18 (1) There is a reduction in telomere length in total T cells during ageing. (2) Continuous antigen exposure results in telomere erosion. Cells specific for CMV (antigen A) have shorter telomeres than those specific for other antigens including Epstein–Barr virus (EBV) and varicella zoster virus (VZV). (Adapted from Akbar AN, Beverley PCL, Salmon M. Nat Rev Immunol 2004;4:737–743. Copyright 2004 with permission from Nature Reviews. www.nature.com/reviews)

Telomere elongation by telomerase

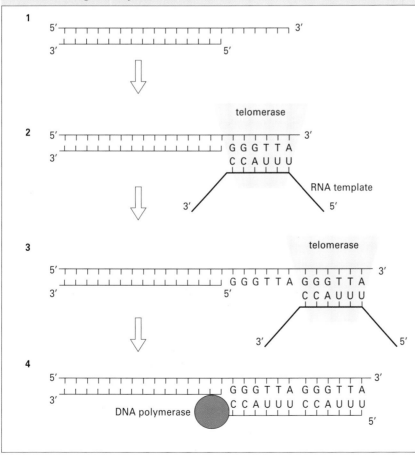

Fig. 11.19 (1) DNA replication results in incomplete transcription of DNA. (2) Telomerase is a ribonucleoprotein. The RNA strand encodes CCAUUU and acts as a template for extension of the telomere. (3) Telomerase translocates along the DNA from a 5′ to 3′ direction with addition of multiple telomeric sequences. (4) Transcription of the opposite strand is then completed by DNA polymerase.

decreases, leading to the telomere erosion observed in memory T cell populations.

Apoptosis maintains homeostasis in the immune system

Apoptosis is a cellular clearance mechanism through which homeostasis is maintained.

Unlike cell damage-induced death (i.e. **necrosis**), which can trigger immune responses, apoptosis maintains intracellular structures within the cell.

Apoptopic cells undergo nuclear fragmentation and the condensation of cytoplasm, plasma membranes, and organelles into **apoptopic bodies** (Fig. 11.20).

Apoptopic cells are rapidly phagocytosed by macrophages, which prevents the release of toxic cellular components into tissues, so avoiding immune responses to the dead cells.

Apoptosis is programmed cell death

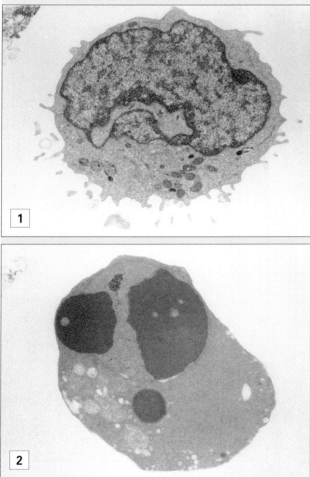

Fig. 11.20 (1) Normal cell. (2) Apoptotic cell. Apoptosis involves nuclear fragmentation, with 'blebbing' often observed. There is also condensation of cytoplasm and plasma membranes.

Apoptosis is:
- involved in clearing cells with a high avidity for antigen in the thymus and is an important mechanism of immunological tolerance (see Chapter 19);
- an important mechanism in maintaining homeostasis in the immune system.

Following resolution of an immune response the majority of antigen-specific cells die by apoptosis. This ensures that no unwanted effector cells remain and also maintains a constant number of cells in the immune system.

A small number of cells are prevented from undergoing apoptosis and enter the memory T cell pool.

Apoptosis is controlled by a number of factors in the cell and depends on expression of the death trigger molecule **CD95 (Fas)**.

Q. How does ligation of Fas lead to apoptosis?

A. It causes activation of a series of inducer and effector caspases (see Chapters 10 and 12 and Fig. 10.9).

Expression of the anti-apoptotic molecule **Bcl-2** makes cells more resistant to cell death. Memory T cells generally express high levels of Bcl-2, which may contribute to the rescue of memory populations from apoptosis.

Different cell populations can express both pro- and anti-apoptotic molecules with the balance of these molecules determining whether a cell survives to participate in immune responses.

SELECTIVE MIGRATION OF LYMPHOCYTE SUBSETS CAN MODULATE THE IMMUNE RESPONSE

Chemokines regulate the migration of lymphocytes

The spatial and temporal production of chemokines by different cell types is an important mechanism of immune regulation.

There is good evidence to suggest that the recruitment of TH1 and TH2 cells is differentially controlled, thereby ensuring the maintenance of locally polarized immune responses.

The expression of different chemokine receptors on TH1 cells (CXCR3 and CCR5) and TH2 cells (CCR3, CCR4, CCR8) allows chemotactic signals to produce the differential localization of T cell subsets to sites of inflammation (see Fig. 6.11).

Chemokines can be induced by cytokines released at sites of inflammation, so providing a mechanism for local reinforcement of particular types of response (Fig. 11.21). Once a response is established the T cells can induce further migration of appropriate effector cells. This is clearly illustrated in TH1 responses where the secondary production of CCL2, CCL3, CXCL10, and CCL5 serves to attract mononuclear phagocytes to the area of inflammation.

The ability of cytokines such as TGFβ, IL-12, and IL-4 to influence chemokine or chemokine receptor expression provides a further level of control on cell migration or recruitment.

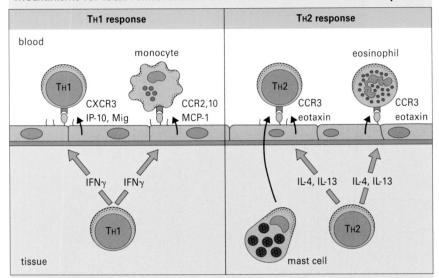

Fig. 11.21 Activated TH1 cells release IFNγ, which induces the chemokines IP-10 and Mig. These act on the chemokine receptors CXCR3, which are selectively expressed on TH1 cells, thereby reinforcing this type of response. Macrophage chemotactic protein-1 (MCP-1), which attracts macrophages and monocytes, is also induced by IFNγ. Mast cells release eotaxin when activated, and endothelial cells and bronchial epithelium can also synthesize this chemokine in response to IL-4 and IL-13 from TH2 cells. Eotaxin acts on CCR3, which is selectively expressed on TH2 cells, thereby reinforcing the TH2 response. Eosinophils and basophils, which mediate allergic responses in airways, also express CCR3. Chemokines can therefore potentiate both the initiation and effector phases of a specific type of immune response.

Immune responses do not normally occur in immune-privileged sites

Immune responses do not normally occur at certain sites in the body such as the anterior chamber of the eye and the testes. These sites are called **immune privileged**.

The failure to evoke immune responses in these sites is partly due to the presence of inhibitory cytokines such as TGFβ and IL-10, which inhibit inflammatory responses. The presence of migration inhibition factor (MIF) in the anterior chamber of the eye also inhibits NK cell activity.

The constitutive expression of FasL in cells of the testes and the eye has been proposed as an additional means of eliminating Fas-expressing lymphocytes that reach these sites through apoptosis.

T cell expression of different molecules can mediate tissue localization

Most studies on the human immune system are performed on blood due to the ethical issues in obtaining tissues. However, only a small proportion of the lymphocyte pool is circulating in the blood, most being resident in lymphoid or effector tissues.

The expression of molecules on T cells can mediate circulation through different tissues. Loss of the **lymph node homing molecules CCR7 and CD62L** on the surface of T cells prevents cells from circulating through

lymphoid tissue – in this way a population of highly differentiated memory cells migrate to non-lymphoid sites where they can exert effector functions.

It has recently been suggested that there are two types of memory cell:

- **central memory cells** express CCR7, home to lymphoid tissues, and do not have immediate effector function;
- **effector memory cells** do not express CCR7, migrate to non-lymphoid tissues, and produce effector cytokines – effector cells in non-lymphoid tissues, such as the skin, can proliferate and senesce and this has a direct effect on the level of local immune responses.

Q. Why do cells that express CCR7 migrate to lymphoid tissues?
A. They respond to **CCL21** expressed only in secondary lymphoid tissues (see Fig. 6.17).

Mucosal surfaces contain specialized cells

Mucosal surfaces are the main point of contact for antigens entering the immune system.

There is an increased proportion of T cells expressing the γδ TCR at mucosal sites, and intraepithelial lymphocytes (IELs) in the gut express CD8 in addition to their γδ TCRs whose repertoire specificity is skewed towards bacterial antigens (see Chapter 5).

T cells and B cells in the lamina propria are thought to play a role in immune surveillance. They also enhance the humoral IgA response, which is an important aspect of mucosal immunity (see Chapter 12).

THE NEUROENDOCRINE SYSTEM INFLUENCES IMMUNE RESPONSES

It is known that stressful conditions can lead to the suppression of immune functions, for example reducing the ability to recover from infection.

The nervous, endocrine, and immune systems are interconnected (Fig. 11.22). There are two routes by which the central nervous system could modulate immune function:

- most lymphoid tissues receive direct sympathetic innervation to the blood vessels passing through the tissues and directly to lymphocytes;
- the nervous system directly and indirectly controls the output of various hormones, in particular corticosteroids, growth hormone, prolactin, α-melanocyte-stimulating hormone, thyroxine, and epinephrine (adrenaline).

Lymphocytes express receptors for many hormones, neurotransmitters, and neuropeptides – expression and responsiveness vary between different lymphocyte and monocyte populations, such that the effect of different transmitters may vary in different circumstances.

Corticosteroids, endorphins, and enkephalins, all of which may be released during stress, are immuno-suppressive in vivo. The precise in-vitro effects of endorphins vary depending on the system and on the doses used – some levels are suppressive and others enhance immune functions.

It is certain, however, that corticosteroids act as a major feedback control on immune responses. It has been found that lymphocytes themselves can respond to corticotrophin releasing factor to generate their own adrenocorticotropic hormone (ACTH), which in turn induces corticosteroid release. Corticosteroids:

- inhibit TH1 cytokine production while sparing TH2 responses; and
- induce the production of TGFβ, which in turn may inhibit the immune response.

The low levels of plasma corticosteroids found in Lewis rats are believed to contribute to the susceptibility of this strain to a variety of induced autoimmune conditions.

The importance of corticosteroids in the overall susceptibility to disease induction is demonstrated in rat models of autoimmune disease where animals normally resistant to EAE become susceptible if adrenalectomized.

The interplay between the neuroendocrine system and the immune system is not unidirectional. Cytokines, in particular IL-1 and IL-6 produced by T cells, neurons, glial cells, and cells in the pituitary and adrenal glands, are bidirectional modulators of neuroendocrine–immune communication. These cytokines are potent stimulators of adrenal corticosteroid production through their influence on corticotrophin releasing hormone (CRH).

Q. In what other ways does IL-1 mediate interactions between the immune and nervous systems?
A. It causes an increase in body temperature, suppresses appetite, and enhances the duration of slow-wave sleep (see Chapter 6).

Neuroendocrine interactions with the immune system

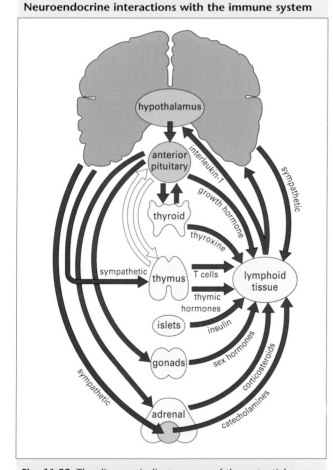

Fig. 11.22 The diagram indicates some of the potential connections between the endocrine, nervous, and immune systems. Blue arrows indicate nervous connections, red arrows indicate hormonal interactions, and white arrows indicate postulated connections for which the effector molecules have not been established.

GENETIC FACTORS INFLUENCE THE IMMUNE SYSTEM

Familial patterns of susceptibility to infectious agents suggest that resistance or susceptibility might be an inherited characteristic. Such patterns of resistance and susceptibility are also shown with autoimmune diseases.

Often many genes are involved in governing susceptibility or resistance to disease and the disease is said to be under polygenic control.

Considerable advances have been made in mapping and identifying the genes governing the response to some diseases as a result of:
- the development of techniques such as microsatellite mapping;
- increased availability of DNA samples; and
- sequencing of the human genome.

In most cases these studies have led to the identification of potential candidate genes, but their real role in disease susceptibility remains to be clarified. In other cases single mutations in genes of known function have been found and the mechanism by which they contribute to disease identified.

MHC haplotypes influence the ability to respond to an antigen

The development of inbred mouse strains conclusively demonstrated that genetic factors have a role in determining immune responsiveness. For example, strains of mice with different MHC haplotypes vary in their ability to mount an antibody response to specific antigens (Fig. 11.23). This function depends on MHC class II molecules (see Chapter 5) and is specific for each antigen – a high

responder strain for some antigens may be a low responder strain for others.

MHC-linked genes control the response to infections

MHC-linked genes (see Chapter 5) are involved in the immune response to infectious agents. In some cases the gene involved is the MHC gene itself, but in others it can be a gene linked to the MHC.

Susceptibility to infection by Trichinella spiralis is affected by the I-E locus in mice

The first observation that genes within the MHC could influence the response to parasites involved the susceptibility to *Trichinella spiralis* infection.

The response of different recombinant mouse strains to infection with *T. spiralis* is affected by the I-E locus. Mouse strains that express I-E (B10.BR, B10.P) appear to be susceptible whereas those that do not (B10.S, B10.M) are resistant to infection (Fig. 11.24). The response to *T. spiralis* is also influenced by the MHC-linked gene *Ts-2*, which maps close to the *TNF* genes.

The I-E locus also influences susceptibility to Leishmania donovani

Using H-2 congenic mice, it was shown that mice expressing the I-E locus were susceptible to visceral leishmaniasis. Parasite clearance was enhanced by anti-I-E antibody, but not by anti-I-A antibody, showing direct involvement of the I-E product. Furthermore, insertion of an I-E transgene into mice lacking the locus prevented effective clearance of parasites from the liver and spleen when compared to the original strain.

Certain HLA haplotypes confer protection from infection

Comparison of HLA haplotypes in humans revealed that certain MHC class I and class II alleles (HLA-B*5301 and DRB1*1302, respectively) are associated with a reduced risk of severe malaria.

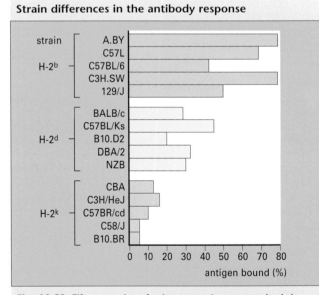

Strain differences in the antibody response

Fig. 11.23 Fifteen strains of mice were given a standard dose of the synthetic antigen (TG)-A-L. Antibody responses are expressed as the antigen-binding capacity of the sera. Animals of the H-2^b haplotype are high responders, whereas those of the H-2^d and H-2^k haplotypes are intermediate and low responders, respectively. However, there is some overlap between the levels of response in different haplotypes, indicating that H-2-linked genes are not the only ones controlling the antibody response.

Susceptibility to Trichinella spiralis

mouse strain	H-2 haplotype	I-E expression	resistance index	resistance phenotype
B10.BR	k	+	0	sus
B10.P	p	+	−22	sus
B10.RIII	r	+	33	sus
B10	b	−	63	res/int
B10.S	s	−	100	res
B10.M	f	−	104	res
B10.Q	q	−	105	res

Fig. 11.24 Association of H-2 haplotype, expression of cell surface I-E molecules, and susceptibility to infection with *T. spiralis*. The resistance index is measured as the number of parasites present after a constant challenge relative to strains B10.BR (susceptible = 0% resistance) and B10.S (resistant = 100% resistance). B10 shows intermediate resistance.

DRB1*1302 binds different peptides from those bound by DRB1*1301 as a result of a single amino acid difference in the β chain. This change is sufficient to influence the response to the malaria parasite.

HLA-DRB1*1302 has also been associated with an increased clearance of the hepatitis B virus and consequently a decreased risk of chronic liver disease.

The MHC class I type, HLA-A*02, is associated with a reduced risk of disease development following human T-lymphotropic virus-1 (HTLV-1) infection. The viral load was lower in HLA-A*02-positive healthy carriers of HTLV-1 correlating with the presence of high levels of virus-specific CTLs.

In HIV-1 infection a selective advantage against disease has been noted in individuals expressing maximal HLA heterozygosity of class I loci (A, B, and C) and lacking expression of HLA-B*35 and HLA-Cw*04.

Polymorphisms in the promoter region of the *TNFα* gene, which lies within the MHC, influence its level of expression through altered binding of the transcription factor OCT-1. One of these polymorphisms, which is commonly associated with cerebral malaria, results in high levels of TNF expression. This may lead to upregulation of intercellular adhesion molecule-1 (ICAM-1) on vascular endothelium, increased adherence of infected erythrocytes, and subsequent blockage of blood flow.

This polymorphism in the TNFα promoter has also been associated with:
- lepromatous leprosy;
- mucocutaneous leishmaniasis; and
- death from meningococcal disease.

Many non-MHC genes also modulate immune responses

Some genes outside the MHC region also govern the immune response. However, these genes are generally less polymorphic than MHC genes and contribute less to variations in disease susceptibility. Nevertheless, their effects are found in autoimmune diseases, allergy, and infection. For example:
- individuals with defects in the complement components C1q, C1r, and C1s (see Chapter 4) are predisposed to develop systemic lupus erythematosus (SLE) and lupus nephritis – the development of SLE-like symptoms in C1q knockout mice parallels the human situation;
- deficiency in C3 leads to an increased susceptibility to bacterial infections and a predisposition to immune complex disease – this is also seen with a deficiency in C2 and C4, both of which are located within the MHC region;
- high IgE production in some allergy-prone families associates with the presence of an 'atopy gene' on human chromosome 11q;
- Biozzi generated two lines of mice based on their responsiveness to erythrocyte antigens. The high responder and low responder Biozzi mice make quantitatively different amounts of antibody in response to antigenic challenge and the basis for these differences has in part been attributed to genetic differences in macrophage activity; the high and low responder strains also differ in their ability to respond to parasitic infections, but this does not correlate with the level of antibody produced.

Q. Why would deficiency in the components of the classical pathway lead to immune complex disease?
A. C3b deposition is required to transport complexes on erythrocytes and their ultimate phagocytosis by macrophages in the liver and spleen (see Chapter 4).

Non-MHC-linked genes affect susceptibility to infection
Genes regulating macrophage activity may determine the outcome of immune responses
Macrophages have a key role in the immune system. Therefore genes regulating their activity may determine the outcome of many immune responses.

The *Lsh/Ity/Bcg* gene provides a good example of such genetic control of macrophage function. This gene governs the early response to infection with *Leishmania donovani*, *Salmonella typhimurium*, *Mycobacterium bovis*, *Mycobacterium lepraemurium*, and *Mycobacterium intracellulare*. Its influence is on the early phase of macrophage priming and activation, and it has wide-ranging effects, including:
- upregulation of the oxidative burst;
- enhanced tumoricidal activity;
- enhanced antimicrobial activity; and
- upregulation of MHC class II molecule expression.

Recent congenic studies have identified the **natural resistance-associated macrophage protein-1 (*Nramp1*)** as the *Bcg* gene. *Nramp1* encodes a membrane protein with homology to known transport proteins and may be implicated in the transport of nitrite (NO_2^-) into the phagolysosome, so facilitating the killing of intracellular organisms.

The human homolog of the mouse gene *Nramp* (*NRAMP1*) has been cloned and several different alleles identified. Polymorphisms in this gene may contribute to resistance to tuberculosis in humans, though the data so far are not as convincing as in the mouse.

Polymorphisms in cytokine and chemokine genes affect susceptibility to infections
Polymorphisms in the genes encoding cytokine receptors have been shown to correlate with an increased susceptibility to:
- infection;
- severe combined immune deficiency (SCID); and
- inflammatory conditions.

The outcome of the mutation is dependent on which cytokine gene is affected.

Q. What effect would you expect a deficiency in the IL-7 receptor (IL-7R) to produce?
A. It causes a reduction in T cell numbers because IL-7 is required for early thymocyte development (see Fig. 2.29).

For example, humans with:
- mutations in the IL-7R α chain have a reduced number of T cells;
- whereas those with deficiency in the common cytokine receptor γ chain (γc), a component of IL-2, IL-4, IL-7, IL-9, and IL-15 receptors, have reduced numbers of T and NK cells and impaired B cell function, in part attributable to the lack of T cell help (Fig. 11.25).

Further examples are the mutations in the IFNγ receptor (IFNγR) or IL-12 receptor (IL-12R), which increase susceptibility to mycobacterial infection.

A list of genetic defects that contribute to impaired immune responses is given in Fig. 11.26.

Mutations in the cytokine promoters influence the levels of expression of cytokines. Polymorphisms such as these have been linked to certain autoimmune conditions and also to susceptibility to infections.

Susceptibility to severe malaria is under complex genetic control with other genes in addition to MHC genes playing an important role. Recent studies have linked the development of cerebral malaria to a polymorphism in the promoter region of the *TNFα* gene. Other studies have implicated polymorphisms in the promoter region of the inducible NO synthase gene (*NOS2*).

Some genes involved in immune responses affect disease susceptibility, but do not affect immune responsiveness. For example, disease progression to AIDS has been shown to be associated with polymorphisms in the chemokine receptor gene-5 (CCR5).

CCR5 is a co-receptor used in the entry of macrophage-tropic strains of HIV-1 into cells. A mutation that inactivates this receptor is found in some individuals of European origin, but is rare in populations of Asian or sub-Saharan African descent. Individuals homozygous for this CCR5 mutation are very resistant to HIV-1 infection. In this case resistance is related to the reduced primary spread of the virus rather than an enhanced immune response against it.

Role of mutations in cytokine receptor genes in severe combined immune deficiency (SCID)

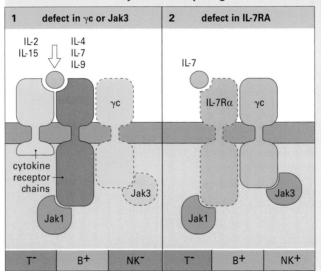

Fig. 11.25 (**1**) A defect in the common chain (γc) of the cytokine receptors IL-2, IL-15, IL-4, IL-7, and IL-9 leads to a SCID, with loss of both T and NK cells. A similar deficiency results from mutation in the janus kinase (Jak3), which transduces signals from the γc chain. Note that IL-2 and IL-15 have three chains in their high-affinity receptor, whereas IL-4, IL-7, and IL-9 have only two chains. (**2**) Absence of the specific IL-7R chain also produces a severe immunodeficiency, but this primarily affects T cell development.

Genetic defects associated with immune deficiency or abnormalities

condition	defective gene	result
SCID	γc	failure of signal transduction by cytokines
	IL-2Rα	failure of IL-2 signal in activation and development
	IL-7Rα	failure of IL-7 signal in lymphocyte development
	Jak3	lack of signal transduction by cytokines
	CD3γ	no signal transduced from TCR
	CD3ε	no signal transduced from TCR
	ZAP70	no signal transduced from TCR
	ADA	T cell toxicity
	RAG1/2	failure in TCR and BCR gene recombination
T cell deficiency	PNP	T cell development failure
class II deficiency	CIIT	failure to express MHC class II molecules
class I deficiency	TAP1/2	failure to load MHC class I molecules
X-linked hyper-IgM	CD40L	no maturation of antibody response
X-linked-agamma-globulinemia	Btk	failure of B cell development
X-linked lymphoproliferative syndrome	SH2DIA/SAP	impaired negative signals to B cells
Autoimmune lymphoproliferative syndrome	Fas(CD95) or FasL	extended lymphocyte life span due to reduced apoptosis
mycobacterial infection	IFNγR1/2, IL-12R	impaired T H1 responses

ADA, adenosine deaminase gene; BCR, B cell receptor; *Btk*, Bruton's tyrosine kinase gene; TCR, T cell receptor; *PNP*, purine nucleoside phosphorylase gene; *RAG*, recombination activating gene

Fig. 11.26 Genetic defects associated with immune deficiency or abnormalities. Based on a review by Leonard, Curr Opin Immunol 2000;12:465–467. See also Chapter 16.

FURTHER READING

Agnello D, Lankford CS, Bream J, et al. Cytokines and transcription factors that regulate T helper cell differentiation: new players and new insights. J Clin Immunol 2003;23:147–161.

Akbar AN, Beverley PCL, Salmon M. Will telomere erosion lead to a loss of T-cell memory. Nat Rev Immunol 2004;4:737–743.

Blalock JE, Bost KL, eds. Shared ligands and receptors as a molecular mechanism for communication between immune and neuro-endocrine systems. Ann NY Acad Sci 1994;741:292–298.

Biron C, Nguyen KB, Pien GC, et al. Natural killer cells in antiviral defense: function and regulation by innate cytokines. Annu Rev Immunol 1999;17:189–220.

Bodnar AG, Ouellette M, Frolkis M, et al. Extension of lifespan by introduction of telomerase into normal human cells. Science 1998;279:349–352.

Chess L, Jiang H. Resurrecting CD8+ suppressor cells. Nat Immunol 2004;5:569–571.

Cottrez F, Groux H. Specialization in tolerance: innate CD4+CD25+ versus acquired Tr1 and TH3 regulatory T cells. Transplantation 2004;1:S12–S15.

Heymann B. Regulation of antibody responses via antibodies, complement, and Fc receptors. Annu Rev Immunol 2000;18:709–738.

Lenardo M, Chan FK-M, Hornung F, et al. Mature T lymphocyte apoptosis–immune regulation in a dynamic and unpredictable antigenic environment. Annu Rev Immunol 1999;17:221–253.

Leonard WJ. Genetic effects on immunity. Curr Opin Immunol 2000;12:465–467.

Metzler B, Wraith DC. Inhibition of experimental autoimmune

encephalomyelitis by inhalation but not oral administration of the encephalitogenic peptide: influence of MHC binding affinity. Int Immunol 1993;5:1159–1165.

Mills KHG, McGuirk P. Antigen-specific regulatory T cells – their induction and role in infection. Semin Immunol 2004;16:107–117.

Reed JR, Vukmanovic-Stejic M, Fletcher JM, et al. Telomere erosion in memory T cells induced by telomerase inhibition at the site of antigenic challenge in vivo. J Exp Med 2004;199:1433–1443.

Romagnani S. Th1/Th2 cells. Inflamm Bowel Dis 1999;5:285–294.

Van der Vliet HJJ, Molling JW, von Blomberg BM, et al. The immunoregulatory role of CD1d-restricted natural killer T cells in disease. Clin Immunol 2004;112:8–23.

Zlotnik A, Yoshie O. Chemokines: a new classification system and their role in immunity. Immunity 2000;12:121–127.

Critical thinking: Regulation of the immune response (see p. 496 for explanations)

1 Why is there a need to regulate the extent of immune activation and lymphocyte proliferation?

2 In what ways can antibody regulate the immune response?

3 How would you use regulatory T cells to modulate aberrant immune responses?

4 What is the advantage of inducing replicative senescence in lymphocytes that are excessively stimulated?

Immune Responses in Tissues

SUMMARY

- **A tissue can influence local immune responses,** promoting some classes of immunity and suppressing others. The tissue can accomplish this by producing cytokines that influence both T cells and APCs. Direct interactions between cells of the tissue can also modulate immune responses.

- **Certain sites in the body are immunologically privileged** and fully allogeneic tissue can be transplanted into them without risk of rejection. These sites, which include the anterior chamber of the eye, the brain, and the testes, are able to promote certain kinds of beneficial classes of immune responses while suppressing classes that can do irreparable local damage.

- **Immune responses in gut, lung, and skin distinguish between pathogens and innocuous organisms and antigens.** Gut enterocytes influence the local immune response. Intraepithelial lymphocytes (IELs) respond to stress-induced class Ib molecules and produce many immunomodulatory cytokines.

- **Endothelium controls which populations of lymphocytes enter a tissue.** Endothelium within each tissue provides signals for the selective accumulation of specific tissue-resident lymphocytes, many of which do not recognize foreign antigens, but are activated by stress-induced self molecules.

- **A number of principles govern the immunological characteristics of each tissue.** As well as the principles outlined in the summary points above, cells of the tissue can promote the accumulation of tissue-resident lymphocytes and exert their effects via cytokines or by direct cell–cell interactions. A tissue can have several microenvironments, each of which has its own physiology and preferred immune response, and the local immune response can produce systemic changes.

A TISSUE CAN INFLUENCE LOCAL IMMUNE RESPONSES

Any immune system faced with a potential threat must answer two questions:

- The first question is 'Shall I respond?', and the mechanisms used to determine that answer are the topics of much of this book.
- Once made, however, there is a second question – 'What type of response shall I make?'

What determines whether an immune response should be comprised of, for example, activated cytotoxic T lymphocytes (CTLs) or a particular class of antibodies?

Although it has long been taught that the effector class of an immune response is tailored to the pathogen being fought, accumulating evidence suggests that there may also be a strong influence from the local tissue milieu (Fig. 12.1).

This chapter focuses on:

- the features of immune responses that are unique to individual tissues; and
- the mechanisms by which the tissues influence local and systemic characteristics.

There are several reasons why a particular organ may need to modify local immunity.

Q. Herpes simplex virus infects sensory neurons and causes cold sores. Why might a CTL response be inappropriate for controlling such an infection?

A. An effective cytotoxic response would kill the infected neuron, which cannot be replaced. This would be worse for the host than the moderate inconvenience caused by the sporadically reactivating viral infection.

This is an example of how an immune response summoned to clear an infection can interfere with a tissue's physiology as seriously as the infection itself.

A similar outcome can occur in both the eye and the gut, which may be damaged by cytokines such as tumor necrosis factor-α (TNFα) and interferon-γ (IFNγ) produced locally during cell-mediated immune reactions.

Indeed, when TNFα and IFNγ reach high systemic levels, they can result in shock and rapid death. An example is seen in Dengue shock syndrome. Individuals who are immune to the Dengue virus or infants with maternal antibodies may develop rapid circulatory collapse. It is thought that interaction between activated T cells and macrophages causes the release of TNFα, which acts on endothelium leading to an increase in capillary permeability and consequent fall in blood pressure.

Factors controlling the characteristic immune response of a tissue

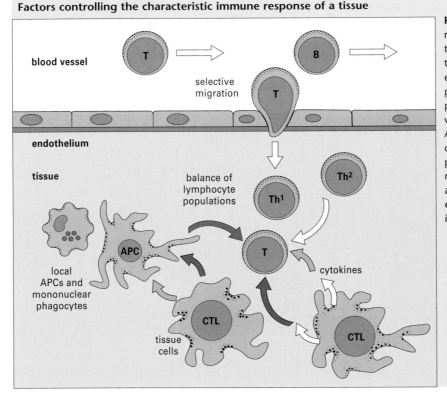

Fig. 12.1 The characteristic immune response of a tissue is controlled both by the leukocyte populations present and by the direct and indirect signals from the endogenous cells of the tissue. The population of lymphocytes that enter a particular tissue is controlled by the vascular endothelium in that tissue. Antigen presentation within the tissue depends on the populations of antigen-presenting cells (APCs), which include resident mononuclear phagocytes. APCs and T cells are influenced directly by endogenous cells of the tissue, and indirectly via cytokines.

Another reason for specific local immune responses is that certain types of immune response are more effective in some tissues than in others.

Q. What type of immune response is suited to the gut and mucosal surfaces?

A. The production of IgA antibodies, promoted by a TH2-type immune response. Accumulation and recirculation of IgA-producing B cells within submucosal tissues means that IgA antibodies are produced near the point of secretion (Fig. 12.2 and see Fig. 3.11)

These observations suggest that the immune system might normally receive guidance from each tissue to make a response that is both appropriate for and effective at that site.

Consequently, tissues have evolved regulatory mechanisms that influence the immune response that occurs within them. The detailed study of these regulatory mechanisms is in its infancy, but we will attempt to assemble some of the broad operating rules, and provide examples of the types of immune response seen in different tissues.

IgA synthesis in the lamina propria

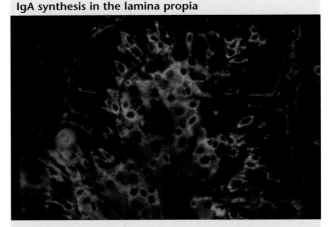

Fig. 12.2 Lymphoid cells in the epithelium and lamina propria fluoresce green using antibody to leukocyte common antigen (CD45). Red cytoplasmic staining is obtained with anti-IgA antibody, which detects plasma cells in the lamina propria and IgA in the mucus. (Courtesy of Professor G Janossy)

CERTAIN SITES IN THE BODY ARE IMMUNOLOGICALLY PRIVILEGED

There are certain sites in the body where fully allogeneic tissue can be transplanted without risk of rejection. These include the:
- anterior chamber of the eye (Fig. 12.3);
- brain;
- testes; and
- (oddly) the hamster cheek pouch.

Several factors may contribute to the **immunological privilege** of these sites, some of which affect the initiation of the immune response and some affect the effector phase. Some of the factors that limit the development of

Corneal allografts

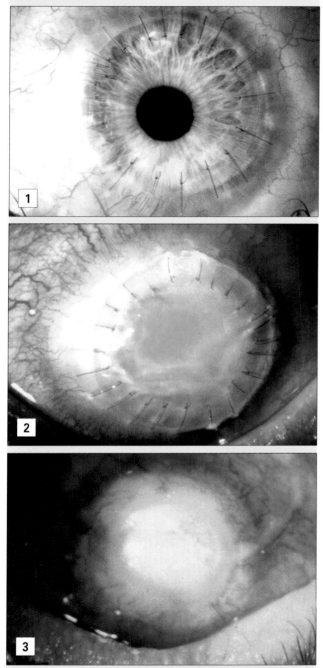

Fig. 12.3 (1) A successful corneal allograft. More than 90% of such grafts remain clear after 1 year. The sutures are still visible in the periphery. Note that vascularization does not extend into the graft. (2) An acutely rejected graft. (3) A chronically rejected graft. The rejected grafts indicate that effective cell-mediated responses can develop within the eye. Note the increased vascularization in the rejected grafts. (With permission from the University of Aberdeen)

immune reactions in the central nervous system (CNS) include the following:

- the blood–brain barrier (endothelium plus astrocytes) prevents the movement of over 99% of large serum proteins into the brain tissue (IgG, complement, etc.);
- low levels of MHC molecule expression, and co-stimulatory molecules result in inefficient antigen presentation;
- there is no conventional lymphatic drainage system from brain tissue to local lymph nodes;
- there are low levels of leukocyte traffic into the CNS in comparison with other tissues;
- neurons have direct immunosuppressive actions on glial cells;
- astrocytes and neurons produce immunosuppressive cytokines.

Similar factors apply in other privileged sites.

The 'privileged sites' were long thought to be locations where adaptive immune responses are so dangerous that the immune system is either not allowed entry, is destroyed upon arrival, or is prevented from functioning.

From an evolutionary point of view, however, this explanation for the acceptance of grafts seems rather unlikely because an unprotected tissue that is warm, wet, and full of nutrients would quickly become a haven for parasites.

Recent evidence suggests that the concept of privileged sites may have been a misconception based on the limitations of the experimental assay systems. Once the experiments were expanded to include a wider variety of assays it became apparent that privileged sites are not immunologically impaired. They are simply sites that are able to promote certain kinds of beneficial classes of immune responses while suppressing classes that can do irreparable local damage.

The eye has very limited self-regenerative capacity and can be completely destroyed by a cell-mediated immune response with the concomitant local production of TNFα and IFNγ (see Fig. 12.3). The same response to the same antigen within the skin does not have such a severe effect. The principal difference is the regenerative capacities of the two organs. The eye has therefore evolved two major mechanisms to actively suppress cell-mediated responses:

- first, the epithelial cells lining the anterior chamber express Fas ligand;
- second, the fluid of the anterior chamber contains cytokines such as transforming growth factor-β (TGFβ).

Q. What would be the functional effect of epithelial cells lining the anterior chamber expressing Fas ligand and the fluid of the anterior chamber containing TGFβ have on an immune response?

A. Expression of Fas ligand (CD178) on the epithelial cells permit engagement of incoming cells (e.g. T cells) that express Fas (CD95) and thereby induce their apoptosis (see Figs 10.8 and 10.9) — a case of the tables being turned on the lymphocytes. Production of TGFβ limits T cell proliferation and tends to induce TH2 and possibly Treg lymphocytes. Additionally, the expression of Fas ligand may also favor a switch to a TH2-type response because Fas ligand has been shown to induce the death of TH1 cells more easily than TH2 cells.

Local immune privilege may extend to other systems

When first discovered, the features of immune privilege described above were thought to fit with the idea of the eye as a privileged site. However, an ingenious set of experiments by Streilein and his colleagues showed that the eye actually does something much more interesting than merely suppress local immunity and shift immune responses into a class of immunity that is non-destructive to the eye. In their experiments they transplanted tumors into the eye, which grew unhindered as expected. Unexpectedly, however, the tumor recipients subsequently became more generally tolerant of any other tissue that shared some of the tumor antigens, no matter the site of transplantation (Fig. 12.4).

Following up on this finding, it was discovered that spleen APCs that had been incubated with fluid from the anterior chamber of the eye were no longer able to induce T cell proliferative responses, but instead promoted production of IL-4, IL-10, and TGFβ. Streilein called this switch anterior chamber associated immune deviation (ACAID) and it was found to be controlled by the cells of the iris and ciliary body, which secrete immunomodulatory cytokines, including TGFβ, vasoactive intestinal peptide (involved in control of the synthesis of the secretory piece of IgA), γ-melanocyte-stimulating hormone (γMSH), and calcitonin gene-related peptide.

These cytokine and molecular controls on immunity are underpinned by the cellular organization of the eye, which has barriers that limit the movement of molecules into the retina, anterior chamber, and vitreous (Fig. 12.5).

Altogether, the picture that emerged is of an organ that actively promotes a type of immunity that is protective and beneficial (the IgA response) while suppressing a type of immunity that can be destructive.

Three principles are illustrated by ACAID:
- a tissue can influence its local immune responses, promoting some classes and suppressing others;
- the tissue can accomplish this by directly producing cytokines that influence both T cells and APCs;
- local influence can cause systemic changes.

The blood–brain barrier shields the CNS from immune reactions

Many of the factors that lead to limited immune responses in the eye also occur in the CNS. Indeed the blood–retinal barrier described in Fig. 12.5 is related to the blood–brain barrier present in most areas of the CNS.

The blood–brain barrier is a composite structure formed by the specialized brain endothelium and the foot processes of astrocytes. Astrocytes are required to induce the special properties of brain endothelial cells, which have continuous belts of tight junctions connecting them to other endothelial cells.

The blood–brain barrier has many physiological properties, but of interest to immunologists is the very low permeability of the endothelium to serum proteins (Fig. 12.6).

For example, the level of IgG found in the CNS is normally approximately 0.2% of the level found in serum. The level may rise during an immune reaction as the endothelial barrier becomes more permeable in response to inflammatory cytokines. Additionally, in some conditions, such as multiple sclerosis, there is often local synthesis of antibody within the CNS, which may contribute to the immune reaction.

Nevertheless, even in the most severe immune reactions, the levels of antibody, complement components, and other serum molecules is much lower in the brain than in other tissues.

Tolerance to allografts transplanted into the eye

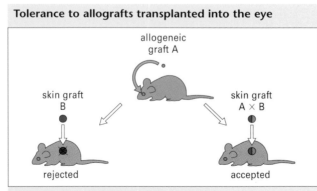

Fig. 12.4 Tumor cells of tissue type A transplanted into the eye are tolerated. Subsequently skin grafts of tissue type A × B are also tolerated in these animals. Tolerance to A, induced within the eye, extends to other tissues, and can turn off the normal immune response that would be expected against a type B skin allograft.

Anatomic and immunological basis of immune privilege in the eye

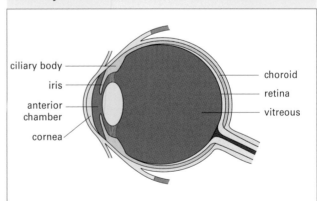

Fig. 12.5 The uvea, consisting of the iris, ciliary body, and chorea, is highly vascularized, but lacks draining lymphatic vessels. Tight junctions between the vessels in the iris and between non-pigmented ciliary epithelial cells maintain a blood–aqueous barrier. Similar junctions on the retinal pigment epithelium and the retinal endothelium maintain a blood–retinal barrier. The iris and ciliary body secrete immunomodulatory cytokines.

The blood–brain barrier

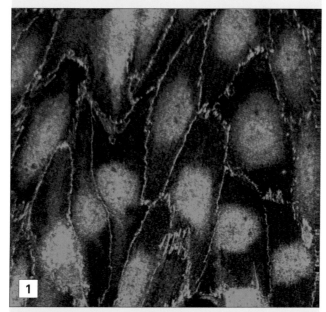

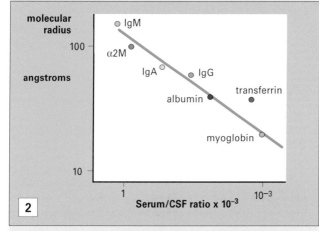

Fig. 12.6 (1) Brain endothelial cells have a continuous ring of tight junctions, identified in this micrograph by the junctional marker ZO-1. The resulting permeability barrier excludes serum proteins from the brain tissue. (2) The graph shows the serum/cerebrospinal fluid (CSF) ratio for different proteins. There is an inverse relationship between molecular size and the level in CSF. Molecules such as transferrin, which are transported into the brain, are present at higher levels than would be expected from their size. Immunoglobulins are not transported.

Neurons suppress immune reactivity in neighboring glial cells

When researchers first started to examine individual populations of cells from the CNS in vitro (e.g. astrocytes), they found that astrocytes would respond to IFNγ by increasing their expression of MHC class I molecules and inducing expression of the normally absent MHC class II molecules. However, in vivo, astrocytes rarely respond in this way. It appeared that the local environ-

ment of the CNS could in some way suppress the ability of astrocytes to respond to IFNγ.

Subsequently it was found that when neurons are co-cultured in contact with astrocytes, then the ability to induce MHC molecules was suppressed, but if the cells were not in contact, they were not repressed (Fig. 12.7).

Q. How do you interpret the repression of MHC induction described in Fig. 12.7?

A. Because repression of MHC induction requires contact between the cells it implies that the effect is not caused by a cytokine.

The results are even more interesting because it subsequently became clear that electrically active neurons are required. This means that:

- neurons that are functioning normally can suppress their neighboring glial cells (and downregulate their own MHC molecules); whereas
- damaged neurons will lift the local immunosuppression to allow an immune response to develop.

The examples of the eye and the CNS illustrate a number of mechanisms that lead to immune privilege. In practice, a combination of mechanisms is active in each tissue.

IMMUNE RESPONSES IN GUT, LUNG, AND SKIN DISTINGUISH BETWEEN PATHOGENS AND INNOCUOUS ANTIGENS

The gut, lung, and skin are examples of tissues that are continuously in contact with high levels of harmless

Immunosuppression by neurons

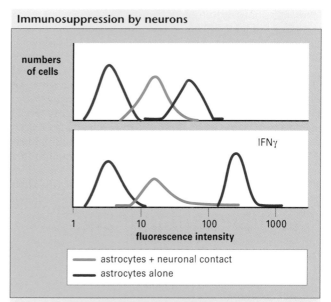

astrocytes + neuronal contact
astrocytes alone

Fig. 12.7 The top fluorescence graph shows the expression of MHC class I molecules on astrocytes cultured in contact with or separate from neurons. Note that neurons suppress MHC class I expression. If IFNγ is added to the cultures (lower graph), astrocytes cultured alone increase their expression of MHC class I molecules, but those cultured with neurons are still suppressed. (Based on data from Tonsch U, Rott O. Immunology 1993;80:507)

commensal organisms and innocuous antigens as well as potential pathogens. The responses in these tissues are concerned not just with whether an immune response takes place, but also on the quality of that response.

Q. What factors allow the immune system to distinguish between pathogens and innocuous organisms and antigens?
A. Many pathogenic organisms have components that are recognized by **pathogen-associated molecular patterns (PAMP) receptors** (see Chapter 6 and Figs 6.22–6.24), which when ligated can lead to efficient antigen presentation. Additionally, pathogenic organisms cause tissue damage. The proteins released from damaged cells can directly activate APCs, while released enzymes such as tissue plasminogen activator (see Fig. 6.19) and tissue kallikrein (see Fig. 6.18) lead to activation of the plasmin and kinin systems.

Oral tolerance or regional immunity in the gut?

Occasionally we hear that a native American Indian child has eaten poison ivy but has not developed the cell-mediated hypersensitivity reaction that normally follows within 48 hours of contact with the plant. This is **oral tolerance**.

Oral tolerance, and the related phenomenon of nasal tolerance, illustrate two points:

- it is systemic in that it can influence responses at non-mucosal sites;
- it is dominant in that it is transferable to naive individuals by CD4 (or occasionally CD8) T cells.

Tolerance is not the only form of immunity that arises from ingestion of antigens. **Oral vaccination** has been recognized since 1919 when Besredka noticed that rabbits were protected from fatal dysentery by oral immunization with killed shigellae. The attenuated polio vaccine that was developed in the 1950s was also given as an oral vaccination. In both case these vaccines would not be viewed as a harmless antigen by the immune system:

- shigellae contain antigens that activate the intracellular PAMP receptor NOD-1 (see Fig. 9.24);
- the attenuated polio vaccine proliferates in the gut and lymphoid tissue, and therefore induces some tissue damage.

In each case, however, the vaccine is effective in protecting the host against disease.

Q. Can you give another example of tolerance induced by administration of antigen across mucosal tissues?
A. Tolerance in mice administered myelin basic protein (MBP) by aerosol can suppress the induction of experimental allergic encephalomyelitis (EAE) in response to the same antigen given intradermally in adjuvant (see Fig. 11.2).

Oral vaccination and tolerance are two sides of the same coin

In essence, they are very similar responses – the main difference lies with the assays used to measure them.

Antigens introduced orally tend to invoke an immune response that is appropriate for the gut and other mucosal surfaces, namely the production of local IgA, and some systemic IgG. There is generally little production of TH1 cells or CTLs, and no cell-mediated immune response.

Measurement of the IgA response would lead to the conclusion that oral antigens induce immunity. However, if the cell-mediated response (lymphocyte proliferation in response to antigen) is measured, one can erroneously conclude that the animal has become tolerant.

The success of the polio vaccine was measured by its ability to protect against the virally induced disease and was therefore labeled 'vaccination'. In contrast, reducing the autoimmune reaction in EAE (a model of multiple sclerosis) is viewed as a success, and this procedure is therefore labeled 'tolerance'. These outcomes – vaccination and tolerance – are, however, merely two sides of the same coin.

Gut enterocytes influence the local immune response

The enterocytes of the gut considerably influence the local immune response by secreting a variety of immuno-modulatory factors such as TGFβ, VIP, IL-1, IL-6, IL-7, CXCL8, and CCL3.

Structure of the villi and crypts of the small intestine

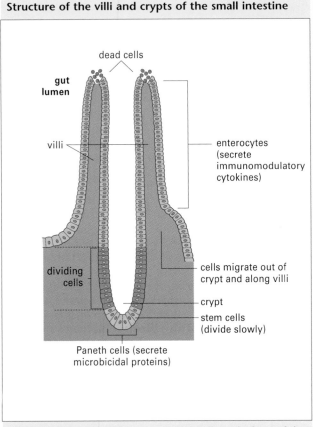

Fig. 12.8 Stem cells give rise to Paneth cells at the base of the crypt, which secrete antimicrobial peptides. The enterocytes are derived from the rapidly dividing transit-amplifying population and will eventually be shed from the tips of the villi. These cells secrete immunomodulatory cytokines.

The Paneth cells at the bottoms of the crypts meanwhile produce several natural antibiotic peptides (Fig. 12.8), which help prevent bacterial overgrowth in these sensitive sites of cellular differentiation.

Enterocytes may also promote migration of intraepithelial lymphocyte (IEL) populations.

Q. What are the characteristics of IELs?

A. IELs have a dendritic morphology and express the γδ form of the T cell receptor (TCR) and often CD8 (see Fig. 2.22).

By expressing E-**cadherin**, a ligand for **αEβ7-integrin**, and by secreting TGFβ, which upregulates the expression of αEβ7, enterocytes may provide a signal for the selective accumulation of IELs that express this integrin. In this way, the tissue cells invite the residency of cells that promote certain types of immunity and aid in repair (see below).

IELs respond to stress-induced class Ib molecules

Many IELs have an activated or memory phenotype and recognize the ancient conserved MHC class I-like molecules, **MICA** and **MICB**, which are upregulated by cellular stress.

When activated by MICA and MICB some of the mucosa-associated lymphocytes secrete epidermal cell growth factor (ECGF) and may therefore function to repair and renew damaged intestinal epithelial cells.

Hence, by expressing molecules, the tissue cells can activate their local resident lymphocytes regardless of the specific antigen that is the target of the immune response. In this way the tissue can influence local immunity against many different antigens.

IELs produce many immunomodulatory cytokines

IELs also produce a wealth of immunomodulatory cytokines, such as IL-1, TGF, lymphotoxin (LT), IFNγ, and TNFα.

Although the conditions under which each set of cytokines is produced have not yet been elucidated, it is clear that certain cytokines, and their attendant antibody subclasses, are associated with certain intestinal diseases.

For example in ulcerative colitis, celiac disease, and Crohn's disease there is some associated production of TNFα and IFNγ, as there is in some other mucosal diseases such as chronic gastritis, chronic rhinitis, and chronic sialadenitis (i.e. situations where there is dysregulation of the normal mucosal immune responses).

ENDOTHELIUM CONTROLS WHICH POPULATIONS OF LYMPHOCYTES ENTER A TISSUE

Migration of leukocytes into different tissues of the body is dependent on the vascular endothelium in each tissue.

For many years, it was thought that the endothelium in different tissues was essentially similar, with the possible exception of tissues such as the brain and retina, which have barrier properties.

It was also acknowledged that the endothelium in lymphoid tissues – high endothelial venules (HEVs) – was specialized to support lymphocyte traffic specific for different areas.

Despite this common belief, it was well known that inflammation in different tissues had different characteristics, even when the inducing agents were similar. Compare the two type IV hypersensitivity reactions seen in the CNS and dermis (Figs 12.9 and 12.10):

- in the brain the lymphocyte infiltrate is confined to the region around the venules and there is little overt tissue disruption;
- in the dermis there is extensive infiltration with macrophages and lymphocytes, which is accompanied by severe edema and tissue disruption.

It has recently become clear that a major element controlling inflammation and the immune response is the vascular endothelium in each tissue, which has its own characteristics. Different endothelia produce distinctive blends of chemokines (Fig. 12.11).

In normal lung there is a high level of macrophage migration, which may be related to the high expression of CCL2 (macrophage chemotactic protein-1) by lung endothelium.

Type IV hypersensitivity in CNS

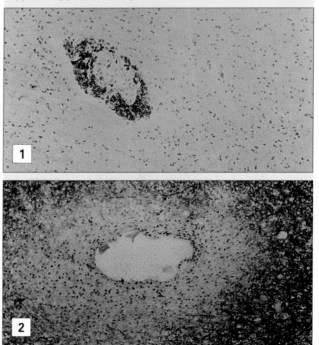

Fig. 12.9 (1) The perivenous infiltrations of lymphocytes in parainfectious encephalomyelitis are confined to the area around the venule top. There is little disruption of the tissue, but a stain for myelin shows that demyelination (2) extends out beyond the initial area of infiltration. (Courtesy of Dr N Woodroofe and Dr H Okazaki)

Type IV hypersensitivity in dermis

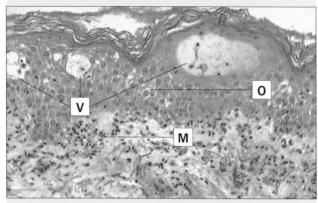

Fig. 12.10 A histological section of a cell-mediated immune reaction (type IV hypersensitivity) in the dermis. Mononuclear cells (M) infiltrate both dermis and epidermis. The epidermis is pushed out and microvesicles (V) form within it due to edema (O). × 130.

Histological section of an airway from a case of fatal asthma

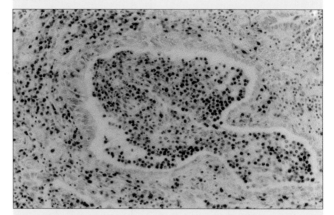

Fig. 12.12 The lumen of an alveolus of the lung is heavily infiltrated with inflammatory exudates, fibrin, and cellular debris. Immunohistochemical staining with monoclonal antibody against EG2 indicates that the majority of cells are eosinophils. × 275. (Courtesy of Arshad SH. Allergy: An Illustrated Colour Text. Philadelphia: Churchill Livingstone, 2002. With permission from Elsevier)

Production of chemokines by endothelium derived from different human tissues

	endothelium		
	lung	dermis	brain
CXCL8	++	++	+++
CXCL10	+	+	+++
CCL2	+++	++	+
CCL5	+	++	+

Fig. 12.11 Brain endothelium produces high levels of CXCL8 and CXCL10 associated with a TH1-type immune response. Dermal endothelium produces high levels of CCL5 associated with T cell migration, whereas lung endothelium produces high levels of CCL2, a chemokine that causes macrophage migration.

Q. How would you expect the high production of CXCL10 to affect immune reactions in the CNS?

A. CXCL10 is induced in response to IFNγ and acts on CXCR3, which is selectively expressed on TH1 cells (see Fig. 6.11). Therefore brain endothelium produces chemokines that promote a TH1-type reaction.

The cellular infiltrate in the CNS can be contrasted with that seen in the bronchus during allergic asthma where eosinophils predominate (Fig. 12.12). In this case the production of IL-5 and CCL3 (eotaxin) are characteristic of both the TH2 response and this particular tissue.

A NUMBER OF PRINCIPLES GOVERN THE IMMUNOLOGICAL CHARACTERISTICS OF EACH TISSUE

Knowledge of the distinctive immunological characteristics of each tissue is only just emerging. Nevertheless a number of principles can be discerned as follows.

- A tissue can influence the local immune response, promoting some classes of immunity and suppressing others.
- The local endothelium plays a major role in determining which leukocytes will enter the tissue by the secretion of distinct blends of chemokines.
- Cells of the tissue can promote the accumulation of tissue-resident lymphocytes, many of which do not recognize foreign antigens, but instead bind to stress-induced self molecules.
- Cells in the tissue can exert their effects via cytokines or by direct cell–cell interactions. In effect, cells of the tissue can signal damage or distress.
- A tissue can have several microenvironments, each of which has its own physiology and preferred immune response.
- The local immune response can produce systemic changes.

FURTHER READING

Brandtzaeg P. History of oral tolerance and mucosal immunity. Ann NY Acad Sci 1996;778:1–27.

Cheroutre H. Starting at the beginning: new perspectives on the biology of mucosal T cells. Annu Rev Immunol 2004;22:217–246.

Debendictis C, Joubeh S, Zhang G, et al. Immune functions of the skin. Clin Dermatol 2001;19:573–585.

Engelhardt B, Ransohoff RM. The ins and outs of T-lymphocyte trafficking to the CNS: anatomical sites and molecular mechanisms. Trends Immunol 2005;26:485–495.

Greenwood J, Begley DJ, Segal MB, eds. New concepts of a blood brain barrier. New York: Plenum Press; 1995.

Mowat AM, Viney JL. The anatomical basis of intestinal immunity. Immunol Rev 1997;156:145–166.

Spellberg B. The cutaneous citadel: a holistic view of skin and immunity. Life Sci 2002;67:477–502.

Wayne Streilein J. Regional immunology of the eye. In: Pepose JS, Holland GN, Wilhelmus KR, eds. Ocular infection and immunity. Oxford: Elsevier; 1996:19–33.

Weiler-Normann C, Rehermann B. The liver as an immunological organ. J Gastroenterol Hepatol 2004;19:S279–S283.

Wilbanks GA, Streilein JW. Fluids from immune privileged sites endow macrophages with the capacity to induce antigen-specific immune deviation via a mechanism involving transforming growth factor-β. Eur J Immunol 1992;22:1031–1036.

Williams IR, Kupper TS. Immunity at the surface: homeostatic mechanisms of the skin immune system. Life Sci 1996;58:1485–1507.

Zhang X, Brunner T, Carter L, et al. Unequal death in T helper cell (Th)1 and Th2 effectors: Th1, but not Th2, effectors undergo rapid Fas/FasL-mediated apoptosis. J Exp Med 1997;185:1837–1849.

Critical thinking: Immune reactions in the gut (see p. 496 for explanations)

Oyster poisoning occurs when an individual eats an oyster that has concentrated bacteria or Protoctista in itself from sea water. Often an individual who has eaten an infected oyster will then be unable to eat oysters again – even good oysters make them ill. Construct a logical explanation for this observation, based on your understanding of immune reactions in the gut.

Defence Against Infectious Agents

Immunity to Viruses

SUMMARY

- **Innate immune mechanisms (interferon, NK cells, and macrophages) restrict the early stages of infection and delay spread of virus.** Interferons exert antiviral activity by a variety of mechanisms. NK cells are cytotoxic for virally infected cells. Macrophages act at three levels to destroy virus and virus-infected cells. DC2 dendritic cells produce IFNα in herpesvirus and influenza virus infection.

- **As a viral infection proceeds, the adaptive (specific) immune response unfolds.** Antibodies and complement can limit viral spread or reinfection. T cells mediate viral immunity in several ways – CD8$^+$ CTLs destroy virus-infected cells; CD4$^+$ T cells are a major effector cell population in the response to many virus infections.

- **Viruses have evolved strategies to evade the immune response.** Virus latency and antigenic variation are the most effective mechanisms. Many viruses deviate the immune response by the production of cytokine analogs and cytokine receptor analogs. Many DNA viruses have strategies to control the expression of MHC molecules.

- **Responses to viral antigens can cause tissue damage** from the formation of immune complexes and by causing immunosuppression, immunodeficiency, or autoimmunity.

EARLY IMMUNE DEFENSES AGAINST VIRUSES INCLUDE INTERFERON, NK CELLS, AND MACROPHAGES

The early stage of a viral infection is often a race between the virus and the host's defense system. The initial defense against virus invasion is the integrity of the body surface. Once breached, early 'non-specific' or innate immune defenses such as interferon (IFN), natural killer (NK) cells, and macrophages become active.

Interferons exert antiviral activity by a variety of mechanisms

There are two major families of IFN – type I and type II IFNs.

Type I IFNs include:
- **IFNα** (leukocyte IFN) – a family of 13 genes on chromosome 9 – produced following virus infection of cells;
- **IFNβ** (fibroblast IFN) – a single gene on chromosome 9 – produced following virus infection of cells;
- **IFNτ/ε** (trophoblast IFN); and
- two new families, IFNλ and IFNκ.

Type II IFN or **IFNγ** – a single gene on chromosome 12 – is only produced following antigenic or mitogenic stimulation of T and NK cells.

Virus infection of a cell leads to the production of IFNα/β, which activates antiviral mechanisms in neighboring cells enabling them to resist virus infection (Fig. 13.1).

Interferons activate a number of genes with direct antiviral activity. A key mechanism involves the dsRNA-dependent protein kinase R (PKR), which:
- phosphorylates the α-subunit of eIF-2 leading to a block in the translation of viral mRNA;
- triggers apoptosis via Bcl-2 and caspase-dependent mechanisms thereby short circuiting virus infection through suicide of the infected cell.

Another mechanism activated by dsRNA involves 2′,5′-oligoadenylate synthetase, which activates a latent endonuclease (RNaseL) involved in degrading viral RNA.

Q. What role does dsRNA play in the normal metabolism of a mammalian cell?

A. dsRNA is formed as part of the replication/transcription of RNA viruses. However, because the mammalian genome is DNA, dsRNA is not produced during transcription of mRNA; consequently dsRNA is a signature of viral replication. At least, this was the view until recently. It is now known that dsRNA is formed in eukaryotic cells as part of the process that controls mRNA activity by small inhibitory RNAs (siRNA). Mammalian cells therefore have an intrinsic normal mechanism that leads to the recognition and degradation of dsRNA.

A third mechanism for controlling viral infection involves Mx proteins, which inhibit viral transcription of a range of RNA viruses, but have little effect on DNA viruses.

The molecular basis of interferon action

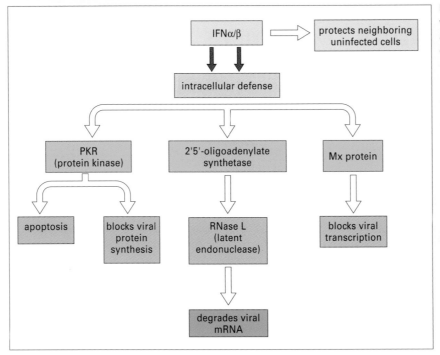

Fig. 13.1 The antiviral state develops within a few hours of interferon stimulation and involves various intracellular antiviral defenses.

Other mechanisms of IFN-mediated intracellular defense exist because mice deficient in *PKR*, *RnaseL*, and *Mx* genes (triple knockouts) still retain antiviral activity.

In addition to the direct inhibition of virus replication, IFNγ and IFNα/β enhance the efficiency of the adaptive immune response by stimulating increased expression of MHC class I and II, along with the antigen processing machinery. These IFNs also activate macrophages and NK cells, promoting their antiviral activity (see below).

The importance of IFNs in vivo is underlined by the increased susceptibility of mice lacking the IFNα/β receptor to virus infection. Similarly, depletion of IFNs by specific antibody treatment also augments virus infection.

NK cells are cytotoxic for virally infected cells

Active NK cells are detected within 2 days of a virus infection. They have been identified as major effector cells against herpesviruses and, in particular, murine cytomegalovirus (MCMV). An absence or reduction of NK cell activity, as seen in beige mutant mice or following depletion with antibodies against NK1.1 and asialo GM1, correlates with an increased susceptibility to MCMV infection.

During the initial stages of infection, NK cells undergo non-specific proliferation mediated by type I IFN and interleukin-15 (IL-15). In MCMV infection there then follows:

* a selection for NK cells expressing Ly49H (an activator of NK cell function); and
* expansion following interaction with the viral protein m157 present on infected cells.

This interaction is the basis of resistance to MCMV infection in resistant mouse strains.

In susceptible mouse strains the activating Ly49H is absent and instead m157 interacts with Ly49I (an inhibitory receptor) that inhibits NK cell responses. In these mice m157 acts as a decoy protein mimicking the host inhibitory receptors, thereby favoring survival of the virus.

The MCMV NK cell model represents a paradigm of how we envisage NK cells operating in other virus infections where an inverse correlation exists between MHC class I expression and NK cell killing. This is an interesting feature because a number of viruses are now known to downregulate MHC class I expression – presumably a strategy to evade T cell recognition.

In executing the antiviral response, NK cells function by:
* mediating direct cytolysis of infected cells through a perforin–granzyme mechanism (see Chapter 10); and
* through the production of IFNγ, which protects cells from infection and activates macrophage antiviral mechanisms.

NK cells are also one of the main mediators of antibody-dependent cellular cytotoxicity (ADCC).

Macrophages act at three levels to destroy virus and virus-infected cells

Macrophages are ever present in the tissues of the body and act as a first line of defense against many pathogens. In virus infection they act at three levels to destroy virus and virus-infected cells:
* phagocytosis of virus and virus-infected cells;
* killing of virus-infected cells; and

• production of antiviral molecules such as tumor necrosis factor-α (TNFα), nitric oxide, and IFNα.

Phagocytosis of infected cells and virus complexes is part of the normal housekeeping role of macrophages at a site of infection.

As with many pathogens the phagolysosome represents a hostile environment for viruses in which oxygen-dependent and oxygen-independent destructive mechanisms prevail. The induction of nitric oxide synthetase and the generation of nitric oxide is a potent inhibitor of herpesvirus and poxvirus infection.

DC2 dendritic cells produce IFNα in herpesvirus and influenza virus infection

A major producer of IFNα in herpesvirus and influenza virus infection is the macrophage-like plasmacytoid-derived DC2 dendritic cell. In influenza virus infection DC2 dendritic cells make large amounts of interferon following the endosomal recognition of viral RNA.

Q. How can macrophages recognize dsRNA?

A. Toll-like receptor-3 (TLR-3) (and TLR-7) recognizes dsRNA (see Fig. 6.23). These cells, along with type I IFN production from infected cells, act as major coordinators of innate immune responses during the early stages of a virus infection. This network is summarized in Fig. 13.2.

AS A VIRAL INFECTION PROCEEDS THE ADAPTIVE (SPECIFIC) IMMUNE RESPONSE UNFOLDS

An absence of T cells renders the host highly susceptible to virus attack. For example, cutaneous infection of congenital athymic 'nude' mice (which lack mature T cells) with herpes simplex virus (HSV) results in a spreading lesion – the virus eventually travels to the central nervous system, resulting in death of the animal.

The transfer of HSV-specific T cells shortly after infection is sufficient to protect the mice.

Antibodies and complement can limit viral spread or reinfection
Antibodies can neutralize the infectivity of viruses

As a viral infection proceeds, the adaptive (specific) immune response unfolds, with the appearance of:
• cytotoxic T lymphocytes (CTLs);
• helper T (TH) cells; and
• antiviral antibodies.

Antibodies provide a major barrier to virus spread between cells and tissues and are particularly important in restricting virus spread in the blood stream. IgA production becomes focused at mucosal surfaces where it serves to prevent reinfection.

An alternative mechanism of IgA-mediated neutralization occurs intracellularly as IgA passes from the luminal to the apical surface. During this transcytosis vesicles containing IgA interact with those containing virus, leading to neutralization.

Antibodies may be generated against any viral protein in the infected cell.

Q. Which proteins are likely to be the most important targets of antibody-mediated defenses?

A. Only antibodies directed against glycoproteins that are expressed on the virion envelope or on the infected cell membrane are of importance in controlling infection.

Antibody-mediated immunity can be achieved in a number of ways, involving quite diverse mechanisms.

Defense against free virus particles involves neutralization of infectivity, which can occur in various ways (Fig. 13.3). Such mechanisms are likely to operate in vivo because injection of neutralizing monoclonal antibodies is highly effective at inhibiting virus replication. Clearly the

Interferon activates NK cells and macrophages

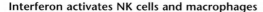
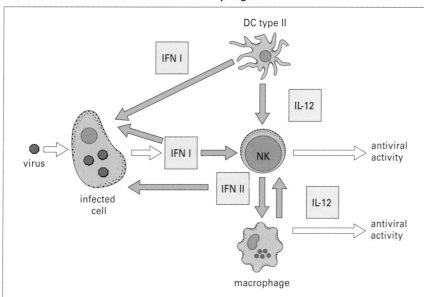

Fig. 13.2 Interferon (IFN) has an important role in orchestrating innate antiviral defenses. (DC type II, plasmacytoid-derived DC2 dendritic cell; IFN I, type I IFN; IFN II, type II IFN)

Antiviral effects of antibody

target	agent	mechanism
free virus	antibody alone	blocks binding to cell blocks entry into cell blocks uncoating of virus
	antibody + complement	damage to virus envelope blockade of virus receptor
virus-infected cells	antibody + complement	lysis of infected cell opsonization of coated virus or infected cells for phagocytosis
	antibody bound to infected cells	ADCC by NK cells, macrophages, and neutrophils
ADCC, antibody-dependent cellular cytotoxicity		

Fig. 13.3 Antibody acts to neutralize virus or kill virally infected cells.

presence of circulating virus-neutralizing antibodies is an important factor in the prevention of reinfection.

Complement is involved in the neutralization of some free viruses

Complement can also damage the virion envelope, a process known as **virolysis**, and some viruses can directly activate the classical and alternative complement pathways. However, complement is not considered to be a major factor in the defense against viruses because individuals with complement deficiencies are not predisposed to severe viral infection.

This should be contrasted with those herpesviruses and poxviruses that carry viral homologs of complement regulatory proteins (CD46, CD55) which regulate complement activation. Presumably these viruses perceive complement to be a threat.

Antibodies mobilize complement and/or effector cells to destroy virus-infected cells

Antibodies are also effective in mediating the destruction of virus-infected cells. This can occur by antibody-mediated activation of the complement system, leading to the assembly of the membrane attack complex and lysis of the infected cell (see Chapter 4). This process requires a high density of viral antigens on the membrane (about 5×10^6/cell) to be effective. In contrast, ADCC mediated by NK cells can recognize as few as 10^3 IgG molecules in order to bind and kill the infected cell.

Q. **How can NK cells use antibody to recognize and destroy virus-infected cells?**

A. The IgG-coated target cells are bound using the NK cell's FcγRIII (CD16; see Chapter 3), and are rapidly destroyed by a perforin-dependent killing mechanism (see Figs 10.1 and 10.12).

Just how important these mechanisms for destroying virus-infected cells are in vivo is difficult to resolve. The best evidence in favor of ADCC comes from studying the protective effect of non-neutralizing monoclonal antibodies in mice. Although these antibodies fail to neutralize virus in vivo, they can protect C5-deficient mice from a high-dose virus challenge. (C5-deficient mice are used in this study to eliminate the role of the late complement components.)

T cells mediate viral immunity in several ways

T cells exhibit a variety of functions in antiviral immunity:
- most of the antibody response is T-dependent, requiring the presence of CD4+ T cells for class switching and affinity maturation;
- CD4+ T cells also help in the induction of CD8+ CTLs and in the recruitment and activation of macrophages at sites of virus infection;
- CD8+ T cells are effective in the prevention of reinfection (following vaccination) by viruses such as influenza virus and respiratory syncytial virus – however, even memory T cells need time to evolve a response to a reinfection virus, and therefore antibodies assume a more dominant role by neutralizing incoming virus and containing the infection by preventing spread to other tissues (see above).

Q. **How do CD4+ T cells help induce and recruit CD8+ T cells?**

A. Cytokines, including IL-2 released by CD4+ T cells, are required for division of CD8+ T cells. CD4+ T cells can recruit CD8+ T cells to sites of infection by the release of chemokines.

CD8+ CTLs destroy virus-infected cells

The principal T cell surveillance system operating against viruses is highly efficient and selective. MHC class I-restricted CD8+ CTLs cells focus at the site of virus replication and destroy virus-infected cells.

CD8+ T cells:
- not only kill infected cells through the release of perforin and granzymes or through Fas–FasL interactions; but

- can 'cure' some types of persistent virus infection (e.g. hepatitis B virus) involving the release of IFNγ and/or TNF, resulting in clearance of the virus without death of the cell.

Virtually all cells in the body express MHC class I molecules, making this an important mechanism for identifying and eliminating or curing virus-infected cells.

Because of the central role played by MHC class I in targeting CD8+ T cells to infected cells, some viruses have evolved elaborate strategies to disrupt MHC class I expression, thereby interfering with T cell recognition and favoring virus persistence (see below).

Virtually any viral protein can be processed in the cytoplasm to generate peptides, which are then transported to the endoplasmic reticulum where they interact with MHC class I molecules.

Q. Why might it be advantageous to the host to present viral peptides that are produced early in the replication cycle, and which may not be part of the assembled virus?

A. Viral proteins expressed early in the replication cycle can be targeted on infected cells, enabling T cell recognition to occur long before new viral progeny are produced. For example, CD8+ T cell-mediated immunity against murine cytomegalovirus (CMV) is mediated predominantly by immediate early protein pp89 (80–90% of the T cell response is directed against pp89). The epitope has been identified as a nonamer peptide presented by the MHC class I molecule L^d. Immunization of mice with a recombinant vaccinia virus containing pp89 is sufficient to confer complete protection from murine CMV-induced disease; deletion of the DNA sequence encoding the nonapeptide abolishes the protective effect of the protein.

The importance of T cell mechanisms in vivo has been identified using various techniques:

- the adoptive transfer of specific T cell subpopulations or T cell clones to infected animals and monitoring of viral clearance;
- depletion of T cell populations in vivo using monoclonal antibodies to CD4 or CD8;
- creation of 'gene knockout' mice, in which genes encoding cell surface receptors (CD8, CD4), transcription factors (T-bet), and signal transduction molecules (STAT) are removed from the germline.

The continued ability of knockout mice that lack particular lymphocyte populations to mount a response against virus infections is a good illustration of the redundancy that can occur in the immune system. For example, in the absence of CD8+ T cells, CD4+ T cells or other mechanisms are able to compensate and bring the infection under control.

CD4+ T cells are a major effector cell population in the response to many virus infections

CD4+ T cells have now been identified as a major effector cell population in the immune response to many virus infections. A good example is in HSV-1 infection of epithelial surfaces. In this instance recruitment of macrophages occurs in delayed-type hypersensitivity (see Chapter 26), resulting in an accelerated clearance of virus. Macrophages are an important component in this process,

inhibiting virus infection probably through the generation and action of nitric oxide (Fig. 13.4). Key cytokines in this response include IFNγ, important in the activation of monocytes, and tumour necrosis factor (TNFα).

TNFα has several antiviral activities, including the induction of intracellular interferon defense mechanisms and apoptotic cell death following interaction with the apoptotic TNF receptor.

In measles virus and Epstein–Barr virus (EBV) infection, CD4+ CTLs are generated that recognize and kill MHC class II-positive cells infected with the virus. This suggests that measles virus and EBV peptides are generated by normal pathways of antigen presentation (i.e. following phagocytosis and degradation, see Chapter 7). However, other pathways have been implicated in which some measles proteins/peptides enter class II vesicles from the cytosol.

A summary of antiviral defense mechanisms is illustrated in Fig. 13.5, and the kinetics of their induction is shown in Fig. 13.6.

Resistance to cutaneous HSV infection

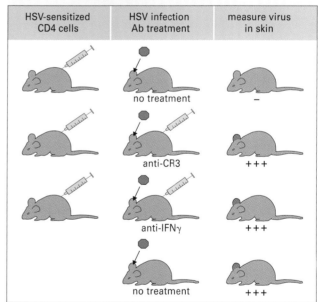

HSV-sensitized CD4 cells	HSV infection Ab treatment	measure virus in skin
	no treatment	–
	anti-CR3	+++
	anti-IFNγ	+++
	no treatment	+++

Fig. 13.4 CD4+ T cells, macrophages, and IFNγ all have a protective role in cutaneous infections with HSV-1. CD4+ T cells were obtained from mice infected with HSV-1 8 days previously. The cells were transferred to syngeneic mice infected with HSV-1 in the skin. These mice were treated with anti-CR3 (to block macrophage migration to the site of infection), or anti-IFNγ (to block the activation of macrophages), or were untreated. An additional control group was infected, but did not receive CD4+ T cells. The amount of infectious virus remaining after 5 days was then determined. The results demonstrate that the protective effects of CD4+ T cells are mediated by macrophages and IFNγ.

Effector mechanisms against virus and virus-infected cells

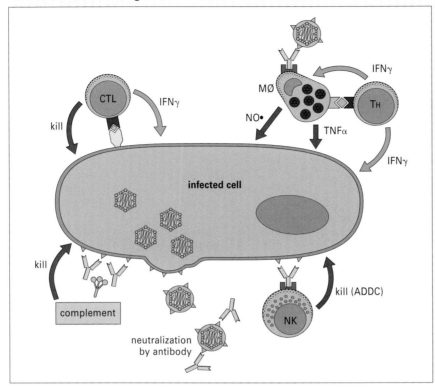

Fig. 13.5 Entry of virus at mucosal surfaces is inhibited by IgA. Following the initial infection, the virus may spread to other tissues via the blood stream. Interferons produced by the innate (IFNα and IFNβ) and adaptive (IFNγ) immune responses make neighboring cells resistant to virus infection. Antibodies are important in controlling free virus, whereas T cells and NK cells are effective at killing infected cells.

Response to a typical acute virus infection

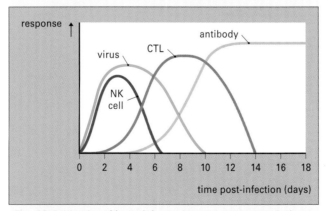

Fig. 13.6 Kinetics of host defenses in response to a typical acute virus infection. Following an acute virus infection (e.g. by influenza or herpes virus), NK cells and interferon are detected in the blood stream and locally in infected tissues. CTLs then become activated in local lymph nodes or spleen, followed by the appearance of neutralizing antibodies in serum. Although activated T cells are absent by the second to third week, T cell memory is established and may last for many years.

VIRUSES HAVE EVOLVED VARIOUS STRATEGIES TO EVADE RECOGNITION BY ANTIBODY AND T CELLS

Virus latency and antigenic variation are the most effective mechanisms

Antigenic variation involves mutating regions on proteins that are normally targeted by antibody and T cells. Antigenic variation is seen in human immunodeficiency virus (HIV) and in foot and mouth disease virus, and is responsible for the antigenic shift and drift seen with influenza virus (Fig. 13.7). Humoral immunity to such diseases lasts only until the new virus strain emerges, making effective longlasting vaccinations difficult to produce.

In HIV infection, sequence changes (mutations) can arise in those viral peptides that bind to MHC class I molecules to which the initial T cell response arose. This results in a failure of T cell surveillance and the emergence of new pathogenic variant viruses.

All viruses trigger an interferon response and consequently most viruses have evolved a strategy for disrupting the interferon system. This occurs at three levels:

- disruption of PKR or 2′,5′-oligoadenylate synthetase activity (adenovirus and herpesviruses);
- production of soluble interferon receptors (pox viruses); and
- interference with interferon signaling (paramyxoviruses).

Antigenic shift in influenza virus

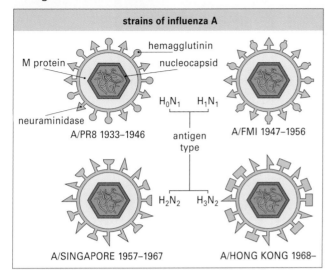

Fig. 13.7 The major surface antigens of influenza virus are hemagglutinin and neuraminidase. Hemagglutinin is involved in attachment to cells, and antibodies to hemagglutinin are protective. Antibodies to neuraminidase are much less effective. The influenza virus can change its antigenic properties slightly (antigenic drift) or radically (antigenic shift). Alterations in the structure of the hemagglutinin antigen render earlier antibodies ineffective and new virus epidemics therefore break out. The diagram shows strains that have emerged by antigenic shift since 1933. The official influenza antigen nomenclature is based on the type of hemagglutinin (H_1, H_2, etc.) and neuraminidase (N_1, N_2, etc.) expressed on the surface of the virion. Note that, although new strains replace old strains, the internal antigens remain largely unchanged.

Viruses also:
- encode other cytokine homologs such as vIL-10 and vIL-6 (herpesviruses); as well as
- receptors to interfere with TNF function.

Q. From this observation, what can you infer about an effective immune response to herpesviruses?

A. The vIL-10 will deviate the immune response, inhibiting a T_H1-type reaction with macrophage activation. One can therefore infer that this type of immune response is the key to anti-herpes immunity and the type of response the viruses aims to deflect.

Chemokines represent an important traffic-light system for cell migration and viruses have evolved elaborate strategies for disrupting the chemokine network. The herpesviruses encode:
- chemokine homologs (e.g. CCL3);
- chemokine receptor homologs; and
- chemokine-binding proteins, which have powerful effects on delaying or inhibiting cell migration during inflammation.

Additionally herpes and pox viruses encode homologs not only for CD46 and CD55 – complement regulatory proteins that block C3 activation – but also for CD59.

HIV makes use of cellular CD59, which is incorporated in the viral envelope, thereby blocking complement-mediated lysis of the virion.

Many DNA viruses have strategies to control the expression of MHC molecules

MHC class I expression can be disrupted by:
- blocking peptide uptake into the endoplasmic reticulum (e.g. HSV-1); and
- preventing maturation assembly and migration of the trimolecular MHC complex (e.g. human CMV).

Similar mechanisms apply for MHC class II molecules where:
- some herpesviruses block transcription; whereas
- other mechanisms involve premature targeting of MHC class II for degradation.

Downregulation of MHC class I may disrupt CD8$^+$ T cell recognition, but NK cells are more efficient killers in the absence of MHC class I. Human and murine CMV have tried to redress the balance by encoding their own MHC class I homolog, which is expressed on infected cells and can inhibit NK cell activation.

Examples of virus-encoded homologs of the host defense system are shown in Fig. 13.8.

RESPONSES TO VIRAL ANTIGENS CAN CAUSE TISSUE DAMAGE
Damage may result from the formation of immune complexes

Immune complexes may arise in body fluids or on cell surfaces and are most common during persistent or chronic infections (e.g. with LCMV or hepatitis B virus). Antibody is ineffective (non-neutralizing) in the presence of large amounts of the viral antigen; instead, immune complexes form and are deposited in the kidney or in blood vessels, where they evoke inflammatory responses leading to tissue damage (e.g. as in glomerulonephritis, see Chapter 25).

An unusual pathological consequence of some virus interactions with weakly neutralizing antibody is **antibody-dependent enhancement of virus infection (ADE)**. This involves Fc receptor-mediated uptake of antibody–virus complexes by macrophages and subsequent enhancement of virus infectivity. This is seen in many persistent or viremic virus infections where the common target for replication is the macrophage. An example is Dengue virus infection where cross-reactive antibodies from different Dengue virus subtypes can result in ADE with the consequence of initiating:
- Dengue hemorrhagic fever; and
- Dengue shock syndrome, which results in excessive procoagulant release by monocytes.

CTL responses can cause severe tissue damage

In any virus infection some tissue damage is likely to arise from the activity of infiltrating T cells. However, in some situations this damage may be considerable, resulting in

Examples of viral products that interfere with host defenses

host defense affected	virus	virus product	mechanism
IFN	EBV	EBERS (small RNAs)	blocks protein kinase R activation
	vaccinia	IFNα/β receptor homolog	secreted and binds to IFNα/β
	SV5 – paramyxovirus	V protein	targets STAT-1 degradation
complement	KSHV	ORF-4-RCA homolog	inhibition of C3 activation
	HVS	CD59 homolog	inhibits formation of membrane attack complex
cytokines	EBV	IL-10 homolog	interferes with IFNγ function
	coxpox	TNF receptor homolog	secreted, binds TNF
chemokines	KSHV	MIP-1 homolog	CCR8 agonist and attracts TH2 cells
	HCMV	US29-CK receptor homolog	binds CC CK, mediates cell migration
	MHV-68	M3-CK binding protein	binds C, CC, CXC, CX3C CK blocks cell migration
MHC	adenovirus	E3	blocks transport of MHC class I to surface
	HSV	ICP-47	stops peptide binding to TAP
	HIV	Nef protein	interferes with MHC class II processing
apoptosis	MHV-68	Bcl-2 homolog	inhibits apoptosis
NK cells	HCMV	UL18-MHC class I homolog	inhibits NK cell lysis

Fig. 13.8 Viruses use diverse strategies to outwit host defenses. (CC, chemokine; CXCR and CCR, chemokine receptors; CK, chemokine; HCMV, human cytomegalovirus; HVS, herpesvirus Saimiri; KSHV, Kaposi's sarcoma-associated herpesvirus; MHV-68, murine gammaherpesvirus)

the death of the animal. The best example of this is the CTL responses to LCMV in the central nervous system (Fig. 13.9). Removal of T cells protects the animal from death, indicating that they, rather than the virus, are damaging the brain.

A similar mechanism has been postulated for chronic active hepatitis in humans, whereby CTLs target hepatitis B virus-infected cells and may also participate in a non-viral autoimmune disease.

Viruses can infect cells of the immune system

Some viruses (e.g. HIV) directly infect lymphocytes or macrophages, resulting in pathogenic effects.

Immunocompetent cells are also favored sites of virus persistence. To facilitate persistence in cells of the lymphoid system, some herpesviruses carry a Bcl-2 homolog.

Q. Where have you encountered Bcl-2 previously, and what effect does it have on lymphocytes?

A. Bcl-2 is induced in germinal center B cells and is required to protect the cell from apoptosis (see Fig. 8.12).

In this case the Bcl-2 homolog also prevents apoptosis thereby preserving the life of the infected cell and favoring virus persistence/latency (see above). In the resting state, leukocytes harbor the virus in a non-infectious form, but on activation of the infected cells the virus may also be reactivated to produce infectious virus particles. Example of viruses infecting B cells, T cells, and macrophages are shown in Fig. 13.10.

HIV infects CD4+ cells

Many of the points raised above are illustrated by HIV, the retrovirus that causes AIDS. Infection with HIV is characterized by:

- prolonged clinical latency;
- ineffective immunity;
- continuous virus mutation;
- neuropathology; and
- a tendency to infect bone marrow-derived cells and lymphocytes (see Chapter 19).

HIV is taken up by CD4+ T cells and macrophages following binding of a viral glycoprotein (gp120) to CD4 and certain chemokine receptors (CXCR4 and CCR5). It also enters other antigen-presenting cells by this route. However, entry into cells bearing Fc and complement

Lymphocytic choriomeningitis virus infection (LCMV) in mice

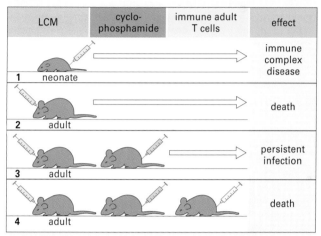

Fig. 13.9 The different effects of LCMV are related to differences in immune status. Infection of neonatal mice (1) produces chronic virus shedding and immune complex disease, manifesting itself as glomerulonephritis and vasculitis. Intracerebral infection of adult mice (2) results in death. This is due to a T cell reaction because suppression of immunity with cyclophosphamide (3) leads to persistent infection, but prevents death. This 'protective' effect produced by cyclophosphamide can be reversed by T cells from an immune animal (4).

Virus infection of immunocompetent cells

B lymphocytes	Epstein–Barr virus murine gammaherpesvirus infectious bursal disease virus
T lymphocytes	human T lymphotropic virus types 1 and 2 HIV measles virus herpesvirus Saimiri human herpesvirus 6
macrophages	Visna virus HIV lactate dehydrogenase virus cytomegalovirus

Fig. 13.10 Some viruses persist indefinitely in immunocompetent cells. Periodically, this infection may lead to pathological consequences, involving the death of the cell (HIV) or transformation leading to neoplasia (Epstein–Barr virus, HTLV-1).

receptors can be enhanced by antibody (ADE), suggesting that this provides an alternative route into phagocytic cells or enhances entry when CD4 is scarce.

There is a long but variable period of clinical latency, and in about 50% of patients progression to AIDS does not occur for 10 years. During this latent period, HIV can exist as a provirus, integrated within the host's genomic DNA, without any transcription occurring.

Numerous factors can lead to the activation of transcription. In vitro both TNF and IL-6 cause increased production of infectious virus from latently infected T cell lines. This may be important in vivo because monocytes from individuals carrying HIV tend to release abnormally large quantities of these cytokines. It is possible that there is a cycle of TNF and IL-6 release leading to enhanced virus transcription (Fig. 13.11). This could lead to infection of further cells, and release of more cytokine. Production is increased in vitro by other cytokines and lymphokines, and by mitogens and phorbol esters.

Elimination of the HIV virus does not occur for a variety of reasons, including:
- latency;
- viral mutation (giving rapid antigenic drift); and
- progressive immunodeficiency.

Viral infection may provoke autoimmunity

Viruses may trigger autoimmune disease in a number of ways, as follows.
- Virus-induced damage – during the course of some virus infections tissues become damaged, provoking an inflammatory response during which 'hidden' antigens become exposed and can be processed and presented to the immune system. Examples of this include Theiler's virus (a murine picornavirus) and murine hepatitis virus infection of the nervous system, in which the constituents of myelin (the insulating material of axons) become targets for antibody and T cells.

Infection of lymphocytes and macrophages by HIV

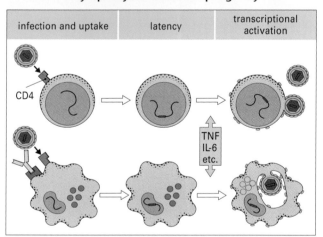

Fig. 13.11 The gp120 on the surface of HIV virions binds to CD4 and chemokine receptors on the lymphocyte membrane, and this triggers uptake. The virus can enter macrophages, which express relatively low levels of CD4, but this may be assisted by binding through antibody to Fc receptors. The virus remains latent, integrated in the host cell's genomic DNA, until some stimulus (e.g. cytokines) causes transcriptional activation. Assembled viruses bud from the outer membrane of T cells or into intracytoplasmic vacuoles of macrophages, where a large reservoir of potentially infectious particles can accumulate.

- Molecular mimicry – a sequence in a viral protein that is homologous to a 'self' protein can become recognized, leading to a breakdown in immunological tolerance to cryptic self antigens in the consequent attack on host tissues by the immune system (see Chapter 26). A good example is Coxsackie B virus-induced myocarditis. Patients with inflammatory cardiomyopathy have antibodies that cross-react with peptides derived from coxsackie B3 protein and with peptides derived from cellular adenine nucleotide translocator.

FURTHER READING

Alcami A, Koszinowski UH. Viral mechanisms of immune evasion. Immunol Today 2000;21:36–50.

Arase H, Mocarski ES, Campbell AE, et al. Direct recognition of cytomegalovirus by activating and inhibitory NK cell receptors. Science 2002;296:1323–1326.

Biron CA, Nguyen KB, Pien GC, et al. Natural killer cells in antiviral defence: function and regulation by innate cytokines. Annu Rev Immunol 1999;17:189–220.

Clements JE, Gidovin SL, Montelaro RC, et al. Antigenic variation in lentiviral disease. Annu Rev Immunol 1988;6:139–159.

Doherty PC, Allan W, Eichelberger M, et al. Roles of α/β and γ/δ T cell subsets in viral immunity. Annu Rev Immunol 1992;10:123–151.

Douek DC, Picker LJ, Koup RA. T cell dynamics in HIV-1 infection. Annu Rev Immunol 2003;21:265–304.

Goodbourn S, Didcock L, Randall RE. Interferons: cell signaling, immune modulation, antiviral responses and virus counter measures. J Gen Virol 2000;81:2341–2364.

Guidotti LG, Chisari FV. Noncytolytic control of viral infections by the innate and adaptive immune response. Annu Rev Immunol 2001;19:65–91.

Klasse PJ, Sattentau QJ. Occupancy and mechanism in antibody-mediated neutralization of animal viruses. J Gen Virol 2002;83:2091–2108

Koszinowski UH, del Val M, Reddehasse MJ. Cellular and molecular basis of the protective immune response to cytomegalovirus infection. Curr Top Microbiol Immunol 1990:154:189–220.

Levy JA. Pathogenesis of human immunodeficiency virus infection. Microbiol Rev 1993;57:183–289.

McMichael A. How viruses hide from T cells. Trends Microbiol 1997;5:211–214.

Mims CA. Interactions of viruses with the immune system. Clin Exp Immunol 1986;66:1–16.

Nash AA, Cambouropoulos P. The immune response to herpes simplex virus. Semin Virol 1993;4:181–186.

Schwimmbeck PL, Fitzgerald NA, Schulze K, et al The humoral immune response in viral heart disease: characterization and pathophysiological significance of antibodies. Med Microbiol Immunol (Berl) 2004;193:115–119.

Tirado SMC, Yoon K-J. Antibody-dependent enhancement of virus infection and disease. Virol Immunol 2003;16:69–86.

Tortorella D, Gewurz BE, Furman MH, et al. Viral subversion of the immune system. Annu Rev Immunol 2000;18:861–926.

Critical thinking: Virus–immune system interactions (see p. 496 for explanations)

1 What are the features of a virus that enable it to evade host defense mechanisms?

A series of IgG monoclonal antibodies were developed against glycoprotein D of herpes simplex virus. When tested in vitro for virus neutralizing activity the antibodies could be divided into two groups: those capable of neutralizing virus infectivity and non-neutralizing antibodies. However, when individual neutralizing or non-neutralizing antibodies were injected into mice infected with herpes simplex virus, both sets of antibodies protected the animals from an overwhelming infection.

2 How do you explain the protection achieved by the non-neutralizing monoclonal antibodies?

3 What experiments would you propose to support some of your conclusions?

Immunity to Bacteria and Fungi

SUMMARY

- **Mechanisms of protection from bacteria can be deduced from their structure and pathogenicity.** There are four main types of bacterial cell wall and pathogenicity varies between two extreme patterns. Non-specific, phylogenetically ancient recognition pathways for conserved bacterial structures trigger protective innate immune responses and guide the development of adaptive immunity.

- **Lymphocyte-independent bacterial recognition pathways have several consequences.** Complement is activated via the alternative pathway. Release of proinflammatory cytokines increases the adhesive properties of the vascular endothelium. Pathogen recognition generates signals that regulate the lymphocyte-mediated response.

- **Antibody provides an antigen-specific protective mechanism.** Neutralizing antibody may be all that is needed for protection if the organism is pathogenic only because of a single toxin or adhesion molecule. Opsonizing antibody responses are particularly important for resistance to extracellular bacterial pathogens. Complement can kill some bacteria, particularly those with an exposed outer lipid bilayer, such as Gram-negative bacteria.

- **Ultimately most bacteria are killed by phagocytes** following a multistage process of chemotaxis, attachment, uptake, and killing. Macrophage killing can be enhanced on activation. Optimal activation of macrophages is dependent on TH1 CD4 T cells. Persistent macrophage recruitment and activation can result in granuloma formation, which is a hallmark of cell-mediated immunity to intracellular bacteria.

- **Successful pathogens have evolved mechanisms to avoid phagocyte-mediated killing** and have evolved a startling diversity of mechanisms for avoiding other aspects of innate and adaptive immunity.

- **Infected cells can be killed by CTLs.** Other T cell populations and some tissue cells can contribute to antibacterial immunity.

- **The response to bacteria can result in immunological tissue damage.** Excessive release of cytokines caused by microorganisms can result in immunopathological syndromes, such as endotoxin shock and the Schwartzman reaction.

- **Fungi can cause life-threatening infections.** Immunity to fungi is predominantly cell mediated and shares many similarities with immunity to bacteria.

MECHANISMS OF PROTECTION FROM BACTERIA CAN BE DEDUCED FROM THEIR STRUCTURE AND PATHOGENICITY

Bacterial infections have had an enormous impact on human society and despite the discovery of antibiotics continue to be a major threat to public health.

Plague caused by *Yersinia pestis* is estimated to have killed one-quarter of the European population in the Middle Ages, whereas infection with *Mycobacterium tuberculosis* is currently a global health emergency.

The immune defense mechanisms elicited against pathogenic bacteria are determined by their:
- surface chemistry;
- mechanism(s) of pathogenicity; and
- whether they are predominantly extracellular or also have the ability to survive inside mammalian cells.

There are four main types of bacterial cell wall

The four main types of bacterial cell wall (Fig. 14.1) belong to the following groups.
- Gram-positive bacteria;
- Gram-negative bacteria;
- mycobacteria;
- spirochetes.

The outer lipid bilayer of Gram-negative organisms is of particular importance because it is often susceptible to lysis by complement. However, killing of most bacteria usually requires uptake by phagocytes. The outer surface of the bacterium may also contain fimbriae or flagellae, or it may be covered by a protective capsule. These can impede the functions of phagocytes or complement, but they also act as targets for the antibody response, the role of which is discussed later.

Bacterial cell walls

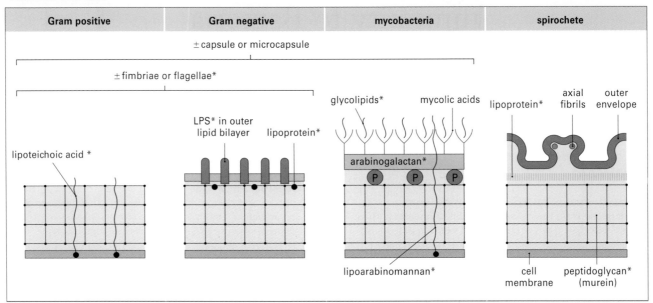

Fig. 14.1 Different immunological mechanisms have evolved to destroy the cell wall structure of the different groups of bacteria. All types have an inner cell membrane and a peptidoglycan wall. Gram-negative bacteria also have an outer lipid bilayer in which lipopolysaccharide (LPS) is embedded. Lysosomal enzymes and lysozyme are active against the peptidoglycan layer, whereas cationic proteins and complement are effective against the outer lipid bilayer of the Gram-negative bacteria. The compound cell wall of mycobacteria is extremely resistant to breakdown, and it is likely that this can be achieved only with the assistance of the bacterial enzymes working from within. Some bacteria also have fimbriae or flagellae, which can provide targets for the antibody response. Others have an outer capsule, which renders the organisms more resistant to phagocytosis or to complement. The components indicated with an asterisk (*) are recognized by the innate immune system as a non-specific 'danger' signal that selectively boosts some aspects of immune activity. (Gram staining is a method that exploits the fact that crystal violet and iodine form a complex that is more abundant on Gram-positive bacteria. The complex easily elutes from Gram-negative bacteria.)

Pathogenicity varies between two extreme patterns

The two extreme patterns of pathogenicity are:
- toxicity without invasiveness;
- invasiveness without toxicity (Fig. 14.2).

However, most bacteria are intermediate between these extremes, having some invasiveness assisted by some locally acting toxins and spreading factors (tissue-degrading enzymes).

Corynebacterium diphtheriae and *Vibrio cholerae* are examples of organisms that are toxic, but not invasive. Because their pathogenicity depends almost entirely on toxin production, neutralizing antibody to the toxin is probably sufficient for immunity, though antibody binding to the bacteria and so blocking their adhesion to the epithelium could also be important.

In contrast, the pathogenicity of most invasive organisms does not rely so heavily on a single toxin, so immunity requires killing of the organisms themselves.

The first lines of defense do not depend on antigen recognition

The body's first line of defense against pathogenic bacteria consists of simple barriers to the entry or establishment of the infection. Thus, the skin and exposed epithelial surfaces have non-specific or innate protective systems, which limit the entry of potentially invasive organisms (see Fig. 1.2).

Intact skin is impenetrable to most bacteria. Additionally, fatty acids produced by the skin are toxic to many organisms. Indeed, the pathogenicity of some strains correlates with their ability to survive on the skin. Epithelial surfaces are cleansed, for example, by ciliary action in the trachea or by flushing of the urinary tract.

Many bacteria are destroyed by pH changes in the stomach and vagina, both of which provide an acidic environment. In the vagina, the epithelium secretes glycogen, which is metabolized by particular species of commensal bacteria, producing lactic acid.

Commensals can limit pathogen invasion

Commensals can limit pathogen invasion through the production of antibacterial proteins termed **colicins**. Commensals may therefore occupy an ecological niche that would otherwise be occupied by something more unpleasant.

When the normal flora are disturbed by antibiotics, infections by *Candida* spp. or *Clostridium difficile* can occur,

Mechanisms of immunopathogenicity

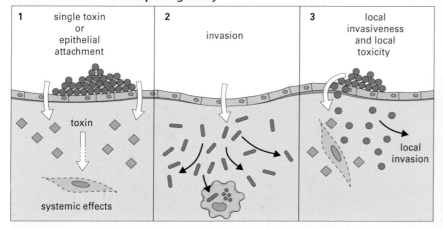

Fig. 14.2 (**1**) Some bacteria cause disease as a result of only a single toxin (e.g. *Corynebacterium diphtheriae, Clostridium tetani*) or because of an ability to attach to epithelial surfaces (e.g. in group A streptococcal sore throat). Immunity to such organisms may require only antibody to neutralize this critical function. (**2**) At the other extreme there are organisms that are not toxic, and cause disease by invasion of tissues and sometimes cells, where damage results mostly from the bulk of organisms or from immunopathology (e.g. lepromatous leprosy). Where organisms invade cells, they must be destroyed and degraded by the cell-mediated immune response. (**3**) Most organisms fall between the two extremes, with some local invasiveness assisted by local toxicity and enzymes that degrade extracellular matrix (e.g. *Staphylococcus aureus, Clostridium perfringens*). Antibody and cell-mediated responses are both involved in resistance.

and the latter is a major cause of antibiotic-induced colitis and diarrhea.

Several studies suggest that the reintroduction of non-pathogenic 'probiotic' organisms such as lactobacilli into the intestinal tract can alleviate the symptoms, presumably by replacing those killed by the antibiotics.

In practice, only a minute proportion of the potentially pathogenic organisms around us ever succeed in gaining access to the tissues.

The second line of defense is mediated by recognition of bacterial components

If organisms do enter the tissues, they can be combated initially by further elements of the innate immune system.

Numerous bacterial components are recognized in ways that do not rely on the antigen-specific receptors of either B cells or T cells. These types of recognition are phylogenetically ancient 'broad-spectrum' mechanisms that evolved before antigen-specific T cells and immunoglobulins, allowing protective responses to be triggered by common microbial components bearing so-called **'pathogen-associated molecular patterns' (PAMPs)**. The host molecules that recognize these microbial components are referred to as the **'pattern recognition molecules'** of the innate immune system.

Q. List some examples of soluble molecules, cell surface receptors, and intracellular molecules that recognize PAMPs.

A. Collectins and ficolins (see Fig. 6.23), the Toll-like receptors (see Fig. 6.24), the mannose receptor (see Fig. 9.18), and the NOD proteins (see Fig. 9.24) all recognize PAMPs.

Many organisms, such as non-pathogenic cocci, are probably removed from the tissues as a consequence of these pathways, without the need for a specific adaptive immune reaction. Fig. 14.3 shows some of the microbial components involved and the host responses that are triggered.

The immune system has selected these structures for recognition because they are not only characteristic of microbes, but are essential for their growth and cannot be easily mutated to evade discovery (though, as might be predicted, there are increasing examples of pathogen strategies that attempt to subvert this process).

It is interesting to note that the 'Limulus assay', which is used to detect contaminating lipopolysaccharide (LPS) in preparations for use in humans, is based on one such recognition pathway found in an invertebrate species. In *Limulus polyphemus* (the horseshoe crab), tiny quantities of LPS trigger fibrin formation, which walls off the LPS-bearing infectious agent.

Bacterial PAMPs activate cells via Toll-like receptors

Many bacterial PAMPs activate cells via Toll-like receptors (TLRs). These are homologs of a receptor mediating antimicrobial immune responses in the fruit fly (*Drosophila* spp.).

The TLR family is made up of at least ten different TLR molecules which differ in the microbial structures they recognize. The most prominent TLRs involved in recognition of bacterial components are TLR1, 2, 4, 5, 6, and 9 (see below).

TLRs are preferentially expressed on phagocytes, dendritic cells, and epithelial cells at sites of bacterial entry

Protective mechanisms not involving antigen-specific B or T cells

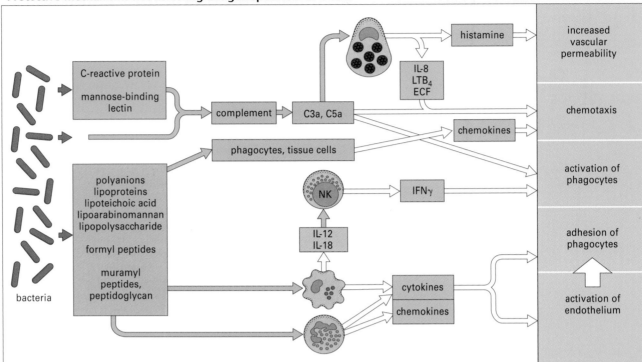

Fig. 14.3 Several common bacterial PAMPs are recognized by molecules present in serum and by receptors on cells. These recognition pathways result in activation of the alternative complement pathway (factors C3, B, D, P), with consequent release of C3a and C5a; activation of neutrophils, macrophages, and NK cells; triggering of cytokine and chemokine release; mast cell degranulation, leading to increased blood flow in the local capillary network; and increased adhesion of cells and fibrin to endothelial cells. These mechanisms, plus tissue injury caused by the bacteria, may activate the clotting system and fibrin formation, which limit bacterial spread.

to the host. Each cell type can express a different combination of receptors and this repertoire can be altered by inflammatory stimuli, allowing the greatest possible recognition coverage to a diverse range of pathogens.

Other important pattern recognition receptors include:
- the mannose receptor; and
- scavenger receptors.

Of course, recognition of bacteria also occurs in the absence of cells via:
- complement;
- C-reactive protein (CRP);
- mannose-binding lectin in the blood;
- surfactant protein A in the lungs.

LPS is the dominant activator of innate immunity in Gram-negative bacteria

Injection of pure LPS into mice or even humans is sufficient to mimic most of the features of acute Gram-negative infection, including massive production of proinflammatory cytokines, such as interleukin-1 (IL-1), IL-6, and tumor necrosis factor (TNF), leading to severe shock.

Q. How does release of proinflammatory cytokines cause shock?

A. These proinflammatory cytokines act directly on endothelium to increase vascular adhesiveness, and indirectly activate other plasma enzyme systems to release vasoactive peptides and amines leading to a drop in blood pressure.

Recognition of LPS is a complex process involving molecules that bind LPS and pass it on to cell membrane-associated receptors on leukocytes, and endothelial and other cells, which initiate this proinflammatory cascade; these events are illustrated in Fig. 14.4.

Binding of LPS to TLR4 is a critical event in immune activation. TLR4 knockout mice are resistant to LPS-induced shock and there is some evidence that polymorphisms in human TLR4 may influence the course of infection with these bacteria.

Other bacterial components are also potent immune activators

Gram-positive bacteria do not possess LPS yet still induce intense inflammatory responses and severe infection.

Effects of lipopolysaccharide

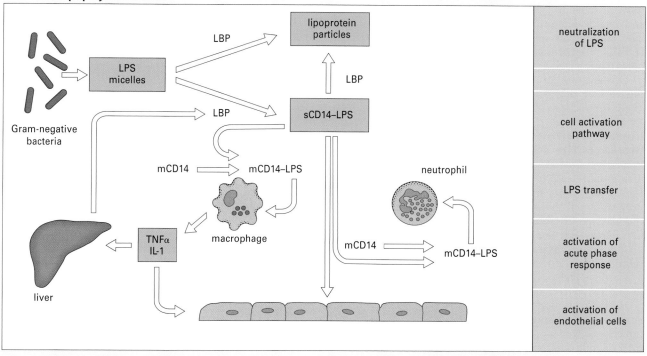

Fig. 14.4 LPS released from Gram-negative bacteria becomes bound to LPS-binding protein (LBP) which promotes transfer of LPS to either soluble CD14 (sCD14) or to a GPI-linked membrane form of the protein (mCD14) expressed on neutrophils and macrophages. LBP then dissociates and the mCD14–LPS complex, in association with Toll-like receptor 4 (TLR4) and MD2, transduces signals that cause increased expression of integrins (adhesion molecules) and increased release of many proinflammatory cytokines including TNFα and IL-1. These in turn activate endothelial cells and drive the acute phase response in the liver. One product of the acute phase response is further LBP.

Most capsular polysaccharides are not potent activators of inflammation (though some can activate macrophages) and instead attempt to shield the bacterium from host immune defenses.

Components of the cell wall, including peptidoglycans and lipoteichoic acids, are the dominant activators of innate immunity, and TLR2, often in cooperation with TLR1 or TLR6, is the major TLR involved.

The LBP and CD14, which bind LPS, are also involved in recognition of lipid-containing bacterial components from mycoplasmas, mycobacteria, and spirochetes.

Other molecules that trigger innate immunity include mycoplasma lipoproteins (via TLR 2/6), flagellin (via TLR5), and DNA (due to its distinct **CpG motifs**) via TLR9.

Most pattern recognition receptors are expressed on the plasma membrane of cells, making contact with microbes during the process of binding and/or phagocytosis.

However, others are designed to detect intracellular pathogens and their products inside phagosomes (such as TLR9) or in the cytosol.

Epithelial cells of the gut and lung have few TLRs on their luminal surface, but can be triggered by pathogens that:
- actively invade the cell (such as *Listeria* spp.);
- inject their components (such as *Helicobacter pylori*); or
- actively reach the basolateral surface (e.g. *Salmonella* spp.).

This may explain why constant exposure to non-pathogenic microbes in the intestine and airways does not induce a chronic state of inflammation – the host waits until they move beyond the lumen, signifying the presence of a real pathogenic threat.

LYMPHOCYTE-INDEPENDENT BACTERIAL RECOGNITION PATHWAYS HAVE SEVERAL CONSEQUENCES
Complement is activated via the alternative pathway
Complement activation can result in the killing of some bacteria, particularly those with an outer lipid bilayer susceptible to the **lytic complex (C5b–9)**.

Q. Which proteins can recognize pathogens in the cytosol, and which pathogen components?

A. NOD-1 and NOD-2 proteins recognize peptidoglycans of both Gram-positive and Gram-negative bacteria (see Fig. 9.24).

Q. To which strains of bacteria are individuals with C9 deficiency more susceptible?

A. *Neisseria* spp. (see Fig. 4.16).

Perhaps more importantly, complement activation releases C5a, which attracts and activates neutrophils and causes degranulation of mast cells (see Chapter 3). The consequent release of **histamine** and **leukotriene (LTB$_4$)** contributes to further increases in vascular permeability (see Fig. 14.3).

Opsonization of the bacteria, by attachment of **cleaved derivatives of C3**, is also critically important in subsequent interactions with phagocytes.

Release of proinflammatory cytokines increases the adhesive properties of the vascular endothelium

The rapid release of cytokines such as TNF and IL-1 (see Fig. 14.4) from macrophages increases the adhesive properties of the vascular endothelium and facilitates the passage of more phagocytes into inflamed tissue. Combined with the release of chemokines such as CCL2, CCL3, and CXCL8 (see Chapter 6), this directs the recruitment of different leukocyte populations.

Epithelial cells, neutrophils, and mast cells are also important sources of proinflammatory cytokines.

IL-1, TNF, and IL-6 also initiate the **acute phase response**, increasing the production of complement components as well as other proteins involved in scavenging material released by tissue damage and, in the case of CRP, an opsonin for improving phagocytosis of bacteria.

When NK cells are stimulated by the phagocyte-derived cytokines **IL-12** and **IL-18** they rapidly release large quantities of interferon-γ (IFNγ). This response happens within the first day of infection, well before the clonal expansion of antigen-specific T cells, and provides a rapid source of IFNγ to activate macrophages. This T cell-independent pathway helps to explain the considerable resistance of mice with SCID (severe combined immune deficiency, a defect in lymphocyte maturation) to infections such as with *Listeria monocytogenes*. In mice, CD1d-restricted NK T cells also secrete IFNγ in response to IL-12 and IL-18 and other ligands, and help to further activate both NK cells and macrophages.

Pathogen recognition generates signals that regulate the lymphocyte-mediated response

The signals generated following the recognition of pathogens not only generate a cascade of innate immune events, but also regulate the development of the appropriate lymphocyte-mediated response.

Dendritic cells (DCs) are crucial for the initial priming of naive T cells specific for bacterial antigens. Contact with bacteria in the periphery induces immature DCs to migrate to the draining lymph nodes and augments their antigen-presenting ability by increasing their:

- display of MHC molecule–peptide complexes;
- expression of co-stimulatory molecules (such as CD40, CD80, and CD86); and
- secretion of T cell differentiating cytokines.

Some of this DC activation occurs secondary to their production of cytokines such as type I IFN.

Activated macrophages also act as antigen-presenting cells (APCs), but probably function more at the site of infection, providing further activation of effector rather than naive T cells.

Binding of bacterial components to pattern recognition receptors such as TLRs induces a local environment rich in cytokines such as IFNγ, IL-12, and IL-18, which promote T cell differentiation down the TH1 rather than TH2 pathway.

Immunologists have made use of these effects for many decades (even without knowing their true molecular basis) in the use of **adjuvants** in vaccination. 'Adjuvant' is derived from the Latin *adiuvare*, to help. When given experimentally, soluble antigens evoke stronger T and B cell-mediated responses if they are mixed with bacterial components that act as adjuvants. Components with this property are indicated in Fig. 14.1. This effect probably reflects that the antigen-specific immune response evolved in a tissue environment that already contained these pharmacologically active bacterial components.

With the exception of proteins such as **flagellin**, which itself stimulates TLR5 and is also a strong T cell immunogen, the response to pure bacterial antigens, injected without adjuvant-active bacterial components, is essentially an artificial situation that does not occur in nature.

The best known adjuvant in laboratory use, **complete Freund's adjuvant**, consists of killed mycobacteria suspended in oil, which is then emulsified with the aqueous antigen solution.

New-generation adjuvants based on bacterial components (and safe to use in humans, unlike Freund's adjuvant) include synthetic TLR activators such as CpG motifs and monophosphoryl lipid A (MPL) as well as recombinant cytokines such as IL-12, IL-1, and IFNγ.

ANTIBODY PROVIDES AN ANTIGEN-SPECIFIC PROTECTIVE MECHANISM

The relevance to protection of interactions of bacteria with antibody depends on the mechanism of pathogenicity.

Antibody clearly plays a crucial role in dealing with bacterial toxins:

- it neutralizes diphtheria toxin by blocking the attachment of the binding portion of the molecule to its target cells;
- similarly it may block locally acting toxins or extracellular matrix-degrading enzymes, which act as spreading factors;

Antibody can also interfere with motility by binding to flagellae.

An important function on external and mucosal surfaces, often performed by secretory IgA (sIgA, see Chapter 3), is to stop bacteria binding to epithelial cells – for instance, antibody to the M proteins of group A streptococci gives type-specific immunity to streptococcal sore throats.

It is likely that some antibodies to the bacterial surface can block functional requirements of the organism such as binding of iron-chelating compounds or intake of nutrients (Fig. 14.5).

An important role of antibody in immunity to non-toxigenic bacteria is the more efficient targeting of complement.

The antibacterial roles of antibody

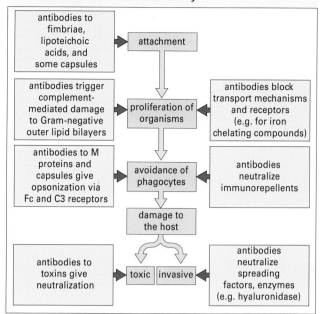

Fig. 14.5 This diagram lists the stages of bacterial invasion (blue) and indicates the antibacterial effects of antibody (yellow) that operate at the different stages. Antibodies to fimbriae, lipoteichoic acid, and some capsules block attachment of the bacterium to the host cell membrane. Antibody triggers complement-mediated damage to Gram-negative outer lipid bilayers. Antibody directly blocks bacterial surface proteins that pick up useful molecules from the environment and transport them across the membrane. Antibody to M proteins and capsules opsonizes the bacteria via Fc and C3 receptors for phagocytosis. Bacterial factors that interfere with normal chemotaxis or phagocytosis are neutralized. Bacterial toxins may be neutralized by antibody, as may bacterial spreading factors that facilitate invasion (e.g. by the destruction of connective tissue or fibrin).

Naturally occurring IgM antibodies, which bind to common bacterial structures such as phosphorylcholine, are important for protection against some bacteria (particularly streptococci) via their complement fixing activity.

Specific, high-affinity IgG antibodies elicited in response to infection are most important – children with primary immune deficiencies in B cell development or in T cell help have increased susceptibility to extracellular rather than intracellular bacteria.

With the aid of antibodies, even organisms that resist the alternative (i.e. innate) complement pathway (see below) are damaged by complement or become coated with C3 products, which then enhance the binding and uptake by phagocytes (Figs 14.6 and 14.7).

Q. How do C3 products attach to pathogens?
A. Following activation by cleavage the larger fragment, **C3b**, attaches covalently to hydroxyl and amine groups on the target (see Fig. 4.6).

Effect of antibody and complement on rate of clearance of virulent bacteria from the blood

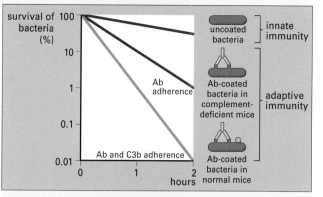

Fig. 14.6 Uncoated bacteria are phagocytosed rather slowly (unless the alternative complement pathway is activated by the strain of bacterium); on coating with antibody (Ab), adherence to phagocytes is greatly increased. The adherence is somewhat less effective in animals temporarily depleted of complement.

The interaction between bacteria and phagocytic cells

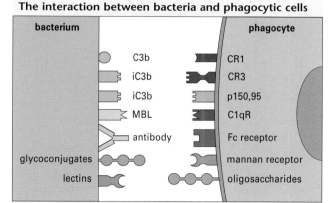

Fig. 14.7 A variety of molecules facilitate the binding of the organisms to the phagocyte membrane. These are in addition to the TLR system (e.g. TLR4 for LPS, TLR5 for flagellin, and TLR2 [plus TLR1/TLR6] for bacterial lipoproteins and peptidoglycans). The precise nature of the interaction will determine whether uptake occurs and whether cytokine secretion and appropriate killing mechanisms are triggered. Recognition invariably involves combinations of different receptor families. Note that apart from complement, antibody, and mannose-binding lectin (MBL), which bind to the bacterial surface, the other components are constitutive bacterial molecules.

The most efficient **complement-fixing antibodies** in humans are IgM, then IgG3 and to a lesser extent IgG1, whereas IgG1 and IgG3 are the subclasses with the highest affinity for Fc receptors.

Pathogenic bacteria may avoid the effects of antibody

Neisseria gonorrhoeae is an example of a pathogenic bacterium that uses several immune evasion strategies

Mechanisms used by *Neisseria gonorrhoeae* to avoid the effects of antibody

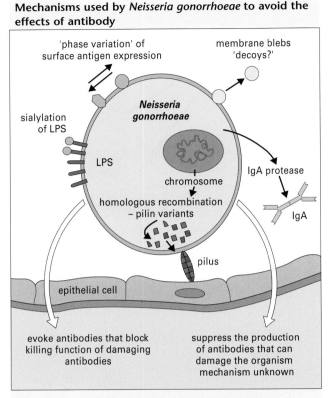

Fig. 14.8 *N. gonorrhoeae* is an example of a bacterium that uses several strategies to avoid the damaging effects of antibody. First, it fails to evoke a large antibody response, and the antibody that does form tends to block the function of damaging antibodies. Second, the organism secretes an IgA protease to destroy antibody. Third, blebs of membrane are released, and these appear to adsorb and so deplete local antibody levels. Finally, the organism uses three strategies to alter its antigenic composition: (i) the LPS may be sialylated, so that it more closely resembles mammalian oligosaccharides and promotes rapid removal of complement; (ii) the organism can undergo phase variation, so that it expresses an alternative set of surface molecules; (iii) the gene encoding pilin, the subunits of the pilus, undergoes homologous recombination to generate variants. *N. gonorrhoeae* also impairs T cell activation by engaging a co-inhibitory receptor CEACAM-1 on the lymphocyte surface by one of its OPA proteins.

Avoidance of complement-mediated damage

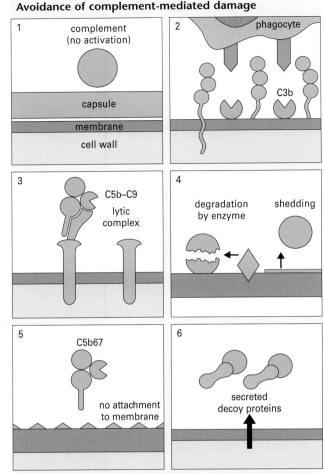

Fig. 14.9 Bacteria avoid complement-mediated damage by a variety of strategies. (**1**) An outer capsule or coat prevents complement activation. (**2**) An outer surface can be configured so that complement receptors on phagocytes cannot obtain access to fixed C3b. (**3**) Surface structures can be expressed that divert attachment of the lytic complex (MAC) from the cell membrane. (**4**) Membrane-bound enzyme can degrade fixed complement or cause it to be shed. (**5**) The outer membrane can resist the insertion of the lytic complex. (**6**) Secreted decoy proteins can cause complement to be deposited on them and not on the bacterium itself.

(Fig. 14.8) and humans can be repeatedly infected with *N. gonorrhoeae* with no evidence of protective immunity.

Antibodies may also be important for effective immunity against some intracellular bacteria such as *Legionella* and *Salmonella* spp.

Pathogenic bacteria can avoid the detrimental effects of complement

Some bacterial capsules are very poor activators of the alternative pathway (Fig. 14.9).

For other bacteria, long side chains (O antigens) on their LPS may fix C3b at a distance from the otherwise vulnerable lipid bilayer. Similarly, smooth-surfaced Gram-negative organisms (*Escherichia coli*, *Salmonella* spp.,

Pseudomonas spp.) may fix but then rapidly shed the C5b–C9 membrane lytic complex.

Other organisms exploit the physiological mechanisms that block destruction of host cells by complement. When C3b has attached to a surface it can interact with factor B leading to further C3b amplification or it can become inactivated by factors H and I. Capsules rich in sialic acid (as host cell membranes are) seem to promote the interaction with factors H and I.

Neisseria meningitidis, *E. coli* K1, and group B streptococci all resist complement attachment in this way.

The M protein of group A streptococci acts as an acceptor for factor H, thus potentiating C3bB dissociation. These bacteria also have a gene for a C5a protease.

Q. What value is a C5a protease to bacteria?

A. C5a is a major chemotactic molecule generated by complement activation that acts on specific receptors on macrophages, neutrophils, and mast cells (see Fig. 4.13).

ULTIMATELY MOST BACTERIA ARE KILLED BY PHAGOCYTES

A few, mostly Gram-negative, bacteria are directly killed by complement. However, immunity to most bacteria, whether considered as extracellular or intracellular pathogens, ultimately needs the killing activity of phagocytes. This process involves several steps.

Bacterial components attract phagocytes by chemotaxis

Unlike neutrophils, which in the uninfected host are found almost entirely in the blood, resident macrophages are constitutively present in tissues where exposure to pathogens first occurs (such as alveolar macrophages in the lung and Kupffer cells in the liver). These macrophages have some killing activity, but invariably need to be supplemented by recruitment of neutrophils and/or monocytes across the blood vessel wall.

Phagocytes are attracted by:
- bacterial components such as **f-Met-Leu-Phe** (which is chemotactic for leukocytes);
- complement products such as C5a; and
- locally released chemokines and cytokines derived from resident macrophages and epithelial cells (see Chapter 6).

The cellular composition of this inflammatory response varies according to the pathogen and the time since infection. For instance:
- acute infection with encapsulated bacteria such as *Streptococcus pyogenes* give rise to tissue lesions rich in neutrophils (typical of so-called pyogenic or pus-forming infections);
- at the other extreme, chronic infections with *M. tuberculosis* result in granulomas rich in macrophages, macrophage-derived multinucleated giant cells, and T cells;
- other organisms, such as *Listeria* and *Salmonella* spp., result in lesions of more mixed composition.

The choice of receptors is critical

The choice of receptors used for attachment of the phagocyte to the organism is critical and will determine:
- the efficiency of uptake;
- whether killing mechanisms are triggered;
- whether the process favors the pathogen by subverting immunity.

The binding can be mediated by lectins on the organism (e.g. on the fimbriae *of E. coli*), but receptors on the phagocyte are the most important. These either bind directly to the bacterium or indirectly via host complement and antibody deposited on the bacterial surface (**opsonization**).
- direct binding is mediated by pattern recognition molecules including Toll-like receptors and scavenger receptors (such as SRA, MARCO), mannose receptor, and dectin-1b;

- opsonization is mediated through complement receptors such as CR1, CR3, and CR4, which recognize complement fragments deposited on the organism via the alternative or classic complement pathways.

Complement can also be fixed by MBL present in serum, which can itself bind to **C1q receptors** and CR1.

Additionally, Fc receptors on the phagocyte (**FcγRI, FcγRII, and FcγRIII**, see Chapter 3) bind antibody that has coated bacteria (see Fig. 14.7), whereas various integrins can bind **fibronectin** and **vitronectin** opsonized particles.

Uptake can be enhanced by macrophage-activating cytokines

The binding of an organism to a receptor on the macrophage membrane does not always lead to its uptake. For example, zymosan particles (derived from yeast) bind via the glucan-recognizing lectin-like site on the CR3 of the macrophage and are taken up, whereas erythrocytes coated with iC3b are not, even though the iC3b also binds to CR3. This can, however, be enhanced by macrophage-activating cytokines such as **granulocyte–macrophage colony stimulating factor (GM-CSF)**.

Different membrane receptors vary in their efficiency at inducing a microbicidal response

Just as the binding of an organism to membrane receptors does not guarantee uptake, so different membrane receptors vary in their efficiency at inducing a microbicidal response – for example, mannose receptors and Fc receptors are particularly efficient at inducing the respiratory burst, but complement receptors are not, providing an evasion strategy for some organisms.

Phagocytic cells have many killing methods

The killing pathways of phagocytic cells can be:
- oxygen dependent (see Chapter 9); or
- oxygen independent.

In summary, one oxygen-dependent pathway involves the reduction of oxygen to superoxide anion (which is molecular oxygen to which a single unpaired electron has been added). This then interacts with numerous other molecules to give rise to a series of free radicals and other toxic derivatives, which can kill bacteria and fungi.

Recent studies in neutrophils suggests that the oxidative burst may also act indirectly, by promoting the flux of K^+ ions into the phagosome and activating microbicidal proteases.

A second oxygen-dependent pathway involves the creation of nitric oxide ($NO^{\bullet}$) from the guanidino nitrogen of L-arginine. This in turn leads to further toxic substances such as the peroxynitrites, which result from interactions of $NO^{\bullet}$ with the products of the oxygen reduction pathway.

Q. What pathway leads to the production of NO by macrophages?

A. Cytokine activation by IFNγ and TNFα leads to production of inducible NO synthase, which generates NO from L-arginine (see Fig. 9.31).

Oxygen-independent killing mechanisms may be more important than previously thought. Many organisms can be killed by cells from patients with chronic granulomatous disease (CGD), which cannot produce reactive oxygen intermediates, and from patients with myeloperoxidase (MPO) deficiency, which cannot produce hypohalous acids. Some of this killing may be due to NO[•], but many organisms can be killed anaerobically, so other mechanisms must exist. Some have been identified and are discussed below.

Some cationic proteins have antibiotic-like properties

The **defensins** (Fig. 14.10) are cysteine- and arginine-rich cationic peptides of 30 to 33 amino acids found in phagocytes such as neutrophils, where they comprise 30–50% of the granule proteins.

Q. Which other cells secrete antimicrobial peptides?

A. Paneth cells of the intestine (see Fig. 12.8) and airway epithelial cells (i.e. sites of primary contact with pathogens).

Defensins evolved early in evolution and similar molecules are found in insects. They act by integrating into microbial lipid membranes (in some cases forming ion-permeable channels) and disrupting membrane function and structure, resulting in lysis of the pathogen. Defensins can kill organisms as diverse as *Staphylococcus aureus*, *Pseudomonas aeruginosa*, *E. coli*, *Cryptococcus neoformans*, and the enveloped virus herpes simplex.

Defensins also have important immunostimulatory properties including:
- promoting chemotaxis and phagocytosis;
- regulating cytokine production; and
- acting as adjuvants for adaptive immunity.

Other antibacterial peptides include the **cathelicidins** and **protegrins**, which can bind LPS and also form membrane pores.

There are also cationic proteins with different pH optima, including **cathepsin G** and **azurocidin**, both of which are related to elastase, but have activity against Gram-negative bacteria – this is unrelated to their enzyme activity.

Other antimicrobial mechanisms also play a role

Following lysosome fusion there is a transient rise in pH before acidification (a fall in pH) of the phagolysosome takes place. This occurs within 10–15 minutes.

The acidification of phagosomes containing bacteria following their fusion with lysosomes is an important step in the killing process and is related to the low pH optima of lysosomal enzymes.

Certain Gram-positive organisms may be killed by **lysozyme**, which is active against their readily exposed peptidoglycan layer.

The availability of intracellular iron is another important factor in the interplay between host and pathogen. Iron is essential for the growth of many bacteria and also influences their expression of key virulence genes. Sequestration of iron can therefore be an effective antimicrobial strategy, particularly for intracellular bacteria.

Lactoferrin is a mammalian iron-binding protein released by degranulating neutrophils that sequesters iron from pathogens, inhibiting their growth, and in the case of *P. aeruginosa* also reducing biofilm formation, a key event in the pathogenesis of infection in cystic fibrosis patients. **Lactoferricin**, an antimicrobial peptide derived from lactoferrin, kills other bacteria.

Iron is also required for many host immune functions including the respiratory burst, the generation of NO[•], and the development of pathogen-specific T cells.

Both iron excess and iron deficiency can therefore have complex effects on the outcome of infection. For example, individuals with iron overload syndromes resulting from genetic defects (such as thalassemia or hemochromatosis), nutritional excess, or following iron or red cell supplementation (such as in the treatment of anemias) have increased susceptibility to infection with *Yersinia* and *Salmonella* spp., and *M. tuberculosis*.

Macrophage killing can be enhanced on activation

Unlike neutrophils, which have a short life span but are efficient killers even in their normal state, macrophages are long-lived cells that without appropriate activation can actually provide a haven for microbial growth.

Cationic host defense peptides in immunity to fungi and bacteria

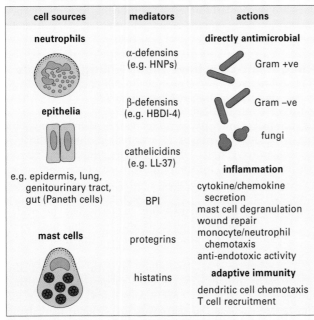

cell sources	mediators	actions
neutrophils	α-defensins (e.g. HNPs)	**directly antimicrobial**
		Gram +ve
epithelia	β-defensins (e.g. HBDI-4)	Gram –ve
		fungi
	cathelicidins (e.g. LL-37)	
e.g. epidermis, lung, genitourinary tract, gut (Paneth cells)	BPI	**inflammation** cytokine/chemokine secretion mast cell degranulation wound repair monocyte/neutrophil chemotaxis anti-endotoxic activity
mast cells	protegrins	
	histatins	**adaptive immunity** dendritic cell chemotaxis T cell recruitment

Fig. 14.10 Numerous cationic host defense peptides are produced by neutrophils, epithelia, and mast cells. Their synthesis is usually constitutive but is also enhanced by proinflammatory cytokines such as TNF generated following infection. Originally defined by their direct killing activity against pathogens, they are now known also to act on immune cells, having multiple immunomodulatory effects on inflammation and adaptive immunity.

Macrophage activation occurs most effectively by the combination of exposure to:
- microbial products (through the receptors described above); and
- cytokines (particularly IFNγ) derived from cells of the innate and adaptive immune system.

Optimal activation of macrophages is dependent on TH1 CD4 T cells

Microbial products can directly activate monocytes and resident macrophages to secrete proinflammatory cytokines and thus initiate the immune process. However, complete activation, including the ability to kill intracellular microbes, requires the action of IFNγ – IFNγ knockout mice are extremely susceptible to infection and children with deficiencies in either the IFNγ receptor or the cytokines necessary for its production (such as IL-12, IL-18, and IL-23) have increased susceptibility to intracellular bacteria such as bacille Calmette–Guérin (BCG), *Salmonella* spp., and atypical mycobacteria.

IFNγ is so potent because it enhances several different microbicidal pathways, including both the respiratory burst and the generation of NO•.

As described above, NK cells, NK T cells, and even macrophages themselves can produce IFNγ during the innate immune response. However, the additional actions of antigen-specific T cells are necessary for optimal cell-mediated immunity.

The most important source of IFNγ during the adaptive immune response to intracellular bacteria is from TH1 CD4+ T cells (Fig. 14.11).

Patients who have AIDS and a reduced CD4 T cell number and function have dramatically increased susceptibility to *M. tuberculosis* as well as other bacteria such as *Mycobacterium avium* and atypical salmonella.

As mentioned above, many bacterial components activate the TLR pattern recognition system, ensuring the preferential expression of TH1 rather than TH2 CD4+ T cell responses in most cases.

TH1 T cells provide both IFNγ for macrophage activation and B cell help to produce IgG subclasses for opsonization of bacteria, rather than the eosinophilia and IgE responses typical of helminth infections.

There is mutual antagonism between the TH1 and TH2 pathways at the level of both T cell differentiation and also directly on the macrophage:

Overview of CD4+ T cell-mediated immunity to bacteria and fungi

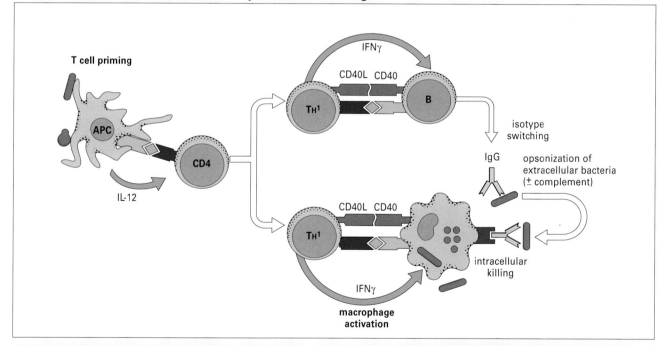

Fig. 14.11 Naive CD4+ T cells are stimulated by class II MHC positive antigen-bearing dendritic cells (DCs) via the TCR, in conjunction with co-stimulatory molecules such as CD80/86 and CD28, which induce T cell activation and proliferation. Differentiation into either TH1 or TH2 effector cells is strongly influenced by the cytokine environment during this interaction – microbial pattern recognition events that favor production of IL-12 promote TH1 development, whereas low IL-12 favors TH2 responses. Although not shown here, conditions with high levels of IL-10 or TGFβ can induce regulatory T cells, rather than TH1 or TH2. Optimal T cell help for either B cells or macrophage responses involves T cell-derived cytokines and direct cell contact. TH1 cells also promote opsonizing antibody production, which complements their activation of phagocytes by IFNγ.

- IFNγ upregulates induced NO• synthetase expression; whereas
- IL-4 and 13 promote the expression of arginase, which inhibits NO• production, reducing the macrophage killing potential and diverting it to a profibrotic phenotype.

Other cytokines such as GM-CSF and TNF can also contribute to macrophage activation.

Macrophage activation is also promoted by direct contact with CD4 T cells via **CD40–CD40L interactions**.

Thus T cell-mediated help for macrophages and B cells shares the common themes of soluble and cell-contact mediated activation by CD4 TH1 cells.

Persistent macrophage recruitment and activation can result in granuloma formation

If intracellular pathogens are not quickly eliminated, the persistent recruitment and activation of macrophages and T cells to an infected tissue can result in the formation of **granulomas**. These are generally associated with chronic bacterial infections such as tuberculosis and syphilis, but similar (although not identical) structures are also induced in parasitic diseases such as schistosomiasis and in response to non-infectious materials such as asbestos.

In the classical example of tuberculosis, granulomas are composed of a core of infected (and uninfected) macrophages, epithelioid cells, and multinucleated giant cells (derived from the fusion of activated macrophages), and a peripheral accumulation of T cells. Neutrophils and dendritic cells can also be found in granulomas, along with extracellular matrix components such as collagen. In human tuberculosis, the center of granulomas undergoes caseating necrosis. The presence of activated macrophages and the fibrosis that ensues is believed to control bacterial growth and prevent dissemination to other organs. Generating these new immunological structures is a highly complex event involving multiple adhesion molecules, chemokines, and cytokines. Once formed, their continued existence also requires active immunological input.

AIDS and diabetes mellitus are important risk factors for loss of control of *M. tuberculosis* growth. TNF is also critical for granuloma maintenance – some patients given TNF-blocking antibodies to alleviate the symptoms of rheumatoid arthritis rapidly reactivate tuberculosis that had otherwise been controlled for many years.

SUCCESSFUL PATHOGENS HAVE EVOLVED MECHANISMS TO AVOID PHAGOCYTE-MEDIATED KILLING

Because most organisms are ultimately killed by phagocytes, it is not surprising that successful pathogens have evolved an array of mechanisms to counteract this risk (Fig. 14.12).

Intracellular pathogens may 'hide' in cells

Some organisms may thrive inside metabolically damaged host phagocytes, or escape killing by moving out of phagosomes into the cytoplasm.

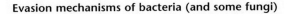

Evasion mechanisms of bacteria (and some fungi)

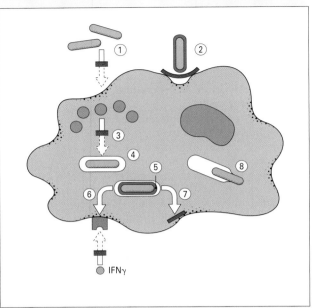

Fig. 14.12 Evasion mechanisms of bacteria (and some fungi), particularly those that are successful intracellular parasites, have evolved the ability to evade different aspects of phagocyte-mediated killing. (**1**) Some can secrete repellents or toxins that inhibit chemotaxis. (**2**) Others have capsules or outer coats that inhibit attachment by the phagocyte (e.g. *Streptococcus pneumoniae* or the yeast *C. neoformans*. (**3**) Others permit uptake, but release factors that block subsequent triggering of killing mechanisms. Once ingested, some, such as *M. tuberculosis*, inhibit lysosome fusion with the phagosome. They also inhibit the proton pump that acidifies the phagosome, so the pH does not fall. (**4**) They may also secrete catalase (e.g. staphylococci), which breaks down hydrogen peroxide. (**5**) Organisms such as *M. leprae* have highly resistant outer coats. *M. leprae* surrounds itself with a phenolic glycolipid, which scavenges free radicals. (**6**) Mycobacteria also release a lipoarabinomannan, which blocks the ability of macrophages to respond to the activating effects of IFNγ. (**7**) Cells infected with *Salmonella enterica*, *M. tuberculosis*, or *Chlamydia trachomatis* have impaired antigen-presenting function. (**8**) Several organisms (e.g. *Listeria* and *Shigella* spp.) can escape from the phagosome to multiply in the cytoplasm. Finally, the organism may kill the phagocyte via either necrosis (e.g. staphylococci) or induction of apoptosis (e.g. *Yersinia* spp.).

Listeria monocytogenes, *Shigella* spp., and *Burkholderia pseudomallei* achieve this by releasing enzymes that lyze the phagosome membrane. These organisms also illustrate the point that bacteria are not just inert particles, but have evolved strategies for taking control of functions of the host cell.

Other organisms, such as *M. leprae* and salmonellae, cause themselves to be taken up by cells that are not normally considered phagocytic and have little antibacterial potential such as Schwann cells, hepatocytes, and epithelial cells.

Before they can be taken up by activated phagocytes or exposed to other killing mechanisms, the organisms may need to be released from such cells.

INFECTED CELLS CAN BE KILLED BY CTLs

CD8$^+$ cytotoxic T lymphocytes (CTLs) can release intracellular organisms by killing the infected cell.

Even macrophages may be targets of CTLs because when infected with intracellular bacteria they can become refractory to activation and less able to kill the organism themselves.

Mice become strikingly susceptible to *M. tuberculosis* if class I MHC genes are knocked out so that antigen-specific CD8$^+$ T cells do not develop.

This is consistent with an essential role for CTLs in resistance to intracellular bacteria, and inducing these responses is now a primary goal of new vaccines against bacteria such as *M. tuberculosis* as well as other pathogens.

Dendritic cells appear to be particularly important in the generation of strong CD8 T cell responses to bacteria such as *L. monocytogenes* and *Salmonella* spp.

Although antigen processing and presentation via the class I MHC pathway (see Chapter 5) is most efficient for microbial antigens derived from the cytosol, nevertheless, CTLs are also clearly induced by bacteria that never escape the phagosome such as *M. tuberculosis*, salmonellae, and chlamydiae. This occurs either by **cross-presentation** of antigens within the same cell or by **cross-priming** where antigens are released from infected cells undergoing apoptosis and then transferred to nearby DCs for efficient presentation via the MHC I pathway. In some cases, lysis of infected host cells by CTLs can result in killing of the organism inside. This can be due to the action of **granulysin** – an antibacterial peptide stored in the cytotoxic granules and released during the cytotoxic process.

CTLs can also secrete IFNγ when they recognize infected targets, providing an additional pathway of macrophage activation and protective immunity (Fig. 14.13).

Other T cell populations can contribute to antibacterial immunity

In addition to the classical MHC class I- and MHC class II-mediated recognition of bacterial proteins by αβ CD4 and CD8 T cells, other 'non-conventional' T cell populations allow the host to respond to other microbial chemistries.

Pathways of CD8 T cell activation and function

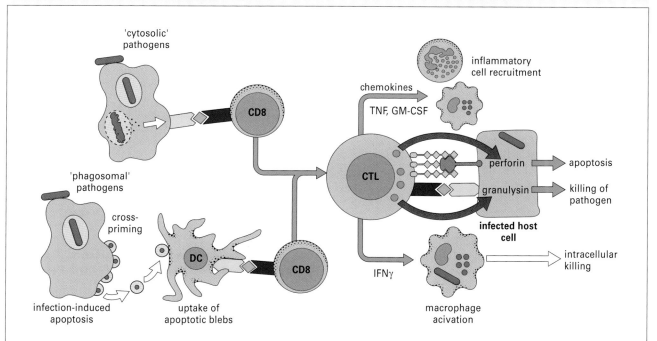

Fig. 14.13 Naive CD8 T cells are activated by peptides presented via MHC class I molecules, primarily derived from microorganisms that reside in the cytoplasm, such as viruses and some intracellular bacteria that escape the phagosome such as *Listeria* spp. Other pathogens that do not escape the phagosome (such as *M. tuberculosis*) can still induce CD8 T cell responses via cross-priming, in which infected and apoptotic host cells release antigenic fragments that are taken up by dendritic cells (DCs). Effector CD8 T cells (CTLs) provide protection by releasing proinflammatory and macrophage-activating cytokines and killing infected host cells via perforin release and Fas (see Figs 10.9 and 10.12). In some cases, the release of granulysin from the CTL can also result in killing of the pathogen.

T cells bearing γδ (rather than αβ) receptors (see Chapter 5) proliferate in response to bacterial infection.

Q. Where in the body are γδ T cells located?
A. They preferentially home to epithelial surfaces (see Chapter 2).

Some γδ T cells recognize small phospholigands derived from *M. tuberculosis* and possibly other bacteria, whereas others are triggered in an antigen-independent manner by the presence of pathogen-activated dendritic cells expressing high levels of co-stimulatory molecules and IL-12.

There are also αβ T cells (either CD4 or CD8) that recognize not proteins, but microbial glycolipids such as the **lipoarabinomannan** from *M. tuberculosis* or the capsular LPS of *H. influenzae*. These are presented via CD1a/b/c molecules, which are non-polymorphic homologs of MHC class I molecules that specialize in the binding of lipophilic antigens.

Such γδ and CD1-restricted αβ T cells have cytotoxic activity and can also secrete IFNγ suggesting a potential role in host defense. In animal models of infection these non-conventional T cells can be protective or immuno-regulatory, but their relative importance in human immunity is not resolved.

Some tissue cells can express antimicrobial mechanisms

Tissue cells that are not components of the immune system can also harbor bacteria such as *M. leprae*, invasive *Shigella* and *Salmonella* spp., and *Rickettsia* and *Chlamydia* spp. As mentioned earlier, these infected cells may be sacrificed by CTLs. On the other hand, intracellular organisms such as *Rickettsia* and *Chlamydia* spp. may be starved by reduction in the availability of L-tryptophan, due to increased expression of indoleamine 2,3-dioxygenase in response to inflammatory cytokines such as IFNγ.

The secretion of antimicrobial peptides such as defensins by epithelial cells also provides an example of the protective effects of cells not strictly considered as part of the immune system.

THE RESPONSE TO BACTERIA CAN RESULT IN IMMUNOLOGICAL TISSUE DAMAGE

The events described so far are generally beneficial to the host and critical for resistance against pathogenic bacteria. However, all immune responses designed to kill invading pathogens have the potential for causing collateral damage to the host.

Excessive cytokine release can lead to endotoxin shock

If cytokine release is sudden and massive, several acute tissue-damaging syndromes can result and are potentially fatal.

One of the most severe examples of this is **endotoxin (septicemic) shock**, when there is massive production of cytokines, usually caused by bacterial products released during septicemic episodes. Endotoxin (LPS) from Gram-negative bacteria is usually responsible, though Gram-positive septicemia can cause a similar syndrome. There can be life-threatening fever, circulatory collapse, diffuse intravascular coagulation, and hemorrhagic necrosis, leading eventually to multiple organ failure (Fig. 14.14).

Paradoxically, individuals who recover from the initial life-threatening phase often overcompensate and switch from a hyper- to a hyporesponsive phase, in which excessive production of endogenous immune regulators such as IL-10 and TGFβ (and possibly other mechanisms) results in immune paralysis, making them susceptible to secondary infection.

The Schwartzman reaction is a form of cytokine-dependent tissue damage

Schwartzman observed that if Gram-negative organisms were injected into the skin of rabbits, followed by a second dose given intravenously 24 hours later, hemorrhagic necrosis occurred at the prepared skin site. This is known as the **Schwartzman reaction** (Fig. 14.15).

Many other organisms are now known to 'prepare' the skin in the same way, including streptococci, mycobacteria, *Haemophilus* spp., corynebacteria, and vaccinia virus.

Schwartzman also noted that two intravenous injections 24 hours apart caused a systemic reaction, commonly involving circulatory collapse and bilateral necrosis of the renal cortex. Sanarelli had made similar observations and this is now known as the systemic Schwartzman, or Sanarelli–Schwartzman, reaction.

These reactions can also be accompanied by necrosis in the pancreas, pituitary, adrenals, and gut. There is marked diffuse intravascular coagulation and thrombosis.

Endotoxin (LPS) is the active component of the intravenous 'triggering' injection.

Early work implicated endothelial changes, fibrin deposition, neutrophil accumulation and degranulation, and platelets as mediating the damage. This is correct, but it is now clear that tissues are primed by the induction of IFNγ (involving IL-12) derived from either NK cells or NK T cells, whereas TNF is critical in the effector phase of systemic tissue damage.

These phenomena may contribute to the characteristic hemorrhagic rash seen in children with meningococcal meningitis and the systemic effects observed in Gram-negative septic shock.

The Koch phenomenon is necrosis in T cell-mediated mycobacterial lesions and skin test sites

The **Koch phenomenon** is a necrotic response to antigens of *M. tuberculosis*, originally demonstrated by Robert Koch in tuberculous guinea pigs (Fig. 14.16). It may be related to the necrosis that also occurs in the lesions in tuberculosis. It is at least partly due to the release of cytokines into a T cell-mediated inflammatory site (**delayed hypersensitivity site**). Such sites can be extremely sensitive to the tissue-damaging effects of cytokines, as seen in the Schwartzman reaction, particularly when there is mixed TH1 and TH2 activity.

Examples to illustrate the relationship between the nature of an organism, the disease, and immunopathology

Endotoxin shock

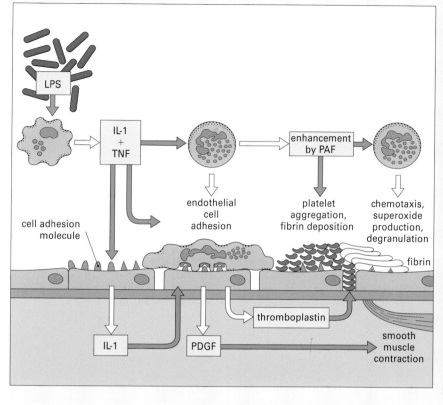

Fig. 14.14 Excessive release of cytokines, often triggered by the endotoxin (LPS) of Gram-negative bacteria, can lead to diffuse intravascular coagulation with consequent defective clotting, changes in vascular permeability, loss of fluid into the tissues, a fall in blood pressure, circulatory collapse, and hemorrhagic necrosis, particularly in the gut. This figure illustrates some important parts of this pathway at the cellular level. The cytokines TNF and IL-1 cause endothelial cells to express cell adhesion molecules and tissue thromboplastin. These promote adhesion of circulating cells and deposition of fibrin, respectively. Platelet activating factor (PAF) enhances these effects. In experimental models, shock can be blocked by neutralizing antibodies to TNF, and greatly diminished by antibodies to tissue thromboplastin, or by inhibitors of PAF or of nitric oxide production, but these have not been successful clinically. Gram-positive bacteria can induce shock, for example by massive release of cytokines mediated by superantigens. (PDGF, platelet-derived growth factor, produced by both platelets and endothelium)

The Schwartzman reaction

induction in rabbit	human clinical equivalent
endotoxin injected into skin	a minor septicemic episode results in dissemination of meningococci to the skin
24 h later endotoxin given intravenously	24 h later a further larger septicemic episode results in systemic release of cytokines and activation of leukocytes
hemorrhagic necrosis in the 'prepared' skin site	this results in necrosis in the sites where bacteria lodged after the first episode

Fig. 14.15 In the Schwartzman reaction there is cytokine-mediated tissue damage in a site of previous inflammation. This phenomenon is related to several clinical situations in humans. The first injection into the skin prepares the site by inducing inflammation and upregulating cytokine receptors, which are now the target for systemic cytokines released by the later intravenous injection of endotoxin (LPS).

caused, and the mechanism of immune response that leads to protection, are given in Fig. 14.17.

Some individuals suffer from excessive immune responses

Why some individuals suffer from excessive immune responses and others control infection with little or no damage is still unclear. The host constantly attempts to regulate immune responses to avoid the scenarios described above. For instance, immunoregulatory cytokines such as IL-10 and transforming growth factor-β (TGFβ) are produced from:

- macrophages during episodes of inflammation; and
- regulatory T cells during adaptive immunity (see Chapter 11).

The influence of both 'natural' and 'inducible' regulatory T cell populations has been reported in infections with bacteria such as *L. monocytogenes*, *Helicobacter* spp.,

The Koch phenomenon

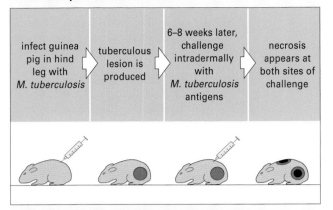

Fig. 14.16 Robert Koch observed that injection of *M. tuberculosis* or soluble antigens from *M. tuberculosis* into the skin of tuberculous guinea pigs resulted in a necrotizing reaction both at the challenge site and in the original tuberculous lesion. This is at least partly due to the fact that the delayed hypersensitivity reaction to mycobacterial antigens can, like the LPS-injected site in the Schwartzman reaction, be very sensitive to the toxicity of cytokines. These may be released locally in the skin test site. A similar reaction is seen in humans who have or have had tuberculosis. Responses to the same antigen in individuals who are skin-test positive as a result of BCG (bacille Calmette–Guérin) vaccination do not usually show necrosis.

Bordetella pertussis, and *M. tuberculosis*. Their presence may be beneficial to the host in preventing unwanted tissue damage, but can also be subverted by pathogens as a means of immune evasion. For example, filamentous hemagglutinin and adenylate cyclase toxin, two known virulence factors of *B. pertussis*, promote the induction of

IL-10-secreting regulatory T cells in mice, dampening protective TH1 immunity and promoting persistence in the host.

Excessive immune responses can occur during treatment of severe bacterial infections

Paradoxically, excessive immune responses can also occur during treatment of humans with severe bacterial infections.

The simultaneous destruction of large numbers of organisms by antibiotics can cause increased cytokine production and systemic pathology following treatment of relapsing fever, Lyme disease, and tuberculosis.

Also, when patients who have AIDS and underlying infections such as tuberculosis and cryptococcal meningitis are treated with effective antiretroviral drugs (highly active antiretroviral therapy – HAART), the recovering T cells induce an '**immune reconstitution inflammatory syndrome**' with severe tissue damage.

THE TOXICITY OF SUPERANTIGENS RESULTS FROM MASSIVE CYTOKINE RELEASE

Certain bacterial components called **superantigens** bind directly to the variable regions of β chains (Vβ) of antigen receptors on subsets of T cells, and cross-link them to the MHC molecules of APCs, usually outside the normal antigen-binding groove.

Q. What effect do superantigens have on T cells?

A. All T cells bearing the relevant Vβ gene product are activated without the processing and presentation of the antigen as peptides in the cleft of the MHC molecule that is normally required for T cell activation (see Fig. 7.22).

Immunity in some important bacterial infections

infection	pathogenesis	major defense mechanisms
Corynebacterium diphtheriae	non-invasive pharyngitis – toxin	neutralizing antibody
Vibrio cholerae	non-invasive enteritis – toxin	neutralizing and adhesion-blocking antibodies
Neisseria meningitidis (Gram-negative)	nasopharynx →bacteremia →meningitis →endotoxemia	killed by antibody and lytic complement; opsonized and phagocytosed
Staphylococcus aureus (Gram-positive)	locally invasive and toxic in skin, etc.	osponized by antibody and complement; killed by phagocytes
Mycobacterium tuberculosis	invasive, evokes immunopathology	macrophage activation by cytokines from T cells, CTLs
Mycobacterium leprae	invasive, space-occupying and/or immunopathology	

Fig. 14.17 This table provides examples of how a knowledge of the organism, and the mechanism of disease, can lead to a prediction of the relevant protective mechanism.

Between them staphylococci and streptococci have some 21 different superantigens and these molecules can also be found in other bacteria such as mycoplasmas. The full biological significance of this bacterial adaptation is not yet clear – it could be to the organism's advantage to exhaust or deplete T cells that would otherwise be protective.

One certain effect is the toxicity of the massive release of cytokines (including IL-2, TNFα, and TNFβ, together with IL-1β from activated macrophages) due to the simultaneous stimulation of up to 20% of the entire T cell pool.

The staphylococcal toxins responsible for the **toxic shock syndrome** (toxic shock syndrome toxin-1 [TSST-1], etc.) operate in this way, though not all shock syndromes caused by staphylococci are the result of T cell activation.

Recent evidence suggests that streptococcal M protein, a known virulence factor of *S. pyogenes*, forms a complex with fibrinogen, which then binds to β-integrins on neutrophils, causing the release of inflammatory mediators, which also result in massive vascular leakage and shock.

Heat-shock proteins are prominent targets of immune responses

Heat-shock proteins (HSPs or stress proteins) are found in all eukaryotic and prokaryotic cells, where they have essential roles in the assembly, folding, and transport of other molecules.

Mammalian cells exposed to abnormally elevated temperatures (or to other stresses including infection) express higher levels of these proteins, which reflects their role in the stabilization of protein structure.

Bacteria also increase HSP expression, particularly as they adapt to the intracellular environment of the host.

Immune responses are generated against both mammalian and pathogen-derived HSPs during infection.

Mammalian (and probably also bacterial) HSPs are able to activate innate immunity via multiple cell surface receptors including the α-globulin receptor CD91, CD40, CD14, and TLRs 2 and 4.

HSPs can enhance the presentation of antigens via the class I MHC/CD8 pathway (see Chapter 5) and are themselves immunogenic for both CD4 and CD8 T cells.

Because the amino acid sequences of HSPs are very highly conserved between humans and bacteria there is still considerable speculation about their role in the initiation of autoimmunity, though it seems their contribution is more complicated than simply antigenic mimicry.

The 'hygiene hypothesis'

Several groups of diseases, all characterized by defects in the regulation of the immune system, are becoming more common, particularly in developed countries. These diseases include:
- allergies;
- inflammatory bowel diseases (Crohn's disease and ulcerative colitis); and
- autoimmune conditions such as multiple sclerosis.

This may have many causes but the 'hygiene hypothesis' suggests that increasing immunological dysregulation correlates with decreasing exposure to environmental microorganisms. Decreased exposure could be due to hygiene, vaccines, and antibiotic use. If proved correct, the solution would clearly not be the abandonment of the most important achievements of medicine (hygiene, vaccines, antibiotics), but rather the identification of the environmental factors that are lacking from the modern lifestyle so that they can be replaced as vaccines or probiotics.

However, recent data suggest that the correlation does not always hold true – some viral infections (such as influenza and respiratory syncytial virus) seem to promote rather than decrease allergy and asthma in animal models.

Whatever their cause, prevention or treatment of these diseases will need to address:
- the balance of TH1/TH2 responses; and
- manipulation of the regulatory T cell circuits that normally control allergy and autoimmunity.

FUNGI CAN CAUSE LIFE-THREATENING INFECTIONS

Fungi are eukaryotes with a rigid cell wall enriched in complex polysaccharides such as chitin, glucans, and mannan.

Among the 70 000 or so species of fungi, only a small number are pathogenic for humans. However, because there are no approved vaccines and antifungal drugs often have severe side effects, fungi can cause serious and sometimes life-threatening infections.

Q. Why has it been more difficult to identify antifungal antibiotics than antibacterial antibiotics?

A. Fungi are eukaryotic organisms and therefore have similar protein synthesis machinery and mechanisms to organize and replicate the genome as mammalian cells.

Fungi can exist as:
- single cells (yeasts) small enough to be ingested by host phagocytes; or
- long slender, branching hyphae, which may require extracellular killing processes.

Some pathogenic fungi are dimorphic, in that they switch from a hyphal form in the environment to a yeast form as they adapt to life in the host. Both phases possess important virulence determinants and pose different problems to the immune system.

There are four categories of fungal infection

Although some fungi can cause disease in otherwise healthy individuals, severe fungal infections are a growing problem because of the markedly increased numbers of immunologically compromised hosts. Fungal infections are therefore regularly seen in:
- patients with untreated AIDS;
- patients with cancer and undergoing chemotherapy;
- patients with transplants on immunosuppressive agents; and
- some patients taking long-term corticosteroids.

These clinical findings point to the key roles of neutrophils and macrophage activating TH1 cell responses in antifungal immunity.

Human fungal infections fall into the following four major categories:

- **superficial mycoses** caused by fungi known as dermatophytes, usually restricted to the non-living keratinized components of skin, hair and nails, and including infection by *Trichophyton* and *Microsporum* spp. (which cause ringworm and athlete's foot) and *Malassezia* spp. (which causes pityriasis);
- **subcutaneous mycoses** in which saprophytic fungi cause chronic nodules or ulcers in subcutaneous tissues following trauma (e.g. chromomycosis, sporotrichosis, and mycetoma);
- **systemic mycoses** caused by soil saprophytes, which are inhaled from the environment and produce subclinical or acute lung infections that can disseminate to almost any tissue in the immunocompromised host – *Histoplasma*, *Blastomyces*, *Coccidioides*, and *Paracoccidioides* spp. can all cause primary disease in otherwise immunocompetent individuals, whereas *Aspergillus* spp., *Pneumocystis carinii*, and *C. neoformans* act more as opportunists;
- **candidiasis** caused by *Candida albicans*, a ubiquitous commensal and the most common opportunistic fungal pathogen – disturbance of normal physiology by immunosuppressive drugs, of normal flora by antibiotics, or T cell function (as in severe combined immune deficiency, thymic aplasia, and AIDS), results in superficial infections of the skin and mucous membranes, and systemic disease can occur in intravenous drug users and patients with lymphoma or leukemia.

Innate immune responses to fungi include defensins and phagocytes

The basic protective features of the skin and normal commensal flora described against bacterial infections above are also important in resistance to fungi.

Defensins have antifungal as well as antibacterial properties, and collectins such as MBL and the surfactant proteins A and D can bind, aggregate, and opsonize fungi for phagocytosis.

Phagocytes, particularly neutrophils (Fig. 14.18) and macrophages, are essential for killing fungi, either by:

Evidence for neutrophil-mediated immunity to mucormycosis

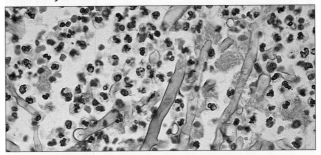

Fig. 14.18 This is a section from the lung of a patient suffering from mucormycosis – an opportunistic infection in an immunosuppressed subject. The inflammatory reaction consists almost entirely of neutrophil polymorphs around the fungal hyphae. The disease is particularly associated with neutropenia (lack of neutrophils). Silver stain. × 400. (Courtesy of Professor RJ Hay)

- degranulation and release of toxic materials onto large indigestible hyphae; or
- ingestion of yeast or conidia.

The oxidative burst plays a crucial role in some antifungal responses, as seen in the susceptibility to severe aspergillosis by patients with CGD who have defects in the NADPH oxidase system. However, phagocytes from such patients with defective oxygen reduction pathways nevertheless kill other yeast and hyphae with near normal efficiency, so demonstrating the role of other killing mechanisms (Fig. 14.19). For instance, NO$^{\bullet}$ and its derivatives are important for resistance to *C. neoformans*.

These responses rely on the recognition of PAMPs in the fungal cell wall by either soluble or cell-bound pattern recognition molecules. The TLR family again plays an important role in this process, along with the mannose receptor and complement receptors:

- TLR2 (which can cooperate with the β-glucan receptor dectin-1) recognizes fungal phospholipomannans, *C. albicans* yeasts, and *A. fumigatus* hyphae and conidia;

Monocyte/macrophage killing of fungi

organism	source of monocytes/macrophages		
	normal	**CGD**	**MPO deficiency**
Candida albicans	killed	sometimes killed	sometimes killed
Candida parapsilosis	killed	not killed	unknown
Cryptococcus neoformans	killed	unknown	killed
Aspergillus fumigatus conidia	killed	sometimes killed	killed
Aspergillus fumigatus hyphae	killed	killed	killed

Fig. 14.19 Many fungi are killed by monocytes or macrophages. Individuals with chronic granulomatous disease (CGD) are highly susceptible to *Aspergillus* spp. infections whereas myeloperoxidase (MPO) deficiency does not usually lead to opportunistic infection, suggesting that non-oxygen-dependent mechanisms are also important in host defense.

- TLR4/CD14 recognizes *C. albicans*, *Aspergillus fumigatus*, and the glucuronoxylomannan capsule of *C. neoformans*.

Not all of these events are to the host's advantage, for example recognition of *Candida albicans* mannan via TLR4 induces proinflammatory chemokine responses, whereas ligation of candidal phospholipomannan and glucans with TLR2/dectin-1 generates a strong IL-10 response, which may inhibit immune function.

T cell-mediated immunity is critical for resistance to fungi

Most fungi are highly immunogenic and induce strong antibody and T cell-mediated immune responses, which can be detected by serology and delayed-type (type IV) hypersensitivity skin reactions (see Chapter 26).

Considerable evidence points to the dominant protective role of TH1 T cells and macrophage activation, rather than antibody-mediated responses.

Patients with T cell deficiencies, rather than defects in antibody production, are more at risk of disseminated fungal disease, and antibody titers, though useful as an epidemiological tool to determine exposure, do not necessarily correlate with prognosis. Nevertheless, fungi can elicit both protective and non-protective antibodies and the protection afforded by some experimental vaccines can be adoptively transferred by immune sera.

Resistance to most pathogenic fungi (including dermatophytes and most systemic mycoses including *C. neoformans*, *Histoplasma capsulatum*, etc., but not *Aspergillus* spp.) is clearly dependent upon T cell-mediated immunity, particularly CD4$^+$ TH1 cells secreting IFNγ (Fig. 14.20). As in the case of bacteria, dendritic cells are necessary for this response and produce IL-12 after engulfing fungi.

The clinical relevance of TH1 versus TH2 responses is also clear for some human mycoses, for example:

- individuals with mild paracoccidioidomycosis have TH1-biased immune responses; whereas

- individuals with severe, disseminated infection have high levels of TH2 cytokines such as IL-4 and IL-10, and eosinophilia.

Children with the primary immunodeficiency hyper IgE syndrome with defects in the production of IFNγ also have increased susceptibility to fungal infections.

An increased level of IL-10 (with concomitant reductions in IFNγ) is also a marker of impaired immunity to systemic mycoses, *C. albicans*, and in neutropenia-associated aspergillosis.

Fungi possess many evasion strategies to promote their survival

Evasion strategies used by fungi to promote their survival include the following:

- *Cryptococcus neoformans* produces a polysaccharide capsule, which inhibits phagocytosis (similar in principle to that of encapsulated bacteria), though this can be overcome by the opsonic effects of complement and antibodies;
- *Histoplasma capsulatum* is an obligate intracellular pathogen that evades macrophage killing by entering the cell via CR3 and then altering the normal pathways of phagosome maturation, in parallel to the strategies of intracellular bacteria such as *M. tuberculosis*;
- dermatophytes suppress host T cell responses to delay cell-mediated destruction.

Immune responses to fungi are therefore as complex and interesting as those against bacteria and for many infections (such as the subcutaneous mycoses) these responses remain poorly understood.

New immunological approaches are being developed to prevent and treat fungal infections

Unlike many antibiotics, which are directly microbicidal, antifungal drugs need significant assistance from the immune system to be most effective.

Reducing the underlying immunosuppression that leads to susceptibility to fungi is an important goal and generic immunotherapies such as cytokine administration (using IFNγ in patients with CGD and granulocyte colony stimulating factor [G-CSF] therapy to reduce neutropenia in patients with cancer) have had some success. There is also considerable interest in dendritic cell-based vaccine strategies to promote TH1-mediated immunity.

FURTHER READING
Bacteria

Collins HL, Kaufmann SH. Prospects for better tuberculosis vaccines. Lancet Infect Dis 2001;1:21–28.

De Gregorio E, Rappuoli R. Inside sensors detecting outside pathogens. Nat Immunol 2004;5:1099–1100.

Harty JT, Tvinnereim AR, White DW. CD8$^+$ T cell effector mechanisms in resistance to infection. Annu Rev Immunol 2000;18:275–308.

Kaufmann SH. How can immunology contribute to the control of tuberculosis? Nat Rev Immunol 2001;1:20–30.

Kaufmann SH, Schaible UE. Antigen presentation and recognition in bacterial infections. Curr Opin Immunol 2005;17:79–87.

Evidence for T cell immunity in chromomycosis

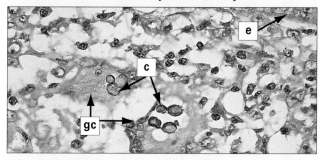

Fig. 14.20 The pigmented fungal cells of chromomycosis (a subcutaneous mycosis) (c) are visible inside giant cells (gc) in the dermis of a patient. The area is surrounded by a predominantly mononuclear cell infiltrate. The basal layer of epidermis (e) is visible at the top of the frame. H & E stain. × 400. (Courtesy of Professor RJ Hay)

MacLennan C, Fieschi C, Lammas DA, et al. Interleukin (IL)-12 and IL-23 are key cytokines for immunity against *Salmonella* in humans. J Infect Dis 2004;190:1755–1757.

Merrell DS, Falkow S. Frontal and stealth attack strategies in microbial pathogenesis. Nature 2004;430:250–256.

Monack DM, Mueller A, Falkow S. Persistent bacterial infections: the interface of the pathogen and the host immune system. Nat Rev Microbiol 2004;2:747–765.

Philpott DJ, Girardin SE. The role of Toll-like receptors and Nod proteins in bacterial infection. Mol Immunol 2004;41:1099–1108.

Reis e Sousa C. Toll-like receptors and dendritic cells: for whom the bug tolls. Semin Immunol 2004;16:27–34.

Rouse BT, Suvas S. Regulatory cells and infectious agents: detentes cordiale and contraire. J Immunol 2004;173:2211–2215.

Schaible UE, Kaufmann SH. Iron and microbial infection. Nat Rev Microbiol 2004;2:946–953.

Stewart GR, Young DB. Heat-shock proteins and the host–pathogen interaction during bacterial infection. Curr Opin Immunol 2004;16:506–510.

Umetsu DT. Revising the immunological theories of asthma and allergy. Lancet 2005;365:98–100.

van de Vosse E, Hoeve MA, Ottenhoff TH. Human genetics of intracellular infectious diseases: molecular and cellular immunity against mycobacteria and salmonellae. Lancet Infect Dis 2004;4:739–749.

Voyich JM, Musser JM, DeLeo FR. *Streptococcus pyogenes* and human neutrophils: a paradigm for evasion of innate host defense by bacterial pathogens. Microbes Infect 2004;6:1117–1123.

Weber JR, Moreillon P, Tuomanen EI. Innate sensors for Gram-positive bacteria. Curr Opin Immunol 2003;15:408–415.

Wills-Karp M, Santeliz J, Karp CL. The germless theory of allergic disease: revisiting the hygiene hypothesis. Nat Rev Immunol 2001;1:69–75.

Fungi

Netea MG, Van der Graaf C, Van der Meer JW, Kullberg BJ. Recognition of fungal pathogens by Toll-like receptors. Eur J Clin Microbiol Infect Dis 2004;23:672–676.

Romani L. Immunity to fungal infections. Nat Rev Immunol 2004;4:1–23.

Critical thinking: Immunoendocrine interactions in the response to infection (see p. 497 for explanations)

Humans subclinically infected with tuberculosis (about one-third of the world's population) may harbor live organisms for the rest of their lives. Similarly tuberculosis can establish a latent non-progressive infection in mice. If animals with such latent infection are subjected to a period of restraint stress (placed in a tube that limits movement) each day for several days, the infection may reactivate. This also happens if cattle with latent disease are transported in trucks. Similarly tuberculosis increases in human populations in war zones, probably due to reactivation of latent disease.

1 What is the physiology of this reactivation?

When American military trainees were subjected to an extremely stressful training schedule their serum IgE levels rose and they lost their previously positive delayed hypersensitivity skin-test responses. The levels of mRNA encoding IFNγ in the peripheral blood mononuclear cells of medical students were lower during the examination period than at other times of the year.

2 Do these observations suggest changes in cytokine profile? If so, why did it happen?

Immunity to Protozoa and Worms

SUMMARY

- Parasites stimulate a variety of immune defense mechanisms.

- **Parasitic infections are often chronic and affect many people.** They are generally host specific and most cause chronic infections. Many are spread by invertebrate vectors and have complicated life cycles. Their antigens are stage specific.

- **Innate immune responses are the first line of immune defense.**

- **T and B cells are pivotal in the development of immunity.** Both CD4 and CD8 T cells are needed for protection from some parasites, and cytokines, chemokines, and their receptors have important roles.

- **Effector cells such as macrophages, neutrophils, eosinophils, and platelets can kill both protozoa and worms.** They secrete cytotoxic molecules such as reactive oxygen radicals and nitric oxide (NO•). All are more effective when activated by cytokines. Worm infections are usually associated with an increase in eosinophil number and circulating IgE, which are characteristic of TH2 responses. TH2 cells are necessary for the elimination of intestinal worms.

- **Parasites have many different escape mechanisms.** Evasion of the host's immune response by parasites occurs in various ways. Some exploit the host response for their own development. It is becoming clear that many parasites, in particular helminths, are able to modulate the host immune response.

- **Inflammatory responses can be a consequence of eliminating parasitic infections.**

- **Parasitic infections have immunopathological consequences.** Parasitic infections are associated with pathology, which can include autoimmunity, splenomegaly, and hepatomegaly. Much immunopathology may be mediated by the adaptive immune response.

- **Vaccines against human parasites are not yet available.**

PARASITES STIMULATE A VARIETY OF IMMUNE DEFENSE MECHANISMS

Parasitic infections typically stimulate a number of immune defense mechanisms, both antibody and cell mediated, and the responses that are most effective depend upon the particular parasite and the stage of infection. Some of the more important parasitic infections of humans (Fig. 15.1) affect the host in diverse ways.

Parasitic protozoa may live:
- in the gut (e.g. amebae);
- in the blood (e.g. African trypanosomes);
- within erythrocytes (e.g. *Plasmodium* spp.);
- in macrophages (e.g. *Leishmania* spp., *Toxoplasma gondii*);
- in liver and spleen (e.g. *Leishmania* spp.); or
- in muscle (e.g. *Trypanosoma cruzi*).

Parasitic worms that infect humans include trematodes or flukes (e.g. schistosomes), cestodes (e.g. tapeworms), and nematodes or roundworms (e.g. *Trichinella spiralis*, hookworms, pinworms, *Ascaris* spp., and the filarial worms).

Tapeworms and adult hookworms inhabit the gut, adult schistosomes live in blood vessels, and some filarial worms live in the lymphatics (Fig. 15.2). It is clear that there is widespread potential for damaging pathological reactions.

Many parasitic worms pass through complicated life cycles, including migration through various parts of the host's body:
- hookworms and schistosome larvae invade their hosts directly by penetrating the skin;
- tapeworms, pinworms, and roundworms are ingested; and
- filarial worms depend upon an intermediate insect host or vector to transmit them from person to person.

Most protozoa rely upon an insect vector, apart from *Toxoplasma* and *Giardia* spp. and amebae, which are transmitted by ingestion. Thus:
- malarial parasites are spread by mosquitoes;
- trypanosomes by tsetse flies;
- *T. cruzi* by triatomine bugs; and
- *Leishmania* by sandflies.

Important parasitic infections of humans

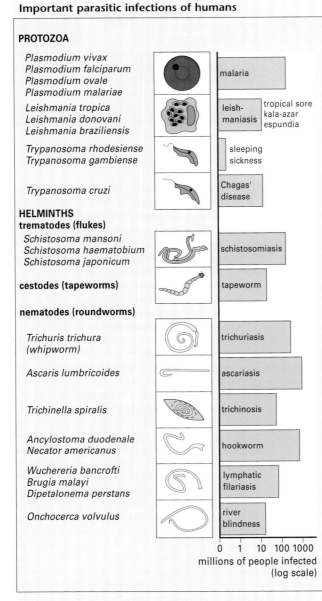

Fig. 15.1 Important parasitic infections, including data from the World Health Organization (1993).

Sites of infection of medically important parasites

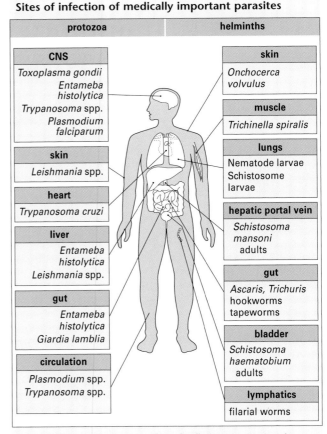

Fig. 15.2 Sites of infection of medically important parasites.

PARASITIC INFECTIONS ARE OFTEN CHRONIC AND AFFECT MANY PEOPLE

Parasitic infections present a major medical problem, especially in tropical countries (see Fig. 15.1), for example:

- malaria kills 1–2 million people every year;
- intestinal worms infect one-third of the world's population – the severity of disease depends upon the worm burden, but in children even moderate intensities of infection may be associated with stunted growth and slow mental development.

Anemia and malnutrition are also associated with parasitic disease.

Over millions of years of evolution, parasites have become well adapted to their hosts and show marked host specificity. For example, the malarial parasites of birds, rodents, or humans can each multiply only in their own particular kind of host.

There are some exceptions to this general rule, for example:

- the protozoan parasite *T. gondii* is not only able to invade and multiply in all nucleated mammalian cells, but can also infect immature mammalian erythrocytes, insect cell cultures, and the nucleated erythrocytes of birds and fish;
- similarly, the tapeworm of the pig can also infect humans.

Protozoan parasites and worms are considerably larger than bacteria and viruses (Fig. 15.3), and have very different strategies for avoiding the host immune response.

Q. Apart from size, what is the basic biological difference between bacterial pathogens and parasites, and how would this affect they way they are recognized by the immune system?

A. Bacteria are prokaryotes, whereas parasites are eukaryotes. The plasma membrane and cell wall structures in bacteria are different, so they have distinct **pathogen-associated molecular patterns** (PAMPs, see Chapter 6). In addition, protein synthesis (initiated with formyl methionine) is different in prokaryotes.

Comparative size of various parasites

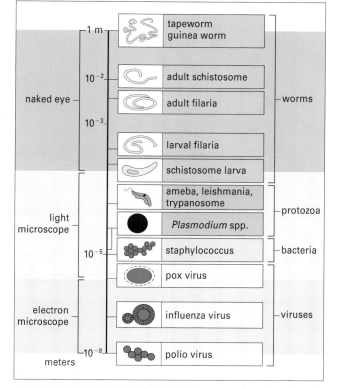

Fig. 15.3 Comparative size of various parasites.

Some species can also change their surface antigens, a process known as **antigenic variation** (see below).

Parasites that have complicated life histories may express certain antigens only at a particular stage of development, giving rise to a stage-specific response. Thus, the protein coat of the sporozoite (the infective stage of the malarial parasite transmitted by the mosquito) induces the production of antibodies that do not react with the erythrocytic stages. The different stages of the worm *T. spiralis* also display different surface antigens.

Protozoa that are small enough to live inside human cells have evolved a special mode of entry:

- the merozoite, the invasive form of the blood stage of the malarial parasite, binds to certain receptors on the surface of the erythrocyte and uses a specialized organelle, the rhoptry, to enter the cell;
- *Leishmania* spp. parasites, which inhabit macrophages, use complement receptors to encourage the cells to engulf them.

Leishmania can also gain entry to the cell by using the mannose receptor (see Fig. 9.18) on the macrophage surface.

Host resistance to parasite infection may be genetic

The resistance of individual hosts to infection varies, and may be controlled by a number of genes. These may be MHC, non-MHC, or other genes (Fig. 15.4).

One should not assume that host genetic background is the only reason determining the outcome of infection. There may be many factors involved. In most helminth infections, for example, a heavy worm burden occurs in comparatively few individuals, but may cluster in families, implying a genetic basis. On the other hand, studies have shown that human behavior can account for large variation in exposure between families.

Many parasitic infections are long-lived

It is not in the interest of a parasite to kill its host, at least not until transmission to another host has been ensured. During the course of a chronic infection the type of immune response may change and immunosuppression and immunopathological effects are common.

Host defense depends upon a number of immunological mechanisms

The development of immunity is a complex process arising from the activation of both adaptive and innate immune responses and the switching on of many different kinds of cell over a period of time. Effects are often local and many cell types secreting different mediators may be present at sites of immune rejection. Moreover, the

Human gene polymorphisms that affect the outcome of parasite infection

parasite	genetic trait
Plasmodium spp.	sickle cell hemoglobin (HbS) protects from malaria certain MHC genes common in West Africans, but rare in Caucasians, protect from malaria (e.g. HLA-B53) Duffy blood group antigen (Fy/Fy)-negative erythrocytes protect from *Plasmodium vivax*
Leishmania spp.	polymorphisms in *Nramp1* govern susceptibility to macrophage invasion
Schistosoma spp.	candidate polymorphic genes on chromosome 5q31-q33, a region that includes key cytokines IL-4 and IL-5
Ascaris spp.	candidate polymorphic genes on chromosomes 1 and 13, a region that includes the TNF family of cytokines

Fig. 15.4 Human gene polymorphisms that affect the outcome of parasite infection.

processes involved in controlling the multiplication of a parasite within an infected individual may differ from those responsible for the ultimate development of resistance to further infection.

In some helminth infections a process of 'concomitant immunity' occurs, whereby an initial infection is not eliminated, but becomes established, and the host then acquires resistance to invasion by new worms of the same species.

In very general terms, humoral responses are important to eliminate extracellular parasites such as those that live in blood (Fig. 15.5), body fluids, or the gut.

However, the type of response conferring most protection varies with the parasite. For example, antibody, alone or with complement, can damage some extracellular parasites, but is better when acting with an effector cell.

As emphasized above, within a single infection different effector mechanisms act against different developmental stages of parasites. Thus in malaria:

- antibody against extracellular forms blocks their capacity to invade new cells;
- cell-mediated responses prevent the development of the liver stage within hepatocytes.

Protective immunity to malaria does not correlate simply with antibody levels and can even be induced in the absence of antibody.

INNATE IMMUNE RESPONSES ARE THE FIRST LINE OF IMMUNE DEFENSE

The innate and adaptive immune responses are co-evolving to allow mammals to identify and eliminate parasites.

The innate immune system provides the first line of immune defense by detecting the immediate presence and nature of infection.

Many different cells are involved in generating innate responses including phagocytic cells and NK cells. It is also becoming clear that early recognition of parasites by

Adult schistosome worm pairs in mesenteric blood vessels

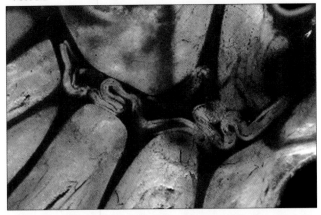

Fig. 15.5 Although very exposed to immune effectors, adult schistosomes are highly resistant and can persist for an average of 3–5 years. (Courtesy of Dr Alison Agnew)

antigen-presenting cells (APCs), for example dendritic cells, determines the phenotype of the adaptive response (Fig. 15.6).

Innate immune recognition relies on a growing number of receptors, termed **pattern recognition receptors (PRRs)** that have evolved to recognize pathogen-associated molecular patterns (PAMPs).

Q. Which groups of receptors and soluble molecules recognize PAMPs?
A. Toll-like receptors (see Fig. 6.24), the mannose receptor (see Fig. 9.18), and scavenger receptors (see Fig. 9.16) allow phagocytes to directly recognize pathogens. Ficolins, collectins, and pentraxins act as soluble opsonins by binding to pathogen surfaces (see Chapter 6 and Fig. 6.23).

Development of the immune response to protozoan and helminth infection

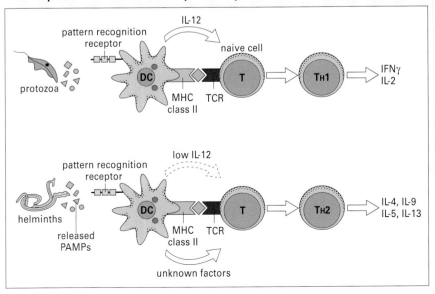

Fig. 15.6 The cytokines secreted by the different subsets of T cells are shown. Note the importance of dendritic cell (DC)-derived IL-12 in driving maturation of helper T cell subsets.

A unifying feature of these targets is their highly conserved structures, which are invariant between parasites of a given class.

Although many parasites are known to activate the immune system in a non-specific manner shortly after infection, it is only recently that attention has been given to the mechanisms involved.

While major advances are being achieved in the area of microbial recognition by PRRs, a small but growing number of studies show that parasites also possess specific molecular patterns capable of engaging PRRs. Examples of some parasite PAMPs along with their receptors are given in Fig. 15.7.

TLR domain-containing PRRs

The discovery of the TLR family (see Fig. 15.7), an evolutionarily conserved group of thirteen mammalian PRRs involved in antimicrobial immunity, has enriched our understanding of how innate and adaptive immunity are mutually dependent.

Very few studies have examined the role of TLRs in immunity to parasites.

Lyso-phosphatidylserine (lyso-PS) from *S. mansoni*, glycophosphatidylinositol (GPI) anchors, and Tc52 from *T. cruzi* are capable of signaling through TLR2. Interestingly, TLR2 triggering by these diverse parasite patterns leads to different immune outcomes:

- with *S. mansoni*, triggering leads to the development of fully mature dendritic cells capable of inducing a Treg response (see Chapter 11), characterized by elevated IL-10 levels;
- with *T. cruzi*, mature dendritic cells induce a TH1 response (see Chapter 7) with raised levels of IL-12.

This dichotomous response could, in part, be explained by the cooperation between TLR2 and other TLRs, including TLR1 and TLR6.

The formation of heterodimers comprising TLR2 and either TLR1 or TLR6 has not yet been observed, but could explain the observed differences in T cell phenotypes.

Innate immune receptors involved in parasite recognition

family	member	parasite ligand(s)
collectins (see Fig. 6.23)	MBL	mannose-rich sugars from numerous protozoans and helminths
pentraxins	CRP	phospholipids and phosphosugars
		Leishmania spp. LPG
C-type lectins (see Fig. 9.18)	macrophage mannose receptor, DC-SIGN	*Trypanosoma cruzi*, *Schistosoma* spp. (LewisX)
scavenger receptors (see Fig. 9.16)	SR-B (CD36)	*Plasmodium falciparum* (PfEMP1)
complement receptors	CR1/CR3	*Leishmania* spp. LPG
		Necator NIF
		Plasmodium PfEMP1
Toll-like receptors (see Fig. 6.24)	TLR2 (with TLR1/TLR6)	GPI anchors from many protozoa
		lyso-PS from *Schistosoma* spp.
	TLR3	double-stranded RNA from *Schistosoma* spp.
	TLR4 (with CD14)	LPS-like molecules from the filarial endosymbiont *Wolbachia* spp.
	TLR9	protozoal DNA
		malarial pigment hemozoin

CRP, C-reactive protein; GPI, glycosylphosphatidylinositol; LPG, lipophosphoglycan; lyso-PS, lyso-phosphatidylserine; MBL, mannose-binding lectin; NIF, neutrophil inhibition factor (NIF); PfEMP1, *P. falciparum* erythrocyte membrane protein-1

Fig. 15.7 Innate immune receptors involved in parasite recognition.

TLR9 mediates innate immune activation by the malaria pigment hemozoin.

Classical human PRRs

Classical PRRs play important roles in the innate response to parasite infection (see Fig. 15.7) and include:

- **collectins** (e.g. MBL);
- **pentraxins** (e.g. CRP);
- **C-type lectins** (e.g. macrophage mannose receptor); and
- **scavenger receptors** (e.g. CD36).

For example MBL binds mannose-rich LPG from *Leishmania*, *Plasmodium*, trypanosomes, and schistosomes; and polymorphisms in the *MBL* gene are associated with increased susceptibility to severe malaria.

Complement receptors are archetypal PRRs

Complement receptors, in particular CR3, are archetypal PRRs involved in innate immune responses (see Fig. 15.7). They are truly multifunctional, being involved in phagocyte adhesion, recognition, migration, activation, and microbe elimination.

Accumulating evidence indicates that complement has pivotal roles to play in diverse biological processes, ranging from early hematopoiesis to skeletal, vascular, and reproductive development.

Why then is CR3, a linchpin of phagocyte responses, the favored portal of entry for diverse intracellular parasites, including leishmania via LPG?

- first, CR3 offers a multiplicity of binding sites, enabling opsonic or non-opsonic binding;
- second, phagocytosis by CR3 alone does not generate an oxidative burst in phagocytic cells;
- third, binding of CR3 suppresses the secretion of IL-12.

Q. What effect would suppression of IL-12 secretion have on the immune response?

A. Because IL-12 promotes the development of the TH1 response, reduced expression will tend to reduce macrophage-mediated immunity.

In isolation, CR3 is not an activating receptor. It requires cooperation from other receptors, most notably Fc receptors, for pathogen killing. Helminths have also exploited this chink in the immune armoury. Hookworm NIF has been shown to bind a domain in the α subunit of CR3, presumably to downregulate cell-mediated immunity.

T AND B CELLS ARE PIVOTAL IN THE DEVELOPMENT OF IMMUNITY

In most parasitic infections, protection can be conferred experimentally on normal animals by the transfer of spleen cells, especially T cells, from immune animals.

The T cell requirement is also demonstrable because nude (athymic) or T-deprived mice fail to clear otherwise non-lethal infections of protozoa such as *T. cruzi* or *Plasmodium yoelii*, and T cell-deprived rats fail to expel the intestinal worm *Nippostrongylus brasiliensis* (Fig. 15.8).

Counter-intuitively, many parasites require signals from immune cells to thrive – for example, schistosomes fail to develop in the absence of hepatic CD4$^+$ lymphocytes.

B cells also play key roles in regulating and controlling immunity to parasites. For example:

- B cells and antibodies are required for resistance to the parasitic gastrointestinal nematode *Trichuris muris*; and
- passive transfer of IgG can protect people from malaria.

Both CD4 and CD8 T cells are needed for protection from some parasites

The type of T cell responsible for controlling an infection varies with the parasite and the stage of infection, and depends upon the kinds of cytokine they produce. For example, CD4$^+$ and CD8$^+$ T cells protect against different phases of *Plasmodium* infection:

- CD4$^+$ T cells mediate immunity against blood-stage *P. yoelii*;
- CD8$^+$ T cells protect against the liver stage of *Plasmodium berghei*.

The action of CD8$^+$ T cells is twofold:

- they secrete IFNγ, which inhibits the multiplication of parasites within hepatocytes;
- they are able to kill infected hepatocytes, but not infected erythrocytes.

Q. By what mechanism are the hepatocytes killed, and why do the CD8$^+$ cells not recognize infected erythrocytes?

A. The CD8$^+$ T cells recognize parasite antigens presented by MHC class I molecules and induce apoptosis in the target, via Fas ligand, tumor necrosis factor (TNF), lymphotoxin, and granzymes. Erythrocytes do not express MHC molecules.

The immune response against *T. cruzi* depends not only upon CD4$^+$ and CD8$^+$ T cells, but also on NK cells and antibody production; the same is true for the immune response against *T. gondii*.

CD8$^+$ T cells confer protection in mice depleted of CD4$^+$ T cells, both through their production of IFNγ and because they are cytotoxic for infected macrophages.

NK cells, stimulated by IL-12 secreted by the macrophages, are another source of IFNγ.

Chronic infections are associated with reduced production of IFNγ.

These observations probably underlie the high incidence of toxoplasmosis in patients with AIDS, who are deficient in CD4$^+$ T cells.

CD4$^+$ T cells are critical for the expulsion of intestinal nematodes and as immunity to *T. muris* can be transferred to a SCID (severe combined immune deficiency) mouse by the transfer of CD4$^+$ T cells alone there is no evidence for a role of CD8$^+$ T cells.

The cytokines produced by CD4$^+$ T cells can be important in determining the outcome of infection. Helper T cells have been phenotypically divided into TH1 and TH2 and more recently regulatory T cell subsets based on the cytokines produced.

As TH1 and TH2 cells have contrasting and cross-regulating cytokine profiles, the roles of TH1 or TH2 cells

Parasitic infections in T cell-deprived mice

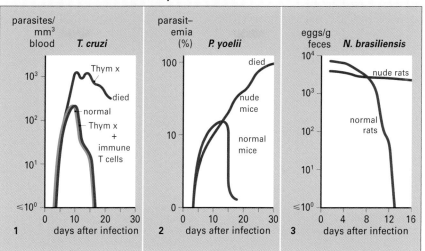

Fig. 15.8 The first two graphs plot the increase in number of blood-borne protozoa (parasitemia) following infection. (1) *T. cruzi* multiplies faster (and gives fatal parasitemia) in mice that have been thymectomized and irradiated to destroy T cells (Thym x). In normal mice, parasites are cleared from the blood by day 16. Reconstitution of T cell-deprived mice with T cells from immune mice restores their ability to control the parasitemia. In these experiments both thymectomized groups were given fetal liver cells to restore vital hematopoietic function. (2) *P. yoelii* causes a self-limiting infection in normal mice and the parasites are cleared from the blood by day 20. In nude mice the parasites continue to multiply, killing the mice after about 30 days. (3) This graph illustrates the time course of the elimination of the intestinal nematode *N. brasiliensis* from the gut of rats. In normal rats the worms are all expelled by day 13, as determined by the number of worm eggs present in the rats' feces. T cells are necessary for this expulsion to occur, as shown by the establishment of a chronic infection in the gut of nude rats.

in determining the outcome of parasitic infections have been extensively investigated.

As a result of early studies, predominantly in mouse infections, certain dogmas have arisen suggesting that:
- TH1 responses mediate killing of intracellular pathogens; and
- TH2 responses eliminate extracellular ones.

However, this is very much an oversimplification of the true picture.

Although the TH1/TH2 paradigm may be a useful tool in some situations, it is probably more realistic to consider that TH1 and TH2 phenotypes represent the extremes of a continuum of cytokine profiles and that perhaps it may be more accurate to look at the role of the cytokines themselves in the resolution of infectious disease.

Regulatory T cells are able to modulate the extremes of both TH2 and TH1 responses.

Cytokines, chemokines, and their receptors have important roles

Q. What experimental methods can be used to elucidate whether a particular cytokine is needed to clear a parasite infection?

A. Experiments with cytokine-knockout animals or cytokine blocking with specific antibody can determine whether a particular cytokine is required. This can be confirmed by observing whether exogenously administered cytokine speeds recovery.

Cytokines not only act on effector cells to enhance their cytotoxic or cytostatic capabilities, but also act as growth factors to increase cell numbers, while chemokines attract cells to the sites of infection. Thus in malaria, the characteristic enlargement of the spleen is caused by an enormous increase in cell numbers.

Other examples include:
- the accumulation of macrophages in the granulomas that develop in the liver in schistosomiasis;
- the eosinophilia characteristic of helminth infections; and
- the recruitment of eosinophils and mast cells into the gut mucosa that occurs in worm infections of the gastrointestinal tract.

Mucosal mast cells and eosinophils are both important in determining the outcome of some helminth infections and proliferate in response to the products of T cells – IL-3 and granulocyte–macrophage colony stimulating factor (GM-CSF), and IL-5, respectively.

However, an increase in cell number can itself harm the host. Thus administration of IL-3 to mice infected with *Leishmania major* can exacerbate the local infection and increase the dissemination of the parasites, probably through the proliferation of bone marrow precursors of the cells the parasites inhabit.

IL-10 and transforming growth factor-β (TGFβ), the regulatory cytokines (see Chapter 11), downregulate the proinflammatory response and thus minimize pathological damage.

Chemokines are key molecules in recruiting immune cells by chemotaxis, but also act in leukocyte activation, hematopoiesis, inflammation, and antiparasite immunity.

Protozoan parasites have been most studied in the context of chemokines and their diverse roles in the parasite–host relationship. For example, *T. gondii* possesses cyclophilin-18, which binds to the chemokine receptor CCR5 and induces IL-12 production by dendritic cells.

T cell responses to protozoa depend on the species

T cell-mediated immunity operating to control protozoan parasites depends on the species of animal infected and the location and complexity of the parasite life cycle within the host.

For example, in mouse models, the induction of TH1 cells with concomitant upregulation of IFNγ and nitric oxide (NO•) is crucial for protection of mice from leishmania. Strains of mice driving TH2 responses on infection, manifested by high levels of IL-4, IL-13, IL-10, and antibody, develop progressive and ultimately lethal disease (Fig. 15.9).

The polarization of helper T cell responses in murine models does not conveniently translate to humans, where both TH1 and TH2 responses appear to be involved in protection.

The importance of TH1 cells to protection from toxoplasmosis is also evident in murine models.

For malaria, the TH1/TH2 paradigm is also somewhat contradictory and less helpful in understanding immunity. This is because the type of immune response mounted and the ensuing risk of pathology depends on whether the first exposure to the parasite occurs during infancy or adulthood.

As a consequence immunity to malaria is best thought of in the context of regulated TH1 responses. Thus, in endemic populations, primary malaria infections in infants induce low levels of IFNγ and TNFα via an innate pathway (potentially involving dendritic cells), which leads to T cell priming.

The infection induces minimal pathology and the parasites can be cleared, either immunologically via maternal antibody or because parasites fail to thrive in fetal hemoglobin.

On reinfection, the malaria-primed T cells produce massive amounts of IFNγ and TNFα leading to an increased risk of unwanted pathology, including cerebral malaria.

Development of the immune response to *Leishmania major* and *Trichuris muris* infection

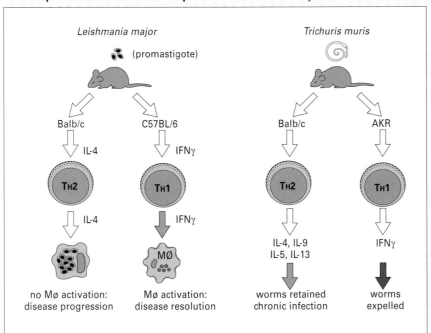

Fig. 15.9 The cytokines secreted by the different subsets of T cells and their effect on the resolution of the disease are shown. Note that resolution of infection is dependent on mouse strain. (Mø, macrophage)

Q. What effects will IFNγ and TNFα have on cerebral blood vessels?

A. These cytokines cause an increase in adhesion molecules (ICAM-1, VCAM-1) and synthesis of inflammatory chemokines (CCL2, CXCL10) producing leukocyte migration into the brain (see Chapter 6). They also cause an increase in the permeability of the vessels so that large serum molecules enter the CNS, and ionic equilibria are disturbed. This is referred to as a breakdown in the blood–brain barrier.

Further infections induce effective anti-parasite immunity principally through the development of an individual's own repertoire of high-affinity antibodies, which inhibit parasite development.

This change in immune environment ultimately leads to a switch in T cell phenotype from TH1 to a regulatory T cell phenotype in which raised levels of IL-10 and TGFβ can be detected.

By contrast, non-immune individuals who contract malaria for the first time in adulthood are unable to control their infections and are more likely to develop severe pathology.

This is believed to arise from cross-reactively primed T cells generated against other microbes that appear to contribute to the development of severe disease.

The immune response to worms depends upon TH2-secreted cytokines

IgE and eosinophilia are the hallmarks of the immune response to worm infections, and depend upon cytokines secreted by TH2 cells (see Fig. 15.9).

In humans schistosomiasis and infection with gastro-intestinal nematodes, resistance to reinfection after drug treatment is correlated with the production of IgE and high pre-treatment levels of TH2 cytokines such as IL-4, IL-5, and IL-13.

The primary stimuli for TH2 development in schistosomiasis are egg antigens. Similarly the excretory and secretory products of nematodes have been shown to polarize cells towards TH2 responses. Again the control of T cell phenotype seems to be exerted by the dendritic cell after exposure to these substances.

The mechanisms of induction of TH2 responses are less well understood than TH1 responses.
- one hypothesis, the default hypothesis, suggests that unless the triggers for TH1 responses are received (including high IL-12), TH2 responses occur;
- more recent evidence, however, suggests that specific signals induce the T cell to make TH2 cytokines, probably including cell–cell interactions.

The pattern of cytokine production in infected hosts may be different from that in vaccinated hosts. For example:
- in mice infected with *S. mansoni*, IL-5-producing TH2 cells predominate;
- in mice that have been immunized, IgE levels and eosinophil numbers are low and TH1 cells predominate.

IFNγ activates effector cells that destroy lung stage larvae, via the production of NO•.

Q. How does IFNγ lead to the production of NO•?

A. It causes the production of inducible NO synthase in macrophages (see Fig. 9.31).

However, when adult worms start to produce eggs, a soluble egg antigen is released that has an effect only in susceptible mice. The antigen reduces levels of IFNγ and increases production of IL-5.

TH2 cytokines control effector mechanisms important in controlling intestinal worm infections. Perhaps the example that demonstrates this most clearly is *T. muris* infection in mice.
- animals normally resistant to infection develop persistent infections in IL-4 and/or IL-13 knockout mice;
- conversely, susceptible mice expel the worms if IL-4 activity is promoted by administration of neutralizing antibody against IFNγ.

The role of IFNγ in promoting chronic infection is again shown by the administration of IL-12 to mice soon after infection with the intestinal worm *Nippostrongylus brasiliensis* (Fig. 15.10).

N. brasiliensis stimulates IFNγ production, which delays expulsion of the worms.

IL-12 acts by inhibiting the production of TH2 cytokines – in particular IL-4 and IL-5, thereby preventing the production of IgE, eosinophilia, and mast cell hypertrophy. IL-9 is another TH2 cytokine that seems to be important in resistance to intestinal nematode infection

Course of infection with *Nippostrongylus brasiliensis* in mice

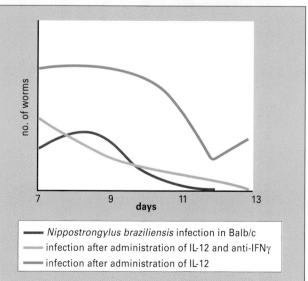

Fig. 15.10 The normal course of infection in Balb/c mice is that worms will be expelled by day 11. This is associated with a TH2 response. If IL-12 is administered straight after infection a TH1 response is promoted and as a result more worms establish and the infection is maintained for longer. If IL-12 is administered, but IFNγ is neutralized, this result is reversed.

and is involved in the production of mucosal mast cell responses and the production of IgE.

IL-9 transgenic mice that produce higher levels of this cytokine have enhanced expulsion of *T. muris*.

What is clear from a number of studies is that there is no single mechanism by which a TH2 response mediates expulsion of all intestinal worms.

The species of worm, its anatomical position within the gut, and the immune status of the host are all factors likely to influence whether a particular immune mechanism will be effective at promoting worm loss.

The host may isolate the parasite with inflammatory cells

In some parasitic infections, the immune system cannot completely eliminate the parasite, but reacts by isolating the organism with inflammatory cells. The host reacts to locally released antigen, which stimulates the production of cytokines that recruit cells to the region. An example of this has been shown in mice vaccinated with radiation-attenuated schistosome cercariae. Infiltrating cells, which are mostly TH1-type lymphocytes, surround the lung-stage larvae as early as 24 hours after intravenous challenge infection. This prevents subsequent migration to the site necessary for development into the adult parasite.

The schistosome egg granuloma in the liver is another example of the host reacting by 'walling off' the parasite. This reaction is a chronic cell-mediated response to soluble antigens released by eggs that have become trapped in the liver. Macrophages accumulate and release fibrogenic factors, which stimulate the formation of granulomatous tissue and, ultimately, fibrosis. Although this reaction may benefit the host, in that it insulates the liver cells from toxins secreted by the worm eggs, it is also the major source of pathology, causing irreversible changes in the liver and the loss of liver function. In the absence of T cells, there is no granuloma formation and no subsequent fibrous encapsulation.

Different mechanisms may affect:
- worms that inhabit different anatomical sites, such as the gut (e.g. *T. trichura*) or the tissues (e.g. *Onchocerca volvulus*); and
- different stages of the life cycle (e.g. schistosome larvae in the lungs and adult worms in the veins).

Parasites induce non-specific and specific antibody production

Many parasitic infections provoke a non-specific hyper-gammaglobulinemia, much of which is probably due to substances released from the parasites acting as B cell mitogens.

Levels of total immunoglobulins are raised:
- IgM in trypanosomiasis and malaria;
- IgG in malaria and visceral leishmaniasis.

The relative importance of antibody-dependent and antibody-independent responses varies with the infection and host (Fig. 15.11).

Relative importance of antibody-dependent and antibody-independent responses in protozoal infections

parasite and habitat		antibody-dependent			antibody-independent	
		importance	mechanism	means of evasion	importance	mechanism
T. brucei free in blood		+ + + +	lysis with complement, which also opsonizes for phagocytosis	antigenic variation	–	
Plasmodium spp. inside red cell		+ + +	blocks invasion, opsonizes for phagocytosis	intracellular; antigenic variation	liver stage + + + blood stage + + +	cytokines macrophage activation
T. cruzi inside macrophage		+ +	limits spread in acute infection, sensitizes for ADCC	intracellular	+ + + (chronic phase)	macrophage activation by IFNγ and TNFα, and killing by NO• and metabolites of O_2
Leishmania spp. inside macrophage		+	limits spread	intracellular	+ + + +	

Fig. 15.11 This table summarizes the relative importance of the two immune responses, the mechanisms involved, and, for antibody, the means by which the protozoon can evade damage by antibody. Antibody is the most important part of the immune response against those parasites that live in the blood stream, such as African trypanosomes and malarial parasites, whereas cell-mediated immunity is active against those like leishmania that live in the tissues. Antibody can damage parasites directly, enhance their clearance by phagocytosis, activate complement, or block their entry into their host cell and so limit the spread of infection. Once inside the cell the parasite is safe from the effects of antibody. *Trypanosoma cruzi* and *Leishmania* spp. are both susceptible to the action of oxygen metabolites release by the respiratory burst of macrophages, and to NO•. Treating macrophages with cytokines enhances release of these products and diminishes the entry and survival of the parasites. (ADCC, antibody-dependent cell-mediated cytotoxicity)

Mechanisms by which specific antibody controls some parasitic infections

parasite	*Plasmodium* spp. sporozoite, intestinal worms, trypanosome	*Plasmodium* spp. sporozoite and merozoite, *T. cruzi*, *T. gondii*	*Plasmodium* spp. trypanosome	schistosomes, *T. spiralis*, filarial worm larvae
mechanism	**1** complement protein	**2**	**3**	**4** Toxic mediators being secreted / larval worm
effect	direct damage or complement-mediated lysis	prevents spread by neutralizing attachment site, prevents escape from lysosomal vacuole, prevents inhibition of lysosomal fusion	enhancement of phagocytosis	antibody-dependent cell-mediated cytotoxicity (ADCC)

Fig. 15.12 **(1)** Direct damage. Antibody activates the classical complement pathway, causing damage to the parasite membrane and increasing susceptibility to other mediators. **(2)** Neutralization. Parasites such as *Plasmodium* spp. spread to new cells by specific receptor attachment; blocking the merozoite binding site with antibody prevents attachment to the receptors on the erythrocyte surface and prevents further multiplication. **(3)** Enhancement of phagocytosis. Complement C3b deposited on the parasite membrane opsonizes it for phagocytosis by cells with C3b receptors (e.g. macrophages). Macrophages also have Fc receptors. **(4)** Eosinophils, neutrophils, platelets, and macrophages may be cytotoxic for some parasites when they recognize the parasite via specific antibody (ADCC). The reaction is enhanced by complement.

The mechanisms by which specific antibody can control parasitic infections and its effects are summarized in Fig. 15.12. Antibody:

- can act directly on protozoa to damage them, either by itself or by activating the complement system (Fig. 15.13);
- can neutralize a parasite directly by blocking its attachment to a new host cell, as with *Plasmodium* spp., whose merozoites enter red blood cells through a special receptor – their entry is inhibited by specific antibody (Fig. 15.14);
- may prevent spread (e.g. in the acute phase of infection by *T. cruzi*);
- can enhance phagocytosis by macrophages – phagocytosis is increased even more by the addition of complement; these effects are mediated by Fc and C3 receptors on macrophages, which may increase in number as a result of macrophage activation;
- is involved in antibody-dependent cell-mediated cytotoxicity (ADCC), for example in infections caused by *T. cruzi*, *T. spiralis*, *S. mansoni*, and filarial worms – cytotoxic cells such as macrophages, neutrophils, and eosinophils adhere to antibody-coated worms by means of their Fc and C3 receptors and degranulate, spilling their toxic contents onto the worm.

Different antibody isotypes may have different effects. In individuals infected with schistosomes, parasite-specific IgE and IgA are associated with resistance to infection and there is an inverse relationship between the amount of IgE in the blood and reinfection.

Direct effect of specific antibody on sporozoites of malaria parasites

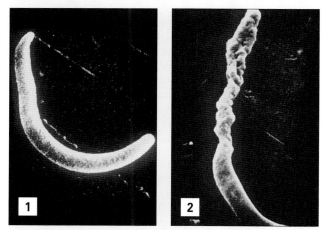

Fig. 15.13 These scanning electron micrographs show a sporozoite of *P. berghei*, which causes malaria in rodents, before **(1)** and after **(2)** incubation in immune serum. The surface of the sporozoite is damaged by the antibody, which perturbs the outer membrane, causing leakage of fluid. Specific antibody protects against infection with *Plasmodium* spp. at several of the extracellular stages of the life cycle. The antibody is stage specific in each case. (Courtesy of Dr R Nussenzweig)

287

Effect of antibody on malarial parasites

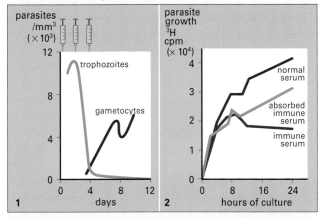

Fig. 15.14 (1) Transfer of γ-globulin from immune adults to a child infected with *Plasmodium falciparum* caused a sharp drop in parasitemia. Specific antibody acts at the merozoite stage in the life of the parasite and prevents the initiation of further cycles of multiplication in the blood. The development of gametocytes from existing intracellular forms is unaffected. (2) In culture, the presence of immune serum blocks the continued increase in number of *Plasmodium knowlesi* (a malarial parasite of monkeys), as measured by incorporation of ³H-leucine. It stops multiplication at the stage after schizont rupture by preventing the released merozoites from invading fresh red blood cells. The inhibitory activity of the immune serum can be reduced by prior absorption of the specific antibody with free schizonts.

Q. What roles does IgE have in immune defense?

A. IgE mediates inflammation by binding to mast cells and basophils, sensitizing them to parasite antigens. Additionally it can act as an opsonin for eosinophils (see Chapter 3).

IgG4 appears to block the action of IgE; reinfection is more likely in children who have high levels of IgG4. Class switching to IgG4 appears to occur in the context of a modified TH2 response involving the induction of Tregs.

The development of immunity seems to depend upon a switch from IgG4 to IgE that occurs with age – infection rates are highest in 10–14-year-olds when IgG4 levels are also at their highest.

In many infections it is difficult to distinguish between cell-mediated and antibody-mediated responses because both can act in concert against the parasite. This is illustrated in Fig. 15.15, which summarizes the immune reaction that can be mounted against schistosome larvae.

EFFECTOR CELLS SUCH AS MACROPHAGES, NEUTROPHILS, EOSINOPHILS, MAST CELLS, AND PLATELETS CAN ATTACK PARASITES

Antibody and cytokines produced specifically in response to parasite antigens enhance the anti-parasitic activities of all these effector cells, though tissue macrophages, monocytes, and granulocytes have some intrinsic activity

before enhancement. The point of entry of the parasite is obviously important, for example:

- the cercariae of *S. mansoni* enter through the skin – experimental depletion of macrophages, neutrophils, and eosinophils from the skin of mice increases their susceptibility to infection;
- trypanosomes and malarial parasites entering the blood are removed from the circulation by phagocytic cells in the spleen and liver;
- comparison of strains of mice with various immunological defects for their resistance to infection by *Trypanosoma rhodesiense* shows that the African trypanosomes are destroyed by macrophages, and later in infection, when opsonized with antibodies and complement C3b, they are taken up by macrophages in the liver more quickly still.

Before acting as APCs initiating an immune response, macrophages act as effector cells to inhibit the multiplication of parasites or even to destroy them. They also secrete molecules that regulate the inflammatory response:

- some of these molecules – IL-1, IL-12, TNFα, and the colony stimulating factors (CSFs) – enhance immunity by activating other cells or stimulating their proliferation;
- others, like IL-10, prostaglandins, and TGFβ, may be anti-inflammatory and immunosuppressive.

Macrophages can kill extracellular parasites

Phagocytosis by macrophages provides an important defense against the smaller parasites. Macrophages also secrete many cytotoxic factors, enabling them to kill parasites without ingesting them.

When activated by cytokines, macrophages can kill both relatively small extracellular parasites, such as the erythrocytic stages of malaria, and also larger parasites, such as the larval stages of the schistosome. Macrophages also:

- act as killer cells through ADCC – specific IgG and IgE, for instance, enhance their ability to kill schistosomules;
- secrete cytokines, such as TNFα and IL-1, which interact with other types of cell, for example rendering hepatocytes resistant to malarial parasites.

Reactive oxygen intermediates (ROIs) are generated by macrophages and granulocytes following phagocytosis of *T. cruzi*, *T. gondii*, *Leishmania* spp., and malarial parasites, for instance. Filarial worms and schistosomes also stimulate the respiratory burst.

When activated by cytokines, macrophages release more superoxide and hydrogen peroxide than normal resident macrophages, and their oxygen-independent killing mechanisms are similarly enhanced.

Nitric oxide, a product of L-arginine metabolism, is one of the potent oxygen-independent toxins. Its synthesis by macrophages in mouse experimental systems is induced by the cytokines IFNγ and TNFα and is greatly increased when they act synergistically. NO• can also be produced by endothelial cells. It contributes to host resistance in leishmaniasis, schistosomiasis, and malaria, and is probably important in the control of most parasitic infections (see Fig. 15.15). For instance, the innate resistance to infection by *T. gondii* that is lost in immuno-

Possible effector responses to schistosomules

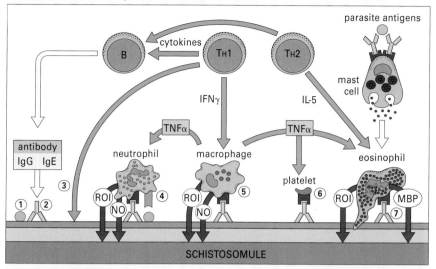

Fig. 15.15 The various effector mechanisms damaging schistosomes in vitro are shown. Complement alone damages worms (**1**) and also does so in combination with antibody (**2**). TH1 cells may act directly, reducing the number of larvae in the lungs (**3**). Antibody sensitizes neutrophils (**4**), macrophages (**5**), platelets (**6**), and eosinophils (**7**) for ADCC. Neutrophils and macrophages probably act by releasing toxic oxygen and nitrogen metabolites, whereas eosinophils damage the worm tegument by the release of major basic protein (MBP) plus reactive oxygen intermediates (ROI). The response is potentiated by cytokines (e.g. TNFα). IgE antibody is important in sensitizing both eosinophils and local mast cells, which release a variety of mediators, including those that activate the eosinophils.

compromised individuals appears to be due to the inhibition of parasite multiplication by such an oxygen-independent mechanism.

Activation of macrophages is a feature of early infection

All macrophage effector functions are enhanced soon after infection. Although their specific activation is by cytokines secreted by T cells (e.g. IFNγ, GM-CSF, IL-3, and IL-4), they can also be activated by T cell-independent mechanisms, for example:

- NK cells secrete IFNγ when stimulated by IL-12 produced by macrophages;
- macrophages secrete TNFα in response to some parasite products (e.g. phospholipid-containing antigens of malarial parasites and some *T. brucei* antigens) – this TNFα then activates other macrophages.

Although TNFα may be secreted by several other cell types, activated macrophages are the most important source of TNFα, which is necessary for protective responses to several species of protozoa (e.g. *Leishmania* spp.) and helminths. Thus TNFα activates macrophages, eosinophils, and platelets to kill the larval form of *S. mansoni*, its effects being enhanced by IFNγ.

TNFα may have harmful as well as beneficial effects on the infected host, depending upon the amount produced and whether it is free in the circulation or locally confined. Serum concentrations of TNFα in falciparum malaria correlate with the severity of the disease. Administration of TNFα cures a susceptible strain of mice infected with the rodent malarial parasite *Plasmodium chabaudi*, but kills a genetically resistant strain. Presumably the latter can already make enough TNFα to control parasite replication, and any more has toxic effects.

Neutrophils can kill large and small parasites

The effector properties displayed by macrophages are also seen in neutrophils. Neutrophils are phagocytic and can kill by both oxygen-dependent and oxygen-independent mechanisms, including NO•. They produce a more intense respiratory burst than macrophages and their secretory granules contain highly cytotoxic proteins.

Q. Which groups of cytotoxic protein are found in neutrophil granules?

A. Defensins, seprocidins, and cathelicidins (see Chapter 2).

Neutrophils can be activated by cytokines, such as IFNγ, TNFα, and GM-CSF.

Extracellular destruction by neutrophils is mediated by hydrogen peroxide, whereas granular components are involved in the intracellular destruction of ingested organisms.

Neutrophils are present in parasite-infected inflammatory lesions and probably act to clear parasites from bursting cells.

Like macrophages, neutrophils bear Fc and complement receptors and can participate in antibody-dependent cytotoxic reactions to kill the larvae of *S. mansoni*, for example. In this mode, they can be more destructive than eosinophils against several species of nematode, including *T. spiralis*, though the relative effectiveness of the two types of cell may depend upon the isotype and specificity of antibody.

Eosinophils are characteristically associated with worm infections

It has been suggested that:
- the eosinophil evolved specifically as a defense against the tissue stages of parasites that are too large to be phagocytosed; and
- the IgE-dependent mast cell reaction has evolved primarily to localize eosinophils near the parasite and enhance their anti-parasitic functions.

The importance of eosinophils in vivo has been shown by experiments using antiserum against eosinophils. Mice infected with *T. spiralis* and treated with the antiserum develop more cysts in their muscles than the controls – without the protection offered by eosinophils, the mice cannot eliminate the worms and so encyst the parasites to minimize damage.

However, recent work has shown that although eosinophils can help the host to control a worm infection, particularly by limiting migration through the tissues, they do not always do so. For instance, their removal does not abolish the immunity of mice infected with *S. mansoni*, nor does this increase the parasite load in a tapeworm infection.

Removal of IL-5, which is important in the generation and activation of eosinophils, did not change the outcome of *T. spiralis* or *T. muris* infection. In contrast the infectivity of *Strongyloides venezuelensis* is enhanced in IL-5-deficient mice. Although *T. spiralis* worm burdens were not affected in a primary infection of IL-5 deleted mice, the worm numbers were significantly higher after challenge infection.

The role of IL-5 and therefore eosinophils has also been suggested from human epidemiological studies on gastrointestinal nematode infections where, after drug treatment, low reinfection worm burdens were associated with high pre-treatment levels of IL-5.

Elevated eosinophilia is often associated with high levels of IgE, both of which are hallmarks of infection with parasites. Although eosinophils express FcεR1, most of the protein is confined to the cytoplasm, and there is little evidence for IgE-dependent function.

Eosinophils can kill helminths by oxygen-dependent and independent mechanisms

Eosinophils are less phagocytic than neutrophils. They degranulate in response to perturbation of their surface membrane and their activities are enhanced by cytokines such as TNFα and GM-CSF. Most of their activities, however, are controlled by antigen-specific mechanisms. Thus their binding in vitro to the larvae of worms coated with IgE or IgA (e.g. *S. mansoni* and *T. spiralis*) increases the release of their granular contents onto the surface of the worms (see Fig. 15.15).

Damage to schistosomules can be caused by the major basic protein (MBP) of the eosinophil crystalloid core. MBP is not specific for any particular target, but because it is confined to a small space between the eosinophil and the schistosome, there is little damage to nearby host cells.

Eosinophils and mast cells can act together

The killing of *S. mansoni* larvae by eosinophils is enhanced by mast cell products, and when studied in vitro eosinophils from patients with schistosomiasis are found to be more effective than those from normal subjects. The antigens released cause local IgE-dependent degranulation of mast cells and the release of mediators. These selectively attract eosinophils to the site and further enhance their activity. Other products of eosinophils later block the mast cell reactions. These effector mechanisms may function in vivo, as has been shown in monkeys, where schistosome killing is associated with eosinophil accumulation.

Mast cells control gastrointestinal helminths

In the case of *T. spiralis* and *Heligmosomoides polygyrus* there is good evidence to suggest the involvement of mucosal mast cells (Fig. 15.16).

Section through the gut of a mouse infected with
Heligmosomoides polygyrus

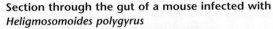

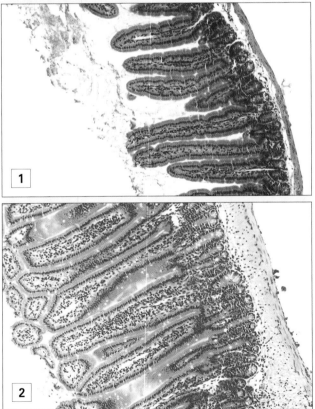

Fig. 15.16 (1) Gut of an uninfected mouse. (2) Gut of an infected mouse. The crypts have shortened and a large influx of mast cells can be clearly seen.

Mast cells contain a number of lipid mediators, such as prostaglandins, proteases, and histamine. In addition, they also represent a source of cytokines such as IL-3, IL-4, IL-5, GM–CSF, and TNFα.

Following mast cell activation, the mast cell contents are released resulting in changes to the permeability of the intestinal epithelium and ultimately an environment that appears hostile for continued *T. spiralis* survival. By contrast, expulsion of *N. brasiliensis* and *T. muris* still proceeds normally following depression of mastocytosis, suggesting that the mast cell is not the major effector cell type.

Therefore, although TH2 cytokines are critical for the elimination of worms from the gut, the exact effector mechanism operating may vary.

Platelets can kill many types of parasite

Potential targets for platelets include the larval stage of flukes, *T. gondii*, and *T. cruzi*.

Like other effector cells, the cytotoxic activity of platelets is enhanced by treatment with cytokines (e.g. IFNγ and TNFα). In rats infected with *S. mansoni*, platelets become larvicidal when acute phase reactants appear in the serum but before antibody can be detected. Incubation of normal platelets in such serum can cause their activation.

Platelets, like macrophages and the other effector cells, also bear Fcε receptors on their surface membrane, by which they mediate antibody-dependent cytotoxicity associated with IgE.

PARASITES HAVE MANY DIFFERENT ESCAPE MECHANISMS

It is a necessary characteristic of all successful parasitic infections that they can evade the full effects of their host's immune responses. Parasites have developed many different ways of doing this. Some even exploit cells and molecules of the immune system to their own advantage – *Leishmania* parasites, by using complement receptors to effect their entry into macrophages, avoid triggering the oxidative burst and thus destruction by its toxic products.

Despite their protective role in the immune response to many different parasites:
- host TNFα actually stimulates egg production by adult worms of *S. mansoni*;
- IFNγ is used as a growth factor by *T. brucei*.

Parasites can resist destruction by complement

In the case of *Leishmania*, resistance correlates with virulence:
- *L. tropica*, which is easily killed by complement, causes a localized self-healing infection in the skin; whereas
- *L. donovani*, which is ten times more resistant to complement, becomes disseminated throughout the viscera, causing a disease that is often fatal.

The mechanisms whereby parasites can resist the effect of complement differ:
- the lipophosphoglycan (LPG) surface coat of *L. major* activates comple-ment, but the complex is then shed so the parasite avoids lysis;

- the trypomastigotes of *T. cruzi* bear a surface glycoprotein that has activity resembling the decay accelerating factor (DAF) that limits the complement reaction.

The resistance that schistosomules acquire as they mature is also correlated with the appearance of a surface molecule similar to DAF.

Intracellular parasites can avoid being killed by oxygen metabolites and lysosomal enzymes

Intracellular parasites that live inside macrophages have evolved different ways of avoiding being killed by oxygen metabolites and lysosomal enzymes (Fig. 15.17):
- *T. gondii* penetrates the macrophage by a non-phagocytic pathway and so avoids triggering the oxidative burst;
- *Leishmania* spp. can enter by binding to complement receptors – another way of avoiding the respiratory burst.

Leishmania organisms also possess enzymes such as superoxide dismutase, which protects them against the action of oxygen radicals.

It can be demonstrated that the vacuole in which *Leishmania* organisms survive is lysosomal in nature (Fig. 15.18), but the parasites have evolved mechanisms that protect it against enzymatic attack. The LPG surface coat not only acts as a scavenger of oxygen metabolites and affords protection against enzymatic attack, but a glycoprotein, Gp63 (Fig. 15.19), inhibits the action of the macrophage's lysosomal enzymes.

Leishmania spp. can also downregulate the expression of MHC class II molecules on the macrophages they inhabit, thus reducing their capacity to stimulate TH cells.

These escape mechanisms, however, are less efficient in the immune host.

Q. Why would reduction in MHC molecule expression be less effective in an immune host?

A. In immune hosts, the release of IFNγ enhances MHC molecule expression by APCs. In addition the level of stimulation required by a primed T cell is less than for a naive T cell, due in part to its enhanced level of receptors for co-stimulatory signals (see Chapter 7).

Parasites can disguise themselves

Parasites that are vulnerable to specific antibody have evolved different methods of evading its effects.

The African trypanosome undergoes antigenic variation

The molecule that forms the surface coat of the African trypanosome, the variable surface glycoprotein (VSG), changes to protect the underlying surface membrane from the host's defense mechanisms. New populations of parasites are antigenically distinct from previous ones (Figs 15.20 and 15.21).

Several antigens of malarial parasites also undergo antigenic variation.

For example, the *P. falciparum* erythrocyte membrane protein-1 (PfEMP1) is extremely polymorphic and

The different ways by which protozoa that multiply within macrophages escape digestion by lysosomal enzymes

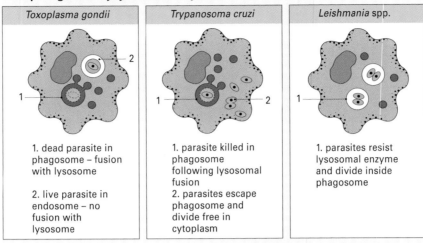

Toxoplasma gondii	*Trypanosoma cruzi*	*Leishmania* spp.
1. dead parasite in phagosome – fusion with lysosome	1. parasite killed in phagosome following lysosomal fusion	1. parasites resist lysosomal enzyme and divide inside phagosome
2. live parasite in endosome – no fusion with lysosome	2. parasites escape phagosome and divide free in cytoplasm	

Fig. 15.17 *T. gondii* – Live parasites enter the cell actively into a membrane-bound vacuole. They are not attacked by enzymes because lysosomes do not fuse with this vacuole. Dead parasites, however, are taken up by normal phagocytosis into a phagosome (by interaction with the Fc receptors on the macrophage if they are coated with antibody) and are then destroyed by the enzymes of the lysosomes that fuse with it. *T. cruzi* – Survival of these parasites depends upon their stage of development; trypomastigotes escape from the phagosome and divide in the cytoplasm whereas epimastigotes do not escape and are killed. The proportion of parasites found in the cytoplasm is decreased if the macrophages are activated. *Leishmania* spp. – These parasites multiply within the phagosome and the presence of a surface protease helps them resist digestion. If the macrophages are first activated by cytokines, the number of parasites entering the cell and the number that replicate diminish.

The leishmanial vacuole is lysosomal in nature

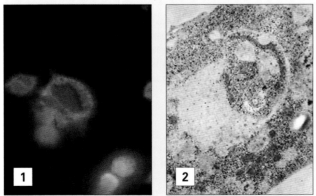

Fig. 15.18 (1) Immunofluorescence of *Leishmania mexicana*-infected murine macrophages probed with a rhodamine-conjugated anti-tubulin antibody to illustrate the parasite (stained yellow/red) and a fluorescein-conjugated monoclonal antibody, which reacts with the late endosomal/lysosomal marker LAMP-1 (stained green). (2) Immunoelectron micrograph of *L. mexicana*-infected murine macrophage probed with gold-labeled anti-cathepsin D demonstrating the lysosomal aspartic proteinase in the leishmanial vacuole. (Courtesy of Dr David Russell)

variable between different strains of the parasite because it is perpetually exposed to the immune system by its location on the red cell membrane.

Other parasites acquire a surface layer of host antigens

Other parasites, such as schistosomes, acquire a surface layer of host antigens so that the host does not distinguish them from 'self'.

Schistosomules cultured in medium containing human serum and red blood cells can acquire surface molecules containing A, B, and H blood group determinants. They can also acquire MHC molecules and immuno-globulins. However, schistosomules maintained in a medium devoid of host molecules also become resistant to attack by antibody and complement, as mentioned above.

Some extracellular parasites hide from immune attack

Some species of protozoa (e.g. *Entameba histolytica*) and helminths (e.g. *T. spiralis*) form protective cysts, while adult worms of *Onchocerca volvulus* in the skin induce the host to surround them with collagenous nodules.

Intestinal nematodes and tapeworms are preserved from many host responses simply because they live in the gut.

Two surface antigens of *Leishmania*

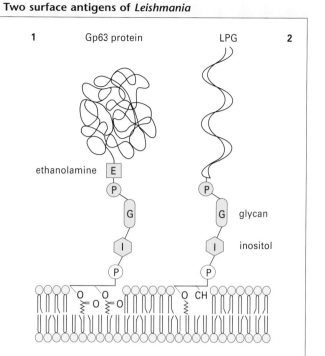

Fig. 15.19 Schematic representation of two surface antigens of *Leishmania* that are anchored to the membrane by phosphatidylinositol tails (GPI anchors). (**1**) This protein antigen, Gp63, has protease activity. That of *L. mexicana*, together with lipophosphoglycan (LPG), binds complement. This enables the promastigote to enter the macrophage through the C3 complement receptor. (**2**) This glycolipid antigen, a LPG, imparts resistance to complement-mediated lysis. That of *L. major* binds C3b, the third component of complement, enabling the promastigote to enter through the CR1 complement receptor. Antibodies to both antigens confer protection against murine cutaneous leishmaniasis. Note that many coat proteins of parasites, such as the variable surface glycoprotein (VSG) of *T. brucei*, are now known to be bound to the surface membrane by a GPI anchor.

Antigenic variation in trypanosomes

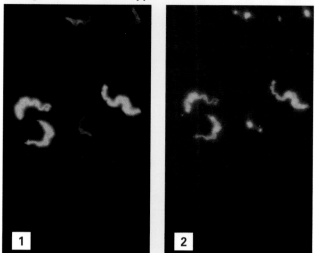

Fig. 15.20 Immunofluorescent labeling of trypanosomes with a variant antigen-type specific monoclonal antibody (**1**). Panel (**2**) shows the same field of view where the nuclei and kinetoplasts of all the parasites are stained with a dye that binds to DNA. Only some of the parasites express a given antigen variant. (Courtesy of Dr Mike Turner)

Some extracellular parasites can withstand immune attack

There are numerous examples of simple, physical, protective strategies in parasites:

- nematodes have a thick extracellular cuticle, which protects them from the toxic effects of an immune response;
- the tegument of schistosomes thickens during maturation to offer similar protection;
- the loose surface coat of many nematodes may slough off under immune attack;
- tapeworms actually prevent attack by secreting an elastase inhibitor, which stops them attracting neutrophils.

Many parasitic worms have evolved methods of resisting the oxidative burst. For instance, schistosomes have surface-associated glutathione S-transferases, and *Onchocerca* spp. can secrete superoxide dismutase.

Some nematodes and trematodes have evolved an elegant method of disabling antibodies by secreting proteases, which cleave immunoglobulins, removing the Fc portion, and preventing their interaction with Fc receptors on phagocytic cells; for example, schistosomes can cleave IgE.

Most parasites interfere with immune responses for their benefit
Parasites produce molecules that interfere with host immune function

Parasites produce molecules that can affect the phenotype of the adaptive response, which may be to their own advantage (Figs 15.22 and 15.23).

In leishmaniasis, T cells from patients infected with *L. donovani* when cultured with specific antigen do not secrete IL-2 or IFNγ. Their production of IL-1 and expression of MHC class II molecules is also decreased, whereas secretion of prostaglandins is increased. IL-2, characteristic of TH1 responses, is also deficient in other protozoal infections including malaria, African trypanosomiasis, and Chagas' disease. In mice infected with *T. cruzi*, a parasite product appears to interfere with expression of the IL-2 receptor.

Filarial worms secrete a protease inhibitor that has been shown to affect the proteases critical in the processing of antigens to peptides resulting in the reduction of class II molecule presentation in filariasis. Onchocystatin – one such protease inhibitor – is also able to modulate T cell proliferation and elicit the upregulation of IL-10

Antigenic variation in African trypanosomes

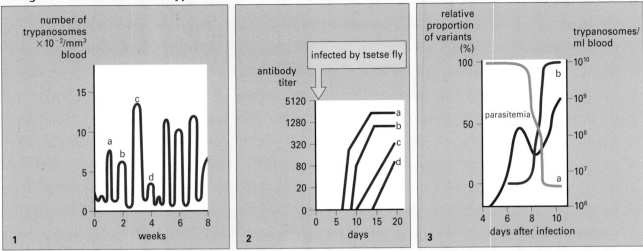

Fig. 15.21 Trypanosome infections may run for several months giving rise to successive waves of parasitemia. Graph (**1**) shows a chart of the fluctuation in parasitemia in a patient with sleeping sickness. Although infection was initiated by a single parasite, each wave is caused by an immunologically distinct population of parasites (a, b, c, d); protection is not afforded by antibody against any of the preceding variants. There is a strong tendency for new variants to appear in the same order in different hosts. Variation does not occur in immunologically compromised animals (i.e. animals treated to deprive them of some aspect of immune function). Graph (**2**) shows the time course of production of antibody against four variants in a rabbit bitten by a tsetse fly carrying *Trypanosoma brucei*. Antibody to successive variants appears shortly after the appearance of each variant and rises to a plateau. The appearance of antibody drives the parasite towards another variant type. Graph (**3**) shows the kinetics of one cycle of antigenic variation. A rat was infected with a homogeneous population of one variant (a) of *T. brucei*. The second wave of parasitemia develops as the new variant (b) emerges and predominates.

expression and is therefore able to modulate the T cell phenotype. Prostaglandins (PGs) produced by helminth parasites may also perform a similar role by modulating APC function. PGE_2 is produced by filarial parasites and tapeworms and blocks the production of IL-12 by dendritic cells and thus may direct responses towards TH2.

Phosphorylcholine (PC)-containing molecules are commonly found in infectious organisms and experiments using a nematode PC-bearing glycoconjugate, ES-62, have been shown to desensitize APCs to subsequent exposure to LPS and may therefore also skew against a TH1 response (LPS is a classical inducer of TH1 responses). ES-62 is also able to inhibit proliferation by both T cells and B cells, causes a decrease in the level of protein kinase C rendering both B and T cells anergic.

Parasites also produce cytokine-like molecules mimicking TGFβ, migration inhibitory factor (MIF), and a histamine-releasing factor.

Genes encoding possible cytokine homologs are being found as part of the genome sequencing projects that are under way for many parasites. Although the sequences are related to cytokines or cytokine receptors, their functions remain to be established.

Soluble parasite antigens released in huge quantities may impair the host's response by a process termed **immune distraction**. Thus the soluble antigens (S or

heat-stable antigens) of *P. falciparum* are thought to mop up circulating antibody, providing a 'smokescreen' and diverting the antibody from the body of the parasite.

Many of the surface antigens that are shed are soluble forms of molecules inserted into the parasite membrane by a GPI anchor, including the VSG of *T. brucei*, the LPG or 'excreted factor' of *Leishmania* (see Fig. 15.19), and several surface antigens of schistosomules. These are released by endogenous phosphatidylinositol-specific phospholipases.

The hypergammaglobulinemic immunoglobulins produced by malaria parasites can bind to FcγRIIB, which may benefit the parasite.

Q. Which cells express FcγRIIB and what effect does ligation of this receptor have on them?

A. B cells express the receptor and ligation inhibits antibody synthesis.

INFLAMMATORY RESPONSES CAN BE A CONSEQUENCE OF ELIMINATING PARASITIC INFECTIONS

Immunosuppression is a common feature of chronic helminth infections, both parasite-specific and general-

Some mechanisms by which parasites avoid host immunity

parasite	habitat	main host effector mechanism	method of avoidance
Trypanosoma brucei	blood stream	antibody + complement	antigenic variation
Plasmodium spp.	hepatocyte bloo dstream	T cells, antibody	antigenic variation, sequestration
Toxoplasma gondii	macrophage	ROI, NO•, lysosomal enzymes	suppresses IL-12, inhibits fusion of lysozymes
Trypanosoma cruzi	many cells	ROI, NO•, lysosomal enzymes	escapes to cytoplasm so avoiding digestion
Leishmania spp.	macrophage	ROI, NO•, lysosomal enzymes	induction of Tregs, resists digestion by phagolysosome
Schistosoma spp.	skin, blood, lungs, portal veins	myeloid cells antibody + complement	acquisition of host antigens (e.g. IgG), proteolytic cleavage of immune proteins, inhibition of dendritic cell maturation
filariasis	lymphatics	myeloid cells	induction of Tregs, secretion of cytokine mimics, interference with antigen processing

NO•, nitric oxide; ROI, reactive oxygen intermediates

Fig. 15.22 A summary of the various methods that parasites have evolved to avoid host defense mechanisms.

ized. For example, patients with schistosomiasis and filariasis have diminished responsiveness to antigens from the infecting parasite. Studies have also shown diminished responses to bystander infections and vaccinations. This spillover suppression may in fact be beneficial to the host in some situations. Reduced inflammatory responses have been observed in *Helicobacter pylori* infection and malaria.

Parasites have co-evolved with humans over millions of years and until recently it was normal for people to carry worms, a fact that argues for their importance in the **'hygiene hypothesis'**, which proposes that the rise in immune disorders, including allergies and autoimmune illness, is due to cleaner living conditions and the almost complete elimination of parasitic infections in westernized societies.

The ability of parasites to suppress hyperactive immune responses is believed to be due to the induction of regulatory T cells (see Fig. 15.23). Understanding how regulatory T cells, also known as suppressor T cells, are induced and how they dampen immune responses is the focus of intensive research. It seems to be the dendritic cell that polarizes the T cell towards a regulator phenotype after exposure to parasite extracts. The schistosome lyso-PS with acyl chains not present on mammalian lyso-PS was shown to activate dendritic cells via TLR2, which when incubated with T cells induced IL-10-producing regulatory T cells.

PARASITIC INFECTIONS HAVE IMMUNOPATHOLOGICAL CONSEQUENCES

Apart from the directly destructive effects of some parasites and their products on host tissues, many immune responses themselves have pathological effects.

In malaria, African trypanosomiasis, and visceral leishmaniasis, the increased number and heightened activity of macrophages and lymphocytes in the liver and spleen lead to enlargement of those organs. In schistosomiasis much of the pathology results from the T cell-dependent granulomas forming around eggs in the liver. The gross changes in individuals with elephantiasis are probably caused by immunopathological responses to adult filariae in the lymphatics.

The formation of immune complexes is common – they may be deposited in the kidney, as in the nephrotic syndrome of quartan malaria, and may give rise to many other pathological changes. For example, tissue-bound immunoglobulins have been found in the muscles of mice infected with African trypanosomes and in the choroid plexus of mice with malaria.

Some immunomodulatory effects of parasites

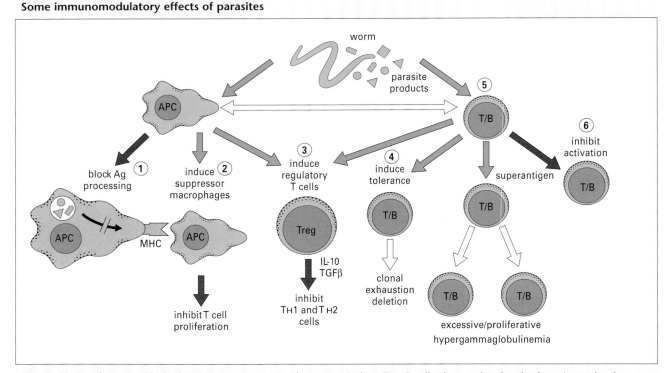

Fig. 15.23 Interference with the host's immune response by molecules released by protozoa or worms. Parasite products act via the APC to (**1**) interfere with antigen processing or presentation (e.g. protease inhibitors from filarial parasites interfere with proteases in the MHC signaling pathway and block antigen presentation); (**2**) induce suppressor macrophages, which can inhibit T cell proliferation; (**3**) induce regulatory T cells (e.g. lyso-PS from schistosomes acts via TLR2 on dendritic cells to induce T cells that secrete IL-10, which inhibits the inflammatory response). Parasite products may also affect lymphocytes to (**3**) make them become regulatory; (**4**) induce T or B cell tolerance by clonal exhaustion or by the induction of anergy; (**5**) cause polyclonal activation (many parasite products are mitogenic to T or B cells, and the high serum concentrations of non-specific IgM [and IgG] commonly found in parasitic infections probably result from this polyclonal stimulation – its continuation is believed to lead to impairment of B cell function, the progressive depletion of antigen-reactive B cells, and thus immunosuppression); (**6**) directly inhibit the activation of T or B cells (e.g. ES-62, a secreted product of a filarial parasites, is able to inhibit the proliferation of both T and B cells).

The IgE of worm infections can have severe effects on the host due to release of mast cell mediators. Anaphylactic shock may occur when a hydatid cyst ruptures. Asthma-like reactions occur in *T. canis* infections and in tropical pulmonary eosinophilia when filarial worms migrate through the lungs.

Autoantibodies, which probably arise as a result of polyclonal activation, have been detected against red blood cells, lymphocytes, and DNA (e.g. in trypanosomiasis and in malaria).

Antibodies against the parasite may cross-react with host tissues. For example, the chronic cardiomyopathy, enlarged esophagus, and megacolon that occur in Chagas' disease are thought to result from the autoimmune effects on nerve ganglia of antibody and cytotoxic T cells that cross-react with *T. cruzi*. Similarly *O. volvulus*, the cause of river blindness, possesses an antigen that cross-reacts with a protein in the retina.

Excessive production of cytokines may contribute to some of the manifestations of disease. Thus the fever, anemia, diarrhea, and pulmonary changes of acute malaria closely resemble the symptoms of endotoxemia and are probably caused by TNFα. The severe wasting of cattle with trypanosomiasis may also be mediated by TNFα.

A single parasite protein may produce multiple pathological effects, as seen with PfEMP1, coded by the *var* genes, and expressed on the surface of infected erythrocytes (Fig. 15.24).

Lastly, the non-specific immunosuppression that is so widespread probably explains why people with parasitic infections are especially susceptible to bacterial and viral infections (e.g. measles). It may also account for the association of Burkitt's lymphoma with malaria because malaria-infected individuals are less able to control infection with the Epstein–Barr virus that causes Burkitt's lymphoma.

Malarial pathology resulting from interactions with PfEMP1

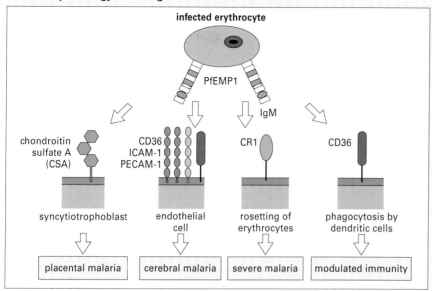

Fig. 15.24 Malaria-infected erythrocytes cause disease through many mechanisms involving the interaction between *P. falciparum* erythrocyte membrane protein-1 (PfEMP1) and diverse host receptors.

VACCINES AGAINST HUMAN PARASITES ARE NOT YET AVAILABLE

Some vaccines composed of attenuated living parasites have proved successful in veterinary practice. However, so far there is none in use against human parasites, though much effort has been directed towards the development of subunit vaccines against malarial parasites and schistosomes in particular. Some clinical trials of vaccines against malaria, based on combinations of putatively protective peptides, are in progress (see Chapter 18).

Parasite genome sequencing ventures and analysis of whole parasite proteomes are highlighting novel targets for both drug and vaccine design. These modern technologies are providing startling insights into how parasite and host immune systems interact. For example, the malaria protein PfEMP1 encoded by *var* genes, known to be expressed in the red blood cell stage within the human host and implicated in immune evasion, has been identified in the mosquito sporozoite stage, indicating that it may have several alternative functions (see Fig. 15.24).

FURTHER READING

Crabb BS, Cooke BM. Molecular approaches to malaria. Trends Parasitol 2004;20:547–614.

Maizels RM, Yazdanbakhsh M. Immune regulation by helminth parasites: cellular and molecular mechanisms. Nat Rev Immunol 2003;3:733–744.

McGuiness DH, Dehal PK, Pleass RJ. Pattern recognition molecules and innate immunity to parasites. Trends Parasitol 2003;19:312–319.

Scott P. Immunoparasitology. Immunol Rev 2004;201:5–8.

Sher A, Pearce E, Kaye P. Shaping the immune response to parasites: role of dendritic cells. Curr Opin Immunol 2003;15:421–429.

Websites

Various newsgroups on the www (though not all dedicated to immunology) can be accessed by exploring keywords

Several discussion groups operate through the bionet, for example http://www.bio.net/archives.html (a parasitology mail newsgroup) and http://www.parasitology.org.uk (British Society for Parasitology)

Critical thinking: Immunity to protozoa and helminths (see p. 497 for explanations)

1 In general, protozoa and helminths adopt different strategies for survival and for transmission to the subsequent host. How do they differ?

2 Many parasites have evolved to live in host cells. Consider the advantages and disadvantages to this mode of existence. Consider the different cell types and how parasites have to adapt this environment to their advantage. In particular *Toxoplasma gondii*, *Trypanosoma cruzi*, and *Leishmania* spp. have adapted to live in the macrophage and can escape destruction by lysosomal enzymes, but the way in which they do this differs. How have these adaptations helped parasite survival?

3 Extracellular parasites have evolved sophisticated mechanisms to avoid the immune response. Consider examples of how they do this.

Primary Immunodeficiency

CHAPTER 16

SUMMARY

- **Primary immunodeficiency diseases** result from intrinsic defects in immune system cells, complement components, and phagocytic cells.

- **Defects in B cell function** result in recurrent pyogenic infections. Defective antibody responses are due to failure of B cell function, as occurs in X-linked agammaglobulinemia, or failure of proper T cell signals to B cells, as occurs in hyper-IgM (HIgM) syndrome, common variable immunodeficiency (CVID), and transient hypogammaglobulinemia of infancy.

- **Poor T cell function** results in susceptibility to opportunistic infections. Defective cell-mediated immunity is due to failure of T cell function, seen for example in severe combined immunodeficiency (SCID), MHC class II deficiency, ataxia telangiectasia (AT), the Wiskott–Aldrich syndrome (WAS), and the DiGeorge anomaly.

- **Hereditary complement component defects** are found in a number of clinical syndromes, the most common of which is that of the C1 inhibitor, which results in hereditary angiedema (HAE). Hereditary complement deficiencies of the terminal complement components (C5, C6, C7, and C8) and the alternative pathway proteins (factor H, factor I, and properdin) lead to extraordinary susceptibility to infections with the two *Neisseria* species, *N. gonorrheae* and *N. meningitidis*.

- **Genetic defects of phagocytes** can result in overwhelming infection. Defects in the oxygen reduction pathway of phagocytes, such that the phagocytes cannot assemble NADPH oxidase and produce the hydrogen peroxide and oxygen radicals that kill bacteria, are the basis of chronic granulomatous disease (CGD). The resulting persistence of bacterial products in phagocytes leads to abscesses or granulomas, depending on the pathogen.

- **Leukocyte adhesion deficiency (LAD)** is associated with a persistent leukocytosis because phagocytic cells with defective integrin molecules cannot migrate through the vascular endothelium from the blood stream into the tissues.

PRIMARY IMMUNODEFICIENCY RESULTS FROM INTRINSIC DEFECTS IN IMMUNE SYSTEM CELLS

Immunodeficiency disease results from the absence or failure of normal function of one or more elements of the immune system:

- specific immunodeficiency diseases involve abnormalities of T or B cells (the cells of the adaptive immune system);
- non-specific immunodeficiency diseases involve abnormalities of elements such as complement or phagocytes, which act non-specifically in immunity.

Primary immunodeficiency diseases are due to intrinsic defects in cells of the immune system and are for the most part genetically determined.

Immunodeficiency diseases cause increased susceptibility to infection in patients.

- the infections encountered in patients who are immunodeficient fall, broadly speaking, into two categories: patients with defects in immunoglobulins, complement proteins, or phagocytes are very susceptible to recurrent infections with encapsulated bacteria such as *Haemophilus influenzae*, *Streptococcus pneumoniae*, and *Staphylococcus aureus* – these are called **pyogenic infections**, because the bacteria give rise to pus formation;
- patients with defects in cell-mediated immunity (i.e. in T cells) are susceptible to overwhelming, even lethal, infections with microorganisms that are ubiquitous in the environment and to which normal people rapidly develop resistance – for this reason, these are called **opportunistic infections**, and opportunistic microorganisms include yeast and common viruses such as chickenpox.

B CELL DEFICIENCIES
Defects in B cell function result in recurrent pyogenic infections

Patients with common defects in B cell function (Fig. 16.1) have recurrent pyogenic infections such as:

- pneumonia;
- otitis media; and
- sinusitis.

Primary B cell deficiencies

X-linked agammaglobulinemia (X-LA)
IgA deficiency
IgG subclass deficiency
immunodeficiency with increased IgM (HIgM)
common variable immunodeficiency (CVID)
transient hypogammaglobulinemia of infancy

Fig. 16.1 The range of B cell deficiencies varies from a delayed maturation of normal immunoglobulin production, through single isotype deficiencies to X-linked agammaglobulinemia, where affected male children have no B cells and no serum immunoglobulins.

If untreated, they develop severe obstructive lung disease (bronchiectasis) from recurrent pneumonia, which destroys the elasticity of the airways.

Early B cell maturation fails in X-LA

X-linked agammaglobulinemia (X-LA) is the model B cell deficiency and was the first immunodeficiency disease to be understood in detail, the underlying deficiency being discovered in 1952.

Affected males have few or no B cells in their blood or lymphoid tissue – consequently their lymph nodes are very small and their tonsils are absent. Their serum usually contains no IgA, IgM, IgD, or IgE, and only small amounts of IgG (less than 100 mg/dl).

For the first 6–12 months of life, affected males are protected from infection by the maternal IgG that crossed the placenta into the fetus. As this supply of IgG is exhausted, they develop recurrent pyogenic infections. If they are infused intravenously with large doses of gammaglobulin they remain healthy.

The X-LA gene lies on the long arm of the X chromosome (Fig. 16.2). This is the site of many other hereditary immunodeficiency diseases and the localization of these genes facilitates prenatal diagnosis.

The gene that is defective in X-LA has recently been identified as a B cell cytoplasmic tyrosine kinase (*btk*) belonging to the *src* oncogene family. Its role in B cell maturation is not yet understood, but it is obviously vital for the process. The bone marrow of males with X-LA contains normal numbers of pre-B cells, but as a result of mutations in the *btk* gene these cells cannot mature into B cells (Fig. 16.3).

Terminal differentiation of B cells fails in IgA and IgG subclass deficiency

IgA deficiency is the most common immunodeficiency. One in 700 Caucasians has the defect, but it is not found, or is found only rarely, in other ethnic groups.

People with IgA deficiency tend to develop immune complex disease (type III hypersensitivity).

The X-linked immunodeficiencies

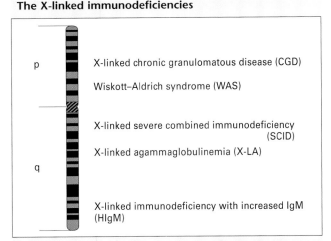

Fig. 16.2 The genes for many immunodeficiency diseases are located on the X chromosome. The genetic defects have been identified for all these diseases. (Adapted from Schwaber J, Rosen FS. X chromosome linked immunodeficiency. Immunodefic Rev 1990;2:233–251)

About 20% of IgA-deficient individuals also lack IgG2 and IgG4, and are therefore susceptible to pyogenic infections. In humans, most antibodies to the capsular polysaccharides of pyogenic bacteria are in the IgG2 subclass. A deficiency in IgG2 alone therefore also results in recurrent pyogenic infections. Individuals with deficiency of only IgG2 are also susceptible to recurrent infections.

These class and subclass deficiencies result from failure in the terminal differentiation of B cells (see Fig. 16.3).

Isotype switching does not occur in HIgM

A peculiar immunodeficiency – **immunodeficiency with increased IgM (hyper-IgM, HIgM)** – results in a situation where individuals are IgG and IgA deficient, but synthesize large amounts (more than 200 mg/dl) of polyclonal IgM.

People with HIgM are susceptible to pyogenic infections and should be treated with intravenous gammaglobulin. They tend to form IgM autoantibodies to neutrophils, platelets, and other elements of the blood, as well as to tissue antigens, thereby adding the complexities of autoimmune disease to the immunodeficiency. The tissues, particularly of the gastrointestinal tract, become infiltrated with IgM-producing cells (Fig. 16.4).

In 70% of cases, HIgM is inherited as an X-linked recessive condition that results from mutations in the **CD40 ligand**, whose gene maps to precisely the same location on the long arm of the X chromosome as HIgM.

Q. What is the function of CD40 and the CD40 ligand (CD154)?

A. Interaction between the CD40 molecule on the B cell surface and the CD40 ligand on activated T cells is a potent co-stimulatory signal required for class switching and affinity maturation (see Fig. 8.8).

B cell maturation in X-linked immunodeficiencies

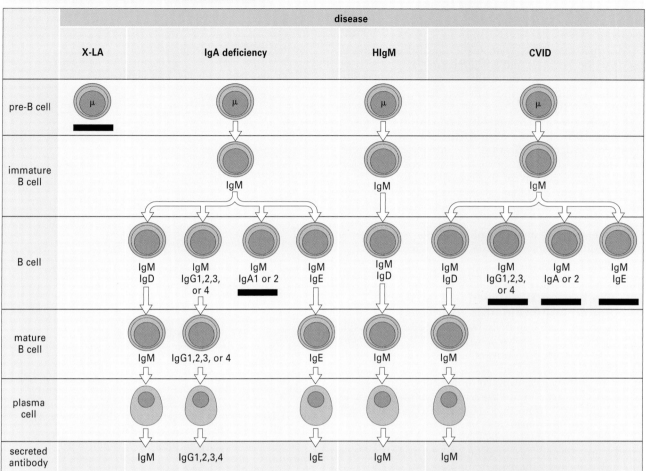

Fig. 16.3 In X-LA, affected male infants have no B cells and no serum immunoglobulins, except for small amounts of maternal IgG. In IgA deficiency, IgA-bearing B cells, and in some cases IgG2- and IgG4-bearing B cells, are unable to differentiate into plasma cells. People with HIgM lack IgG and IgA. In CVID, B cells of most isotypes are unable to differentiate into plasma cells. Black bars denote points of inhibition.

Gall bladder from a patient with HIgM

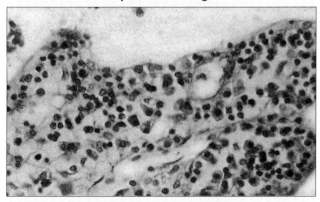

Fig. 16.4 The submucosa is filled with cells with pink-staining cytoplasm and eccentric nuclei. The cells are synthesizing and secreting IgM.

In HIgM the B cells cannot make the switch from IgM to IgG, IgA, and IgE synthesis that normally occurs in B cell maturation.

HIgM may also be transmitted as an autosomal recessive trait, affecting females as well as males. Autosomal recessive HIgM is due to a genetic defect in a B cell enzyme called **activation-induced cytidine deaminase (AID)**. This enzyme, activated in stimulated B cells, converts cytidine to uridine in single-stranded DNA. The uridine is further degraded to uracil and this causes breaks in the DNA strand, allowing downstream recombination in the heavy chain genes – or class switch recombination.

T cell signaling to B cells is defective in CVID

Individuals with **common variable immunodeficiency (CVID)** have acquired agammaglobulinemia in the second or third decade of life, or later.

Both males and females are equally affected, and the cause is generally not known, but may follow infection with viruses such as Epstein–Barr virus (EBV).

Patients with CVID, like males with X-LA, are very susceptible to pyogenic organisms and to the intestinal protozoon, *Giardia lamblia* (Fig. 16.5), which causes severe diarrhea.

Most patients (80%) with CVID have B cells that do not function properly and are immature. The B cells are not defective; instead, they fail to receive proper signals from the T cells. The T cell defects have not been well defined in CVID.

Patients with CVID should be treated with intravenous gammaglobulin because it provides protection against recurrent pyogenic infections. Many patients develop autoimmune diseases, most prominently pernicious anemia, but the reason for this is not known.

CVID is not hereditary, but is commonly associated with the MHC haplotypes HLA-B8 and HLA-DR3.

Q. In what other immunodeficiency do patients often develop autoantibodies to elements of the blood?
A. In HIgM (see above).

IgG production is delayed in transient hypogammaglobulinemia of infancy

Infants are protected initially by their mother's IgG. The maternal IgG is catabolized, with a half-life of approximately 30 days. By 3 months of age, normal infants begin to synthesize their own IgG, though formation of antibody to bacterial capsular polysaccharides does not commence in earnest until the second year of life. In some infants, the onset of normal IgG synthesis can be delayed for as long as 36 months and, until then, such infants are susceptible to pyogenic infections. The B cells of these infants are normal, but they appear to lack help from CD4+ T cells in synthesizing antibodies.

T CELL DEFICIENCIES
Poor T cell function results in susceptibility to opportunistic infections

The major T cell deficiencies are shown in Fig. 16.6.

Giardia lamblia

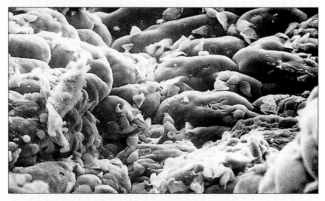

Fig. 16.5 Numerous *Giardia lamblia* parasites can be seen swarming over the mucosa of the jejunum of a patient with CVID.

Primary T cell deficiencies

severe combined immunodeficiency (SCID)
adenosine deaminase deficiency
purine nucleoside phosphorylase deficiency
MHC class II deficiency
DiGeorge anomaly
hereditary ataxia telangiectasia (AT)
Wiskott–Aldrich syndrome (WAS)

Fig. 16.6 There is a wide range of causes for T cell deficiencies, ranging from absence of lymphocytes, to enzyme deficiency, through to MHC deficiency. All affect the ability of T cells to function, which leads to combined T and B cell deficiency.

People with no T cells or poor T cell function are susceptible to opportunistic infections.

Because B cell function in humans is largely T cell dependent, T cell deficiency also results in humoral immunodeficiency, that is, it leads to a combined deficiency of both humoral and cell-mediated immunity.

In SCID there is lymphocyte deficiency and the thymus does not develop

The most profound hereditary deficiency of cell-mediated immunity occurs in infants with **severe combined immunodeficiency (SCID)** who develop recurrent infections early in life (in contrast to X-LA). They:
- have prolonged diarrhea due to rotavirus or bacterial infection of the gastrointestinal tract; and
- develop pneumonia, usually due to the protozoon, *Pneumocystis carinii*.

The common yeast organism *Candida albicans* grows luxuriantly in the mouth or on the skin of patients with SCID (Fig. 16.7).

If patients with SCID are vaccinated with live organisms, such as poliovirus or bacille Calmette–Guérin (BCG) (used for immunization against tuberculosis), they die from progressive infection with these ordinarily benign organisms.

SCID is incompatible with life and affected infants usually die within the first 2 years unless they are rescued with transplants of bone marrow. In this case they become **lymphocyte chimeras** and can survive and live normally.

Infants with SCID have very few lymphocytes in their blood (fewer than 3000/ml). Their lymphoid tissue also contains few or no lymphocytes. The thymus has a fetal appearance (Fig. 16.8), containing the endodermal stromal cells derived embryonically from the third and fourth pharyngeal pouch. Lymphoid stem cells, which normally populate the thymus by 6 weeks of human gestation (see Chapter 2), fail to appear and the thymus does not become a lymphoid organ.

Candida albicans in the mouth of a patient with SCID

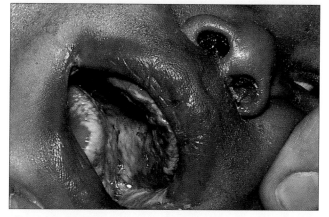

Fig. 16.7 *C. albicans* grows luxuriantly in the mouth and on the skin of patients with SCID.

Thymus of SCID

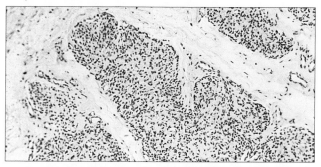

Fig. 16.8 Note that the thymic stroma has not been invaded by lymphoid cells and no Hassall's corpuscles are seen. The gland has a fetal appearance.

Possible role of adenosine deaminase and purine nucleoside phosphorylase deficiency in SCID

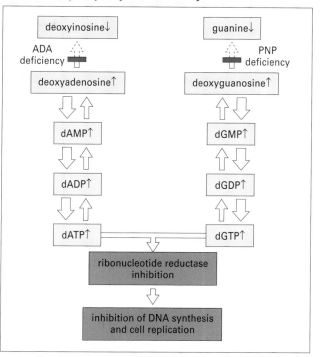

Fig. 16.9 It is thought that deficiencies of ADA and PNP lead to accumulations of dATP and dGTP, respectively. Both of these metabolites are powerful inhibitors of ribonucleotide reductase, which is an essential enzyme for DNA synthesis.

SCID is more common in male than female infants (3:1) because over 50% of cases are caused by a gene defect on the X chromosome. The defective gene encodes the γ chain of the interleukin-2 (IL-2) receptor. This γ chain also forms part of the receptors for IL-4, IL-7, IL-11, and IL-15.

Q. Which of these cytokines is most critically important in early T cell development?
A. Of these, the binding of IL-7 to the IL-7 receptor is most important for T cell maturation. Thus, the lymphoid stem cells are incapable of receiving a number of signals for growth and maturation (see Fig. 2.29).

The remaining cases of SCID are due to recessive genes on other chromosomes. Of these, half have a genetic deficiency of **adenosine deaminase (ADA)** or **purine nucleoside phosphorylase (PNP)**. Deficiency of these purine degradation enzymes results in the accumulation of metabolites that are toxic to lymphoid stem cells, namely dATP and dGTP (Fig. 16.9). These metabolites inhibit the enzyme ribonucleotide reductase, which is required for DNA synthesis and, therefore, for cell replication.

ADA and PNP are found in all mammalian cells, so why should these defects affect only lymphocytes? The explanation appears to lie in the relative deficiency of 5'-nucleotidase in lymphoid cells; in other cells, this enzyme compensates for defective ADA or PNP by preventing dAMP and dGMP accumulation.

An autosomal recessive form of SCID results from a mutation in either of the genes encoding **RAG-1 or RAG-2** .

Q. What are the functions of the genes encoding RAG-1 or RAG-2, and why would loss of function lead to combined immunodeficiency?
A. The two recombinase activation genes, *RAG-1* and *RAG-2*, are absolutely required for cleaving double-stranded DNA before recombination of DNA to form the immunoglobulin genes and the genes encoding the T cell receptor. If these gene rearrangements do not occur, B and T cells do not develop (see Fig. 3.29).

The optimal treatment for SCID is a bone marrow transplant from a completely histocompatible donor, usually a normal sibling. About 70% of patients do not have a histocompatible sibling, in which case parental marrow, which would have one haplotype identical, has been transplanted successfully.

Q. Why is it necessary to match the bone marrow graft in a patient with SCID when the immune system of the SCID recipient is unable to reject the donor bone marrow cells?

A. The donor bone marrow cells are fully immunocompetent and would generate a reaction against the recipient's cells. This is called **graft versus host disease** (see Fig. 21.8).

Recently a retroviral vector, into which the *ADA* gene had been inserted, has been used to transfect the lymphocytes of children who are ADA deficient. This was the first example of successful '**gene therapy**'. Males with X-linked SCID have since been successfully treated by transducing their bone marrow cells with the gene of the common γ chain of the IL-2 receptor incorporated into a viral vector.

Tʜ cell deficiency results from MHC class II deficiency

The failure to express class II MHC molecules on antigen-presenting cells (macrophages and B cells) is inherited as an autosomal recessive characteristic, which is not linked to the MHC locus on the short arm of chromosome 6.

Affected infants have recurrent infections, particularly of the gastrointestinal tract.

Because the development of CD4⁺ helper T cells (Tʜ) depends on positive selection by MHC class II molecules in the thymus (see Chapter 2), MHC class II molecule-deficient infants have a deficiency of CD4⁺ T cells. This lack of Tʜ cells leads to a deficiency in antibodies as well. The MHC class II deficiency results from defects in promoter proteins that bind to the 5′ untranslated region of the class II genes.

The DiGeorge anomaly arises from a defect in thymus embryogenesis

The thymic epithelium is derived from the third and fourth pharyngeal pouches by the sixth week of human gestation. Subsequently the endodermal anlage is invaded by lymphoid stem cells, which undergo development into T cells. The parathyroid glands are also derived from the same embryonic origin.

A congenital defect in the organs derived from the third and fourth pharyngeal pouches results in the **DiGeorge anomaly**. The T cell deficiency is variable, depending on how badly the thymus is affected. Affected infants have distinctive facial features (Fig. 16.10) in that their eyes are widely separated (hypertelorism), the ears are low set, and the philtrum of the upper lip is shortened. They also have congenital malformations of the heart or aortic arch and neonatal tetany from the hypoplasia or aplasia of the parathyroid glands. These infants have **partial monosomy of 22q11-pter** or **10p**.

XLP follows infection with EBV

X-linked proliferative syndrome (**XLP**) results from a failure to control the normal proliferation of cytotoxic T cells following an infection with Epstein–Barr virus (EBV), which causes infectious mononucleosis.

Affected males appear normal until they encounter EBV, when they develop either:

DiGeorge anomaly

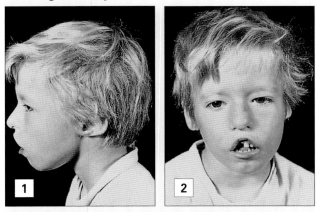

Fig. 16.10 Note the wide-set eyes, low-set ears, and shortened philtrum of upper lip. Congenital malformations of the cardiovascular system may also occur.

- fatal infectious mononucleosis;
- complete destruction of their B cells so that agammaglobulinemia ensues;
- a fatal lymphoid malignancy; or
- aplastic anemia.

The defective gene on the X chromosome encodes an adapter protein of T and B cells called **SAP** or the **SLAM-associated protein**. SLAM is expressed on the surface of T and B cells. Its intracellular tail interacts with the adapter protein, SAP. By a mechanism that is not understood, SAP controls the limitless proliferation of cytotoxic T cells. A genetic defect in SAP results in the destruction of lymphoid and other hematopoietic tissue by uncontrolled proliferation of cytotoxic T cells and maternal killer cells.

Chromosomal breaks occur in TCR and immunoglobulin genes in AT

Hereditary ataxia telangiectasia (**AT**) is inherited as an autosomal recessive trait.

Affected infants with AT develop a wobbly gait (ataxia) at about 18 months. Dilated capillaries (telangiectasia) appear in the eyes and on the skin by 6 years of age.

AT is accompanied by a variable T cell deficiency. About 70% of patients with AT are also IgA deficient and some also have IgG2 and IgG4 deficiency.

Q. In what other ways are IgA, IgG2, and IgG4 related (as opposed to IgM, IgG1, and IgG3)?

A. The IgA1, IgA2, IgG2, and IgG4 heavy chain genes all lie further downstream of the recombined VDJ gene than IgM, IgG1, and IgG3 (see Fig. 8.19). This may account for the selective deficiency in making the class switch to IgA, IgG2, and IgG4. Class switching involves the production and resolution of double-stranded DNA breaks.

The number and function of circulating T cells are greatly diminished, so cell-mediated function is depressed.

Patients develop severe sinus and lung infections. Their cells exhibit chromosomal breaks, usually in chromosome 7 and chromosome 14, at the sites of the T cell receptor (TCR) genes and the genes encoding the heavy chains of immunoglobulins.

The cells of patients with AT, as well as those from patients with AT in vitro, are very susceptible to ionizing irradiation because the defective gene in AT encodes a protein involved in the repair of double-strand breaks in DNA.

T cell defects and abnormal immunoglobulin levels occur in Wiskott–Aldrich syndrome

Wiskott–Aldrich syndrome (WAS) is an X-linked immunodeficiency disease.

Affected males with WAS:
- have small and profoundly abnormal platelets, which are also few in number (thrombocytopenia);
- develop severe eczema as well as pyogenic and opportunistic infections;
- have increased amounts of serum IgA and IgE, normal levels of IgG, and decreased amounts of IgM;
- have T cells with defective function.

The malfunction of cell-mediated immunity gets progressively worse. The T cells have a uniquely abnormal appearance, as shown by scanning electron microscopy, reflecting a cytoskeletal defect. They have fewer microvilli on the cell surface than normal T cells.

During collaboration of T and B cells in antibody formation, the cytoskeleton of the T cells reorientates itself or becomes polarized towards the B cells. This fails to occur in WAS, resulting in faulty collaboration between immune cells.

GENETIC DEFICIENCIES OF COMPLEMENT PROTEINS

The proteins of the complement system and their interactions with the immune system are discussed in Chapter 4. Genetic deficiencies of almost all the complement proteins have been found in humans (Fig. 16.11) and these deficiencies reveal much about the normal function of the complement system (see Figs 4.16 and 4.17).

Immune complex clearance, inflammation, phagocytosis, and bacteriolysis can be affected by complement deficiencies

Deficiencies of the classical pathway components, C1q, C1r, C1s, C4, or C2, result in a propensity to develop immune complex diseases such as systemic lupus erythematosus.

Q. Why should these deficiencies result in immune complex disease?

A. The classical complement pathway is required for the dissolution of immune complexes by covalent binding of C4b and C3b to components of the complex. It is also required for the transport of complexes on erythrocytes in humans (see Fig. 4.6).

Deficiencies of C3, factor H, or factor I result in increased susceptibility to pyogenic infections – this correlates with the important role of C3 in the opsonization of pyogenic bacteria.

Deficiencies of the terminal components, C5, C6, C7, and C8, and of the alternative pathway components, factor D and properdin, result in remarkable susceptibility to infection with the two pathogenic species of the *Neisseria*

Genetic deficiencies of human complement

group	type	deficiency	hereditary		
			AR	AD	XL
I	immune complex disease	C1q	•		
		C1s, or C1r + C1s	•		
		C2	•		
		C4	•		
II	angiedema	C1 inhibitor		•	
III	recurrent pyogenic infections	C3	•		
		factor H	•		
		factor I	•		
IV	recurrent *Neisseria* infections	C5	•		
		C6	•		
		C7	•		
		C8	•		
		properdin			•
		factor D	•		
V	asymptomatic	C9	•		

Fig. 16.11 Genetic deficiencies of human complement. (AR, phenotypically autosomal recessive; AD, autosomal dominant; XL, X-linked recessive)

genus: *N. gonorrhoeae* and *N. meningitidis*. This clearly demonstrates the importance of the alternative pathway and the macromolecular attack complex in the bacteriolysis of this genus of bacteria.

All of these genetic complement component deficiencies are inherited as autosomal recessive traits, except:
- properdin deficiency, which is inherited as an X-linked recessive; and
- C1 inhibitor deficiency, which is inherited as an autosomal dominant.

HAE results from C1 inhibitor deficiency

Clinically, the most important deficiency of the complement system is that of **C1 inhibitor**. This molecule is responsible for dissociation of activated C1, by binding to $\overline{C1r_2C1s_2}$. The deficiency results in the well-known disease, **hereditary angioneurotic edema (HAE)** (Fig. 16.12).

HAE is inherited as an autosomal dominant trait. Patients have recurrent episodes of circumscribed swelling of various parts of the body (angiedema):
- when the edema involves the intestine, excruciating abdominal pains and cramps result, with severe vomiting;
- when the edema involves the upper airway, the patients may choke to death from respiratory obstruction – angiedema of the upper airway therefore presents a medical emergency, which requires rapid action to restore normal breathing.

C1 inhibitor inhibits not only the classical pathway of complement, but also joint elements of the kinin, plasmin, and clotting systems.

The edema is mediated by two peptides generated by uninhibited activation of the complement and surface contact systems:
- a peptide derived from the activation of C2, called C2 kinin; and
- bradykinin derived from the activation of the contact system (Fig. 16.13).

The effect of these peptides is on the postcapillary venule, where they cause endothelial cells to retract, forming gaps that allow leakage of plasma (see Chapter 2).

There are two genetically determined forms of HAE.
- in type I, the C1 inhibitor gene is defective and no transcripts are formed;
- in type II, there are point mutations in the C1 inhibitor gene resulting in the synthesis of defective molecules.

The distinction between type I and type II is important because the diagnosis of type II disease cannot be made by quantitative measurement of serum C1 inhibitor alone. Simultaneous measurements of **C4** must also be done. C4 is always decreased in the serum of patients with HAE because of its destruction by uninhibited activated C1.

C1 inhibitor deficiency may be acquired later in life. In some cases an autoantibody to C1 inhibitor is found. In others, there is a monoclonal B cell proliferation, such as occurs in chronic lymphocytic leukemia, multiple myeloma, or B cell lymphoma. Such patients make an anti-idiotype to their over-produced immunoglobulin; the idiotype–anti-idiotype interaction, for unknown reasons,

Pathogenesis of hereditary angioneurotic edema

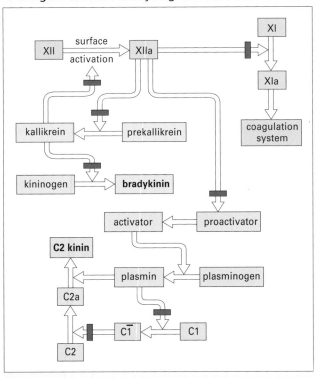

Fig. 16.13 C1 inhibitor is involved in inactivation of elements of the clotting, kinin, plasmin and complement systems, which may be activated following the surface-dependent activation of factor XII (Hageman factor). The points at which C1 inhibitor acts are shown in red. Uncontrolled activation of these pathways results in the formation of bradykinin and C2 kinin, which induce edema formation.

Hereditary angioneurotic edema

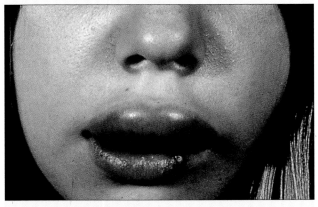

Fig. 16.12 This clinical photograph shows the transient localized swelling that occurs in this condition.

results in consumption of C1, C4, and C2, and C1 inhibitor without formation of an effective C3 convertase (which would cause C3 deposition and removal of the complement complex).

Purified C1 inhibitor is available for treatment of acute attacks of angiedema. Intravenous administration of C1 inhibitor brings about prompt resolution of laryngeal edema or gastrointestinal symptoms. It is not approved for use in the United States.

GENETIC DEFECTS OF PHAGOCYTES CAN RESULT IN OVERWHELMING INFECTION

Phagocytic cells – polymorphonuclear leukocytes and cells of the monocyte/macrophage lineage – are important in host defense against pyogenic bacteria and other intracellular microorganisms.

A severe deficiency of polymorphonuclear leukocytes (**neutropenia**) can result in overwhelming bacterial infection.

Two genetic defects of phagocytes are clinically important in that they result in susceptibility to severe infections and are often fatal:

- **chronic granulomatous disease (CGD)**; and
- **leukocyte adhesion deficiency (LAD)**.

CGD results from a defect in the oxygen reduction pathway

Patients with CGD have defective **NADPH oxidase**, which catalyzes the reduction of O_2 to $^{\bullet}O_2^-$ by the reaction: $NADPH + 2O_2 \rightarrow NADP^+ + 2^{\bullet}O_2^- + H^+$. They are therefore incapable of forming superoxide anions (ΣO_2^-) and hydrogen peroxide in their phagocytes following the ingestion of microorganisms.

Q. What would be the consequence of a failure of superoxide generation?

A. Phagocytes cannot readily kill ingested bacteria or fungi, particularly catalase-producing organisms (see Fig. 9.30 and Chapter 14).

As a result, microorganisms remain alive in phagocytes of patients with CGD. This gives rise to a cell-mediated response to persistent intracellular microbial antigens, and granulomas form.

Children with CGD develop pneumonia, infections in the lymph nodes (lymphadenitis), and abscesses in the skin, liver, and other viscera.

The diagnosis of CGD is made by the inability of phagocytes to reduce **nitroblue tetrazolium (NBT)** dye after a phagocytic stimulus. NBT is a pale, clear, yellow dye taken up by phagocytes when they are ingesting a particle. When NBT accepts H and is reduced as a result of NADPH oxidation it forms a deep purple precipitate inside the phagocytes; precipitation does not occur in the phagocytes of patients with CGD (Fig. 16.14).

The NADPH oxidase reaction is complicated and the enzyme complex has many subunits. In resting phagocytes the membrane contains a phagocyte-specific cytochrome, cytochrome b_{558}. This cytochrome is composed of two chains:

Nitroblue tetrazolium test

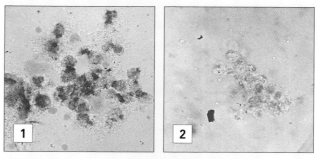

Fig. 16.14 In normal polymorphs and monocytes, reactive oxygen intermediates (ROIs) are activated by phagocytosis, and yellow NBT is converted to purple-blue formazan (**1**). Patients with CGD cannot form ROIs and so the dye stays yellow (**2**). (Courtesy of Professor AR Hayward)

- one of 91 kDa, encoded by a gene on the short arm of the X chromosome; and
- one of 22 kDa, encoded by a gene on chromosome 16.

When phagocytosis occurs, several proteins from the cytosol become phosphorylated, move to the membrane, and bind to cytochrome b_{558}. The complex formed acts as an enzyme, NADPH oxidase, catalyzing the NADPH oxidation reaction and thereby activating oxygen radical production (Fig. 16.15).

The most common form of CGD is X-linked and involves a defect in the 91-kDa chain of cytochrome b_{558}.

Three types of CGD are autosomal recessive and result from defects in the 22-kDa chain of the cytochrome b_{558}, or from defects in one or other of two proteins, called p47^{phox} or p67^{phox}.

LAD is due to integrin gene defects

The receptor in the phagocyte membrane that binds to C3bi on opsonized microorganisms is critical for the ingestion of bacteria by phagocytes. This receptor – an integrin called **complement receptor 3 (CR3)** – is deficient in patients with LAD, who consequently develop severe bacterial infections, particularly of the mouth and gastrointestinal tract.

CR3 is composed of two polypeptide chains:
- an α chain of 165 kDa (CD11b); and
- a β chain of 95 kDa (CD18).

In LAD, there is a genetic defect of the β chain, encoded by a gene on chromosome 21.

Two other integrin proteins share the same β chain as CR3 – namely lymphocyte functional antigen (LFA-1) and p150,95 (see Chapter 3). Although they have unique α chains (CD11a and CD11c, respectively), these proteins are also defective in LAD.

LFA-1 is important in cell adhesion and interacts with intercellular adhesion molecule-1 (ICAM-1) on endothelial cell surfaces and other cell membranes. Because of the defect in LFA-1, phagocytes from patients with LAD cannot adhere to vascular endothelium and cannot therefore migrate out of blood vessels into areas of

NADPH oxidase and its components

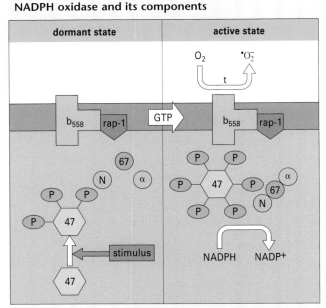

Fig. 16.15 Prevailing knowledge of the NADPH oxidase suggests that in its dormant state some of its component parts are in the membrane (cytochrome b_{558} and possibly rap-1) while others are in the cytosol (p47^{phox}, p67^{phox}, the NADPH-binding component, N, and a putative fourth component, α). The initiation of phagocytosis provides a stimulus for the cytosolic components to associate and move to the membrane, an event possibly mediated by phosphorylation (P) of p47^{phox}. Once the cytosol components are associated with the membrane components, the oxidase becomes catalytically active and p47^{phox} is phosphorylated further. Activation of the cytochrome b_{558} catalyzes the acceptance of an electron by O_2 to form the superoxide anion $^{\bullet}O_2^{-}$. In the different forms of CGD, there are defects in the genes for different components of the oxidase. (phox is an abbreviation for phagocytic oxidase. t, electron) (Adapted from Smith RM, Curnutte JT. Molecular basis of chronic granulomatous disease. Blood 1997;77:673–686)

infection. As a result patients with LAD cannot form pus efficiently and this allows the rapid spread of bacterial invaders.

LAD type 2 results from a failure of normal synthesis of selectin ligands

When leukocytes in the circulation enter an area of inflammation their speed of movement is greatly retarded by the interaction of **selectins** (see Fig. 6.9), which are expressed on the surface of the leukocytes, with ligands that are expressed on the surface of the endothelium in areas of inflammation. The leukocytes start to roll on the endothelial surface before the interaction of the leukocyte integrins with adhesion molecules such as ICAM-1. The ligands with which the selectins interact are glycoproteins that contain fucosylated sugars, such as the blood group sialyl Lewis^x. A genetic defect in the conversion of mannose to fucose results in failure of normal synthesis in these selectin ligands. Consequently the leukocytes of such patients cannot roll on the endothelium. This causes a second form of LAD, called **LAD type 2**.

Macrophage microbicidal activity is impaired by defects in IFNγ signaling

The destruction of intracellular microorganisms that flourish in macrophages depends on the activation of microbicidal activity in macrophages by interferon-γ (IFNγ).

When microorganisms are taken up by macrophages, the macrophages secrete IL-12, which then binds to the IL-12 receptor on T cells and induces secretion of IFNγ.

Children with genetic defects in the genes encoding IL-12, the IL-12 receptor, or the IFNγ receptor sustain recurrent infection with non-pathogenic mycobacteria and, to a lesser extent, with salmonella. These various defects are inherited as autosomal recessive traits and can be fatal unless treated with IFNγ.

FURTHER READING

Buckley RH. Primary immunodeficiency diseases due to defects in lymphocytes. N Engl J Med 2000;343:313.

Conley ME. Molecular approaches to analysis of X-linked immunodeficiencies. Ann Rev Immunol 1992;10:215.

Curnutte JT, Orkin SH, Dinauer MC. Genetic disorders of phagocyte function. In: Stamatoyannopoulos G, Nienhuis AW, Majerus PW, Varmus H, eds. The molecular basis of blood diseases. Philadelphia: PA Saunders; 1994:443.

Lekstrom-Himes JA, Gallin JI. Immunodeficiency diseases caused by defects in phagocytes. N Engl J Med 2000;343:1703.

Rosen FS, Cooper MD, Wedgwood RJP. The primary immunodeficiencies. N Engl J Med 1995;333:43.

Rosen FS, Seligman M, eds. Immunodeficiencies. Switzerland: Harwood Academic Publishers; 1993.

Snapper SB, Rosen FS. The Wiskott–Aldrich syndrome protein (WASP): roles in signaling and cytoskeletal organization. Annu Rev Immunol 1999;17:905–929.

Von Andrian UH, Berger EM, Chambers JD, et al. In vivo behaviour of neutrophils from two patients with distinct inherited leukocyte adhesion deficiency syndromes. J Clin Invest 1993;91:2893.

Critical thinking: Hyper-IgM immunodeficiency (see p. 497 for explanations)

A 3-year-old girl was brought to the emergency room because of fever and rapid respiration. She had had pneumonia once before at age 25 months. She had also had otitis media on ten different occasions, each time successfully treated with antibiotics. A chest radiograph resulted in the diagnosis of left lower lobe pneumonia. Blood and sputum cultures contained *Streptococcus pneumoniae*. The white blood count was 13 500/mcl of which 81% were neutrophils and 14% lymphocytes. Serum IgM was 470 mg/dl, IgG 40 mg/dl, and IgA and IgE were undetectable. Antibody to tetanus toxoid was undetectable. Blood typing was A positive, anti-B 1:320.

1 What clinical and laboratory tests lead to the suspicion that this child has hyper-IgM (HIgM) immunodeficiency and how do you conclude that it is not due to a mutation in CD40 ligand?

2 What further laboratory testing should be done to establish the diagnosis?

3 How do you explain that this child had no response to tetanus immunization and yet has a high titer for her age of antibody to blood group substance B?

4 What treatment would you recommend to the parents for this child and what would you say is her prognosis?

5 If the mother of this baby were to be tested for random X-chromosome inactivation, what results would you expect?

6 What would you tell the parents about this child's prognosis?

AIDS and Secondary Immunodeficiency

SUMMARY

- **Some drugs selectively alter immune function.** Immunomodulatory drugs can severely depress immune functions. Steroids affect cell traffic, induce leukocytopenia, and inhibit cytokine synthesis. Cyclophosphamide, azathioprine, and mycophenolate mofetil act directly on DNA or its synthesis.

- **Nutrient deficiencies are generally associated with impaired immune responses.** Malnutrition increases the risk of infant mortality from infection through reduction in cell-mediated immunity, reduced CD4 helper cells, reduced T cell help, and a reduction of secretory IgA. Trace elements, iron, selenium, copper, and zinc are important in immunity. Lack of these elements can lead to diminished neutrophil killing of bacteria and fungi, susceptibility to viral infections, and diminished antibody responses. Vitamins A, B6, C, E, and folic acid are important in overall resistance to infection.

- **Antioxidant activity.** Carotenoids are antioxidants like vitamin C and E and can enhance NK cell activity, stimulate the production of cytokines and increase the activity of phagocytic cells. Diet and nutrition are powerful innovative tools to reduce illness and death caused by infection.

- **The most significant global cause of immunodeficiency is HIV infection.** AIDS is caused by HIV, which is a double-stranded RNA retrovirus that infects CD4 T cells. Severe CD4 depletion results from a variety of mechanisms, with drastic functional impairment of cell-mediated immunity and death from opportunistic infections.

- **Combination therapy for AIDS** with inhibitors of reverse transcriptase, protease, and viral entry are reasonably successful, but associated with long-term toxicities in almost 50% of persons. An effective vaccine remains an elusive goal.

SOME DRUGS SELECTIVELY ALTER IMMUNE FUNCTION

There have been substantial advances over the past decade in understanding how the immune system is regulated and how drugs may selectively alter function, producing not only **immunodeficiency**, but also, in some circumstances, **immune enhancement**. This chapter examines the most important agents commonly used for systemic immunotherapy.

Corticosteroids are powerful immune modulators

The immune system is regulated by at least four fundamental mechanisms:
- hormones (e.g. glucocorticoids);
- the cytokine system (including interleukins [ILs] and interferons [IFNs]);
- network connectivity (through idiotypic–anti-idiotypic responses); and
- antigens.

Glucocorticoids are among the most powerful naturally occurring modulators of the immune response and have profound effects at most levels and on most components.

As lipid-soluble molecules, steroids gain entry into cells by diffusion through the plasma membrane where they bind to their receptors in the cytoplasm.

The steroid–receptor complex translocates to the nucleus where it binds promoter regions of steroid-responsive genes.

In addition to their direct hormonal action on immune cell traffic and function, steroids have a substantial influence on cytokine synthesis, thereby also exerting a powerful indirect effect.

Significant changes in cell traffic are produced

Administration of steroids causes striking changes in circulating leukocyte populations, even when quite small quantities are used – for example, to produce physiological concentrations in previously adrenalectomized patients. These effects vary between cell types (Fig. 17.1).

Steroid treatment causes circulating **lymphocytopenia**, which is maximal at 4–6 hours and returns to normal by 24 hours. T cells are affected more than B cells, and, within the T cell subsets, CD4 cells are more depleted than CD8 cells. Experimental studies suggest these cells are redistributed to marrow and spleen.

Effects of glucocorticoids on circulating leukocytes

cell type	hours after injection		
	0	6	24
neutrophils	4000	10 000	4000
lymphocytes	2000	500	2000
eosinophils	400	100	400
monocytes	300	50	300
basophils	100	0	100

Fig. 17.1 Effect of a dose of glucocorticoid (40 mg/kg), given once at time zero, on circulating human leukocyte numbers (per mm^3).

Monocytopenia occurs after steroid treatment, is most evident at 2 hours, and recovers by 24 hours, but unlike effects on lymphocyte traffic, further repeated daily dosage does not cause subsequent cycles of depletion.

Neutrophilia is a feature of steroid treatment, due partly to the release of mature stored cells from bone marrow and partly to a reduction in cells leaving the circulation. The rapid and prolonged **decrease in circulating eosinophils and basophils** that occurs after steroid treatment in normal individuals contrasts markedly with the neutrophilia seen at the same time.

T cell activation and B cell maturation are inhibited

T cell activation and proliferation are inhibited by steroids, which make T cells unresponsive to IL-1 and therefore unable to synthesize IL-2, but steroids have little effect on mature B cells.

Q. After prolonged high steroid dosage there is a modest decrease in all immunoglobulin isotypes. Why should this be?
A. Lack of T cell help for B cells will result in a general reduction in the numbers of mature B cells that develop.

Steroids inhibit production of IL-1 and tumor necrosis factor (TNF) by monocytes (see below), but do not block the effect of cytokines on phagocytosis – indeed, they can promote it. Thus the binding of IFNγ and the subsequent expression of HLA-DR molecules and Fc receptors may be increased by low-dose steroids. However, the function of polymorphonuclear leukocytes is resistant to the levels of steroids achievable pharmacologically, as judged by chemotaxis, phagocytosis, and cytotoxicity.

Cytokine synthesis is inhibited

Studies in vitro have shown that physiological and pharmacological concentrations of steroids inhibit the synthesis of cytokines, but have little effect on their function. More impressively, after in-vivo administration, reduced production of IL-1, IL-2, IL-4, IL-6, IL-10, TNFα, and IFNγ has been demonstrated.

Q. What can you infer about which populations of T cells are targeted by steroids?
A. These cytokines are characteristic of different T cell populations, including helper T cells (TH1, TH2) and cytotoxic T cells (CTLs) (see Chapters 2 and 10).

Several different mechanisms may be involved:
- attachment to potential glucocorticoid response elements in the promoter region of the cytokine genes (IL-4, IL-6, and IL-10);
- direct binding, which antagonizes transcription-activating factors for IL-2, IL-8, and TNFα; or
- accelerating breakdown of mRNA (IL-1 and IL-3).

The major consequences of this are inhibition of:
- T cell activation, both TH1 and TH2 cells of the CD4 subpopulation being similarly affected; and
- cells of the monocyte/macrophage system.

Cyclophosphamide acts by covalent alkylation

Together with chlorambucil, cyclophosphamide belongs to the group of immunomodulatory drugs that act by covalent alkylation of other molecules.

Cyclophosphamide has no alkylating ability itself, but many of its metabolites are active, each having two active sites to effect the cross-linking of DNA strands, thereby interfering with strand separation during replication.

The main side effect of cyclophosphamide is marrow toxicity, and so leukopenia must be monitored.

Both T and B cell functions are affected

Cyclophosphamide mainly affects lymphocyte numbers and function, particularly after low-dose daily oral therapy. Polymorphonuclear cell numbers may remain relatively unchanged.

Low-dose oral therapy may have a greater impact on cell-mediated responses, and bolus intermittent treatment more effect on antibody production.

In both humans and experimental animals, after a low-dose bolus (600 mg/m^2 body surface area), the numbers of B lymphocytes are reduced more than T cells and, among T cell subsets, CD8 more than CD4; however, with higher dosage, all cell types are reduced similarly.

Experimental studies have shown that this differential effect of low-dose depletion of CD8 cells allows a paradoxical increase in some CD4-controlled functions, such as antibody production. Evidence that low-dose cyclophosphamide has corresponding clinical relevance in humans remains equivocal.

As cyclophosphamide interferes with both B and T cell function, it is effective in controlling both antibody-mediated and cell-mediated immune responses in experimental animals and humans, and therefore has a major role in the management of both:
- autoantibody-mediated disease; and
- allograft rejection.

Azathioprine is active only on dividing cells

Azathioprine is converted rapidly and non-enzymatically to 6-mercaptopurine in vivo. It exerts its effect after metabolism to thioinosinic acid by competitive inhibition of purine metabolism and by incorporation into DNA as a fraudulent base. Its main effects are therefore on DNA synthesis.

Unlike cyclophosphamide, which is cytotoxic, azathioprine is cytostatic and is active only on dividing cells, exerting maximal effect if given soon after antigenic challenge.

Allopurinol, which inhibits xanthine oxidase, increases the effective dose of azathioprine fourfold. Therefore, if allopurinol is clinically essential (e.g. to treat gout) the dose of azathioprine should be decreased.

T and B cell numbers are reduced

Azathioprine is moderately immunosuppressive and produces modest reductions in both T and B cells after prolonged oral therapy at 2–3 mg/kg daily. Natural killer (NK) cell activity also appears to be suppressed after its use. Humoral immunity and delayed-type hypersensitivity are not affected at the doses given clinically, though there is a reduction in mitogenic responses to pokeweed mitogen in lymphocytes taken from patients receiving the drug.

Mycophenolate inhibits de-novo purine biosynthesis

Mycophenolate mofetil was developed to target selectively the final stage of purine synthesis, along a pathway used specifically by lymphocytes proliferating in response to antigenic challenge. Therefore, unlike nucleoside analogs such as azathioprine, it does not inhibit DNA repair enzymes or incorporate fraudulent purine analogs into DNA.

Mycophenolate is rapidly hydrolyzed in vivo to mycophenolic acid, which is an inhibitor of the enzyme inosine monophosphate dehydrogenase, and therefore results in inhibition of de-novo purine biosynthesis.

Q. In what other circumstances does aberrant purine metabolism selectively damage T cells?
A. Deficiency of purine nucleotide phosphorylase (PNP) or adenosine deaminase (ADA), produces SCID due to the toxic build up of purine metabolites in T cells (see Fig. 16.9).

Lymphocyte proliferation is blocked

Mycophenolate blocks both T and B cell proliferative responses in doses that appear to have no effect on other cell types. It also inhibits glycosylation of adhesion molecules involved in leukocyte traffic, thus restricting amplification of inflammatory injury.

Q. How would inhibiting glycosylation reduce lymphocyte traffic to sites of inflammation?
A. Selectins on the endothelium bind to glycoproteins on lymphocytes to slow them in the circulation before transendothelial migration (see Chapter 6).

Methotrexate blocks DNA synthesis

Methotrexate is a structural analog of folic acid and blocks folic acid-dependent synthetic pathways essential for DNA synthesis.

Immunoglobulin synthesis is reduced after prolonged treatment

Several reports note a reduction in immunoglobulin synthesis, with significantly lowered levels of all isotypes after 3 months of treatment with methotrexate. No consistent change has been noted in T cell subsets, in either the short or long term, or in the function of the monocyte/macrophage system. However, inhibition of dihydrofolate reductase involved in purine synthesis releases adenosine, which is a powerful inhibitor of activated polymorphonuclear leukocytes; hence methotrexate is anti-inflammatory.

Other effects of methotrexate on inflammation may be mediated by its inhibitory effect on arachidonic acid metabolism. More anti-inflammatory actions are indicated by the rapid decrease in indices of inflammatory activity such as C-reactive protein (CRP) and erythrocyte sedimentation rate (ESR), without affecting immune cell function or immunoglobulin synthesis.

Q. Where is CRP synthesized and what is its function?
A. CRP is synthesized primarily in the liver, and it acts as an opsonin by binding to pneumococcal carbohydrates.

Leflunomide inhibits T and B cell proliferation and antibody production

In vivo, **leflunomide** is converted to A77 1726, which non-cytotoxically and reversibly inhibits proliferation of both T and B cells stimulated by a variety of mitogens, and inhibits antibody production. A77 1726 inhibits **dihydro-orotate dehydrogenase**, an enzyme required for pyrimidine nucleotide synthesis.

Ciclosporin, tacrolimus (FK506), and rapamycin affect T cell signaling

Ciclosporin, tacrolimus (FK506), and rapamycin have complicated effects on T cell signaling and hence T cell function. They all bind to a class of cytoplasmic proteins (named **immunophilins**) with peptidyl prolyl isomerase (rotamase) activity, which they inhibit. Immunophilins are believed to have a critical role in transducing signals from the cell surface to the cell nucleus.

Ciclosporin binds to one family of immunophilins, **cyclophilins**, whereas **tacrolimus** and **rapamycin** bind to the **FK binding proteins**.

The ciclosporin–cyclophilin complex targets a serine threonine phosphatase called **calcineurin**, as does the tacrolimus–FK binding protein complex. Both inhibit signal transduction pathways, characteristically producing an increase in intracellular free calcium, and inhibiting transcriptional activation of cytokines and other genes essential for T cell proliferation and function.

Rapamycin blocks T cell proliferation by a different mechanism, through inhibition of IL-2-dependent signal transduction pathways, which function independently of calcium concentration and do not affect cytokine gene transcription (Fig. 17.2). Rapamycin arrests cells in the G_1 phase of the cell cycle, resulting in cell death by apoptosis.

Effects of ciclosporin, tacrolimus, and rapamycin

	ciclosporin	tacrolimus	rapamycin
lymphokine secretion (IL-2, IL-3, IL-4, IL-6, GM–CSF, IFNγ)	↓	↓	– or ↑
IL-2 receptor expression	↓	↓	–
response to IL-2	–	–	↓

GM-CSF, granulocyte–macrophage colony stimulating factor

Fig. 17.2 Differential effects of ciclosporin, tacrolimus, and rapamycin immunophilins on cytokine activity.

T cell proliferation is inhibited

Ciclosporin has:
- a marked inhibitory effect on the early events of T cell proliferation induced by mixed lymphocyte reactions, concanavalin A, or phytohemagglutinin;
- a specific effect on B cells, inhibiting antiglobulin-driven proliferative responses, but not those due to stimulation with lipopolysaccharide;
- effects on antigen presentation by monocytes and Langerhans' cells.

The effect of ciclosporin, while profound on T cells, therefore extends to other cells of the immune system.

It is believed that tacrolimus has a mode of action similar to that of ciclosporin, albeit by attachment to a different immunophilin.

Rapamycin, however, also affects cells of non-hematopoietic origin – for example, it inhibits proliferation of vascular smooth muscle cells after balloon catheter injury and may then be useful in preventing restenosis after angioplasty. Also, because rapamycin inhibits T lymphocyte proliferation at a later stage than ciclosporin or tacrolimus, it may be used synergistically with these agents or as an alternative in conditions refractory to the use of one or the other.

NUTRIENT DEFICIENCIES ARE GENERALLY ASSOCIATED WITH IMPAIRED IMMUNE RESPONSES

The relationship between nutrition and resistance to infection has been suggested by historical accounts of famine and pestilence, clinical observations, and epidemiological data.

Generally, nutrient deficiencies are associated with impaired immune responses. The five aspects of immunity most consistently affected by malnutrition are:
- cell-mediated immunity;
- phagocyte function;
- the complement system;
- secretory antibody; and
- cytokine production.

Worldwide, nutritional deficiency is the most common cause of immunodeficiency.

Economically underprivileged countries have a high prevalence of nutritional deficiencies, as do communities that are economically poor in many industrialized countries.

In addition, nutritional deficiency can result from primary systemic disorders – patients with cancer, chronic renal disease, burns, multiple trauma, and chronic infection show a high prevalence of malnutrition.

Paradoxically, obesity and an excess intake of nutrients are also associated with reduced immune responses.

Infection and malnutrition usually aggravate each other

Nutritional deficiency does not affect all infections equally:
- the clinical course and final outcome of pneumonia, diarrhea, measles, and tuberculosis are affected adversely by nutritional deficiency;
- for some infections (e.g. tetanus and viral encephalitis), the effect of nutritional deficiency is minimal;
- for other infections (e.g. influenza virus and human immunodeficiency virus [HIV]), nutrition exerts a moderate influence.

Many factors predispose to the development of infection in the malnourished individual, including poor sanitation, contaminated food and water, lack of nutritional and health knowledge, illiteracy, and overcrowding.

Lymphoid tissues are damaged by nutrient deficiencies

Lymphoid tissues are very vulnerable to the damaging effects of malnutrition.

The extent and severity of lymphoid dysfunction caused by nutrient deficiencies depend upon several factors, including:
- the rate of cell proliferation;
- the amount and rate of protein synthesis; and
- the role of individual nutrients in critical metabolic pathways.

Numerous enzymes with key roles in immune processes require zinc, iron, vitamin B_6, and other micronutrients to function.

Lymphoid atrophy is a prominent morphological feature of malnutrition.

The thymus, in particular, is a sensitive barometer in young children and the profound reduction in weight and size of the organ in several malnourished subjects has been termed 'nutritional thymectomy'. Histologically:
- the lobular architecture is ill defined;
- there is a loss of corticomedullary demarcation;
- there are fewer lymphoid cells;
- Hassall's corpuscles are enlarged and degenerate – some may be calcified.

Atrophy is observed in the thymus-dependent periarteriolar areas of the spleen and in the paracortical section of the lymph nodes.

Protein–energy malnutrition affects cell-mediated immunity and phagocytosis

Protein-energy malnutrition (PEM) is associated with a significant reduction in cell-mediated immunity, indicated by:
- a reduced number of CD4+ helper T cells; and
- a lower CD4+/CD8+ ratio.

Co-culture experiments indicate a reduction in T cell help available to B cells. Lymphocyte proliferative responses to mitogen are decreased. The immaturity of circulating T cells is reflected in increased leukocyte deoxynucleotidyltransferase activity. Reduced **thymulin** activity may underlie these changes in T cell number and function. There is a reduction in the secretory IgA antibody response to common vaccine antigens, which may contribute to a higher incidence of mucosal infections.

Phagocytosis is affected in PEM:

- opsonization is decreased, largely because of a reduction in levels of various complement components – C3, C5, and factor B;
- ingestion of microorganisms is intact, but the ability of phagocytes to kill intracellular organisms is impaired;
- the production of certain cytokines, such as IL-2 and TNF, is decreased.

Some innate mechanisms of immunity are also affected by nutrition:

- the production of lysozyme is slightly decreased;
- a larger number of bacteria bind to epithelial cells of malnourished subjects;
- wound healing is impaired.

There are very few data on the quality and quantity of mucus produced in PEM.

Zinc and iron deficiencies have a variety of effects on immunity

The profound effect of **zinc deprivation** on immune responses has been documented extensively. There is:

- a reduction in delayed cutaneous hypersensitivity,
- lower CD4+/CD8+ ratios; and
- T cell dysfunction.

A striking and pathognomonic feature of zinc deficiency is reduction in the activity of serum thymulin (a nonapeptide that contains zinc as an integral part of its molecule) and lymphoid atrophy.

There is also an intergeneration effect of zinc on immunity as demonstrated by the surprising finding of the effect in mice of zinc deficiency in pregnancy. Even the third-generation progeny have impaired antibody responses, as shown by diminished numbers of plaque-forming cells (PFC) and lower levels of IgM (Fig. 17.3).

Iron is a double-edged sword:

- it is required by most microorganisms for their growth;
- iron-dependent enzymes have crucial roles in lymphocyte and phagocyte function.

Iron deficiency is therefore generally associated with a reduced ability of neutrophils to kill bacteria and fungi, decreased lymphocyte response to mitogens and antigens, and impaired NK cell activity.

Q. In what ways can neutrophils and macrophages restrict iron availability for microorganisms?

A. Soluble proteins such as lactoferrin produced by neutrophils reduce the availability of free iron in the phagolysosome. Macrophages have ion pumps (e.g. nRAMP) in their phagosomal membrane that remove iron from the phagosome (see Chapter 15).

Intergeneration effects of zinc deficiency on immunity

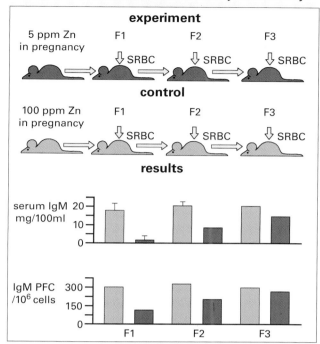

Fig. 17.3 An experimental group of animals was fed a zinc-deficient diet (5 ppm Zn) during the later two-thirds of pregnancy and a control group was fed a zinc-adequate diet (100 ppm Zn) during the same period. The former regimen reduced serum Zn to 60–70% of control values. F1, F2, and F3 generations were fed sufficient zinc throughout. Both the PFC response and serum concentration of IgM were assessed at 6 weeks. Results showed that both were low in at least three generations of offspring.

Selenium and copper are also important for immune responses

An exciting recent observation indicates that viruses can mutate and show altered virulence in malnourished hosts. Coxsackie virus recovered from selenium-deficient mice produced heightened myocardial damage – there were six nucleotide changes between the avirulent input virus strain and the virulent virus recovered from selenium-deficient animals.

The clinical counterpart of coxsackie myocarditis and nutritional deficiency is Keshan disease, which was endemic in some parts of China. Selenium supplementation has virtually eradicated this condition.

Vitamin supplementation is of value in severe measles

Vitamin A deficiency alters epithelial structure, leading to metaplasia and increased binding of bacteria. There is a reduction in the numbers of certain lymphocyte subsets and in the response to mitogen.

Vitamin supplementation is of value in preventing the complications of severe measles and reducing the mortality rate from this disease.

Vitamin B₆ and folate deficiencies reduce cell-mediated immunity, particularly lymphocyte proliferation responses, and also impair antibody production.

Obesity is associated with altered immune responses

Obese subjects and animals show alteration in various immune responses, including:

- cytotoxicity;
- NK activity; and
- the ability of phagocytes to kill ingested bacteria and fungi.

Altered levels of some micronutrients, lipids, and hormones may explain these immunological changes.

Some nutrients in moderate excess enhance immune responses

Some nutrients given in moderate excess enhance selected aspects of immune responses, particularly cell-mediated immunity. These include:

- vitamin E;
- vitamin A;
- zinc; and
- selenium.

However, for most nutrients, there is an upper limit of intake beyond which immune responses are impaired.

Nutritional intervention may prevent infection

There are exciting new possibilities for nutritional intervention for both primary and secondary prevention of infection in high-risk groups.

Hospital inpatients who are malnourished are at high risk of complicated opportunistic infections. Nutrient-enriched feeding formulas:

- enhance immunity; and
- reduce the risk of complications such as sepsis and poor wound healing.

However, the administration of such nutritional supplements, often delivered intravenously, can make the patient susceptible to nosocomial infections associated with indwelling catheters.

In the elderly, respiratory infection is a common cause of illness. Modest amounts of micronutrient supplements improve immune responses and, more significantly, reduce the incidence of respiratory infections and antibiotic usage. Furthermore, post-vaccination immune responses are higher in subjects given nutritional supplements than in untreated controls.

Probiotics benefit health and immunity

In both clinical and veterinary medicine, the value of probiotics is being recognized. These 'desirable' bacteria such as *Lactobacillus acidophilus*, *L. casei*, cocci such as *Enterococcus fecium*, and bifidobacteria are given orally to replace or increase their presence in the gut microflora. Benefits to health and immunity come from:

- the 'barrier effect' in the gut;
- production of bacteriocidins;

- alteration of the local immune response via a change in cytokine profile in the gut mucosa; and
- increased antibody production.

ACQUIRED IMMUNE DEFICIENCY SYNDROME

The most significant global cause of immunodeficiency is HIV infection

HIV is a retrovirus that is transmitted sexually, in blood or blood products, and perinatally. There are two main variants, HIV-1 and HIV-2:

- HIV-2 is endemic in West Africa and appears to be less pathogenic;
- HIV-1 has several subtypes (or clades), which are designated by the letters A through K, and the prevalence of the different clades varies by geographical region – over 90% of people infected with HIV-1 live in developing countries and spread is 80% by the sexual route.

Over 25 million people have died from AIDS since the first cases were described in 1981.

Although sub-Saharan Africa has the highest prevalence of HIV-1 infection in the world (7.4% for the region), the largest increase of new infections is occurring in East Asia, where the number of HIV-positive people increased by 50% between 2002 and 2004.

As of the end of 2004, The World Health Organization (WHO) estimates that, approximately 40 million people are living with HIV infection worldwide, with approximately five million new infections and three million deaths due to AIDS each year.

CD4 antigen is the main receptor for HIV entry

HIV is an enveloped retrovirus that contains two copies of a single-stranded RNA (ssRNA) genome (Fig. 17.4). Upon entry into a cell, the genome is reverse transcribed into complementary DNA (cDNA), which is integrated into the host cell genome (provirus).

The 10-kilobase genome encodes nine genes flanked at each end by long terminal repeat (LTR) sequences, which are:

- essential for integration of viral DNA into the host cell DNA; and
- contain binding sites for regulatory proteins involved in viral replication.

The basic gene structure contains *gag* (core protein), *pol* (reverse transcriptase, protease, and integrase enzymes), and *env* (envelope protein) genes.

In addition to these three main gene products, the virus encodes six regulatory and accessory proteins (Tat, Rev, Vpr, Vpu, Vif, and Nef), which regulate viral protein synthesis.

The viral genes overlap in different reading frames and the proteins are generated by alternative splicing mechanisms.

CD4 antigen is the main receptor for viral entry – it is present on CD4⁺ T lymphocytes, monocytes, dendritic cells (DCs), and brain microglia. The envelope glycoprotein gp120 is also capable of binding DC-SIGN.

Human immunodeficiency virus and its life cycle

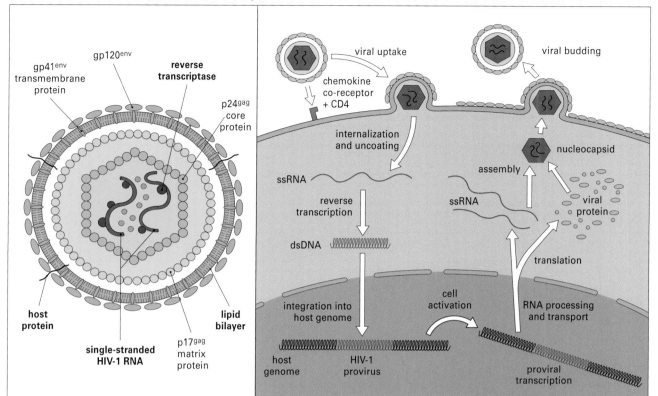

Fig. 17.4 After attachment to CD4 and a chemokine co-receptor (usually CCR5), the virus membrane fuses with the cellular membrane to allow entry into the cell. Following uncoating, reverse transcription of viral RNA results in the production of double-stranded DNA (dsDNA). This is inserted into the host genome as the HIV provirus, by a virally coded integrase enzyme, which is a target for new antiviral medications currently in development. Cell activation leads to transcription and the production of viral mRNAs. Structural proteins are produced and assembled. Free HIV viruses are produced by viral budding from the host cell, after which further internal assembly occurs with the cleavage of a large precursor core protein into the small core protein components by a virally coded protease enzyme, producing mature virus particles, which are released and can go on to infect additional cells bearing CD4 and the chemokine co-receptor.

Q. What is DC-SIGN?
A. DC-SIGN is a type II transmembrane protein on DCs that has a C-type lectin extracellular domain (see Fig. 9.18).

Although HIV-1 does not use DC-SIGN to infect DCs, this interaction allows DCs to internalize HIV-1 at mucosal sites and then migrate to lymph nodes where they deliver HIV-1 to CD4 T cells.

The viral envelope glycoprotein gp120 binds to CD4
The binding of the viral envelope glycoprotein gp120 to CD4 results in conformational changes in gp120 that expose binding sites for chemokine receptors, which serve as co-receptors for viral entry.

The chemokine receptor used largely determines which cell type different HIV-1 variants can infect:
- most primary isolates of HIV-1 use CCR5 as a co-receptor (R5 viruses) – rare individuals with a genetic 32-base pair deletion in CCR5 that results in a frameshift mutation and truncation of the protein are relatively resistant to HIV-1 infection;
- the other major variant of HIV-1 uses CXCR4 as a co-receptor (X4 viruses).

In approximately 50% of individuals the viral phenotype switches from R5 to X4 during the later stages of infection.

Q. How will the switch in the viral phenotype affect which cells are infected?
A. CCR5 is selectively expressed on mononuclear phagocytes. CXCR4 is present on a number of cell types, including naive T cells, B cells, and monocytes; consequently there is a shift towards T cell infectivity (see Chapter 6 and Appendix 4).

Immune dysfunction results from the direct effects of HIV and impairment of CD4 T cells

There is wide-ranging immune dysfunction in HIV-1 infection, with immune suppression within a milieu of immune activation, resulting from:

- direct effects of HIV; and
- depletion and functional impairment of the CD4 T cell subset over time.

How HIV kills its target cells is not well understood. Several different mechanisms have been proposed, including accumulation of RNA and unintegrated DNA in the cell cytoplasm and intracellular binding of CD4 and gp120. Infected cells may bind to uninfected cells by gp120–CD4 linkages, with multinucleate giant cell and syncytium formation.

gp120 bound to the surface of uninfected CD4 T cells also makes them vulnerable to antibody-dependent cell-mediated cytotoxicity (ADCC), while infected cells may be killed by HIV-1-specific CD8 cytotoxic T lymphocytes (CTLs).

HIV proteins may act as superantigens, resulting in vast expansion and then exhaustive depletion of cells. In addition, HIV may induce T cell apoptosis and viral budding may lead to cell membrane weakening and lysis.

The spectrum of immune dysfunction is characterized by:

- depletion of the CD4 T cell subset; and
- decreased responses to antigens, mitogens, alloantigens, and anti-CD3 antibody, associated with decreased IL-2 production and other changes in cytokine production.

The HIV-1 protein Nef selectively downregulates expression of HLA-A and -B alleles, so reducing surface expression of MHC class I molecule–peptide complexes and decreasing detection by CTLs. To avoid killing of infected cells by NK cells, which kill cells devoid of MHC class I molecules, Nef does not decrease expression of HLA-C and HLA-E.

Q. What is the functional significance of the observation that Nef does not decrease HLA-C and HLA-E?

A. HLA-C and HLA-E are inhibitory signals for NK cells. Therefore Nef can decrease cell recognition by CTLs while not increasing susceptibility to NK cells (see Chapter 10).

Nef has also been shown to decrease the expression of CD4 on infected cells such that gp120 on progeny virions is free to bind to CD4 and chemokine receptors on recipient cells.

There is an:

- increase in activated and unresponsive CD8 T cells;
- increased β_2-microglobulin and neopterin in serum;
- polyclonal B cell activation with B cells refractory to T cell-independent B cell activators; and
- an increase in autoantibodies and immune complexes.

Modeling of the plasma virus and CD4 T cell responses to antiviral therapy suggest that the average half-life of the virus and infected cells in the circulation is less than 2 days; 10^9–10^{10} viruses are released from infected cells and similar numbers of new cells are infected and die daily.

Antibody response appears to be ineffective in controlling HIV infection

The development of antibodies is an important component of the adaptive immune response to prevent or modulate infection. However, in the case of HIV-1 infection, neutralizing antibodies appear to be ineffective in controlling infection and viral replication.

Antibody responses to envelope glycoproteins can be detected in the serum of infected individuals 2–3 weeks after infection, though these lack the ability to inhibit viral infection. It is not until several more weeks after virus infection, and usually after the initially high levels of viremia have subsided, that neutralizing antibody responses are detected.

The main targets of neutralizing antibodies are:

- gp41;
- the second and third hypervariable loops (V2 and V3) of gp120; and
- the CD4-binding domain of gp120.

Antibodies to the V2 and V3 loop tend to be isolate-specific and therefore of doubtful use as potential vaccine-elicited antibodies. Furthermore, the genes encoding the V2 and V3 loops of gp120 are highly mutatic.

Q. What is likely to be the effect on the virus of antibodies to V2 and V3 during an HIV infection?

A. Specific antibodies will act as selective pressure on the virus to mutate these segments of the antigen to avoid immune recognition (see Chapter 13).

It is noteworthy that broadly cross-reactive neutralizing V3-specific antibodies have been described later in infection after prolonged antigen exposure, most likely resulting from somatic hypermutation in the variable region immunoglobulin genes.

Furthermore, studies in simian immunodeficiency virus (SIV) infection in macaques have indicated that pre-existing circulating neutralizing antibodies may alter the clinical outcome of infection. This indicates that the induction of high-titre neutralizing antibodies will be an important component in strategies to prevent HIV-1 infection.

Cellular immune responses play a role in controlling HIV viremia

In addition to antibody responses, cellular immune responses are generated in infected individuals and are thought to play an important role in control of viremia, though, like antibody responses, they are unable to eliminate infection.

The importance of virus-specific CD8 T cells in HIV-1 infection has been best demonstrated using an animal model of AIDS, where macaques depleted of CD8 T cells for more than 28 days during primary SIV infection failed to control viremia, experienced an accelerated disease course, and developed an AIDS-like syndrome resulting in death.

In humans, HIV-1-specific CD8 T cells are readily detected in:

- peripheral blood;
- lymph nodes; and
- gastrointestinal mucosal tissues.

HIV-1-specific CTLs have been shown to lyze infected cells and suppress viral replication in vitro. All expressed proteins have been shown to be targeted by HIV-1-specific CTLs, and in some individuals greater than 25% of total CD8 T cells are specific for HIV-1 epitopes.

Despite the presence of high numbers of HIV-1-specific CTLs in peripheral blood, no significant correlations have been established between the total number of IFNγ-producing CTLs and viral load.

HIV-1-specific CTLs in chronic progressive HIV-1 infection are impaired

There is evidence that HIV-1-specific CTLs in chronic progressive infection are functionally impaired because they:

- typically contain low levels of intracellular perforin (see Figs 10.11 and 10.12), a cytotoxic protein; and
- fail to exhibit strong proliferative capacity upon exposure to cognate antigens in vitro in individuals with high viral loads.

HIV-1-specific CTLs do, however, exert strong selection pressure on the virus, resulting in mutations in CTL epitopes that are incapable of binding to specific MHC class I molecules.

In addition, mutations affecting antigen processing have recently been described that interfere with intracellular proteasome processing of viral proteins such that specific epitopes are no longer generated and presented by MHC class I molecules on the surface of infected cells.

Depending on where in the HIV-1 genome these occur:

- mutations may result in loss of recognition of epitopes by HIV-1-specific CTLs and subsequent loss of control of viremia; or
- the mutations may occur in functionally important regions of viral proteins that impose a significant fitness cost to the virus and ultimately result in lower infectivity of the virus.

HIV-1-specific CD4 T cells are preferentially infected by the virus

HIV-1-specific CD4 T cell responses are complicated by the fact that CD4 T cells are the major population of cells infected by HIV-1, and recent evidence indicates HIV-1-specific CD4 T cells are preferentially infected by the virus.

Although HIV-1-specific CD4 T cells are present in peripheral blood at much lower levels than their CD8 counterparts, increasing evidence supports an essential role for these cells in containing viremia.

The major targets of HIV-1-specific CD4 T cells are the Gag and Nef proteins, and an inverse correlation between proliferative responses to Gag p24 antigen and viral load has been described.

Furthermore individuals with low to undetectable viral loads have been shown to have a higher percentage of HIV-1-specific cells capable of secreting both IFNγ and IL-2 in response to cognate antigen, in contrast to CD4 T cells from individuals with higher viral loads who secrete IFNγ only, with little or no detectable IL-2 production.

Evidence that HIV-1 exerts a progressive functional impairment of CD4 T cells over time has come from recent data indicating that autologous CD4 T cells isolated from individuals during acute infection can restore the proliferative capacity of CD8 T cells from chronically infected individuals when added back to in-vitro proliferation assays.

Moreover, vaccine-induced HIV-1-specific CD4 T cell responses have been correlated with restoration of the proliferative capacity of HIV-1-specific CD8 T cells.

The long-term clinical benefits of restored HIV-1-specific CD4 and CD8 T cell function remain to be determined, and such studies will provide important information regarding correlates of immune protection in HIV-1 infection.

Acute HIV infection is associated with a transient depletion of peripheral CD4 T cells

Acute HIV infection is associated with a transient illness similar to glandular fever (infectious mononucleosis) in up to 80% of persons, with clinical symptoms including malaise, muscle pains, swollen lymph nodes, sore throat, and rash. There is:

- transient depletion of peripheral CD4 T cells;
- expansion of CD8 T cells; and
- levels of plasma virus that reach 10 million virus particles per ml of plasma in most persons (Fig. 17.5).

Gut-associated lymphoid tissue is a major site of early virus replication, where there is large percentage of CCR5-positive CD4 cells, which become virtually eliminated in the early weeks following infection.

Because it takes 2–6 weeks on average for antibodies to core and surface proteins to be detectable by enzyme-linked immunoassays (ELISAs, see Method Box 3.2, Fig. 2), acute infection cannot be diagnosed by standard tests. Instead, this early acute phase can be detected only by assays that detect virus, such as plasma viral RNA levels.

Symptoms of acute infection have usually resolved by the time antibodies are detected, and a period of asymptomatic infection ensures.

The rate of disease progression in HIV infection is associated with both viral load and CD4 count at 6 months after infection.

Viral load 6 months after acute infection averages 30 000 RNA copies/ml plasma, with normal CD4 cell numbers in most persons.

AIDS is defined by a CD4 count < 200/μl

On average it takes 10 years to develop AIDS, defined by the presence of an AIDS-defining illness or a CD4 count of less than 200 cells/μl.

Strikingly, some persons progress to AIDS in less than 2 years, whereas other untreated persons have not developed AIDS in over 25 years of documented infection.

In untreated infection, there is a gradual increase in viral load and decline in CD4 count. Early indicators of immune function decline include non-specific constitutional symptoms such as fevers, night sweats, diarrhea, and weight loss.

Natural history of HIV infection

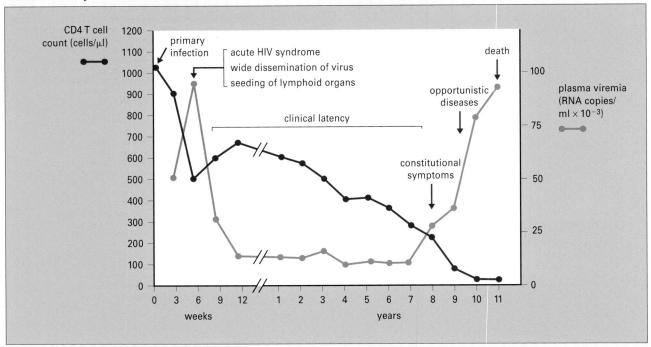

Fig. 17.5 A typical course of HIV infection. (Courtesy of Dr AS Fauci. Modified with permission from Pantaleo G, Graziosi C.

Q. Which mediators lead to the symptoms described above?

A. Inflammatory cytokines, including IL-1, which induces fever, and TNFα, which induces cachexia (weight loss), generate these symptoms (see Chapter 6).

Other less severe conditions that occur largely affect the mucous membranes and skin, for example:
- oral candidiasis (thrush);
- dermatomal varicella-zoster infection (shingles);
- recurrent anogenital herpes simplex virus infection; and
- a variety of other cutaneous skin infections.

These conditions often precede the development of serious opportunistic infections and tumors, which are AIDS-defining illnesses that typically occur when the CD4 count is less than 200/μl.

More severe infections are associated with a low CD4 count

Because of the strong relationship between CD4 count and risk of more severe infections, reflecting severe immune deficiency, AIDS is now also defined on the basis of CD4 count alone even in the absence of symptomatic disease, when the CD4+ T cell count is below 200/ml (see Fig. 17.5).

Kaposi's sarcoma, a multifocal tumor of endothelial cells (Fig. 17.6), is the commonest tumor. Widespread skin, mucous membrane, visceral (gut and lungs), and lymph node disease occurs. Infection with **human herpes virus 8 (HHV8)** is associated with development of the tumor. B cell lymphomas also occur, affecting the brain, gut, and bone marrow.

Most of the opportunistic infections are due to reactivation of latent organisms in the host or, in some cases, ubiquitous organisms to which we are continually exposed. They are difficult to diagnose and treatment often suppresses rather than eradicates them. Relapses are common and continuous suppressive or maintenance treatment is necessary, using drugs that cause side effects. The three main organ systems affected are the:
- gastrointestinal tract;
- respiratory system; and
- nervous system.

Q. Why should these systems be most commonly affected in HIV infection?

A. The respiratory and gastrointestinal systems are sites that are normally colonized by non-pathogenic microbes. A shift in the balance of the immune defense of these systems means that such microbes are not controlled. Immune responses are also limited and viruses are often tolerated in host cells, rather than destroyed. Again a shift in the immune balance can leave such latent infections uncontrolled (see Chapter 6).

Pneumonia is common and ***Pneumocystis carinii*** is the commonest infection (see Fig. 17.6), but bacterial infections, including ***Mycobacterium tuberculosis***, and **fungal infections** also occur.

Common features of late-stage HIV infection

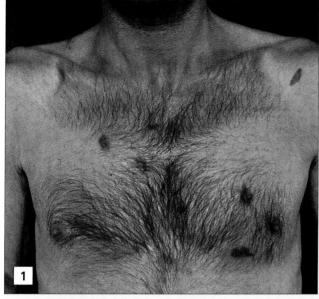

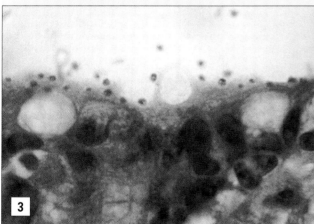

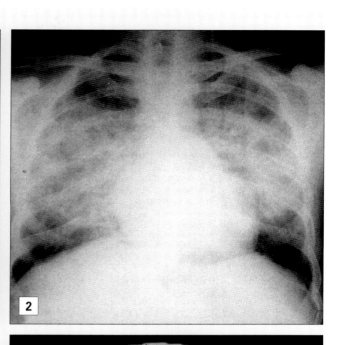

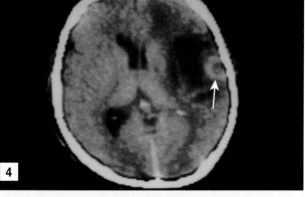

Fig. 17.6 (1) Multiple Kaposi's sarcoma lesions on the chest and abdomen. (2) Chest radiograph of a patient with *Pneumocystis carinii* pneumonia, showing bilateral interstitial shadowing. (3) Small bowel biopsy from a patient with diarrhea caused by cryptosporidia, showing intermediate forms of cryptosporidia (small pink dots) on the surface of the mucosa.

(4) Computed tomography scan of the head of a patient with cerebral toxoplasmosis. The patient presented with a history of fits and weakness of the left arm and leg. Injection of contrast revealed a ring-enhancing lesion in the right hemisphere (arrow), with surrounding edema (dark area).

Discomfort on swallowing is usually caused by **candidiasis** (thrush), but cytomegalovirus can cause esophageal ulceration.

Protozoa (cryptosporidia and microsporidia) are the commonest pathogens isolated in patients with diarrhea and weight loss (see Fig. 17.6), but **enteric bacteria** such as *Salmonella* and *Campylobacter* spp. may also be found.

Neurological complications in AIDS are due to:
- direct effects of HIV infection;
- opportunistic infections; or
- lymphoma.

AIDS-related dementia once affected between 10% and 40% of patients with other manifestations of AIDS, but with more effective antiviral treatment has become less common.

Spinal cord and peripheral nerve disease also occur.

Toxoplasmosis, a protozoal infection, causes cysts in the brain and neurological deficit (see Fig. 17.6).

Cryptococcus neoformans is a fungus that causes meningitis.

Cytomegalovirus may cause inflammation of the retina, brain, and spinal cord and its nerve roots, and a polyomavirus (JC virus), which infects oligodendrocytes in the brain, produces a rapidly fatal demyelinating disease – **progressive multifocal leukoencephalopathy**.

Treatment with highly active antiretroviral therapy (HAART) controls HIV infection

In 1987, zidovudine (AZT) was licensed as the first **nucleoside analog reverse transcriptase inhibitor (NRTI)** to be used in HIV infection. Together with targeted therapies to prevent opportunistic infections, even single drug therapy had an impact on the mortality rate.

Since then there have been considerable advances, with the development of:
* other NRTIs;
* **non-nucleoside reverse transcriptase inhibitors (NNRTIs)**;
* **protease inhibitors**; and
* **entry inhibitors** (see Fig. 17.4).

The introduction of **combination chemotherapy** for the treatment of HIV infection, which occurred in 1996, resulted in a dramatic decrease in deaths due to AIDS. HIV infection became a chronic controllable illness for persons fortunate enough to have access to these medications, which typically consist of:
* two NRTIs; and
* a NNRTI or protease inhibitor.

Treatment with these combinations, termed **highly active antiretroviral therapy (HAART)**, typically results in:
* lowering of plasma viral load to levels below detection by the most sensitive assays (< 50 RNA copies/ml plasma); and
* dramatic increases in CD4 cell counts, though these often do not return to normal levels of greater than 800 cells/μl;
* a decreased risk of opportunistic infections as CD4 counts rise.

The optimal time to start therapy continues to be debated, but most guidelines recommend HAART when:
* CD4 count is below 350 or 200 cells/μl;
* in all patients who have an AIDS defining illness.

Serum HIV RNA levels also influence this decision, though again there is debate on when to act, with some recommending therapy when the viral load is greater than 50 000 RNA copies/ml plasma, and others deferring until viral load is greater than 100 000.

Until recently, the cost of these drugs was so high that they were not accessible in resource-constrained settings, which is where over 90% of global infections are found. The combination of international donor efforts, reduced drug pricing, and generic medications have all contributed to an increasing access to these life-saving medications.

Early studies show that persons living in poverty not only can adhere to the complicated regimens, but that they are quite effective.

An effective vaccine remains an elusive goal

To date there have been clinical trials of numerous candidate HIV vaccines, but most would agree that an effective vaccine remains an elusive goal.

Despite increasing characterization of adaptive immune responses, the correlates of protection remain to be fully defined, and this has left the field with mostly empiric approaches.

Encouraging early reports of persons repeatedly exposed to HIV who never became infected suggested that adaptive immune responses, particularly HIV-specific CD8 T cell responses, might be responsible for apparent protection, but this remains somewhat controversial.

A vaccine that prevents infection altogether will almost certainly require the induction of broadly neutralizing antibody responses, something that is yet to be achieved.

Q. Why is it difficult to identify suitable antigens that could be used in a neutralizing vaccine?

A. The very rapid rate of HIV mutation and the high rate of virus production mean that the virus can readily mutate to evade a specific immune response, and yet may develop variants that retain infectivity.

Many in the field believe that a vaccine that protects from disease progression, while not necessarily protecting from the initial infection, is a more realistic short-term goal. The approaches being used for this goal focus on the induction of cellular immune responses, particularly CD8 T cell responses, though increasing data indicate that robust CD4 T cell responses to HIV will also be needed.

As no cure or vaccine is currently available, our main weapon is prevention through health education and control of infection.

FURTHER READING

Altfeld M, Allen TM, Yu XG, et al. HIV-1 superinfection despite broad CD8+ T cell responses containing replication of the primary virus. Nature 2002;420:434–439.

Brenchley JM, Schacker TW, Ruff LE, et al. CD4+ T cell depletion during all stages of HIV disease occurs predominantly in the gastrointestinal tract. J Exp Med 2004;200:749–759.

Day CL, Walker BD. Progress in defining CD4 helper cell responses in chronic viral infections. J Exp Med 2003;198:1773–1777.

Migueles SA, Laborico AC, Shupert WL, et al. HIV-specific CD8+ T cell proliferation is coupled to perforin expression and is maintained in nonprogressors. Nat Immunol 2002;3:1061–1068.

Piot P, Feachem RG, Lee JW, Wolfensohn JD. Public health. A global response to AIDS: lessons learned, next steps. Science 2004;304:1909–1910.

Robbins GK, De Gruttola V, Shafer RW, et al. Comparison of sequential three-drug regimens as initial therapy for HIV-1 infection. N Engl J Med 2003;349:2293–2303.

Critical thinking: Secondary immunodeficiency (see p. 498 for explanations)

A 52-year-old record producer developed a severe cough with increasing shortness of breath. He also had a fever, chest pain, and malaise. For the week before presentation he complained of pain on swallowing. His past medical history included gonorrhea and genital herpes within the previous 3 years. Over the previous 2 months he had suffered from persistent diarrhea and lost 9 kg in weight from a baseline of 68 kg. He lived with his male partner with whom he had been having unprotected intercourse for several years. There was no history of intravenous drug abuse.

On examination he was underweight and had enlarged lymph nodes in the neck, axillae, and groin. Plaques of *Candida albicans* were visible in his throat. There were abnormal breath sounds in his lungs. The results of his blood tests are shown in Table 1.

Table 1 Results of investigations on presentation

investigation	result (normal range)
hemoglobin (g/dl)	12.8 (13.5–18.0)
platelet count ($\times 10^9$/l)	128 (150–400)
white cell count ($\times 10^9$/l)	6.2 (4.0–11.0)
neutrophils ($\times 10^9$/l)	5.4 (2.0–7.5)
eosinophils ($\times 10^9$/l)	0.24 (0.4–0.44)
total lymphocytes ($\times 10^9$/l)	0.75 (1.6–3.5)
T lymphocytes CD4$^+$ ($\times 10^9$/l)) CD8$^+$ ($\times 10^9$/l)	0.12 (0.7–1.1) 0.42 (0.5–0.9)
B lymphocytes ($\times 10^9$/l)	0.11 (0.2–0.5)
arterial blood gases PaO_2 (kPa) $PaCO_2$ (kPa) pH HCO_3^- base excess	7.8 (> 10.6) 5.52 (4.7–6.0) 7.39 (7.35–7.45) 25.6 −0.9
ECG	normal
chest radiography	bilateral diffuse interstitial shadowing
bronchoscopy with bronchoalveolar lavage	positive for *Pneumocystis carinii*

Because of his sexual history, the patient was counseled about having a human immunodeficiency virus (HIV) test, and consented. An enzyme-linked immunosorbent assay (ELISA, see Method Box 3.2, Fig. 2) was positive for anti-HIV antibodies and a polymerase chain reaction (PCR) demonstrated HIV-1 RNA in the plasma.

Examination of an induced sputum specimen revealed cysts of *Pneumocystis carinii*, which together with the positive HIV ELISA is an AIDS-defining illness. Thus a clear diagnosis of acquired immune deficiency syndrome (AIDS) was made and the patient's *P. carinii* pneumonia was treated with oxygen by mask and parenteral co-trimoxazole. He was discharged from hospital taking oral co-trimoxazole.

Within 3 months he was seen again in accident and emergency with blurred vision and 'flashing lights' in his eyes. He was shown to have an infection of his retina with cytomegalovirus and was treated with injections of ganciclovir. The CD4 count at this time was 0.04×10^9/l. While receiving this treatment the patient became increasingly unwell and semiconscious. Investigations at this time are shown Table 2.

Critical thinking: Secondary immunodeficiency *(Continued)*

Table 2 Results of investigations 3 months after presentation

investigation	result (normal range)	
hemoglobin (g/dl)	10.4 (13.5–18.0)	
platelet count ($\times 10^9$/l)	104 (150–400)	
white cell count ($\times 10^9$/l)	4.1 (4.0–11.0)	
neutrophils ($\times 10^9$/l)	4.2 (2.0–7.5)	
eosinophils ($\times 10^9$/l)	0.24 (0.4–0.44)	
total lymphocytes ($\times 10^9$/l)	0.62 (1.6–3.5)	

T lymphocytes
  CD4$^+$ ($\times 10^9$/l)
  CD8$^+$ ($\times 10^9$/l)
	
	0.03 (0.7–1.1)
	0.40 (0.5–0.9)	

B lymphocytes ($\times 10^9$/l)	0.09 (0.2–0.5)	
chest radiography	minimal areas of diffuse shadowing	
blood culture	negative	
blood glucose (mmol/l)	7.6 (< 10.0)	

CSF from lumbar puncture
  appearance
  white cells (polymorphs/mm^3)
  protein (g/l)
	
	turbid
	2500
	4.2 (0.15–0.45)	

glucose (mmol/l)	4.5 (> 60% blood glucose)	
Indian ink stain	positive for cryptococcus	

A diagnosis of cryptococcal meningitis was made and intravenous amphotericin was started. The patient did not respond to treatment and died shortly afterwards. At autopsy, *P. carinii* was isolated from his lungs and evidence of early cerebral lymphoma was noted.

1 What diagnostic tests are available for HIV infection?
2 Which of these tests should be used if HIV infection is suspected in a mother and her child infected vertically?
3 What serological and cellular indices can be used to monitor the course of HIV infection?

Vaccination

SUMMARY

- **Vaccination applies immunological principles to human health.** Adaptive immunity and the ability of lymphocytes to develop memory for a pathogen's antigens underlie vaccination. Active immunization is known as vaccination.

- **A wide range of antigen preparations are in use as vaccines,** from whole organisms to simple peptides and sugars. Living and non-living vaccines have important differences, living vaccines being generally more effective.

- **Adjuvants enhance antibody production,** and are usually required with non-living vaccines. They concentrate antigen at appropriate sites or induce cytokines.

- **Most vaccines are still given by injection,** but other routes are being investigated.

- **Vaccine efficacy needs to be reviewed from time to time.**

- **Vaccine safety is an overriding consideration.** The MMR controversy resulted in measles epidemics.

- **Vaccines in general use have variable success rates.** Some vaccines are reserved for special groups only and vaccines for parasitic and some other infections are only experimental.

- **Passive immunization can be life-saving.** The direct administration of antibodies still has a role to play in certain circumstances, for example when tetanus toxin is already in the circulation.

- **Non-specific immunotherapy can boost immune activity.** Non-specific immunization, for example by cytokines, may be of use in selected conditions.

- **Immunization against a variety of non-infectious conditions is being investigated.** Recombinant DNA technology will probably be the basis for the next generation of vaccines.

VACCINATION APPLIES IMMUNOLOGICAL PRINCIPLES TO HUMAN HEALTH

Vaccination is the best known and most successful application of immunological principles to human health.

The first vaccine was named after vaccinia, the cowpox virus. Jenner pioneered its use 200 years ago. It was the first deliberate scientific attempt to prevent an infectious disease (smallpox), but it was done in complete ignorance of viruses (or indeed any kind of microbe) and immunology.

It was not until the work of Pasteur 100 years later that the general principle governing vaccination emerged – altered preparations of microbes could be used to generate enhanced immunity against the fully virulent organism.

Thus Pasteur's dried rabies-infected rabbit spinal cords and heated anthrax bacilli were the true forerunners of today's vaccines, whereas Jenner's animal-derived (i.e. 'heterologous') vaccinia virus has had no real successors.

Even Pasteur did not have a proper understanding of immunological memory or the functions of the lymphocyte, which had to wait another half century.

Finally, with Burnet's clonal selection theory (1957) and the discovery of T and B lymphocytes (1965), the key mechanism became clear.

In any immune response, the antigen(s) induces clonal expansion in specific T and/or B cells, leaving behind a population of memory cells. These enable the next encounter with the same antigen(s) to induce a secondary response, which is more rapid and effective than the normal primary response (Fig. 18.1).

While for many infections the primary response may be too slow to prevent serious disease, if the individual has been exposed to antigens from the organism in a vaccine before encountering the pathogenic organism, the expanded population of memory cells and raised levels of specific antibody are able to protect against disease.

Q. Rabies is one of the few diseases in which active immunization may be carried out after the individual becomes infected. What particular feature of rabies infection makes this a reasonable treatment?

A. The time between infection and the development of the disease is long, so an effective immune response has time to develop before virus reaches the CNS to produce symptoms.

Vaccines have two major effects

First, vaccines protect individuals against disease, and second, if there are sufficient immune individuals in a

Principles of vaccination

vaccination stimulates protective adaptive immune response – this priming expands the pool of specific memory cells
subsequent natural infection induces fast, vigorous responses
harmless forms of the immunogen are used to vaccinate – these can be killed or modified living organisms, subcellular fragments, or toxoids
vaccine adjuvants enhance immune responses
vaccines must be safe, affordable, and produce herd immunity

Fig. 18.1 Principles of vaccination.

population, transmission of the infection is prevented. This is known as **herd immunity**.

The proportion of the population that needs to be immune to prevent epidemics occurring depends on the nature of the infection:

- if the organism is highly infectious so that one individual can rapidly infect several non-immune individuals, as is the case for measles, a high proportion of the population must be immune to maintain herd immunity;
- if the infection is less readily transmitted, immunity in a lower proportion of the population may be sufficient to prevent disease transmission.

Effective vaccines must be safe to administer, induce the correct type of immunity, and be affordable by the population at which they are aimed. For many diseases, this has been achieved with brilliant success, but for others there is no vaccine whatsoever. This chapter is mainly concerned with the reasons for this disparity.

A WIDE RANGE OF ANTIGEN PREPARATIONS ARE IN USE AS VACCINES

In general, the more antigens of the microbe retained in the vaccine, the better, and living organisms tend to be more effective than killed organisms (see below). Exceptions to this rule are:

- diseases where a toxin is responsible for the pathology – in this case the vaccine can be based on the toxin alone;
- a vaccine in which microbial antigens are expressed in another type of cell, which acts as a vector.

Fig. 18.2 lists the main antigenic preparations currently available.

Live vaccines can be natural or attenuated organisms

Natural live vaccines have rarely been used

Apart from vaccinia, no other completely natural organism has ever come into standard use. However:

- bovine and simian rotaviruses have been tried in children;
- the vole tubercle bacillus was once popular against tuberculosis; and
- in the Middle East and Russia *Leishmania* infection from mild cases is reputed to induce immunity.

It is possible that another good heterologous vaccine will be found, but the safety problems will be considerable.

Attenuated live vaccines have been highly successful

The preferred strategy has been to attenuate a human pathogen, with the aim of diminishing its virulence while retaining the desired antigens.

This was first done successfully by Calmette and Guérin with a bovine strain (*Mycobacterium bovis*) of *Mycobacterium tuberculosis*, which during 13 years (1908– 1921) of culture in vitro changed to the much less virulent form now known as BCG (bacille Calmette– Guérin), which has at least some protective effect against tuberculosis.

The real successes have been with viruses, starting with the 17D strain of yellow fever virus obtained by passage in mice and chicken embryos (1937), and followed by a roughly similar approach with polio, measles, mumps, and rubella (Fig. 18.3).

Q. Why would passage of a virus in a non-human species be a rational way of developing a vaccine for use in humans?

A. The selective pressure on the virus to retain genes needed for virulence in humans and for human-to-human transfer is removed. Consequently some variants may lose these genes and are at no disadvantage in the animal, but will retain antigenicity for use as attenuated vaccine strains.

Just how successful the vaccines for polio, measles, mumps, and rubella are is shown by the decline in these four diseases between 1950 and 1980 (Fig. 18.4).

ATTENUATED MICROORGANISMS ARE LESS ABLE TO CAUSE DISEASE IN THEIR NATURAL HOST – Attenuation 'changes' microorganisms to make them less able to grow and cause disease in their natural host.

In early attenuated organisms, 'changed' meant a purely random set of mutations induced by adverse conditions of growth.

Vaccine candidates were selected by constantly monitoring for retention of antigenicity and loss of virulence – a tedious process.

When viral gene sequencing became possible it emerged that the results of attenuation were widely

The main antigenic preparations

type of antigen		vaccine examples
living organisms	natural	vaccinia (for smallpox) vole bacillus (for tuberculosis; historical)
	attenuated	polio (Sabin; oral polio vaccine)*, measles*, mumps*, rubella*, yellow fever 17D, varicella-zoster (human herpesvirus 3), BCG (for tuberculosis)*
intact but non-living organisms	viruses	polio (Salk)*, rabies, influenza, hepatitis A, typhus
	bacteria	*pertussis, typhoid, cholera, plague
subcellular fragments	capsular polysaccharides	pneumococcus, meningococcus, *Haemophilus influenzae*
	surface antigen	hepatitis B*
toxoids		tetanus*, diphtheria*
recombinant DNA-based	gene cloned and expressed	hepatitis B (yeast-derived)*
	genes expressed in vectors	experimental
	naked DNA	experimental
anti-idiotype		experimental
*standard in most countries		

Fig. 18.2 A wide range of antigenic preparations are used as vaccines.

Live attenuated vaccines

disease		remarks
viruses	polio	types 2 and 3 may revert; also killed vaccine
	measles	80% effective
	mumps	
	rubella	now given to both sexes
	yellow fever	stable since 1937
	varicella-zoster	mainly in leukemia
	hepatitis A	also killed vaccine
bacteria	tuberculosis	stable since 1921; also some protection against leprosy

Fig. 18.3 Attenuated vaccines are available for many, but not all, infections. In general it has proved easier to attenuate viruses than bacteria.

divergent. An example is the divergence between the three types of live (Sabin) polio vaccine:

- type 1 polio has 57 mutations and has almost never reverted to wild type;
- types 2 and 3 vaccines depend for their safety and virulence on only two key mutations – frequent reversion to wild type has occurred, in some cases leading to outbreaks of paralytic poliomyelitis.

VACCINIA VIRUS IS BEING USED AS A VECTOR FOR ANTIGENS OF MICROORGANISMS SUCH AS HIV AND MALARIA – Vaccinia virus is not an attenuated smallpox virus (present-day vaccinia virus strains being most closely related to rodent pox viruses), nor is vaccination against smallpox carried out. However, vaccinia virus is returning to use as a vector for antigens of other microorganisms such as HIV and malaria and is yielding very interesting information on the effects of attenuation.

Pox viruses contain approximately 200 genes of which about two-thirds are essential for growth in mammalian cells in vitro.

The modified vaccinia Ankara strain (MVA) was grown for a prolonged period in avian cells and has deleted genes required to complete the replicative cycle in mammalian cells, but it can still infect them and is a safe and immunogenic smallpox vaccine. Those genes not essential for replication of the virus are mostly concerned with evasion of host responses and virulence.

Virulence is the ability to replicate efficiently and disseminate widely within the body, with pathological consequences.

All pox viruses contain virulence genes and many of these mimic or interfere with cytokine and chemokine function. Some of these have sequence homology to their mammalian counterparts and others do not. Most vaccinia

327

Effect of vaccination on the incidence of viral disease

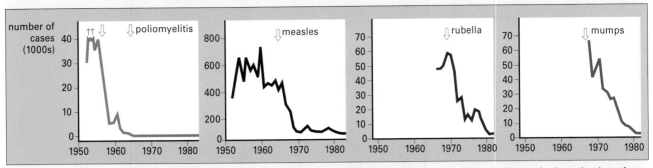

Fig. 18.4 The effect of vaccination on the incidence of various viral diseases in the USA has been that most infections have shown a dramatic downward trend since the introduction of a vaccine (arrows).

strains lack some of these genes while smallpox virus itself contains almost all of them.

It is now possible to use recombinant DNA technology to remove virulence genes completely or to introduce site-directed mutations to inactivate them. A problem remains due to the large size of pox viruses, where deriving an ideal vector is a major enterprise that has not yet been achieved.

Q. It is often found that attenuated viruses that are avirulent do not make good vaccines. Why should this be?
A. Inflammation induced by damage to the host has an adjuvant effect, leading to more effective presentation of the vaccine antigens.

Killed vaccines are intact but non-living organisms

Killed vaccines are the successors of Pasteur's killed vaccines mentioned above:
- some are very effective (rabies and the Salk polio vaccine);
- some are moderately effective (typhoid, cholera, and influenza);
- some are of debatable value (plague and typhus); and
- some are controversial on the grounds of toxicity (pertussis).

Fig. 18.5 lists the main killed vaccines in use today. Some of these will undoubtedly be replaced by attenuated or subunit vaccines.

Inactivated toxins and toxoids are the most successful bacterial vaccines

The most successful of all bacterial vaccines – tetanus and diphtheria – are based on inactivated exotoxins (Fig. 18.6), and in principle the same approach can be used for several other infections.

Subunit vaccines and carriers

Aside from the toxin-based vaccines, which are subunits of their respective microorganisms, a number of other vaccines are in use that make use of antigens either purified from microorganisms or produced by recombinant DNA technology (Fig. 18.7).

Killed (whole organism) vaccines

disease		remarks
viruses	polio	preferred in Scandinavia; safe in immunocompromised
	rabies	can be given post-exposure, with passive antiserum
	influenza	strain-specific
	hepatitis A	also attenuated vaccine
bacteria	pertussis	potential to cause brain damage (controversial)
	typhoid	about 70% protection
	cholera	protection dubious; may be combined with toxin subunit
	plague	short-term protection only
	Q fever	good protection

Fig. 18.5 The principal vaccines using killed whole organisms.

Acellular pertussis vaccine consisting of a small number of proteins purified from the bacterium is available and has been shown to be effective and less toxic.

Although hepatitis B surface antigen is immunogenic when given with alum adjuvant (see below), the bacterial capsular polysaccharides of *Neisseria meningitidis*, *Streptococcus pneumoniae*, and *Haemophilus influenzae B* are relatively poorly immunogenic and often do not induce IgG responses or long-lasting protection.

Q. Why do polysaccharide antigens not induce IgG responses or lasting immunity?
A. Polysaccharide antigens are not presented to helper T cells, so they do not induce class switching, affinity maturation, or generate memory T cells (see Chapters 7 and 8).

A significant improvement in the efficacy of subunit vaccines has been obtained by conjugating the purified

Toxin-based vaccines

organism	vaccine	remarks
Clostridium tetani	inactivated toxin (formalin)	three doses, alum-precipitated; boost every 10 years
Corynebacterium diphtheriae		usually given with tetanus
Vibrio cholerae	toxin, B subunit	sometimes combined with whole killed organisms
Clostridium perfringens	inactivated toxin (formalin)	for newborn lambs

Fig. 18.6 The principal toxin-based vaccines. Note that there are no vaccines against the numerous staphylococcal and streptococcal exotoxins, or against bacterial endotoxins such as lipopolysaccharides.

Subunit vaccines

	organism	remarks
virus	hepatitis B virus	surface antigen can be purified from blood of carriers or produced in yeast by recombinant DNA technology
bacteria	Neisseria meningitidis	capsular polysaccharides or conjugates of group A and C are effective; group B is non-immunogenic
	Streptococcus pneumoniae	84 serotypes; capsular polysaccharide vaccines contain 23 serotypes; conjugates with five or seven bacterial serotypes are being tested
	Haemophilus influenzae B	good conjugate vaccines now available

Fig. 18.7 Conjugate vaccines are replacing pure polysaccharides. *N. meningitidis* type B is non-immunogenic in humans because the capsular polysaccharide cross-reacts with self carbohydrates towards which the host is immunologically tolerant.

polysaccharides to carrier proteins such as tetanus or diphtheria toxoid. These protein carriers are presumed to recruit helper T cells and the conjugates induce IgG antibody responses and more effective protection.

Subunit vaccines are more expensive than conventional killed vaccines so initially their use is likely to be restricted to the developed world.

Antigens can be made synthetically or by gene cloning

Where it can be shown that a small peptide is protective it may be more convenient to make it synthetically. However, although there are animal models of viral infection or tumor immunotherapy where immunization with a synthetic MHC-binding peptide epitope can be effective, so far there is no human vaccine based on this approach.

Q. What fundamental problem associated with a peptide antigen vaccine arises when it is used in humans as opposed to animal models of disease?

A. In an outbred population (e.g. humans) a single peptide will usually be effective as an immunogen in only a proportion of the population because only certain MHC types can present the antigen and some people may not have a suitable MHC molecule (i.e. MHC restriction, see Chapter 7).

So far, therefore, the alternative approach of producing antigens by cloning their genes into a suitable expression vector has been much more useful because all possible MHC-binding epitopes within the antigen are retained:

- this approach has been highly successful with the hepatitis B surface (HBs) antigen, cloned into yeast and now replacing the first-generation HBs vaccine, which was laboriously purified from the blood of hepatitis B carriers; it has also brought down the cost of the vaccine;
- a second example of this approach is the recently tested vaccine against human papilloma virus types 16 and 11 – the L1 capsid antigen is the main component of the vaccine and, when expressed in yeast, the recombinant protein assembles into protein polymers, forming virus-like particles (VLPs) that are highly immunogenic.

An attractive feature of this approach is that further sequences can be added – for example, selected B and T cell epitopes can be combined in various ways to optimize the resulting immune response.

It is important to remember that, whereas B cells respond to the three-dimensional shape of antigens, T cells recognize linear sequences of amino acids (see Chapters 3 and 5). Peptides can therefore function well as T cell epitopes, but cannot readily mimic discontinuous B cell epitopes.

Even where a B cell determinant is linear, antibodies raised against the free flexible peptide, which adopts many configurations, do not bind optimally to the sequence in the way that they do when it is present as a more rigid structure within the native protein molecule.

Anti-idiotype vaccines could be used when the original antigen was unsuitable

Anti-idiotype vaccine is the only type of vaccine for which immunological thinking has been entirely responsible. The idea is to use monoclonal antibody (mAb) technology to make large amounts of anti-idiotype (anti-Id) against the V region (idiotype) of an antibody of proven protective value (Fig. 18.8).

The anti-Id, if properly selected, would then have a three-dimensional shape similar to the original immunizing antigen and could be used in place of it (Fig. 18.8).

Although often dismissed as 'armchair immunology', this strategy could have real value where the original antigen is not itself suitable (i.e. is not immunogenic or is toxic). Polysaccharides are one example, and the lipid A region of bacterial endotoxin (lipopolysaccharide [LPS]) is another. The advantage of the mAb would be that because it is a protein it should induce memory, which polysaccharides and lipids normally do not, unless conjugated to a carrier.

ADJUVANTS ENHANCE ANTIBODY PRODUCTION

During work in the 1920s on the production of animal sera for human therapy, it was discovered that certain substances, notably aluminum salts, added to or emulsified with an antigen, greatly enhance antibody production – that is, they act as adjuvants.

Aluminum hydroxide is still widely used with, for example, diphtheria and tetanus toxoids.

With modern understanding of the processes leading to lymphocyte triggering and the development of memory, considerable efforts have been made to produce better adjuvants, particularly for T cell-mediated responses. Fig. 18.9 gives a list of these, but it should be stressed that none of the new adjuvants is yet accepted for routine human use.

Adjuvants concentrate antigen at appropriate sites or induce cytokines

It appears that the effect of adjuvants is due mainly to two activities:
- the concentration of antigen in a site where lymphocytes are exposed to it (the 'depot' effect); and
- the induction of cytokines that regulate lymphocyte function.

Aluminum salts probably have a predominantly depot function, inducing small granulomas in which antigen is retained.

Newer formulations such as liposomes and immune-stimulating complexes (ISCOMs) achieve the same purpose by ensuring that antigens trapped in them are delivered to antigen-presenting cells (APCs).

Particulate antigens such as virus-like particles (polymers of viral capsid proteins containing no viral DNA or RNA) are highly immunogenic and have the useful property that they may also induce cross-priming (i.e. enter the MHC class 1 processing pathway though not synthesized within the APC, see Chapter 7).

Q. Many bacterial carbohydrates and glycolipids are good adjuvants, even though they are not good immunogens. Why should this be so?

A. The discovery of Toll-like receptors (TLRs, see Fig. 6.24) and other pattern recognition receptors (PRRs, see Chapter 15), such as lectin-like receptors for carbohydrates (see Fig. 9.18), has provided an explanation for the long-known efficacy of many bacterial products as adjuvants. It is clear that they act mainly by binding to PRRs and stimulating the formation of appropriate cytokines by APCs.

Ligation of different PRRs may bias the response toward TH1 or TH2 cytokine production.

Not surprisingly cytokines themselves have been shown to be effective adjuvants, particularly when coupled directly to the antigen. Cytokines may be particularly useful in immunocompromised patients (see below, Fig. 18.11), who often fail to respond to normal vaccines. It is hoped that they might also be useful in directing the immune response in the desired direction – for example in diseases where only TH1 (or TH2) cell memory is wanted.

Anti-idiotype antibodies as vaccines

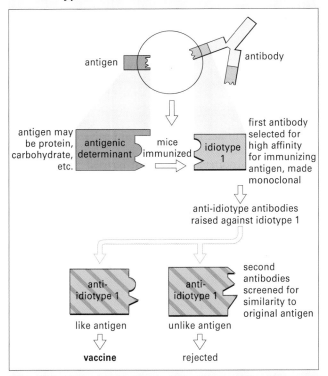

Fig. 18.8 Monoclonal antibody technology and the discovery of the 'idiotype network' have meant that immunoglobulins can now be used as 'surrogate' antigens. In the case of a carbohydrate or lipid antigen, this allows a protein 'copy' to be made, which may have some advantages as a vaccine. Note also that a monoclonal anti-idiotype can act as a mimic of a discontinuous B cell epitope.

Adjuvants

adjuvant type	routinely used in humans	experimental* or too toxic for human use†
inorganic salts	aluminum hydroxide (alhydrogel) aluminum phosphate calcium phosphate	beryllium hydroxide
delivery systems		liposomes* ISCOMs* block polymers slow-release formulations*
bacterial products	*Bordetella pertussis* (with diphtheria, tetanus toxoids)	BCG *Mycobacterium bovis* and oil† (complete Freund's adjuvant) muramyl dipeptide (MDP)†
natural mediators (cytokines)		IL-1 IL-2 IL-12 IFNγ

ISCOMs, immune-stimulating complexes

Fig. 18.9 A variety of foreign and endogenous substances can act as adjuvants, but only aluminum and calcium salts and pertussis are routinely used in clinical practice.

MOST VACCINES ARE GIVEN BY INJECTION

Most vaccines are still delivered by injection, but this is a risky method in developing countries, where re-use of needles and syringes may transmit disease, particularly HIV.

Because most organisms enter via mucosal surfaces, mucosal immunization makes logical sense and the success of oral polio vaccine indicates that it can be made to work. However, although live polio works when delivered orally, most killed vaccines do not.

Q. What key problems would one expect to be associated with oral vaccines?

A. Antigens may be broken down by passage through the stomach and digestive system, but, more problematically, the intestinal immune system is designed to generate tolerance rather than an immune response against food antigens.

Immunization only occurs when pathogenic organisms invade the gut wall. This can be mimicked by providing an adjuvant. Toxins from pathogenic intestinal organisms (cholera and *Escherichia coli*) have been the most studied intestinal adjuvants. Because the native toxins are extremely potent, partially inactivating mutations have been introduced to prevent excessive intestinal stimulation. Although these adjuvants work in experimental models, it is difficult to achieve a reproducible balance between:
- adequate stimulation of an immune response; and
- excessive gut inflammation.

An alternative is to use recombinant bacteria engineered to express antigens of interest, but the same difficulty applies:
- if the bacteria are non-pathogenic they may not immunize;
- if the bacteria are too pathogenic they may cause unpleasant symptoms.

Several recombinant and partially attenuated salmonella strains have been used experimentally to explore this vaccine strategy.

Similar problems relate to nasal immunization, usually tried against upper respiratory infections such as influenza or respiratory syncytial viruses (RSV). No nasal vaccine has entered routine use because of:
- difficulties in balancing attenuation against immunogenicity in the case of live RSV vaccine strains;
- the need for an adjuvant for an inactivated nasal influenza virus;
- safety worries because of the proximity of the nasal mucosa to the brain though the cribriform plate.

More recently the transdermal route has attracted attention. The 'gene gun' propels microscopic gold particles coated with DNA into the epidermis using a pressurized gas device (see below), but can be used with a variety of particles and proteins or other immunogens. The target is epidermal Langerhans' cells. Many antigens are also well absorbed and immunogenic if applied in a suitable vehicle to lightly abraded skin or even through the intact epidermis. As yet these methods are experimental, but it is hoped that eventually injection will be replaced by less invasive and safer methods.

VACCINE EFFICACY NEEDS TO REVIEWED FROM TIME TO TIME

To be introduced and approved, a vaccine must obviously be effective, and the efficacy of all vaccines is reviewed from time to time. Many factors affect it.

An effective vaccine must **induce the right sort of immunity**:

- antibody for toxins and extracellular organisms such as *Streptococcus pneumoniae*;
- cell-mediated immunity for intracellular organisms such as the tubercle bacillus.

Where the ideal type of response is not clear (as in malaria, for instance), designing an effective vaccine becomes correspondingly more difficult.

An effective vaccine must also be:

- **stable on storage** – this is particularly important for living vaccines, which normally require to be kept cold (i.e. a complete 'cold chain' from manufacturer to clinic, which is not always easy to maintain).
- have **sufficient immunogenicity** – with non-living vaccines it is often necessary to boost their immunogenicity with an adjuvant (see above, p. 330).

Live vaccines are generally more effective than killed vaccines.

Induction of appropriate immunity depends on the properties of the antigen

Living vaccines have the great advantage of providing an increasing antigenic challenge that lasts days or weeks, and inducing it in the right site – which in practice is most important where mucosal immunity is concerned (Fig. 18.10).

Live vaccines are likely to contain the greatest number of microbial antigens, but safety is an issue in a time of increasing concern about the side effects of vaccines.

Vaccines made from whole killed organisms have been used, but because a killed organism no longer has the advantage of producing a prolonged antigenic stimulus, killed vaccines now frequently replaced by purified components of the organism (subunit vaccines). These may suffer from several problems:

- purified subunits may be relatively poorly immunogenic and require adjuvants;
- the smaller the antigen, the more histocompatibility complex (MHC) restriction may be a problem (see Chapters 5 and 7); and
- purified polysaccharides are typically thymus independent – they do not bind to MHC and therefore do not immunize T cells.

These problems have been overcome in vaccines that are routinely used in humans by the use of adjuvants and by coupling polysaccharides either to:

- a standard protein carrier such as tetanus toxoid; or
- to a protein from the immunizing organism such as the outer membrane protein of pneumococci.

MHC restriction is probably more of a hypothetical than real difficulty because most candidate vaccines are large enough to contain several MHC-binding epitopes. Nevertheless, even the most effective vaccines often fail to immunize every individual – for example, about 5% of

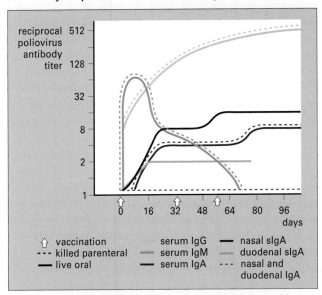

Antibody responses to live and killed polio vaccine

Fig. 18.10 The antibody response to orally administered live attenuated polio vaccine (solid lines) and intramuscularly administered killed polio vaccine (broken lines). The live vaccine induces the production of secretory IgA (sIgA) in addition to serum antibodies, whereas the killed vaccine induces no nasal or duodenal sIgA. As sIgA is the immunoglobulin of the mucosa-associated lymphoid tissue (MALT) system (see Chapter 2), the live vaccine confers protection at the portal of entry of the virus, the gastrointestinal mucosa. (Courtesy of Professor JR Pattison, Ch. 26 in Brostoff J, et al., eds. Clinical immunology. London: Mosby; 1991)

individuals fail to seroconvert after the full course of hepatitis B vaccine.

Most of the vaccines in routine use in humans depend on the induction of protective antibody. However, for many important infections, particularly of intracellular organisms (e.g. tuberculosis, malaria, and HIV infection), cellular immune responses are important protective mechanisms.

In recent years there has therefore been much effort to develop vaccines to induce immunity of both CD4 and CD8 T cells. So far the use of DNA and viral vectors have been the routes most commonly explored because both of these strategies lead to the production of antigens within cells and therefore the display of processed peptide epitopes on MHC molecules.

Although these methods, particularly combined in prime-boost regimens, have been highly effective in experimental animal models, so far in humans it has proved difficult to induce high frequencies of long-lasting antigen-specific T memory cells.

Even in experimental animals the duration of protection may not be long-lasting, perhaps because protection by cellular mechanisms requires activated effector cells rather than resting memory cells. Such cells are not well maintained in the absence of antigen.

VACCINE SAFETY IS AN OVERRIDING CONSIDERATION

Vaccine safety is of course a relative term, with minor local pain or swelling at the injection site, and even mild fever, being generally acceptable. More serious complications may stem from the vaccine or from the patient (Fig. 18.11):

- vaccines may be contaminated with unwanted proteins or toxins, or even live viruses;
- supposedly killed vaccines may not have been properly killed;
- attenuated vaccines may revert to the wild type;
- the patient may be hypersensitive to minute amounts of contaminating protein, or immunocompromised, in which case any living vaccine is usually contraindicated.

Although serious complications are very rare, vaccine safety has now become an overriding consideration, in part because of the very success of vaccines:

- because many childhood infectious diseases have become uncommon in developed countries, the populations of these countries are no longer aware of the potentially devastating effects of infectious diseases;
- unlike most drugs, vaccinations are given to people who have previously been perfectly well;
- the public is becoming increasingly aware of the possibilities of profitable litigation and companies correspondingly more defensive.

Q. Why is vaccine safety perceived as a less important issue when a vaccine is first introduced?

A. At the time of vaccine introduction the prevalence and danger associated with the infection is so great that any risks associated with the vaccine are relatively small.

The MMR controversy resulted in measles epidemics

The difficulties concerning vaccine safety are well illustrated by the recent controversy over MMR (measles, mumps, and rubella triple vaccine), though anti-vaccine movements in the UK date from a few years after the introduction of smallpox vaccination by Jenner in 1796.

In 1998 a paper was published that received wide publicity in the UK media, purporting to support an association between MMR vaccination and the development of autism and chronic bowel disease. Although a large amount of subsequent work failed to substantiate these findings and the interpretation of the original paper was withdrawn, take-up of MMR in the UK and Ireland declined over several years and epidemics of measles occurred because of declining herd immunity.

At the present time, the introduction of a five-valent vaccine containing diphtheria and tetanus toxoids, acellular pertussis, *Haemophilus influenzae* type B, and inactivated polio virus threatens to lead to decreased take-up in the UK. Here the argument seems to be that giving five immunogens simultaneously may be 'too much' for the delicate immune system of infants, though the vaccine has been shown to be safe and effective. Of course, because most of the vaccines within it are subunits, except for inactivated polio, the whole vaccine contains fewer antigens than the live bacteria and other organisms that the infant will encounter every day.

A rotavirus vaccine will prevent many infants from dying in developing countries

The story of a recent rotavirus vaccine is also instructive. In 1998 a live rotavirus vaccine was tested on large numbers of infants in the USA. Approximately 1 in 2500 vaccinated infants developed intussusception (a potentially fatal bowel condition) and the vaccine was withdrawn by the manufacturer. However, although this complication rate was unacceptable in the USA, the vaccine was highly

Safety problems with vaccine

type of vaccine	potential safety problems	examples
attenuated vaccines	reversion to wild type	especially polio types 2 and 3
	severe disease in immunodeficient patients	vaccinia, BCG, measles
	persistent infection	varicella-zoster
	hypersensitivity to viral antigens	measles
	hypersensitivity to egg antigens	measles, mumps
killed vaccines	vaccine not killed	polio accidents in the past
	yeast contaminant	hepatitis B
	contamination with animal viruses	polio
	contamination with endotoxin	pertussis

Fig. 18.11 The potential safety problems encountered with vaccines emphasize the need for continuous monitoring of both production and administration.

effective and would have saved many lives if used in developing countries where as many as 1 in 200 infants die from rotavirus diarrhea.

Complicating the debate further are more recent findings that the real risk of intussusception in vaccinated infants may in fact be much lower than appeared in the original trial and even lower if the vaccine is given in the first 2 months of life. Two newer rotavirus vaccines produced by other manufacturers are now in late-phase trials. Clearly vaccine safety raises many practical and ethical issues.

New vaccines can be very expensive

Although vaccination can safely be considered the most cost-effective treatment for infectious disease, new vaccines may be very expensive. The initial high cost is necessary to recoup the enormous development costs (US$200–400 million).

A good example is the recombinant hepatitis B vaccine, which was initially marketed in 1986 at US$150 for three doses. Although the cost has decreased greatly, even $1 is beyond the health budget of many of the world's poorer nations.

By contrast, the cost of the six vaccines included in the World Health Organization Expanded Program on Immunization (diphtheria, tetanus, whooping cough, polio, measles, and tuberculosis) is less than $1. The actual cost of immunizing a child is several times greater than this because it includes the cost of laboratories, transport, the cold chain, personnel, and research.

The Children's Vaccine Initiative, set up in 1990, is a global forum that aims to bring together vaccine researchers, development agencies, governments, donors, commercial and public sector vaccine manufacturers to seek means of delivering vaccines to the world's poorest populations who most need them.

VACCINES IN GENERAL USE HAVE VARIABLE SUCCESS RATES

The vaccines in standard use worldwide are listed in Fig. 18.12. Four of them – polio, measles, mumps, and rubella – are so successful that these diseases are

earmarked for eradication early in the 21st century. If this happens, it will be an extraordinary achievement, because mathematical modeling suggests that they are all more 'difficult' targets for eradication than smallpox was.

In the case of polio, where reversion to virulence of types 2 and 3 can occur, it has been suggested that it will be necessary to switch to the use of killed virus vaccine for some years, so that virulent virus shed by live virus-vaccinated individuals is no longer produced (as mentioned above, the new five-valent vaccine recently introduced in the UK and elsewhere contains inactivated poliovirus in accordance with this suggestion).

For a number of reasons, other vaccines are less likely to lead to eradication of disease. These include:

- **the carrier state** – eradication of hepatitis B would be a major triumph, but it will require the breaking of the carrier state, especially in the Far East, where mother to child is the normal route of infection;
- **suboptimal effectiveness** – effectiveness of BCG varies markedly between countries, possibly due to variation in environmental mycobacterial species (tuberculosis is increasing, especially in patients with immune deficiency or AIDS), and the pertussis vaccine is only about 70% effective;
- **side effects** – the MMR vaccine was suspected of having side effects, reducing the public's willingness to be vaccinated;
- **free-living forms and animal hosts** – the free-living form of tetanus will presumably survive indefinitely and it will not be possible to eradicate diseases that also have an animal host, such as yellow fever.

One of the future problems is going to be maintaining awareness of the need for vaccination against diseases that seem to be disappearing, while, as the reservoir of infection diminishes, cases tend to occur at a later age, which with measles and rubella could actually lead to worse clinical consequences.

Some vaccines are reserved for special groups only

In the developed world BCG and hepatitis B fall into this category, but some vaccines will probably always be confined to selected populations – travelers, nurses,

Vaccines in general use

disease	vaccine	remarks
tetanus diphtheria pertussis polio (DTPP)	toxoid toxoid killed whole killed (Salk) or attenuated (Sabin)	given together in three doses between 2 and 6 months; tetanus and diphtheria boosted every 10 years
measles mumps rubella	attenuated	given together (MMR) at 12–18 months
Haemophilus influenzae type b	polysaccharide	new; may be given with DTPP

Fig. 18.12 Vaccines that are currently given, as far as is possible, to all individuals.

Vaccines restricted to certain groups

disease	vaccine	eligible groups
tuberculosis	BCG	tropics – at birth; UK – 10–14 years; USA – at-risk only
hepatitis B	surface antigen	at risk (medical, nursing staff, etc.); drug addicts; male homosexuals; known contacts of carriers
rabies	killed	at risk (animal workers); postexposure
meningitis yellow fever typhoid, cholera hepatitis A	polysaccharide attenuated killed or mutant killed or attenuated	travelers
influenza	killed	at risk; elderly
pneumococcal pneumonia	polysaccharide	elderly
varicella-zoster	attenuated	leukemic children

Fig. 18.13 Vaccines that are currently restricted to certain groups.

the elderly, etc. (Fig. 18.13). In some cases this is because of:

- geographical restrictions (e.g. yellow fever);
- the rarity of exposure (e.g. rabies);
- problems in producing sufficient vaccine in time to meet the demand (e.g. each influenza epidemic is caused by a different strain, requiring a new vaccine).

A vaccine effective against all strains of influenza would be of tremendous value. However, both the hemagglutinin and neuraminidase antigens, which together make up the outer layer of the virus and are the antigens of importance in the vaccine, are subject to variation.

Vaccines for parasitic and some other infections are only experimental

Some of the most intensively researched vaccines are those for the major tropical protozoal and worm infections (see Chapter 15). However, none has come into standard use, and some have argued that none will because none of these diseases induces effective immunity and 'you cannot improve on nature'.

Nevertheless, extensive work in laboratory animals has shown that vaccines against malaria, leishmaniasis, and schistosomiasis are perfectly feasible, and there is a moderately effective vaccine against babesia in dogs. In cattle an irradiated vaccine against the lungworm has been in veterinary use for decades.

Q. Why, even with effective vaccines, will it be impossible to eradicate many parasitic diseases?

A. Many parasites have alternative species to humans as their host (see Chapter 15).

It remains possible, however, that the parasitic diseases of humans are uniquely difficult to treat, partly because of the polymorphic and rapidly changing nature of many parasitic antigens. For example:

- none of the small animal models of malaria shows such extensive antigenic variation as *Plasmodium falciparum*,

the protozoon causing malignant tertian malaria in humans;
- similarly, rats appear to be much easier to immunize against schistosomiasis than other animals, including possibly humans.

Part of the problem is that these parasites are usually not in their natural host in the laboratory.

Several trials of clinical malaria vaccine have been published, using antigens derived from either the liver or the blood stage, with only very moderate success. Malaria is unusual in that its life cycle offers a variety of possible targets for vaccination (Fig. 18.14).

A problem with these chronic parasitic diseases is that of immunopathology. For example, the symptoms of *Trypanosoma cruzi* infection (Chagas' disease) are largely due to the immune system (i.e. autoimmunity). A bacterial parallel is leprosy, where the symptoms are due to the (apparent) overreactivity of TH1 or TH2 cells. A vaccine that boosted immunity without clearing the pathogen could make these conditions worse. Another example of this unpleasant possibility is with dengue, where certain antibodies enhance the infection by allowing the virus to enter cells via Fc receptors. Enhancing antibodies have also been reported in an experimental model of a transmission-blocking anti-malarial vaccine.

Some viral and bacterial vaccines are also in the experimental category

Other viral and bacterial vaccines that are also experimental are:

- cholera toxin;
- attenuated shigella;
- Epstein–Barr virus surface glycoprotein.

A recombinant vaccine against human papilloma virus type 16 consisting of virus-like particles has recently undergone trials and appears to be highly effective in preventing genital infection. It remains to be determined whether such a vaccine will also reduce the incidence of cervical carcinoma.

335

Malaria vaccine strategies

stage	vaccine strategy
sporozoites	sporozoite vaccine to induce blocking antibody, already field-tested in humans
liver stage	sporozoite vaccine to induce cell-mediated immunity to liver stage
merozoites	merozoite (antigen) vaccine to induce blocking antibody
asexual erythrocyte stage	asexual stage (antigen) vaccine to induce other responses to red cell stage, and against toxic products ('anti-disease' vaccine)
gametocytes / gametes	vaccines to interrupt sexual stages – 'transmission-blocking' vaccine

Fig. 18.14 A number of different approaches to malaria vaccines are being investigated, reflecting the complexity of both the life cycle of malaria and immunity to it.

For many diseases there is no vaccine available

No vaccine is currently available for many serious infectious diseases (Fig. 18.15). Headed by HIV infection (see Chapter 17), these represent the major challenge for research and development in the coming decade.

PASSIVE IMMUNIZATION CAN BE LIFE-SAVING

Driven from use by the advent of antibiotics, the idea of injecting preformed antibody to treat infection is still valid for certain situations (Fig. 18.16). It can be life-saving when:
- toxins are already circulating (e.g. in tetanus, diphtheria, and snake-bite);
- high-titer specific antibody is required, generally made in horses, but occasionally obtained from recovered patients.

At the opposite end of the scale, normal pooled human immunoglobulin contains enough antibody against common infections for a dose of 100–400 mg IgG to protect hypogammaglobulinemic patients for a month. Over 1000 donors are used for each pool, and the sera must be screened for HIV and hepatitis B and C.

The use of specific monoclonal antibodies, though theoretically attractive, has not yet proved to be an improvement on traditional methods, and their chief application to infectious disease at present remains in diagnosis. This may change as human monoclonal antibodies become more readily available (and less expensive), either through cell culture or protein engineering.

In tumor immunotherapy a monoclonal antibody to CD20 has found a place in the treatment of B cell lymphomas. Immunotherapy using similar means of B cell depletion has also had beneficial effects in rheumatoid arthritis and systemic lupus erythematosus (SLE, see Chapter 20).

Antibody genes can now be engineered to form Fab, single chain Fv, or V_H fragments (see Chapter 3). Libraries of these can be expressed in recombinant phages and screened against antigens of interest. Selected antibody fragments can be produced in bulk in bacteria, yeasts, or mammalian cells, for use in vitro or in vivo.

Differently sized antibody fragments may have different uses – in general the smaller the fragment the better the penetration into tissues, but also the shorter the half-life. Bacteria engineered to produce antibody fragments may in the future be used to target protective antibody to a particular microenvironment, such as the intestine.

NON-SPECIFIC IMMUNOTHERAPY CAN BOOST IMMUNE ACTIVITY

Many of the same compounds that act as adjuvants for vaccines have also been used on their own in an attempt to boost the general level of immune activity (Fig. 18.17). The best results have been obtained with cytokines, and among these IFNα is the most widely used, mainly for its antiviral properties (but also for certain tumours – see below).

Perhaps the most striking clinical effect of a cytokine has been that of granulocyte colony stimulating factor (G-CSF) in restoring bone marrow function after anti-cancer therapy, with benefit to both bleeding and infection.

Finally cytokine inhibitors can be used for severe or chronic inflammatory conditions. Various ways of inhibiting TNF and IL-1 have proved valuable:
- in rheumatoid arthritis; and
- more controversially, in septic (Gram-negative) shock and severe malaria.

In a few years, one would expect the clinical pharmacology of cytokines and cytokine inhibitors to be clarified so that these communication molecules of the immune system can be fully exploited, in the same way as vaccination has exploited the properties of the lymphocyte.

IMMUNIZATION AGAINST A VARIETY OF NON-INFECTIOUS CONDITIONS IS BEING INVESTIGATED

The idea of non-specifically stimulating the immune system to reject tumors goes back almost a century to the work of Coley, who used bacterial filtrates with considerable success, possibly through the induction of

Major diseases for which no vaccines are available

	disease	problems
viruses	HIV	antigenic variation; immunosuppression?
	herpes viruses	risk of reactivation? (but varicella-zoster appears safe)
	adenoviruses, rhinoviruses	multiple serotypes
bacteria	staphylococci group A streptococci	early vaccines ineffective (antibiotics originally better)
	Mycobacterium leprae	(BCG gives some protection)
	Treponema pallidum (syphilis)	ignorance of effective immunity
	Chlamydia spp.	early vaccines ineffective
fungi	*Candida* spp. *Pneumocystis* spp.	ignorance of effective immunity
protozoa	malaria	antigenic variation
	trypanosomiasis – sleeping sickness; Chagas' disease	extreme antigenic variation; immunopathology; autoimmunity; trials encouraging
	leishmaniasis	
worms	schistosomiasis	(trials in animals encouraging)
	onchocerciasis	ignorance of effective immunity

Fig. 18.15 For some serious diseases there is currently no effective vaccine. The predominant problem is the lack of understanding of how to induce effective immunity.

Passive immunization

disease	source of antibody	indication
diphtheria, tetanus	human, horse	prophylaxis, treatment
varicella-zoster	human	treatment in immunodeficiencies
gas gangrene, botulism, snake bite, scorpion sting	horse	post-exposure
rabies	human	post-exposure (plus vaccine)
hepatitis B	human	post-exposure
hepatitis A, measles	pooled human immunoglobulin	prophylaxis (travel), post-exposure

Fig. 18.16 Although not so commonly used as 50 years ago, injections of specific antibody can still be a life-saving treatment in specific clinical conditions.

cytokines such as TNF and IFN. However, attempts to equal his results with purified cytokines or immuno-stimulants (e.g. BCG) have been successful in only a restricted range of tumors, and current efforts are mainly directed at the induction of specific immunity – just as for infectious microbes – encouraged by the evidence that tumors may sometimes be spontaneously rejected as if they were foreign grafts (see Chapter 21).

In principle, conception and implantation can be interrupted by inducing immunity against a wide range of pregnancy hormones. The target of the most successful experimental trials has been human chorionic gonadotro-pin (hCG), the embryo-specific hormone responsible for maintaining the corpus luteum.

Vaccines based on the β chain of hCG, coupled to tetanus or diphtheria toxoid, have been extremely

Non-specific immunotherapy

source		remarks
microbial	filtered bacterial cultures	used by Coley (1909) against tumors
	BCG	some activity against tumors
cytokines	IFNα	effective for chronic hepatitis B, hepatitis C, herpes zoster, wart virus, prophylactic against common cold (also some tumors)
	IFNγ	effective in some cases of chronic granulomatous disease, lepromatous leprosy, leishmaniasis (cutaneous)
	IL-2	leishmaniasis (cutaneous)
	G-CSF	bone marrow restoration after cytotoxic drugs
cytokine inhibitors	TNF antagonists	septic shock
	IL-1 antagonists	severe (cerebral) malaria?
	IL-10	
G-CSF, granulocyte colony stimulating factor; IFN, interferon; IL, interleukin; TNF, tumor necrosis factor		

Fig. 18.17 Non-specific stimulation or inhibition of particular components of the immune system may sometimes be of benefit.

successful in preventing conception in baboons and, more recently, humans. In the human trial, infertility was only temporary, and no serious side effects were observed. Clearly this represents a powerful new means of safely limiting family size, though there are of course cultural and ethical aspects to consider too.

Other uses of immunization that are being explored include:

- the treatment of drug dependency, because it is possible to neutralize the effect of a drug by pre-immunization with the drug coupled to a suitable carrier (the 'hapten–carrier' effect);
- lowering cholesterol by 'neutralizing' lipid-binding proteins; and
- preventing Alzheimer's disease by immunizing against components of amyloid plaque.

So far these vaccines are largely experimental.

Q. What problems can one foresee associated with the types of treatment described above?

A. Breaking tolerance to self molecules raises safety issues. These are well-founded concerns because in some primate and early-phase human trials of Alzheimer's vaccines encephalitis has been observed following immunization.

Future vaccines will use genes and vectors to deliver antigens

Vaccinia is a convenient vector

A development of the use of gene cloning is to insert the desired gene into a vector, which can then be injected into the patient, allowed to replicate, express the gene, and produce the antigen in situ (Fig. 18.18). Vaccinia is a convenient vector that is large enough to carry several antigens. Modified vaccinia Ankara (MVA) may be particularly safe because it does not replicate in human cells (see above, p. 330).

Because immunization against smallpox ceased some years ago, the problem of pre-existing immunity is also decreasing. A number of experimental vaccines using recombinant vaccinia have been tested, though none is yet in routine use. Many other viruses have also been proposed and tested experimentally as vaccine vectors.

BCG and salmonellae have been favored for experimental recombinant bacterial vaccines

Attenuated bacteria have the advantage that they have genomes large enough to incorporate many genes from other organisms. BCG and salmonellae have been favored organisms for experimental recombinant bacterial vaccines.

Mutant salmonellae can be given by mouth and immunize the gut-associated lymphoid tissue before being eliminated – a very useful property because diarrhea is one of the world's major killers in infancy. The mutant bacteria are also capable of inducing systemic immunity. However, as yet no bacterial recombinant vaccines are routinely used.

Transgenic plants can be genetically engineered to express vaccine antigens

An even more innovative approach is to construct transgenic plants expressing vaccine antigens. Mice have been successfully immunized by eating genetically engineered raw potatoes. Many problems with this approach need to be overcome:

- protein antigens may be rapidly degraded in the digestive tract;
- consistency and dosage will be difficult to control;

Generation of recombinant vaccinia virus for expression of a foreign gene

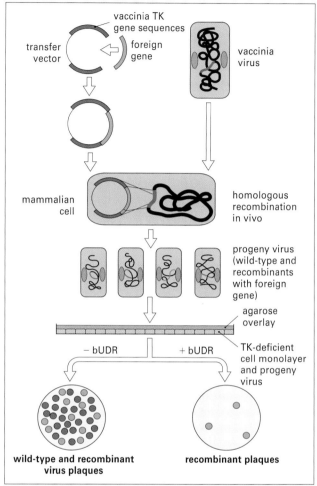

Fig. 18.18 Recombinant vaccinia virus can be generated to express a foreign gene. The foreign gene is inserted into vaccinia's thymidine kinase (TK) gene so that recombinant virus plaques can be distinguished from wild type. TK is used by virus to take up thymidine from the culture medium or intracellular pool for DNA synthesis; the recombinant virus cannot produce TK, because the gene has been interrupted and so must use the separate pathway for de-novo synthesis of thymidine. In the presence of bromodeoxyuridine (bUDR), a thymidine analog that blocks DNA synthesis when it is incorporated into DNA, wild-type virus replication is blocked but recombinant virus replication continues, using de-novo synthesis of thymidine. The cell monolayer must be TK deficient so that recombinant virus cannot use the cells' TK to take up bUDR. (Courtesy of Dr DJ Rowlands, Ch. 26 in Brostoff J., et al., eds. Clinical Immunology, London: Mosby; 1991)

- antigens administered orally often tolerize rather than immunize, and oral adjuvants may need to be incorporated into the plants.

Even if edible plant vaccines present problems, however, recombinant plants may provide a cheap and convenient way of producing vaccine antigens, which may be purified from the leaves or fruit of the plant and used in conventional subunit vaccines.

A recent development is the use of 'naked' DNA

Genes of interest coupled with a suitable promoter are injected directly into muscle or coated onto gold microparticles and 'shot' into the skin by pressurized gas – the **gene gun**. Surprisingly this can induce long-lasting cellular and humoral immunity in experimental animals. The mechanism appears to be through uptake and expression of the DNA in APCs.

This method has the advantage that immunomodulatory genes (cytokines or co-stimuli) can be incorporated into the DNA construct along with the genes coding for antigens, to generate and amplify the desired immune response. It has also been found that bacterial olignucleotide (CpG DNA) sequences have adjuvant properties and these can be included in the plasmids used to produce the DNA.

DNA vaccines have not yet fulfilled in humans the promise they have shown in animal model systems. This may be because doses of DNA used in animals have generally been relatively higher than in humans, and it is clear that different bacterial CpG sequences are needed to stimulate optimally the dendritic cells of experimental animals and humans.

At present DNA immunization is largely being tested in life-threatening situations (tumors, HIV infection) rather than in routine vaccination of infants.

Priming with DNA and boosting with recombinant vaccinia virus is significantly more effective than DNA alone, at least in animals. However, so far clinical trials of a prime boost regimen of DNA followed by MVA for an HIV vaccine have not been particularly encouraging.

Nevertheless DNA vaccines have the important potential advantages of cheapness and stability so that many means of overcoming these difficulties are being tested, such as:

- the use of in-vivo electroporation to increase the efficiency of DNA entry into cells;
- the optimization of immunostimulatory CpG sequences; and
- the incorporation of carrier proteins or adjuvant cytokines into the vaccines.

FURTHER READING

Beverley PCL, Borysiewicz L, Hill AVS, et al., eds. Vaccination. Br Med Bull 2002;62:1–230.

Fife KH, Wheeler CM, Koutsky LA, et al. Dose-ranging studies of the safety and immunogenicity of human papillomavirus type 11 and type 16 virus-like particle candidate vaccines in young healthy women. Vaccine 2004;22:2943–2952.

Mononego A, Weiner HL. Immunotherapeutic approaches to Alzheimer's disease. Science 2003;302:834–838.

Naz RK. Vaccine for contraception targeting sperm. Immunol Rev 1999;171:193–202.

Roberts L. Rotavirus vaccines' second chance. Science 2004;305:1890–1893.

Critical thinking: Vaccination (see p. 499 for explanations)

1 Why have attenuated vaccines not been developed for all viruses and bacteria?

2 'A vaccine cannot improve on nature'. Is this unduly pessimistic?

3 'The smallpox success story is unlikely to be repeated.' Is this true?

4 Will vaccines eventually replace antibiotics?

5 BCG: vaccine, adjuvant, or non-specific stimulant?

6 Why could an anti-worm vaccine do more harm than good?

7 By what means, other than their reaction with antibodies, might you identify antigens that could be used as vaccines?

Immune
Responses
Against Tissues

Immunological Tolerance

SUMMARY

- **Immunological tolerance is a state of unresponsiveness for a particular antigen.** Tolerance mechanisms are needed because the immune system randomly generates a vast diversity of antigen-specific receptors and some of these will be self reactive; tolerance prevents harmful reactivity against the body's own tissues.

- **Immunological tolerance was demonstrated by some key historical experiments.**

- **The study of tolerance involves inducing tolerance experimentally.**

- **Central tolerance takes place during T cell development in the thymus.** Central thymic tolerance to self antigens (autoantigens) results from deletion of differentiating T cells that express antigen-specific receptors with high binding affinity for intrathymic self antigens. Low-affinity self-reactive T cells, and T cells with receptors specific for antigens that are not represented intrathymically, differentiate and join the peripheral T cell pool.

- **A variety of mechanisms maintain tolerance in peripheral lymphoid organs.** Post-thymic tolerance to self antigens has five main mechanisms: (i) self-reactive T cells in the circulation may ignore self antigens, for example when the antigens are in tissues sequestered from the circulation; (ii) their response to a self antigen may be suppressed if the antigen is present in a privileged site; (iii) self-reactive cells may under certain conditions be deleted or (iv) rendered anergic and unable to respond; (v) finally a state of tolerance to self antigens can also be maintained by regulatory T cells.

- **Tolerance is also imposed on B cells.** B cell deletion takes place in both bone marrow and peripheral lymphoid organs. Differentiating B cells that express surface immunoglobulin receptors with high binding affinity for self membrane-bound antigens will be deleted soon after their generation in the bone marrow. A high proportion of short-lived, low-avidity, autoreactive B cells appear in peripheral lymphoid organs. These cells may be recruited to fight against infection.

- **Tolerance can be induced artificially** by various regimens that may eventually be exploited clinically to prevent rejection of foreign transplants and to manipulate autoimmune and allergic diseases.

IMMUNOLOGICAL TOLERANCE IS A STATE OF UNRESPONSIVENESS FOR A PARTICULAR ANTIGEN

Immunological tolerance is a state of unresponsiveness that is specific for a particular antigen; it is induced by previous exposure to that antigen.

Active tolerance mechanisms are required to prevent inflammatory responses to the many innocuous air-borne and food antigens that are encountered at mucosal surfaces in the lung and gut.

The most important aspect of tolerance, however, is **self tolerance**, which prevents the body from mounting an immune attack against its own tissues. There is potential for such attack because the immune system randomly generates a vast diversity of antigen-specific receptors, some of which will be self reactive. Cells bearing these receptors therefore must be eliminated, either functionally or physically, or regulated.

Self reactivity is prevented by processes that occur during development, rather than being genetically preprogrammed. Thus:
- homozygous animals of histoincompatible strains A and B reject each other's skin;
- their F_1 hybrid offspring (which express the antigens of both the A and B parents) reject neither A skin nor B skin;
- the ability to reject A and B skin reappears in homozygotes of the F_2 progeny.

It is therefore clear that self–non-self discrimination is learned during development – immunological 'self' must encompass all **epitopes** (antigenic determinants) encoded by the individual's DNA, all other epitopes being considered as non-self.

Q. Why is it necessary for every individual's immune system to learn self–non-self discrimination – we do not just inherit a library of immune receptors from our parents that recognize non-self?

A. The immediate reason is that each individual's immune system is unique. The diversity of MHC molecules (see Chapter 5) and allogeneic variants of self molecules means that new epitopes are present in each generation as a result of gene reassortment. The ultimate reason is that the immune system has to be able to recognize newly arising non-self antigens as new pathogens evolve to threaten each new generation of individuals.

However it is not the structure of a molecule per se that determines whether it will be distinguished as self or non-self. Factors other than the structural characteristics of an epitope are also important. Among these are:

- the stage of differentiation when lymphocytes first confront their epitopes;
- the site of the encounter;
- the nature of the cells presenting epitopes;
- the number of lymphocytes responding to the epitopes.

IMMUNOLOGICAL TOLERANCE WAS DEMONSTRATED BY SOME KEY HISTORICAL EXPERIMENTS

Soon after the existence of antibody specificity was established, it was realized that there must be some mechanism to prevent autoantibody formation. As early as the turn of the 19th century, Ehrlich coined the term 'horror autotoxicus', implying the need for a 'regulating contrivance' to stop the production of autoantibodies.

In 1938, Traub induced specific tolerance by inoculating mice in utero with lymphocytic choriomeningitis virus, producing an infection that was maintained throughout life. Unlike normal mice, these inoculated mice did not produce neutralizing antibodies when challenged with the virus in adult life.

In 1945, Owen reported an 'experiment of nature' in non-identical cattle twins that showed that cells carrying self and non-self antigens could develop within a single host. These animals exchanged hematopoietic (stem) cells via their shared placental blood vessels and each animal carried the erythrocyte markers of both calves. They exhibited life-long tolerance to the otherwise foreign cells, in being unable to mount antibody responses to the relevant erythrocyte antigens.

Following this observation, Burnet and Fenner postulated that the age of the animal at the time of first encounter was the critical factor in determining responsiveness, and hence recognition, of non-self antigens. This hypothesis seemed logical because the immune system is usually confronted with most self components before birth and only later with non-self antigens.

Experimental support came in 1953, when Medawar and his colleagues induced immunological tolerance to skin allografts (grafts that are genetically non-identical,

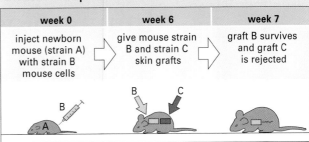

Induction of specific tolerance in mice

week 0	week 6	week 7
inject newborn mouse (strain A) with strain B mouse cells	give mouse strain B and strain C skin grafts	graft B survives and graft C is rejected

Fig. 19.1 The experiment demonstrates the induction of specific tolerance to grafted skin, induced by neonatal injection of spleen cells from a different strain. Mice of strain A normally reject grafts from strain B. However, if newborn mice of strain A receive cells from strain B, they show tolerance to skin grafts from this donor at 6 weeks of age, but reject grafts from other strains (C). This phenomenon is due to immune deviation.

but are from the same species) in mice by neonatal injection of allogeneic cells (Fig. 19.1).

This phenomenon was easily accommodated in Burnet's clonal selection theory (1957), which states that a particular immunocyte (a particular B or T cell) is selected by antigen and then divides to give rise to a clone of daughter cells, all with the same specificity.

According to this theory, antigens encountered after birth activate specific clones of lymphocytes, whereas when antigens are encountered before birth the result is the deletion of the clones specific for them, which Burnet termed 'forbidden clones'. Implicit in the theory is the need for the entire immune repertoire to be generated before birth, but in fact lymphocyte differentiation continues long after birth.

The key factor in determining responsiveness is therefore not the developmental stage of the individual, but rather the state of maturity of the lymphocyte at the time it encounters antigen. This was suggested by Lederberg in 1959, in his modification of the clonal selection theory: immature lymphocytes contacting antigen would be subject to 'clonal abortion', whereas mature cells would be activated.

It is now established that the neonate is in fact immunocompetent. The reason that one can induce tolerance to certain antigens in the neonate is simply that the type of immune response to antigen can be functionally different in the neonate compared with that in the adult. Past descriptions of neonatal tolerance may therefore have been early examples of this type of **'immune deviation'** (see below, p. 355).

Key discoveries in the 1960s established:

- the immunological competence of the lymphocyte;
- the crucial role of the thymus in the development of the immune system; and
- the existence of two interacting subsets of lymphocytes – T and B cells.

This set the scene for a thorough investigation of the cellular mechanisms involved in tolerance.

THE STUDY OF TOLERANCE INVOLVES INDUCING TOLERANCE EXPERIMENTALLY

Transgenic technology has allowed the study of tolerance to authentic self antigens

Until recently, only artificially induced tolerance was amenable to experimental study: antigens or foreign cells were inoculated into an animal and the fate of responding T or B cells was investigated under a variety of circumstances. It was not clear, however, to what extent these experimental models resembled natural self tolerance.

Transgenic methods have now made possible the direct investigation of self tolerance. These methods allow:
- introduction of a specific gene into mice of defined genetic background; and
- analysis of its effects upon the development of the immune system.

Furthermore, if the introduced gene is linked to a tissue-specific promoter, its expression can be confined to specific cell types.

The protein product encoded by a 'transgene' is treated by the immune system essentially as an authentic self antigen (autoantigen), and its effects can be studied in vivo without the trauma and inflammation associated with grafting foreign cells or tissues.

In addition, the parent strain and the transgenic strain are ideal for control experiments and lymphocyte transfer studies because they are congenic – that is, they differ at only one locus.

Transgenic mice can also be created in which all of either their B or T lymphocytes express a single antigen receptor. By increasing the frequency of antigen-specific precursor cells in this way, tolerance mechanisms can be readily dissected.

Finally, the use of targeted mutagenesis has allowed immunologists to 'knock out' specific genes to study the role of their gene products in the process of immunological tolerance.

Ways in which self-reactive lymphocytes may be prevented from responding to self antigen

There are five possible ways in which self-reactive lymphocytes may be prevented from responding to self antigens:
- self-reactive T cells in the circulation may ignore self antigens (e.g. when the antigens are in tissues sequestered from the circulation);
- their response to a self antigen may be suppressed if the antigen is in a privileged site (see Chapter 12 and p. 352);
- self-reactive cells may be deleted at certain stages of development;
- self-reactive cells may be rendered anergic and unable to respond;
- a state of tolerance to self antigens can also be maintained by immune regulation.

Which of these fates awaits the self-reactive lymphocyte depends on numerous factors, including:
- the stage of maturity of the cell being silenced;
- the affinity of its receptor for the self antigen;
- the nature of this antigen;
- its concentration;
- its tissue distribution; and
- its pattern of expression.

CENTRAL TOLERANCE TAKES PLACE DURING T CELL DEVELOPMENT IN THE THYMUS

The process of generating new T cell receptors (TCRs) involves gene rearrangement in addition to N-region modifications. This allows the immune system to generate a vast array of TCRs. Such a broad repertoire is clearly necessary to provide protection against the multitude of different infectious agents that any individual in the species is likely to encounter.

T lymphocytes are not, however, simply effector cells of the immune system. They also function as regulators of the system through provision of help for some and suppression of other responses.

For effective control, lymphocytes must interact with other cells of the immune system and this is one reason why MHC restriction of T cell recognition has evolved. Central tolerance among T lymphocytes revolves around a schooling process in which key cells are educated so that they become dependent on self MHC for survival, while at the same time potentially rebellious lymphocytes are identified and eliminated. This process of central tolerance among T lymphocytes takes place during their development within the thymus and depends on a number of checkpoints through which the cells have to pass in order to develop further.

T cell development involves positive and negative selection and lineage commitment

T lymphocytes develop from precursors in the bone marrow and are derived from a common lymphoid progenitor cell that gives rise to:
- B cells;
- natural killer (NK) cells; and
- both $\alpha\beta$ and $\gamma\delta$ subsets of T lymphocytes (Fig. 19.2).

Signals exchanged between cells via the Notch receptor determine the fate of lymphoid progenitor cells. Thus:
- deletion of Notch 1 leads to a block in T cell development and results in ectopic development of B cells in the thymus;
- conversely, expression of activated forms of Notch leads to selective development of T cells from lymphoid progenitor cells.

The function of $\alpha\beta$ T lymphocytes in the maintenance of self tolerance is now well understood

When immature T cells enter the thymus they express neither CD4 nor CD8 co-receptor molecules (Fig. 19.3). These so-called double-negative (DN) cells constitute approximately 3% of total thymocytes. At this stage the TCR β chain genes start their recombination.

345

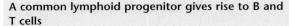

A common lymphoid progenitor gives rise to B and T cells

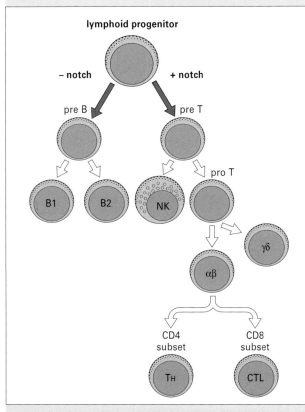

Fig. 19.2 Both B and T cells develop from a common precursor found in the fetal liver or adult bone marrow. T cell progenitors give rise to both the αβ and γδ lineages as well as NK T cells. Recent studies have shown that the decision of lymphocyte precursors to differentiate down the B or T cell pathway depends on ligation of Notch 1. Notch 1 is essential for development of both thymus-dependent and -independent T cells.

Q. What processes are involved in the generation of the diverse genes for the TCR?

A. This process involves sequential rearrangement of variable (V), diversity (D), and junctional (J) region genes within the TCR β chain locus, and expression of a β chain. Subsequently recombination of V and J segments from the TCR α chain locus generates diversity in the α chains (see Figs 5.3–5.5).

First the β chain diversity and junctional genes rearrange and this is followed by rearrangement of the DJ gene with a variable region gene. The VDJ then combines with a constant region by alternative splicing of RNA to give the complete β chain gene.

At this point the α chain genes remain in their genomic configuration, but the transcribed and translated β chain nevertheless appears at the cell surface. This is possible

only because the β chain can pair with a 'surrogate' α chain and other components of the CD3 signaling complex to migrate from the endoplasmic reticulum to the cell surface.

Surface expression of this complex allows DN cells to:

- switch off their *RAG* genes (recombination activating genes);
- begin to proliferate; and
- mature into CD4 and CD8 double-positive (DP) cells (see Fig. 19.3).

There is no evidence that this 'checkpoint' (the β selection checkpoint) involves recognition of antigen.

T cells undergo a degree of 'receptor editing' of the α chain

Newly formed DP cells reactivate *RAG* genes allowing rearrangement of the α chain.

Like the immunoglobulin light chain, the TCR α chain has no D segment and the first event is to direct rearrangement of Vα to Jα region genes. Suitable pairing of α and β chains at the α-selection checkpoint allows T cells to proceed to the next selection stage.

Evidence shows, however, that unlike the β chain, which largely permits rearrangement of only one β gene through allelic exclusion, α chain rearrangement can continue to generate a second chain.

In fact, up to 30% of mature human T cells express more than one rearranged α chain.

This implies that T cells, like B cells, undergo a degree of 'receptor editing' of the α chain to increase the likelihood of positive selection of cells selected to interact with self MHC.

T cells are positively selected for 'usefulness' (MHC restriction)

The potential for α–β pairing in combination with TCR gene rearrangement allows for a massive repertoire of TCR structures. Interestingly, however, some 95% of these structures fail to contribute to the T cell repertoire found in peripheral lymphoid tissues. This is because thymocytes undergo a rigorous education before they exit the thymus.

Education requires preliminary selection of cells for survival and their subsequent commitment to a particular lineage (**positive selection**). This is then followed by death of those cells that interact strongly with MHC (**negative selection**).

In other words, T cells are positively selected for 'usefulness' (MHC restriction) and negatively selected against 'dangerous' autoreactivity.

The controlling element in thymic education is the MHC expressed by antigen-presenting cells (APCs) in the thymus (Fig. 19.4). This is such that T cell development is blocked at the DP stage in a thymus that does not express MHC molecules. In fact, cells at this stage of development need to be nurtured by cells expressing MHC molecules.

Cells whose TCR fails to engage either a class I or a class II MHC molecule undergo programmed cell death (death by neglect), while cells that recognize MHC

Developmental pathways of murine thymocytes

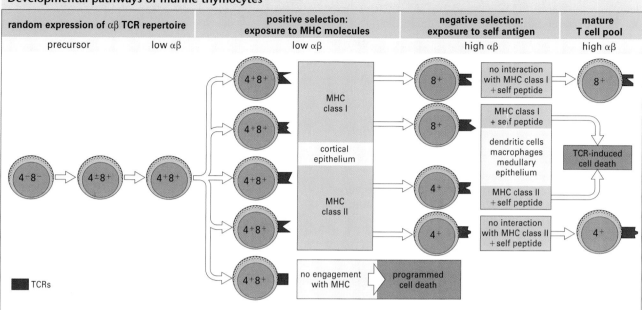

Fig. 19.3 Precursor thymocytes develop into 'double-positive' cells expressing low levels of the αβ TCR. These undergo positive selection for interaction with self MHC class I or class II molecules on cortical epithelium. Unselected cells (the majority) undergo programmed cell death by apoptosis. Cells undergoing positive selection lose one or the other of their co-receptor molecules (CD4 or CD8). Finally, self-reactive cells are eliminated by their interaction with self peptides presented on cells at the corticomedullary junction and in the thymic medulla.

T cell–MHC restriction occurs in the thymus

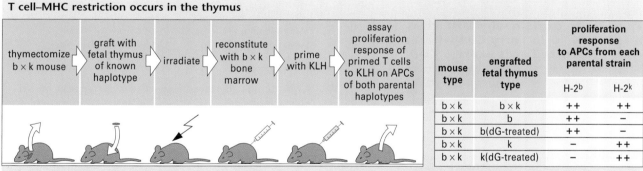

mouse type	engrafted fetal thymus type	proliferation response to APCs from each parental strain	
		H-2ᵇ	H-2ᵏ
b × k	b × k	++	++
b × k	b	++	−
b × k	b(dG-treated)	++	−
b × k	k	−	++
b × k	k(dG-treated)	−	++

Fig. 19.4 Host mice (F₁[H-2ᵇ × H-2ᵏ]) were thymectomized, then engrafted with 14-day fetal thymuses of various genotypes. They were subsequently irradiated to remove their resident T cell populations, then reconstituted with F₁ bone marrow to provide stem cells. After priming with antigen (keyhole limpet hemocyanin, KLH), the proliferative response of lymph node T cells to KLH on APCs from each parental strain was evaluated. In some experiments, thymus lobes were incubated before grafting with deoxyguanosine (dG), which destroys intrathymic cells of macrophage/dendritic cell lineage. The results show (i) that the thymic environment is necessary for T cells to learn to recognize MHC; and (ii) that bone marrow-derived cells (removed by dG treatment) are not required for this process to occur. (Based on data from Lo D, Sprent J. Nature 1986;319:672)

molecules with moderate affinity on cortical epithelial cells survive.

Cells mature from DP cells to the single-positive (SP) cells where they express either CD4 or CD8. It is clear that MHC molecules play a role in this selection process.

Q. What do you predict would occur in mice that lack either MHC class I or class II molecules?

A. Mice lacking MHC class I molecules have few CD8 SP thymocytes; mice that lack MHC class II molecules have few CD4 SP cells.

It is likely that evolution has shaped complementarity-determining regions (CDRs) 1 and 2 of the TCR so that the TCR preferentially matches MHC molecules.

Signaling via CD4 and CD8 drives lineage commitment

Why has the immune system evolved two separate types of T cell? Would it not be more economical to have just one DP cell that could interact with either class I or class II expressing cells?

Selection of cells expressing either CD4 or CD8 has evolved just as the need for two pathways of antigen processing has been driven by the encounter of vertebrates with increasingly sophisticated pathogens.

Class I and class II pathways have evolved to allow the immune system to recognize either cytoplasmic or extracellular/intravacuolar infectious agents, respectively. This has then driven the evolution of two subsets of T cell equipped with the means to help eradicate these infectious agents.

The remaining question is how CD4 and CD8 cells develop from one common precursor?

Q. Transgenic mice that have a TCR that recognizes antigen in association with MHC class I molecules and express a hybrid CD4/CD8 molecule (CD4 intracellular segment/CD8 extracellular domains) generate predominantly CD4⁺ thymocytes. Interpret this experiment.

A. This implies that intracellular signaling via the CD4 intracellular domain leads to selective commitment along the CD4 lineage with inactivation of CD8 expression.

Theories to explain why MHC class II-restricted cells carry CD4 whereas MHC class I-restricted cells express CD8

The mechanisms of thymic selection and CD4/CD8 lineage commitment have many uncertainties. A number of theories have arisen to explain why MHC class II-restricted cells carry CD4 whereas MHC class I-restricted cells express CD8 co-receptors.

Stochastic selection

Lineage choice is independent of MHC–TCR signal, resulting in some thymocytes being mismatched between TCR specificity and co-receptor expression. These mismatched cells subsequently die through lack of an effective survival signal. This theory has been superseded by the following proposals.

Instructional selection

This theory states that coincident engagement of both TCR and co-receptor by MHC leads to lineage choice. Experimental evidence suggests that this is an oversimplified view of selection.

Strength of signal

The instructional model has been extended by experiments suggesting that lineage commitment is influenced by strength or duration of signal. The src family kinase Lck is associated with the cytoplasmic tail of CD4 and CD8, but is known to associate better with CD4 than

---

The kinetic signaling model of lineage commitment in thymic selection

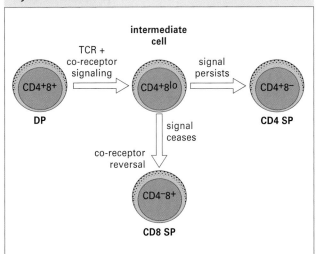

Fig. 19.5 The kinetic signaling model of lineage commitment proposes that cell fate is determined by the duration of signaling during positive selection. The model suggests that double-positive thymocytes are programmed to respond to TCR plus co-receptor signals (regardless of MHC specificity) by terminating CD8 transcription and converting into CD4⁺CD8ˡᵒ 'intermediate' thymocytes. CD4⁺CD8ˡᵒ intermediate thymocytes still have the potential to differentiate into either mature CD4 SP or CD8 SP T cells. Sustained signaling in intermediate thymocytes results in their differentiation into mature CD4 SP T cells, whereas cessation of signaling in intermediate thymocytes results in 'co-receptor reversal' and differentiation into CD8 SP T cells. (Based on the model described by Singer A. Curr Opin Immunol 2002;14:207)

CD8. It was therefore suggested that ligation of MHC plus peptide by TCR plus CD4 leads to more effective, stronger signaling and hence selection of CD4 SP cells, while TCR plus CD8 generates a weaker signal hence leading to CD8 selection. Interestingly, however, CD8 is downregulated in both CD4 and CD8 lineage-committed cells during the process of selection and this has led to revision of the validity of the signal model.

Kinetic signaling

A further model accommodates the observation that TCR signaling initially downregulates CD8 but not CD4 expression. As such, TCR signaling of short duration leads to CD8 commitment with subsequent downregulation of CD4. Longer TCR signaling leads to CD4 commitment and further downregulation of CD8. Clearly the strength of signaling and kinetic signaling models overlaps, because a strong signal will normally be of longer duration (Fig. 19.5).

In mice, the HD mutation causes redirection of class II-restricted thymocytes to the CD8 lineage

Interestingly, a spontaneous mutation in mice, the HD mutation, causes redirection of class II-restricted thymocytes to the CD8 lineage. The mutation lies in the gene *Th-POK*. The expression of *Th-POK* is confined to cells expressing a class II-restricted TCR and CD4 suggesting that it may be induced by strong TCR signaling. Furthermore, the transcription factor GATA-3 is specific for and involved in CD4 lineage differentiation, whereas the transcriptional regulator RUNX3 functions as a CD4-silencing factor during CD8 lineage differentiation.

Antigen recognition is important for development of the T cell repertoire

Do T cells need to see antigen for positive selection and, if so, does this have to be a specific MHC-bound peptide?

Mice deficient in the proteins required to transport peptides into the endoplasmic reticulum (TAP proteins) do not allow selection of CD8 cells. This proves that peptide antigen in conjunction with MHC class I is required for CD8 cell differentiation. But how many peptides are required for a completely functional T cell repertoire?

Q. Transgenic mice that have MHC class II molecules of a single type occupied by a single peptide generate CD4 SP cells and are able to respond to a number of different antigens. T cell numbers are reduced by 50%, but the repertoire of TCRs that can develop in these animals is highly restricted. Interpret this observation.

A. A diverse range of MHC–peptide complexes is required to select a full repertoire of TCRs.

Thymic cells involved in negative selection

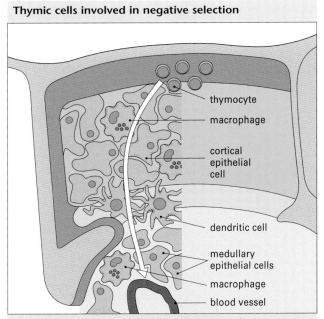

thymocyte

macrophage

cortical epithelial cell

dendritic cell

medullary epithelial cells

macrophage

blood vessel

Fig. 19.6 The deleting population includes bone marrow-derived macrophages and dendritic cells, which are located at the corticomedullary junction. Other cells involved in deletion may be the thymocytes themselves, through their veto function, and some types of thymic epithelial cells, especially those in the medulla.

T cell selection is compartmentalized in the thymus

The thymus is made up of lobes, each of which is organized into outer cortical and inner medullary regions (Fig. 19.6).

Immature lymphocytes are found in the cortical region associated with cortical epithelial cells. Cells in the outer cortex are rapidly proliferating immature cells. Cells in the inner cortex are more mature DP cells probably undergoing positive selection.

The medulla contains:
- mature SP lymphocytes;
- medullary epithelial cells; and
- bone marrow-derived macrophages and dendritic cells.

It is a matter of hot debate as to whether spatial separation of MHC molecules on different APCs and their isolation in different thymic regions influence positive and negative selection. Clearly hematopoietic cells are restricted to the medulla.

Two important considerations are:
- the fact that the thymic cortex is relatively inaccessible to large circulating proteins because of its vascular supply; and
- the observation that cortical epithelial cells are inefficient at presenting exogenous proteins – these cells would thus be predicted to present endogenous antigens only and not antigens carried to the thymus in the blood supply.

Cortical epithelial cells definitely play a role in positive selection because mice expressing MHC class II molecules only on these cells show normal levels of positive selection, but impaired negative selection. By contrast, bone marrow-derived macrophages and dendritic cells account for the removal of at least 50% of all positively selected cells.

Medullary thymic epithelial cells can express antigens whose expression was previously thought to be limited to specific organs

A further question relates to how the thymus could ever possibly express all of the antigens that a T cell might encounter outside the thymus. There seems little doubt that the thymus does not express all potential self antigens. Nevertheless there is clear evidence that medullary thymic epithelial cells (mTECs) can express antigens whose expression was previously thought to be limited to specific organs (Fig. 19.7). Importantly, expression of many of these proteins is controlled by a single gene called autoimmune regulatory (*Aire*).

Aire was first identified by mapping the gene responsible for autoimmune polyendocrinopathy syndrome type 1 (APS-1) in humans. This disease is characterized by the coincidence of two or three major clinical symptoms: Addison's disease, hypoparathyroidism and chronic mucocutaneous candidiasis.

Antibodies against a variety of endocrine glands have been detected in patients with APS-1 and the disease is associated with lymphocytic infiltrates in the affected organs. The comparison of protein expression in wild-type and *Aire*-deficient mTECs shows that expression of organ-specific genes is preferentially downregulated in

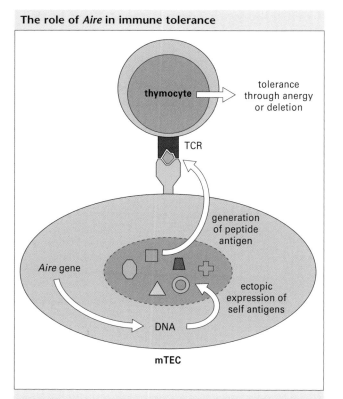

The role of *Aire* in immune tolerance

Fig. 19.7 *Aire* promotes the expression of organ-specific genes in medullary thymic epithelial cells (mTECs). These organ-specific proteins are presented on the surface of mTECs by MHC molecules to T cells developing in the thymus. Thymocytes that recognize these organ-specific proteins in the context of MHC molecules undergo negative selection. The role of *Aire* is therefore to limit the generation of self-reactive T cells. Mutations in the *Aire* gene affect expression of many but not all ectopically expressed proteins, suggesting that other genes may play a similar role. (Based on Su MA, Anderson MS. Curr Opin Immunol 2004;16:746. Copyright 2004 with permission from Elsevier)

Aire-deficient mTECs. Among these are preproinsulin and cytochrome P-4501A2, which are known targets for autoantibodies in APS-1. From this we can conclude that APS-1 and a similar disease found in *Aire*-deficient mice results from the failure to delete or anergize developing thymocytes specific for these organ-specific proteins.

T cell development includes a series of checkpoints

In conclusion, the architecture of the thymus appears to be designed to compartmentalize thymic selection. Cortical epithelial cells present a wide range of endogenous antigens and contribute to positive selection.

Interestingly, it is estimated that a developing thymocyte might only ever interact with a single cortical epithelial cell. The imprint that this leaves on the T cell clearly has a profound effect on the resulting T cell repertoire.

Medullary APCs have access to circulating antigens and are largely responsible for negative selection.

It is now also clear that antigens from a wide variety of tissues are expressed by mTECs where they induce central tolerance.

Furthermore, there is evidence that antigen recognition in the thymus may contribute to the generation of regulatory T lymphocytes, which play such an important role in peripheral tolerance (see below, p. 354).

Checkpoints in central T cell tolerance include:
- β selection checkpoint – only cells with a rearranged β chain mature from DN to DP cells – this process is not dependent on MHC proteins;
- α selection checkpoint – cells expressing an αβ complex must interact with MHC molecules to survive;
- lineage commitment checkpoint – cells are instructed to repress expression of either CD4 or CD8 and to develop into SP cells;
- negative selection checkpoint – cells that interact strongly with MHC molecules and antigen in the thymus are deleted (Fig. 19.8).

It is important to consider how a cell with one TCR can receive signals instructing it to survive and undergo lineage commitment without coincidentally receiving a signal to undergo negative selection. The most likely explanation is that this relies on the avidity of the cell's interaction with MHC and peptide.

Experiments have shown that the decision to undergo positive and negative selection is directly related to the half-life of TCR binding to the MHC–peptide complex (Fig. 19.9).

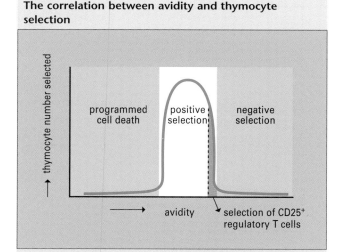

The correlation between avidity and thymocyte selection

Fig. 19.8 The avidity of a T cell's interaction with antigenic peptide presented by an APC will depend on the level of expression of the MHC–peptide complex [MHC + peptide] on the APC and both the affinity and surface expression of TCR on the T cell. [MHC + peptide] depends on the affinity of peptide for MHC and the stability of the complex once formed. Current evidence suggests that CD25+ regulatory T cells are selected in the thymus and have a relatively high affinity for MHC and peptide.

TCR affinity for MHC–peptide complex influences positive selection

nature of peptide	half-life	affinity of complex	thymocyte selection
agonist	++	++	negative
antagonist	±	+	positive
irrelevant	–	–	no effect

Fig. 19.9 The affinity of a soluble TCR for complexes between various peptides and the appropriate MHC restriction element can be measured by biophysical techniques such as surface plasmon resonance. There is a direct correlation between the half-life of TCR binding to the MHC–peptide complex and the response made by mature T cells expressing the same receptor (i.e. agonist > antagonist > irrelevant peptide). In thymocyte organ cultures, however, addition of the agonist peptide causes deletion of the developing cells (negative selection), whereas the antagonist stimulates positive selection. This demonstrates that low-avidity interaction promotes positive selection, whereas high-avidity interaction leads to negative selection. (Data summarized from Alam SM, Travers PJ, Wung JL, et al. Nature 1996;381:616)

Selection also depends on:
- the architecture of the thymus;
- the nature of APCs in the cortex versus the medulla of the thymus; and
- the types of antigen that these cells are able to present.

A VARIETY OF MECHANISMS MAINTAIN TOLERANCE IN PERIPHERAL LYMPHOID ORGANS

There is no doubt that many potentially autoreactive T cells escape central tolerance. This reflects the fact that many antigens are either not present or are present at insufficiently high levels to induce tolerance in the thymus. Thus, for example, peripheral blood lymphocytes from healthy individuals respond vigorously to purified myelin basic protein, a major constituent of myelin in the brain, following their culture in vitro (Fig. 19.10).

So, how are these cells kept at bay in healthy individuals and why are autoimmune diseases directed to such proteins so incredibly rare? This is because various mechanisms have evolved to maintain tolerance in peripheral lymphoid organs (Fig. 19.11).

Sequestration of antigen occurs in some tissues

Both developing and mature lymphocytes may never encounter self antigens. Many of these are sequestered away from the immune system by physical or immunological barriers. In this way, tissue antigens may never be available to T lymphocytes, either because:
- of their location; or
- they may never be processed by functional APCs.

Peripheral blood cells from a healthy individual respond to the self antigen myelin basic protein

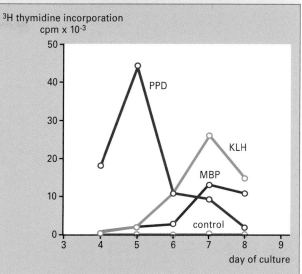

Fig. 19.10 Purified white blood cells can be stimulated in tissue culture with antigens such as purified protein derivative (PPD) from *Mycobacterium tuberculosis* or keyhole limpet hemocyanin (KLH). The rate at which the cells respond (measured by incorporation of 3H-thymidine) reflects whether the response is primary/naive (KLH) or secondary/memory (PPD). Note that blood cells from a healthy individual respond with primary kinetics to purified human myelin basic protein (MBP). This experiment shows how cells that have escaped tolerance induction in the thymus can nevertheless respond to self antigens under artificial conditions. (Based on data from Ponsford M, Mazza G, Coad J, et al. Clin Exp Immunol 2001;124:315)

Privileged sites are protected by regulatory mechanisms

Cells that have escaped tolerance in the thymus can also ignore self antigens if they are expressed in a privileged site.

Q. Name some privileged sites, their characteristics, and the underlying basis of the privilege.

A. Immunologically privileged sites include the brain, anterior chamber of the eye, and testes, because transplanted tissues have an enhanced chance of survival within them. Within these sites proinflammatory lymphocytes are controlled either by apoptosis (Fas ligand [FasL] expression) or by cytokine (transforming growth factor-β/interleukin-10 [TGFβ/IL-10]) secretion (see Chapter 12, p. 236 and Figs 12.3–12.7).

Does immune privilege contribute to self tolerance or is it a phenomenon seen only by the introduction of foreign antigen to the privileged site?

Immune privilege is clearly designed to dampen down inflammatory responses in certain vital organs. The same suppressive mechanisms would equally apply to inflam-

Mechanisms of central and peripheral tolerance

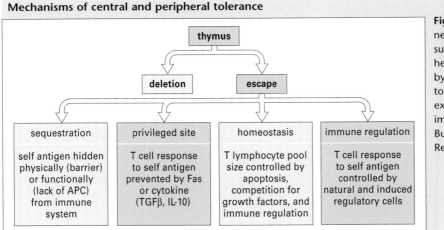

Fig. 19.11 Cells that have escaped negative selection in the thymus are still subject to control in the periphery. Most healthy individuals maintain self tolerance by a variety of mechanisms of peripheral tolerance involving sequestration, expression at a privileged site, deletion or immune regulation. (Based on Anderton S, Burkhart C, Metzler B, Wraith D. Immunol Rev 1999;169:123)

mation caused by an immune response to either an infectious or a self antigen.

Immune privilege does not discriminate and therefore contributes to peripheral tolerance, at least in these particular organs.

T cell death can be induced by persistent activation or neglect

Apoptotic death of lymphocytes is an extremely important mechanism of immune control and is essential for the maintenance of immune homeostasis in healthy individuals. It contributes both to the deletion of cells with high avidity for antigen and to the death of lymphocytes when the immune response is no longer required. These functions are fulfilled by two distinct mechanisms:

- **activation-induced cell death (AICD)**; and
- **programmed cell death (PCD)**.

Fas is the most important death receptor

Cells repeatedly stimulated with antigen undergo AICD by mechanisms involving so-called 'death receptors' of the tumor necrosis factor receptor (TNFR) family (see Fig. 10.8). Among these, the most important molecule is Fas, which on cross-linking by its ligand (FasL) leads to activation of the caspase cascade via caspase-8 and subsequent apoptotic death of the cell (Fig. 19.12 and see Fig. 10.9). This can occur by cell–cell interactions and there is, in addition, evidence that T lymphocytes can kill themselves through 'fratricidal cell death' following the secretion of soluble FasL (Fig. 19.13).

Many activated cells die by PCD

In addition, many activated cells die by PCD because their antigen is simply eliminated, as happens, for example, following clearance of an infection. Removal of the antigen then deprives cells of essential survival stimuli including growth factors. Under these conditions mitochondria in the cell respond by releasing cytochrome c. This, in combination with apoptosis activating factor-1,

leads to activation of the caspase cascade following cleavage and activation of caspase-9 (see Fig. 19.12).

The Fas pathway is required for peripheral tolerance

Presumably, the survival rate of T cells that cross-react with self antigens, but which are generated during the immune response to infection, will be increased in the absence of AICD.

The importance of the Fas pathway for AICD has been revealed by genetic defects in both mouse and human. For example, the lpr mouse has a mutation in Fas and the gld mouse has a mutation in FasL. Both mutations lead to lymphadenopathy (expanded secondary lymphoid tissue). Importantly this lack of regulation also leads to the generation of autoimmunity, autoantibody production, and nephritis with similarities to systemic lupus erythematosus in humans.

Note that thymus selection in the lpr mouse is normal, showing that the Fas pathway is not essential for central tolerance but is clearly required for peripheral tolerance.

Recent studies have shown that analogous mutations lead to a similar form of disease known as human **autoimmune lymphoproliferative syndrome (ALPS)**, characterized by:

- defective lymphocyte apoptosis;
- lymphocyte accumulation; and
- humoral autoimmunity.

The ALPS phenotype is associated with inherited mutations in the Fas gene (ALPS type 1a) or the Fas ligand gene (ALPS type 1b).

Both AICD and PCD are tightly regulated but the two apoptopic pathways are under independent regulation.

Bcl family members, for example, block PCD by inhibiting the release of cytochrome c, but do not affect AICD.

AICD is inhibited by proteins binding to the death receptor complex. Of these, the most important is FLIP (**FLICE inhibitory protein** where FLICE is the FADD-like IL-1β converting enzyme). FLIP binds to the adapter

Two distinct mechanisms of lymphocyte apoptosis

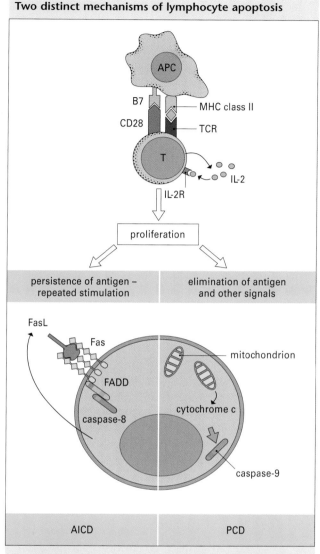

Fig. 19.12 Activated T lymphocytes will die by passive cell death (PCD) when deprived of an antigenic stimulus. This mechanism is designed to maintain homeostasis in the immune system. Activated T lymphocytes will die by activation-induced cell death (AICD) if repeatedly stimulated with antigen. This mechanism is designed to limit hypersensitivity reactions to allergens and autoantigens.

protein FADD or to a precursor form of caspase-8 and blocks generation of the Fas-associated death receptor complex.

AICD is also regulated by IL-2. This cytokine stimulates Fas-mediated AICD by enhancing transcription and expression of FasL while inhibiting transcription of FLIP.

Note that disruption of the genes for IL-2, IL-2Rα, or IL-2Rβ leads to lymphadenopathy and autoimmunity in mice in which any one of these genes has been inactivated. This is consistent with a role for IL-2-driven apoptotic death (**propriocidal death**) in homeostasis and peripheral tolerance.

The role of the Fas system in T cell death

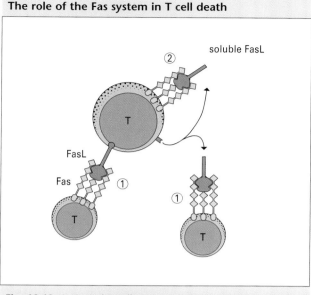

Fig. 19.13 Activated T cells express both Fas (CD95) and the ligand for this molecule (FasL). Fratricide (**1**) can result either from direct cell contact or from cleavage of FasL and the ligation of Fas by soluble FasL. Autocrine suicide (**2**) can result from the interaction of soluble FasL with Fas.

The balance of co-stimulatory signals affects immune homeostasis and self tolerance

Naive T lymphocytes require two signals to proliferate and differentiate:
- the first signal is triggered by TCR recognition of the appropriate peptide–MHC complex;
- the second signal is delivered by CD80 (B7.1) and CD86 (B7.2) co-stimulatory molecules expressed by APCs.

How a T cell interprets co-stimulation depends on which co-stimulation receptor it uses.

The CD28 molecule is constitutively expressed on T cells and signaling via CD28 enhances cell survival, prevents anergy induction, and enhances CD40L expression.

Q. What effect does ligation of CTLA-4 (CD152), the alternative ligand for B7, have on the T cell?

A. CTLA-4 ligation inhibits early T cell activation including expression of the IL-2 receptor α chain and secretion of IL-2 (see Fig. 7.18).

The **CTLA-4 pathway** inhibits IL-2 messenger RNA accumulation and progression through the cell cycle. CTLA-4 has a higher avidity (100 ×) for CD80 and CD86 than CD28, but is normally restricted to the perinuclear Golgi apparatus. On T cell contact with an APC, CTLA-4 traffics to the plasma membrane at the TCR–APC interface (Fig. 19.14).

The role of CTLA-4 in normal homeostasis is revealed in the CTLA-4 knockout mouse. These mice show normal thymus selection, but suffer from polyclonal T cell expansion and die from a fatal lymphoproliferative disease.

Interestingly, CTLA-4 influences CD4 cells more than CD8 cells because depletion of CD4 cells from the CTLA-4 knockout mouse prevents the lymphoproliferative disease in this mouse.

Dendritic cells contribute to peripheral tolerance

Thymic dendritic cells contribute to self tolerance by deleting self antigen-responsive T cells.

Dendritic cells also contribute to tolerance extrathymically. Subsets of dendritic cells are distinguished according to their cell surface phenotype and in mice have been defined as:

- myeloid (precursors shared with macrophages); or
- lymphoid (precursors shared with lymphocytes).

Plasmacytoid dendritic cells are found in various organs and are distinguished by their secretion of type I interferon in response to viruses.

All dendritic cells originate, however, from hematopoietic precursor cells and there is considerable plasticity between the different lineages.

The general rule governing dendritic cells is that they readily take up antigen in the immature state, but present antigen effectively to naive T cells only when they have undergone differentiation to a more mature state (Fig. 19.15):

- mature dendritic cells presenting specific antigen both activate T cells and promote their survival;
- immature dendritic cells presenting antigen activate T cells, but the outcome is different, resulting in apoptosis, anergy, or the generation of regulatory T cells.

In the steady state, the immature dendritic cell can take up self antigens even when these are contained in dying cells and induce tolerance towards these antigens rather than immunity.

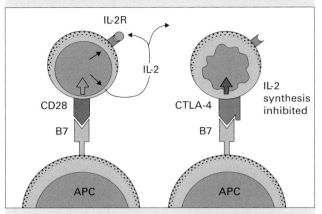

T cell activation is controlled by co-stimulatory signals

Fig. 19.14 Ligation of CD28 stimulates intracellular signals that lead to IL-2 production, IL-2 receptor (IL-2R) expression, and cell cycle progression in activated T cells. Ligation of cell surface CTLA-4 blocks these CD28-dependent responses and inhibits IL-2 synthesis.

The difference between self antigens and the antigens contained in microbes lies in the ability of microbes to induce maturation of the dendritic cell by ligating Toll-like and other receptors (see Chapters 15 and 16).

Targeting of antigens to dendritic cells, either in the form of synthetic peptides or antigens coupled to antibodies, against antigen-uptake receptors of dendritic cells (i.e. DEC-205) will therefore induce peripheral tolerance if the targeted dendritic cell remains in an immature state.

Comparison of immature and mature dendritic cells

inducing agents		properties
		antigen capture
pathogens (e.g. LPS, bacterial DNA, CpG) cytokines (e.g. TNF, GM-CSF) T cells (e.g CD40L) viral dsRNA	**immature DC**	high intracellular MHCII (MIICs) endocytosis phagocytosis high CCR1, CCR5, CCR6 low CCR7 low CD54, 58, 80, 86 low CD40 low CD83 high CD68 no DC-LAMP
	mature DC	**antigen presentation** high surface MHCII low endocytosis low phagocytosis low CCR1, CCR5, CCR6 high CCR7 high CD54, 58, 80, 86 high CD40 high CD83 low CD68/high DC-LAMP high p55

Fig. 19.15 On the left are listed factors known to promote maturation of dendritic cells (DCs). These include baterial and viral products, cytokines, and interaction with T cells expressing CD40L. Immature DCs are dedicated to antigen capture whereas mature DCs take up antigen poorly, but are highly efficient APCs. (Based on Banchereau J, Briere F, Caux C, et al. Annu Rev Immunol 2000;18:767, with permission. Copyright 2000 by Annual Reviews www.annualreviews.org)

Homeostatic balance is required to prevent lymphoproliferative responses

In summary, homeostatic balance in the immune system is required to prevent lymphoproliferative responses. Lymphoproliferative disorders are associated with responses to both foreign and self antigens. Lack of homeostatic control leads to autoimmunity and therefore the molecules involved in homeostatic control are important regulators of peripheral tolerance. These molecules include:

- CTLA-4, which acts as a brake on the normal immune response to both foreign and self antigens;
- members of the TNFR family, particularly Fas and FasL;
- components of the caspase cascade;
- IL-2 and the IL-2 receptor (IL-2R), which together regulate sensitivity to Fas-mediated apoptosis.

Regulatory T cells play a crucial role in controlling autoimmune responses

Peripheral tolerance to antigens can be 'infectious'. The experimentally induced tolerance to one antigen can thus maintain tolerance or suppress the immune response to a second antigen as long as the two antigens are structurally or physically associated (e.g. within the same tissue). This implies that mechanisms other than ignorance and cell death must be involved in tolerance.

One explanation for such phenomena depends on the existence of populations of T lymphocytes that produce distinct cytokines.

Many inflammatory autoimmune diseases are caused by TH1 cells that produce cytokines such as interferon-γ (IFNγ) and tumour necrosis factor-α (TNFα). Cytokines derived from TH2 cells (IL-4, IL-5, IL-6, IL-10) support antibody production. A major additional effect of TH2-derived cytokines such as IL-10, however, is downregulation of macrophage effector functions, including antigen presentation to TH1 and naive T cells. TH2 cells are therefore able to suppress inflammatory (delayed-type hypersensitivity, DTH) responses.

TH1 cell-derived IFNγ can prevent the differentiation of TH0 to TH2 cells. This type of immune deviation was defined more than 30 years ago to describe how an individual animal could respond to the same antigen in two completely different ways:

- guinea pigs primed with antigen in alum produced high levels of IgG1 antibody, but did not support a DTH response;
- animals primed with the same antigen in complete Freund's adjuvant developed strong DTH responses.

It was subsequently suggested that the ability of the same antigen to induce either 'humoral' or 'cellular' immunity could reflect the distinct activation of two mutually antagonistic arms of the immune system.

The results of these experiments were undoubtedly a form of immune deviation resulting from the selective induction of TH2 rather than TH1 cells.

Immune deviation can influence hypersensitivity conditions. Diabetes in the NOD (non-obese diabetic) mouse is known to be caused by TH1 cells and can be prevented by antigen-primed TH2 cells, whereas certain allergic disorders can be treated by induction of TH1 cells.

Q. Transgenic mice that express the antigen influenza hemagglutinin [HA]) in pancreatic islet cells and a TCR on their T cells that recognizes this antigen have been bred into mice with different genetic backgrounds. If bred into a strain that produces high levels of IL-4 and IFNγ, the mice have no inflammatory disease in the pancreas. If bred into a strain that produces predominantly IFNγ and IL-12, the T cells infiltrate the pancreatic islets and cause diabetes. Interpret these observations.

A. Peripheral T cell tolerance depends on the genetic make-up of the individual. Immune deviation is clearly controlled by background genes, many of which combine to control the susceptibility of an individual to autoimmune disease.

In another mouse strain (B10.D2 background), the HA-reactive cells produce only TH1 cytokines. T cell-mediated diseases (such as insulin-dependent diabetes, thyroiditis, and gastritis) can be produced in otherwise normal mice simply by eliminating a subpopulation of CD4⁺ T cells expressing CD5, CD25, or a particular isoform of CD45.

This is best illustrated by the transfer of subsets of murine cells isolated from healthy mice into $Rag^{-/-}$ mice that otherwise do not contain T cells of their own. Naive and activated murine T cells can be distinguished according to the level of cell surface expression of CD45 RB – activated cells have low levels of this isoform and naive cells have high levels. Activated or naive populations are then transferred into recipient $Rag^{-/-}$ mice:

- transfer of naive cells leads to inflammatory bowel disease (IBD) in the $Rag^{-/-}$ recipients; but
- co-transfer of relatively few activated cells prevents disease (Fig. 19.16).

The activated cells either produce or induce production of the immune suppressive cytokine TGFβ.

Another cytokine, IL-10, undoubtedly plays a role in the function of the activated, regulatory cells because transfer of these regulatory cells from an IL-10 knockout mouse fails to suppress the induction of IBD by naive cells.

Regulatory T cells suppress the activation of other T cells

Although the nature of regulatory T cells was discussed extensively in Chapter 11, the subject is of such relevance to tolerance induction that it is worth recapitulating the features of these cells. As described above (Fig. 19.8), a naturally occurring subset of regulatory lymphocytes is distinguished by expression of the α chain of the IL-2R (CD25). Elimination of these cells from normal mice leads to the generation of various organ-specific autoimmune conditions. Similar cells exist in humans and there is clear evidence that they play a role in protecting against autoimmunity. These natural regulatory T cells are anergic to TCR-mediated activation, but potently suppress the activation of other T cells.

CD25⁺ AND IL-10 REGULATORY CELLS CONSTITUTE DISTINCT REGULATORY CELL SUBSETS – CD25⁺ regulatory cells are generated in the thymus. It seems likely

IL-10 is required for regulation of inflammatory bowel disease mediated by activated T cells

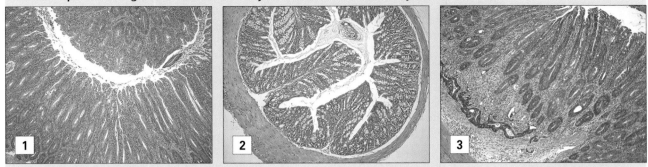

Fig. 19.16 (**1**) Severe colitis in a mouse injected with CD45RB^high CD4^+ T cells from normal mice. (**2**) Normal appearance of the colon in a mouse restored with both CD45RB^high and CD45RB^low cells. This shows that the CD45RB^low population of T cells is able to inhibit inflammation caused by normal CD45RB^high cells. (**3**) Severe colitis in a mouse restored with both CD45RB^high and IL-10^−/− CD45RB^low cells. This experiment demonstrates that CD45RB^low cells that cannot produce IL-10 fail to serve as regulators of disease. (Based on Asseman C, Mauze S, Leach MW, et al. Reproduced from The Journal of Experimental Medicine 1999;190:995 by copyright permission of The Rockefeller University Press)

that the cells destined to become CD25^+ regulatory cells have a relatively high affinity for their MHC restriction element and only just escape negative selection in the thymus (see Fig. 19.8). Indeed their high affinity for MHC molecules could explain their continuous expression of CD25, a marker of T cell activation, as well as their anergic state. There is also evidence that CD25^+ regulatory cells can be generated in peripheral lymphoid tissues.

As discussed previously, the forkhead/winged helix transcription factor FoxP3 appears to control the generation and function of CD25^+ Treg cells (see Figs 11.13 and 11.14).

In mice, FoxP3 is preferentially expressed by CD25^+ cells. Furthermore, mutations of the *FoxP3* gene are associated with a broad range of hypersensitivity conditions in both mouse and humans. Importantly, CD25^+ FoxP3^+ cells from normal mice prevent disease when transferred into the FoxP3 mutant 'scurfy' mouse and it will be recalled from Chapter 11, that point mutations and microdeletions of the *FoxP3* gene were found in the affected members of families with the IPEX (immune dysfunction, polyendocrinopathy, enteropathy, X-linked) syndrome.

Precisely how CD25^+ cells regulate immune function in vivo is not clear. The cells express molecules such as CTLA-4 and this may function by ligating B7 molecules on neighboring T cells.

The ability of CD25^+ regulatory cells to control different types of immune pathology may or may not require them to secrete immunosuppressive cytokines such as TGFβ and IL-10. These cytokines can suppress antigen presentation by professional APCs and have directly suppressive effects on naive T cells.

In addition to the FoxP3^+ CD25^+ regulatory cells there are other important subsets of cells with regulatory properties. These include the CD25^− TGFβ-producing Tr1 cells elicited by oral administration of proteins, and IL-10-secreting regulatory cells (see Fig. 11.14).

IL-10 regulatory cells:
- can be selected in vivo by repeated antigen encounter;
- differentiate from CD25^− precursors; and
- do not necessarily express FoxP3.

CD25^+ and IL-10 regulatory cells therefore constitute distinct regulatory cell subsets (Fig. 19.17).

THE LIGANDS FOR TLRs AND CYTOKINES OVERRIDE SUPPRESSION IN POTENTIALLY OVERWHELMING INFECTION – The balance between immune response and immune suppression must be under fine control to ensure an effective response to infection while preventing an aberrant response to self antigens. How then does the immune system mount an effective response to infection in the face of such immune regulation? Here the non-specific receptors for infectious agents, including the Toll-like receptors (TLRs), may sense the presence of an infectious agent. The ligands for TLRs and cytokines, secreted by both the innate and adaptive immune systems, combine to override suppression in the face of potentially overwhelming infection. When the immune system has eradicated the infection, however, the regulatory cells more than fully recover their suppressive function and hence control autoimmunity (Fig. 19.18).

Q. Which CD25^+ cells are not regulators?
A. The CD25 marker is upregulated on naive T cells in response to antigen as part of an active immune response (see Fig. 7.23).

In conclusion, regulatory lymphocytes play a crucial role in the control of autoimmune responses. Scientists are only just beginning to reveal the mechanisms by which these cells mediate their suppressive activity. Furthermore we know very little about how these cells are generated in the normal immune repertoire of healthy individuals. There is little doubt that clarification of these questions will help in the control of many hypersensitivity conditions including allergic and autoimmune diseases.

CD4⁺ regulatory T cells

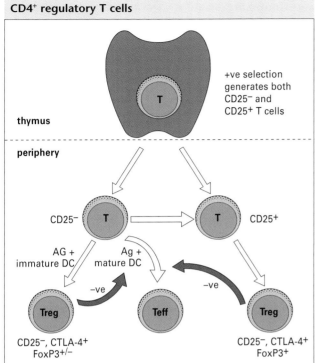

Fig. 19.17 The thymus generates both CD25⁻ and CD25⁺ regulatory T (Treg) cells. T cells respond to antigen presented by mature dendritic cells by differentiating into effector T cells (Teff), secreting cytokines and providing help for cytotoxic T and B cells. Antigen presented by immature dendritic cells drives the differentiation of CD25⁻ cells, such as IL-10⁺ Treg cells that suppress effector cell generation. Thymus-derived CD25⁺ Treg cells block expansion of the effector cell population. CD25⁺ FoxP3⁺ Treg cells can also be generated from CD25⁻ precursors in peripheral lymphoid tissues. Both these and other regulatory populations depend on the production of cytokines, such as IL-10 and TGFβ, for suppression in vivo, although the requirement for cytokines depends on the nature of the effector T cell response. (Based on Wraith DC, Nicolson KS, Whitley NT. Curr Opin Immunol 2004;16:695. Copyright 2004 with permission from Elsevier)

TOLERANCE IS ALSO IMPOSED ON B CELLS

High-affinity IgG production is T cell dependent. For this reason, and because the threshold of tolerance for T cells is lower than that for B cells, the simplest explanation for non-self reactivity by B cells is a lack of T cell help.

Until quite recently it was therefore felt that immunological tolerance should be the responsibility of T lymphocytes alone, the logical argument being: Why evolve a complex process of immunological tolerance among cells such as B cells when they are then allowed to hypermutate? All nature would have to do would be to evolve a system in which T cells never reacted with self antigens; a 'perfect' system would delete all self-reactive T cells. The immune system could then allow the B cell

Stability of the suppressor phenotype

steady state	infection/inflammation	steady state
low TLR ligation low co-stimulation low IL-2 low IL-6, etc.	Treg Treg cells lose suppressive capacity	low TLR ligation low co-stimulation low IL-2 low IL-6, etc.
Treg Treg cells suppress responses to self antigens	high TLR ligation high co-stimulation high IL-2 high IL-6, etc.	Treg Treg cells suppress responses to self antigens

time

Fig. 19.18 Treg cells suppress the response of autoreactive (red) cells to self antigens in the steady state by ensuring that they do not reach the threshold for activation (dashed line). Their ability to suppress responses can be overcome in the face of infection, as a result of TLR ligation or increasing levels of co-stimulation and cytokines secreted in response to infection. This might permit localized activation of some autoreactive (green) cells through bystander activation or molecular mimicry. Their expansion will, however, be prevented by clonal competition from cells specific for antigens carried by the infectious agent. Available evidence suggests that Treg cells retain their suppressive capacity and will therefore continue to suppress the response to self antigens when the infection has been cleared. (Based on Wraith DC, Nicolson KS, Whitley NT. Curr Opin Immunol 2004;16:695. Copyright 2004 with permission from Elsevier)

repertoire to expand widely and generate as many autoreactive B cells as possible by random rearrangement. Without help from T cells these B cells would remain harmless.

Now we appreciate that the immune system is not allowed to be 'perfect'. If it were, it would almost inevitably develop 'holes' in the immunological repertoire through which faster evolving microorganisms would inevitably break. We now appreciate that autoreactive T cells exist in all of us and that the balance between health and autoimmunity is a fine one.

Q. Give one piece of evidence that autoimmunity occurs in normal individuals.

A. It is possible to generate autoimmune conditions in normal animals by injection of self molecules in adjuvant (e.g. experimental autoimmune encephalomyelitis). Autoreactive T cells can be generated in vitro from lymphoid tissues of healthy individuals by appropriate stimulation with antigen–APCs and cytokines.

The B lymphocyte pool is subject to analogous but subtly different mechanisms of immunological tolerance to those that apply to the T lymphocyte pool.

There are clearly circumstances in which B cells must be tolerized directly. For example, some microorganisms have cross-reactive antigens that have both foreign T cell-reactive epitopes and other epitopes that resemble self epitopes and are capable of stimulating B cells. Such antigens could provoke a vigorous antibody response to self antigens (Fig. 19.19).

Furthermore, in contrast to TCRs, the immunoglobulin receptors on mature, antigenically stimulated B cells can undergo hypermutation and may acquire anti-self reactivities at this late stage. Tolerance thus needs to be imposed on B cells both during their development and after antigenic stimulation in secondary lymphoid tissues.

Self-reactive B cells may be deleted or anergized, depending on the affinity of the B cell antigen receptor and the nature of the antigen.

Tolerance induction by self antigens can lead to one of several results, such as deletion or anergy. The outcome depends on:

• the affinity of the B cell antigen receptor; and
• the nature of the antigen it encounters, whether this is an integral membrane protein or a soluble and largely monomeric protein in the circulation.

The fate of self-reactive B cells has been determined using transgenic technology (Figs 19.20 and 19.21).

B cells pass through several developmental checkpoints

B cell development shows similar features to T cell development, but takes place largely in the bone marrow. Development is marked by expression of surrogate receptor molecules.

The first notable event takes place in the late pro-B stage when the CD79a and CD79b (Igα and Igβ) molecules appear at the cell surface (see Figs 8.1 and 8.3). Progression to the pre-B stage is accompanied by VDJ recombination at the heavy chain locus. The rearranged

Breakdown of B cell tolerance caused by cross-reactive antigen

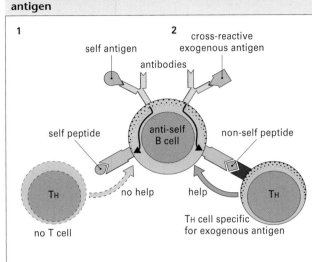

Fig. 19.19 (1) If T$_H$ cells are not available, either because of a hole in the T cell repertoire or because of deletion resulting from self tolerance achieved intrathymically, any B cells that are self-reactive will be unable to mount an anti-self antibody response. (2) Autoantibodies can be produced if an anti-self B cell collaborates with an anti-non-self T$_H$ cell in response to cross-reactive antigens containing both self and non-self determinants.

heavy chain can then appear at the cell surface in combination with both CD79a and CD79b and the V$_{pre-B}$ and λ5 molecules that act as surrogate light chains (see Fig. 8.2).

There are clear analogies with T cell development here – T cells rearrange the heavy chain genes first and

Tolerance induction in peripheral B cells by clonal deletion

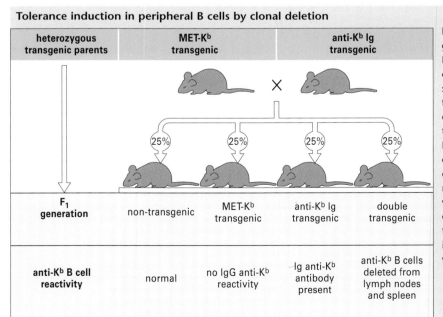

heterozygous transgenic parents	MET-K^b transgenic	anti-K^b Ig transgenic

F$_1$ generation	non-transgenic	MET-K^b transgenic	anti-K^b Ig transgenic	double transgenic
anti-K^b B cell reactivity	normal	no IgG anti-K^b reactivity	Ig anti-K^b antibody present	anti-K^b B cells deleted from lymph nodes and spleen

Fig. 19.20 Non-b haplotype mice were given the gene for H-2K^b, which is a foreign MHC class I molecule. The gene was controlled by the metallothionein promoter, specific for such sites as the liver (MET-K^b transgenic). These mice were crossed with other non-b mice, which had been given the genes for anti-H-2K^b antibodies (anti-K^b Ig transgenic). Double transgenic offspring expressed H-2K^b in the liver and exported B cells specific for H-2K^b from the bone marrow. However, these self-reactive B cells were partially deleted in the spleen and entirely deleted in the lymph nodes and thus no autoantibody was produced – no idiotype corresponding to the anti-K^b Ig was detectable.

B cell tolerance induction to a soluble protein by clonal anergy

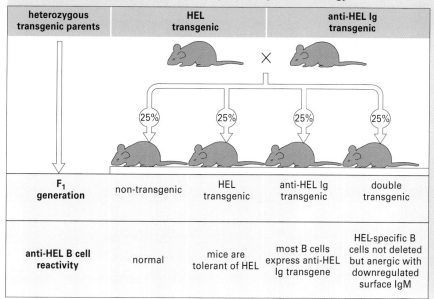

heterozygous transgenic parents	HEL transgenic		anti-HEL Ig transgenic

F₁ generation	non-transgenic	HEL transgenic	anti-HEL Ig transgenic	double transgenic
anti-HEL B cell reactivity	normal	mice are tolerant of HEL	most B cells express anti-HEL Ig transgene	HEL-specific B cells not deleted but anergic with downregulated surface IgM

Fig. 19.21 A mouse was given the hen egg lysozyme gene (HEL) linked to a tissue-specific promoter. The (largely soluble) HEL induced B and T cell tolerance. A second transgenic line (anti-HEL Ig) carried rearranged heavy and light chain genes encoding a high-affinity HEL antibody. An allotypic marker (IgHᵃ) distinguished this from endogenous immunoglobulin (IgHᵇ). The majority of B cells in these transgenics carried IgM and IgD of the 'a' allotype. Double transgenic offspring were highly HEL tolerant, producing neither anti-HEL antibody nor antibody-secreting B cells. HEL-binding (self reactive) B cells were not, however, deleted, but had downregulated surface IgM, but not IgD, receptors. They behaved as anergic cells.

also employ a surrogate light chain. In addition, it appears that expression of the pre-B cell receptor is necessary for successful allelic exclusion at the heavy chain locus.

As pre-B cells develop, recombination at the light chain locus proceeds and the cells become immature B cells. At this point the cells are IgD⁻.

B cells then go through a 'transitional' stage in development becoming IgDˡᵒʷ as well as IgM⁺. Mature B cells express IgD at higher levels than IgM.

Checkpoints in B cell development include:
- successful expression of CD79a and CD79b in late pro-B cells;
- successful rearrangement at the heavy chain locus in pre-B cells;
- successful rearrangement at the light chain locus and receptor editing.

Self tolerance begins when IgM first appears at the surface of the developing cell.

Immature cells are resistant to apoptosis, though the development of immature B cells can still be blocked by interaction with self antigen. However, immature B cells can edit their receptor, thus allowing development to progress.

Receptor editing allows potentially self-reactive B cells to continue development

When the IgM receptor on an immature bone marrow B cell reacts with self antigen further cell differentiation is blocked, but light chain rearrangement can continue.

If the new IgM receptor does not react with a self antigen in bone marrow, B cell development can proceed.

Interestingly the 'immature' B cell is relatively resistant to apoptotic cell death, whereas the later 'transitional' cell is sensitive.

Allowing light chain rearrangement to continue among immature cells permits the B cell to edit its receptor and thus rescue potentially autoreactive cells from inevitable death. This mechanism of altering offending receptors before the B cell becomes sensitive to antigen-mediated cell death clearly allows the immune system to optimize the generation of its repertoire.

In fact it appears that mechanisms have evolved to promote receptor editing in B cells. The κ light chain locus can be inactivated by recombination of a recombining sequence (RS). Recombination of the RS element results in deletion of CK and other sequences required for transcription of the κ allele. It is important to appreciate that 40–60% of IgM⁺λ⁺ B cells carry a VκJκ rearrangement inactivated by this RS recombination. Receptor editing therefore plays an important role in the generation of the normal B cell repertoire.

Self-reactive B cells are usually deleted

As B cells mature through the transitional stage they become poor at reactivating the *RAG* genes. So, if receptor editing has failed to eliminate autoreactive B cells, they are likely to be eliminated by apoptotic death because they can no longer select a new receptor. Interestingly these transitional IgMʰⁱIgDˡᵒ cells can emigrate to the periphery where their high IgM level ensures that apoptotic cell death can still take place.

The spleen eliminates unwanted B cells as effectively as the thymus removes unwanted T cells

Recent studies have shown that the bone marrow exports a higher proportion of new B cells than the thymus does new T cells. Also, unlike T cells leaving the thymus, B cells leaving the bone marrow are relatively immature. These cells express the heat-stable antigen (HSA) and migrate from the bone marrow to the outer T cell zone of the spleen.

It is among these cells that the most significant amount of negative selection takes place. This splenic environment eliminates unwanted B cells as effectively as the thymus removes unwanted T cells (Fig. 19.22). Self-reactive B cells are purged by a process that:

- induces anergy;
- prevents migration into B cell follicles; and
- rapidly leads to cell death.

Anergy in an autoreactive B cell can be overcome by high-avidity antigen

Self-reactive B cells in the outer T cell zone are short-lived (1–3 days), whereas cells selected to enter B cell follicles become long-lived and recirculate for from 1 to 4 weeks.

Short-lived, autoreactive B cells may, however, contribute to immune responses to foreign antigens. Anergy in such an autoreactive B cell can be overcome by high-avidity antigen.

Self-reactive B cells may then be recruited into the functional immune repertoire because their B cell receptor cross-reacts sufficiently strongly with foreign antigen.

At first sight, allowing B cell tolerance to self antigen to be overwhelmed by foreign antigen would seem risky. Why promote a pluripotent B cell repertoire at the risk of autoimmunity? This reflects a balance between the risk of autoimmunity and protection of the species from infectious pandemics.

The immune system has evolved to ensure that among the population there will be individuals equipped to fight almost any infection.

Diversity among T cells is generated by rearrangement of their receptors in concert with MHC polymorphism. MHC polymorphism and TCR selection together provide sufficient diversity across the population to protect against almost any infection. MHC polymorphism has evolved to fill holes in the protective repertoire of the species.

Likewise the fact that the B cell pool permits a proportion of short-lived and potentially autoreactive B cells to emigrate to the periphery provides an additional level of protection from infection. In the absence of an infection these cells die rapidly. This short-lived pool of cells can, however, contribute to broadening the potential B cell repertoire. Such repertoire diversity and further differences between the repertoires of individuals within the population will ensure that there will always be some individuals ready to mount an effective immune response to infection.

A second window of susceptibility to tolerance occurs transiently during the generation of B cell memory. Secondary B cells (derived from memory B cells produced by T cell-dependent stimulation) are highly susceptible to tolerance by epitopes presented multivalently in the absence of T cell help. Such a tolerance-susceptible stage probably ensures that newly derived memory B cells that have acquired self reactivity (as a result of accumulated somatic mutations) are purged from the repertoire.

TOLERANCE CAN BE INDUCED ARTIFICIALLY IN VIVO
Chimerism is associated with tolerance

Tolerance can be induced by the inoculation of allogeneic cells into hosts that lack immunocompetence, for example

Self-reactive B cells die in peripheral lymphoid tissues

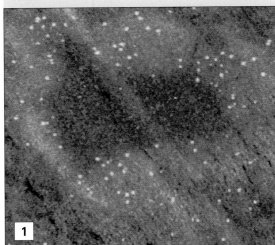

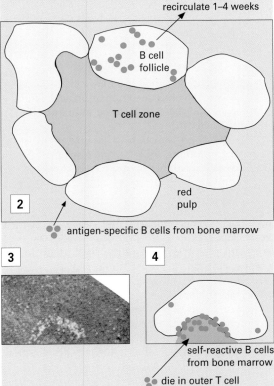

Fig. 19.22 Transgenic B cells expressing a B cell receptor specific for lysozyme were stained green and adoptively transferred into either normal mice (**1** and **2**) or mice expressing soluble lysozyme as a self antigen (**3** and **4**). In the absence of antigen the B cells migrate to B cell follicles. In the presence of the self antigen the B cells are excluded from B cell follicles in the outer T cell zone where they die in 1–2 days. (From Townsend SE, Weintraub BC, Goodnow CC. Immunol Today 1999;20:217. Copyright 1999 with permission from Elsevier)

neonatal hosts or adult hosts after immunosuppressive regimens such as:

- total body irradiation;
- drugs (e.g. ciclosporin);
- anti-lymphocytic antibodies (anti-lymphocyte globulin, anti-CD4 antibodies, etc.).

For tolerance to be maintained, a certain degree of chimerism – the coexistence of cells from genetically different individuals – must be maintained. This is best achieved if the inoculum contains cells capable of self renewal (e.g. bone marrow cells).

If mature T cells are present in the injected cell population, they may react against the histocompatibility antigens of their host and induce a severe and often fatal disease known as graft versus host disease.

Antibodies to co-receptor and co-stimulatory molecules induce tolerance to transplants

Tolerance of transplanted tissues can be achieved in adult animals by monoclonal antibodies directed against the T cell molecules, CD4 and CD8 (the antibodies can be either the T cell-depleting or the non-depleting type). In this situation, tolerance of skin allografts is obtained even in the absence of cellular chimerism.

Q. How could an anti-CD4 antibody have its effect, if it does not deplete CD4 T cell numbers?

A. The antibody may inhibit the interaction of T cells with APCs, and the assembly of the immunological synapse (see Figs 7.19 and 7.20).

Another highly promising approach to transplantation tolerance has arisen through the use of agents designed to blockade co-stimulatory molecules.

As mentioned above, T cells require co-stimulatory signals for effective priming. CD28 and CD154 both play important roles in co-stimulation.

The CD28 pathway of activation can be inhibited by blocking both B7 molecules with a soluble form of CTLA-4 (CTLA-4–Ig). In combination with an antibody to the ligand for CD40 (CD154), CTLA-4–Ig has been shown to block recognition of allografts and allow long-term skin allograft survival in mice.

Antibodies to CD154 alone will prolong renal allograft survival in non-human primates. It is thought that anti-CD154 prevents the three-cell interplay between CD4, CD8, and dendritic cells that is required for the maturation of CD8 cells (Fig. 19.23).

Soluble antigens readily induce tolerance

Tolerance is inducible in both neonatal and adult animals by administering soluble protein antigens in deaggregated form. T and B cells differ in their susceptibility to tolerization by these antigens. Thus:

- tolerance is achieved in T cells from spleen and thymus after very low antigen doses and within a few hours;
- tolerance of spleen B cells requires much more time and higher doses of antigen (Fig. 19.24).

The antigen levels that will produce B cell tolerance in neonates are about one-hundredth of those required in adults.

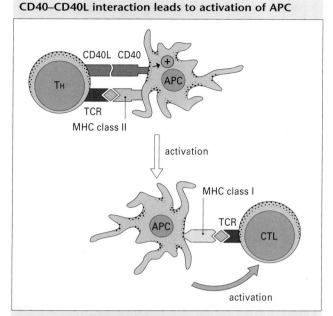

CD40–CD40L interaction leads to activation of APC

Fig. 19.23 CD8 T killer cells will not respond to resting APCs. T helper (TH) cell recognition of antigen is one way that APCs such as dendritic cells can be armed to present antigen to CD8 cells. The molecules responsible for the interaction between CD4 TH cells and dendritic cells are called CD40L and CD40. Ligation of CD40 on the surface of dendritic cells leads to their activation. Blocking this interaction is one way to prevent the presentation of alloantigens to CD8 cells and hence prevent allograft rejection. (Based on Lanzavecchia A. Nature 1998;393:413)

Oral administration of antigens induces tolerance by a variety of mechanisms

High doses of orally administered antigen can cause anergy or deletion; this could be one situation in which the term anergy is being used to describe a state of paralysis preceding cell death.

Lower doses of orally administered antigen can, however, induce the priming of T cells in the gut. As an effective antibody response in the gut requires class switching to the IgA isotype, it is no surprise that antigen feeding induces T cells that support IgA production. These 'Tr1-like' cells produce cytokines including IL-10 and TGFβ, and serve to inhibit inflammatory responses mediated by TH1 cells. TGFβ:

- inhibits the proliferation and function of B cells, cytotoxic T cells, and NK cells;
- inhibits cytokine production in lymphocytes; and
- antagonizes the effects of TNF.

Although the induction of mucosal Tr1 cells is antigen specific, the suppressive activity of cytokines such as TGFβ is not. Hence, the induction of oral tolerance to one antigen is able to suppress the immune response to a second, associated antigen.

The effect of **'bystander suppression'** by mucosal Tr1 cells allows the suppression of complex organ-specific

Relative susceptibilities of B cells and T cells to tolerance induction in vivo

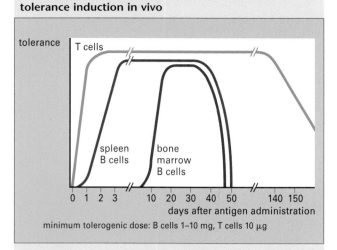

minimum tolerogenic dose: B cells 1–10 mg, T cells 10 μg

Fig. 19.24 A mouse was given a T-dependent antigen (human γ-globulin) at tolerance-inducing doses, and the duration of tolerance was measured. T cell tolerance was more rapidly induced and more persistent than B cell tolerance. Bone marrow B cells may take considerably longer to tolerize than splenic B cells. Typically, much less antigen is needed to tolerize T cells – 10 μg as opposed to 1–10 mg, a 1000-fold difference.

autoimmune diseases by feeding with a single antigen derived from the affected tissue.

Other mucosal surfaces are proving effective routes for inducing antigen-specific tolerance

Other mucosal surfaces are proving equally effective as routes for the induction of antigen-specific tolerance.

Nasal deposition of MHC class II-restricted peptides has been used to control both 'humoral' and 'cellular' immune responses. In addition, administration of aerosolized antigen to the lung can be used to control allergic responses to foreign antigens and autoimmune responses to self antigens.

Q. Why is the treatment described above not an example of immune deviation?

A. The fact that one can inhibit both autoimmune (TH1 type) and allergic (TH2 type) responses argues against immune deviation as the mechanism of tolerance induction.

Recent evidence suggests that other cells producing IL-10 may be responsible for nasal peptide-induced tolerance. It could be that other cell types, including CD8 cells, are responsible for suppressing the immune response that follows the aerosol administration of protein antigens.

Extensive clonal proliferation can lead to exhaustion and tolerance

Tolerance in T cells, and to a lesser extent in B cells, can be due to clonal exhaustion – the end result of a powerful immune response. Repeated antigenic challenge may stimulate all the antigen-responding cells to differentiate into short-lived end cells, leaving no cells that can respond to a subsequent challenge with antigen.

Anti-idiotypic responses can be associated with tolerance

An antibody's combining site may act as an antigen and induce the formation of 'anti-idiotypic antibodies'. By cross-linking immunoglobulin on B cells, these antibodies can block B cell responsiveness of the cell. Because most of the antibodies produced in response to particular antigens in some animals bear a particular idiotype, suppression of this idiotype by anti-idiotypic antibody can significantly alter the response. This type of tolerance will be partial, however, because it affects only those B cells carrying the idiotype.

The idiotype of a T cell is represented by the polymorphic regions of the TCR α and β chains. TCR-specific regulatory cells, induced after vaccination with self-reactive T cells, TCR peptides, and even DNA-encoding TCR molecules, have been shown to prevent autoimmunity in animal models.

Tolerance in vivo relates to persistence of antigen

Persistence of antigen plays a major part in maintaining a state of tolerance to it in vivo – when the antigen concentration decreases below a certain threshold, responsiveness is restored.

If the tolerance results from clonal deletion, recovery of responsiveness is related to the time required to generate new lymphocytes from their precursors. This tolerance can be prevented by measures such as thymectomy.

If, on the other hand, the tolerance is maintained by a suppressive mechanism resulting, for example, from the induction of regulatory T cells, then the state of tolerance can be relatively long-lived.

Tolerance could be used to control damaging immune responses

A better understanding of tolerogenesis could be valuable in many ways. It could be used to:

• promote tolerance of foreign tissue grafts;
• control the damaging immune responses in hypersensitivity states and autoimmune diseases.

The various ways of establishing artificial tolerance in adult animals are being investigated for their potential clinical applications.

Some success has been obtained in the case of transplants associated with chimerism and performed under the umbrella of immunosuppressive agents.

Treatment with monoclonal non-depleting anti-CD4 and anti-CD8 or anti-CD154 antibodies has also been used successfully with foreign tissue or organ transplants.

The possibility that tolerance can be induced either by mucosal administration of the target antigen or through the use of peptide drugs awaits extensive clinical trials in humans.

It is also important to learn how to activate T cells that ignore certain antigens to enable the immune system to mount an appropriate active response. This could be exploited to limit the growth of tumors that may express their own unique tumor-specific genes.

FURTHER READING

Gotter J, Kyewski B. Regulating self-tolerance by deregulating gene expression. Curr Opin Immunol 2004;16:741–745.

Radtke F, Wilson A, MacDonald HR. Notch signaling in T- and B-cell development. Curr Opin Immunol 2004;16:174–179.

Singer A. New perspectives on a developmental dilemma: the kinetic signaling model and the importance of signal duration for the CD4/CD8 lineage decision. Curr Opin Immunol 2002;14:207–215.

Su MA, Anderson MS. Aire: an update. Curr Opin Immunol 2004;16:746–752.

Venanzi ES, Benoist C, Mathis D Good riddance: thymocyte clonal deletion prevents autoimmunity. Curr Opin Immunol 2004;16:197–202.

Verkoczy LK, Martensson AS, Nemazee D. The scope of receptor editing and its association with autoimmunity. Curr Opin Immunol 2004;16:808–814.

Wraith DC, Nicolson KS, Whitley NT. Regulatory CD4+ T cells and the control of autoimmune disease. Curr Opin Immunol 2004;16:695–701.

Zamoyska R, Lovatt M. Signalling in T-lymphocyte development: integration of signalling pathways is the key. Curr Opin Immunol 2004;16:191–196.

Critical thinking: Tolerance (see p. 499 for explanations)

Lineage commitment in thymocyte development

Thymocytes bearing MHC class I-restricted TCRs differentiate into CD8 T cells, while those recognizing MHC class II molecules become CD4 T cells. It was previously thought that this process might be random or 'stochastic', but it now appears that this is an 'instructive' process.

AND mice express a transgenic TCR specific for a peptide derived from pigeon cytochrome c in the context of I-E^k (class II). Normally the majority of thymocytes in these mice develop into CD4 single positive (SP) cells. OT-1 mice bear a transgenic TCR specific for an ovalbumin peptide that is H-2K^b (class I)

restricted. Normally the majority of thymocytes in these mice develop into CD8 SP cells. TCR$^{+/-}$ heterozygotes were crossed with heterozygotes expressing either a constitutively active (dLGF) or catalytically inactive (dLGKR) form of Lck.

Thymocytes from AND, AND/dLGKR, OT-1, or OT-1/dLGF were stained with antibodies specific for CD4 or CD8 and analysed by flow cytometry. Table 1 shows the absolute number of CD4 and CD8 SP cells obtained from three individual experiments (median values) in which littermates were studied.

experimental mouse	CD4 cells	CD8 cells	experimental mouse	CD4 cells	CD8 cells
AND	487	8	OT-1	6	113
AND/dLGKR	4	39	OT-1/dLGF	380	37

Data summarized from Hernandez-Hoyos G, Sohn SJ, Rothenberg EV, Alberola-Ila J. Immunity 2000;12:313–322.

Table 1

1 What drives expression of CD4 cells in a mouse expressing a class I-restricted TCR?
2 What effect does inhibiting the activity of Lck have on thymocyte development?

3 Are the results seen with the four different strains of mice mutually consistent?

The molecular basis of activation-induced cell death (AICD)

The 3A9 transgenic mouse expresses a TCR specific for a peptide derived from hen egg white lysozyme. These mice were crossed onto the lpr, gld, or TNF-R1 knockout background. Remember that the lpr and gld mice have defective Fas and FasL genes, respectively.

Previously activated T cells may undergo AICD on further restimulation in vitro. T cells from the 3A9-backcrossed mice

were activated in vitro and then restimulated with anti-CD3 (to induce AICD), IL-2, or IL-2 with anti-Fas antibody (to induce death via the Fas pathway). The cells were then assayed for apoptosis by propidium iodide staining (Table 2).

Critical thinking: Tolerance (Continued)

mice	apoptotic T cells		
	anti-CD3	IL-2	IL-2 and anti-Fas
3A9	++	–	++
3A9.lpr knockout	–	–	–
3A9.TNF-R1 knockout	++	–	++
3A9.gld knockout	–	–	++
Data summarized from Refaeli Y, Van Parijs L, Abbas AK. Immunol Rev 1999;169:273–282.			

Table 2

4 Is AICD mediated by signaling through the Fas or TNF-R1 pathway?

5 What evidence is there to support your choice?

6 Why are T cells from the gld mouse susceptible to anti-Fas-mediated death?

7 Why has the immune system developed a way of killing off activated T cells?

8 If T cells die on reactivation, how does immune memory arise?

The role of regulatory T cells in peripheral tolerance

Certain mice are congenitally athymic and do not have mature T lymphocytes. The 'nude' mouse carries a mutation in the gene for the Wnt transcription factor. This results in lack of hair and absence of the thymus. Nude mice can, however, be reconstituted with lymphocytes from normal mice. In the experiment for which results are shown in Table 3, either thymocytes or spleen and lymph node (SP/LN) cells from normal mice were treated with various antibodies and complement to deplete cell subsets and then transferred into 'nude' recipients by intravenous injection. The recipient mice were left for 3 months and then examined for histological and serological evidence of autoimmune disease.

inoculated cells	number of mice with autoimmune disease					
	number of mice	OOP	THR	SIAL	ADR	GN
A whole thymocytes	12	0	0	0	0	0
B CD25⁻ thymocytes	12	12	4	3	1	3
C CD4⁺8⁻ thymocytes	5	0	0	0	0	0
D CD25⁻4⁺ thymocytes	5	5	2	1	2	1
E whole SP/LN cells	8	0	0	0	0	0
F CD25⁻ SP/LN cells	8	8	5	5	2	2
G CD25⁻ thymocytes and CD4⁺ SP/LN cells	8	0	0	0	0	0
Data summarized from Itoh M, Takahashi T, Sakaguchi N, et al. J Immunol 1999;162:5317–5326. (ADR, adrenalitis; GN, glomerulonephritis; OOP, oophoritis; SIAL, sialoadenitis; THR, thyroiditis)						

Table 3

9 Why do CD25⁻ lymphocytes cause widespread auto-immunity?

10 Where do CD25⁺ cells arise?

11 Why are certain tissues more susceptible to autoimmune disease than others?

Autoimmunity and Autoimmune Disease

SUMMARY

- **Autoimmunity is associated with disease.** Autoimmune mechanisms underlie many diseases, some organ-specific, others systemic in distribution, and autoimmune disorders can overlap – an individual may have more than one organ-specific disorder, or more than one systemic disease.

- **Genetic factors play a role in the development of autoimmune diseases.** Factors such as HLA type are important, and it is probable that each disease involves several factors.

- **Self-reactive B and T cells persist even in normal subjects.** Autoreactive B and T cells persist in normal subjects, but in disease are selected by autoantigen in the production of autoimmune responses.

- **Controls on the development of autoimmunity can be bypassed.** Microbial cross-reacting antigens and cytokine dysregulation can lead to autoimmunity.

- **In most diseases associated with autoimmunity, the autoimmune process produces the lesions.** The pathogenic role of autoimmunity can be demonstrated in experimental models. Human autoantibodies can be directly pathogenic. Immune complexes are often associated with systemic autoimmune disease. Autoantibody tests are valuable for diagnosis and sometimes for prognosis.

- **Treatment of autoimmune disease has a variety of aims.** Treatment of organ-specific diseases usually involves metabolic control. Treatment of systemic diseases includes the use of anti-inflammatory and immunosuppressive drugs. Future treatment will probably focus on manipulation of the pivotal autoreactive T cells by antigens or peptides, by anti-CD4, and possibly by T cell vaccination.

AUTOIMMUNITY IS ASSOCIATED WITH DISEASE

The immune system has tremendous diversity and, because the repertoire of specificities expressed by the B and T cell populations is generated randomly, it is bound to include many that are specific for self components. The body must therefore establish self-tolerance mechanisms to distinguish between self and non-self determinants to avoid autoreactivity (see Chapter 19). However, all mechanisms have a risk of breakdown. The self-recognition mechanisms are no exception, and a number of diseases have been identified in which there is autoimmunity, due to copious production of autoantibodies and autoreactive T cells.

One of the earliest examples in which the production of autoantibodies was associated with disease in a given organ is Hashimoto's thyroiditis.

Among the autoimmune diseases, thyroiditis has been particularly well studied, and many of the aspects discussed in this chapter will draw upon our knowledge of it. It is a disease of the thyroid that is most common in middle-aged women and often leads to formation of a goiter and hypothyroidism. The gland is infiltrated, sometimes to an extraordinary extent, with inflammatory lymphoid cells. These are predominantly mononuclear phagocytes, lymphocytes and plasma cells, and secondary lymphoid follicles are common (Fig. 20.1).

In Hashimoto's disease, the gland often shows regenerating thyroid follicles, but this is not a feature of the thyroid in the related condition, primary myxedema, in which comparable immunological features are seen and where the gland undergoes almost complete destruction and shrinks.

The serum of patients with Hashimoto's disease usually contains antibodies to thyroglobulin. These antibodies are demonstrable by agglutination and by precipitin reactions when present in high titer.

Most patients also have antibodies directed against a cytoplasmic or microsomal antigen, also present on the apical surface of the follicular epithelial cells (Fig. 20.2), and now known to be thyroid peroxidase, the enzyme that iodinates thyroglobulin.

Hashimoto's thyroiditis and SLE represent the extremes of the spectrum of autoimmune diseases

The antibodies associated with Hashimoto's thyroiditis and primary myxedema react only with the thyroid, so the resulting lesion is highly localized.

By contrast, the serum from patients with diseases such as systemic lupus erythematosus (SLE) reacts with many,

Pathological changes in Hashimoto's thyroiditis

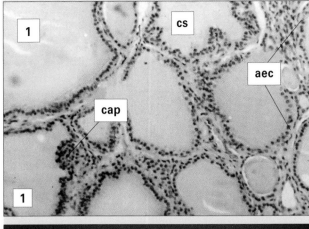

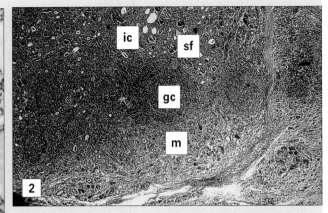

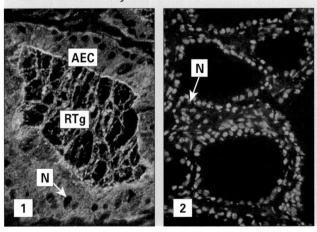

Fig. 20.1 In the normal thyroid gland (1), the acinar epithelial cells (aec) line the colloid space (cs) into which they secrete thyroglobulin, which is broken down on demand to provide thyroid hormones (cap, capillaries containing red blood cells). In the Hashimoto gland (2), the normal architecture is virtually destroyed and replaced by invading cells (ic), which consist essentially of lymphocytes, macrophages, and plasma cells. A secondary lymphoid follicle (sf), with a germinal center (gc) and a mantle of small lymphocytes (m), is present. H&E stain. × 80. (Reproduced from Woolf N. Pathology: basic and systemic. London: WB Saunders; 1998) (3) In contrast to the red color and soft texture of the normal thyroid, the pale and firm gross appearance of the Hashimoto gland reflects the loss of colloid and heavy infiltration with inflammatory cells.

Autoantibodies to thyroid

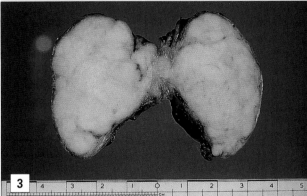

Fig. 20.2 Healthy, unfixed human thyroid sections were treated with patients' serum, and then with fluoresceinated rabbit anti-human immunoglobulin. (1) Some residual thyroglobulin in the colloid (RTg) and the acinar epithelial cells (AEC) of the follicles, particularly the apical surface, are stained by antibodies from a patient with Hashimoto's disease, which react with the cells' cytoplasm but not the nuclei (N). (2) In contrast, serum from a patient with systemic lupus erythematosus (SLE) contains antibodies that react only with the nuclei of acinar epithelial cells and leave the cytoplasm unstained. (Courtesy of Mr G Swana)

if not all, of the tissues in the body. In SLE, one of the dominant antibodies is directed against the cell nucleus (see Fig. 20.2[2]).

Hashimoto's thyroiditis and SLE represent the extremes of the autoimmune spectrum (Fig. 20.3):

- the common target organs in **organ-specific disease** include the thyroid, adrenal, stomach, and pancreas;
- the non-organ-specific diseases, often termed **systemic autoimmune diseases**, which include the rheuma-

tological disorders, characteristically involve the skin, kidney, joints, and muscle (Fig. 20.4).

An individual may have more than one autoimmune disease

Interestingly, there are remarkable overlaps at each end of the autoimmune disease spectrum:

- thyroid antibodies occur with a high frequency in patients with pernicious anemia who have gastric autoimmunity,

The spectrum of autoimmune diseases

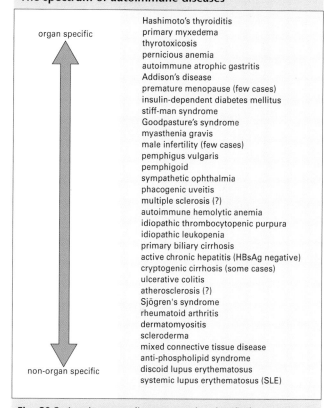

organ specific

Hashimoto's thyroiditis
primary myxedema
thyrotoxicosis
pernicious anemia
autoimmune atrophic gastritis
Addison's disease
premature menopause (few cases)
insulin-dependent diabetes mellitus
stiff-man syndrome
Goodpasture's syndrome
myasthenia gravis
male infertility (few cases)
pemphigus vulgaris
pemphigoid
sympathetic ophthalmia
phacogenic uveitis
multiple sclerosis (?)
autoimmune hemolytic anemia
idiopathic thrombocytopenic purpura
idiopathic leukopenia
primary biliary cirrhosis
active chronic hepatitis (HBsAg negative)
cryptogenic cirrhosis (some cases)
ulcerative colitis
atherosclerosis (?)
Sjögren's syndrome
rheumatoid arthritis
dermatomyositis
scleroderma
mixed connective tissue disease
anti-phospholipid syndrome
discoid lupus erythematosus
systemic lupus erythematosus (SLE)

non-organ specific

Fig. 20.3 Autoimmune diseases may be classified as organ-specific or non-organ-specific depending on whether the response is primarily against antigens localized to particular organs or against widespread antigens.

Two types of autoimmune disease

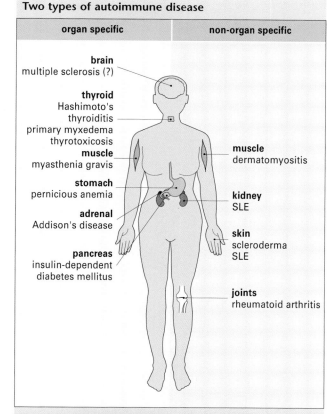

organ specific | non-organ specific

brain
multiple sclerosis (?)

thyroid
Hashimoto's
thyroiditis
primary myxedema
thyrotoxicosis

muscle
myasthenia gravis

stomach
pernicious anemia

adrenal
Addison's disease

pancreas
insulin-dependent
diabetes mellitus

muscle
dermatomyositis

kidney
SLE

skin
scleroderma
SLE

joints
rheumatoid arthritis

Fig. 20.4 Although the non-organ-specific diseases characteristically produce symptoms in the skin, joints, kidney, and muscle, individual organs are more markedly affected by particular diseases, for example the kidney in SLE and the joints in rheumatoid arthritis.

and these patients have a higher incidence of thyroid autoimmune disease than the normal population;

- similarly, patients with thyroid autoimmunity have a high incidence of stomach autoantibodies and, to a lesser extent, the clinical disease itself, namely pernicious anemia.

The cluster of rheumatological disorders at the other end of the spectrum also shows considerable overlap. Features of rheumatoid arthritis, for example, are often associated with the clinical picture of SLE. In these diseases immune complexes are deposited systemically, particularly in the kidney, joints, and skin, giving rise to widespread lesions.

By contrast, overlap of diseases from the two ends of the spectrum is relatively rare.

The mechanisms of immunopathological damage vary depending on where the disease lies in the spectrum:

- where the antigen is localized in a particular organ, type II hypersensitivity (e.g. autoimmune hemolytic anemia) and type IV cell-mediated reactions, as in type 1 insulin-dependent diabetes, are most important (see Chapters 24–26);
- in non-organ-specific autoimmune disorders such as SLE, type III immune complex deposition leads to inflammation through a variety of mechanisms, includ-

ing complement activation and phagocyte recruitment (see Chapters 24 and 25).

GENETIC FACTORS PLAY A ROLE IN THE DEVELOPMENT OF AUTOIMMUNITY

There is an undoubted familial incidence of autoimmunity. This is largely genetic rather than environmental, as may be seen from studies of identical and non-identical twins, and from the association of thyroid autoantibodies with abnormalities of the X chromosome.

Within the families of patients with organ-specific autoimmunity, not only is there a general predisposition to develop organ-specific antibodies, it is also clear that other genetically controlled factors tend to select the organ that is mainly affected.

Thus, although relatives of patients with Hashimoto's thyroiditis and families of patients with pernicious anemia both have a higher than normal incidence and titer of thyroid autoantibodies, the relatives of patients with pernicious anemia have a far higher frequency of gastric autoantibodies (Fig. 20.5), indicating that there are genetic factors that differentially select the stomach as the target within these families.

Overlap between thyroid and gastric autoimmunity

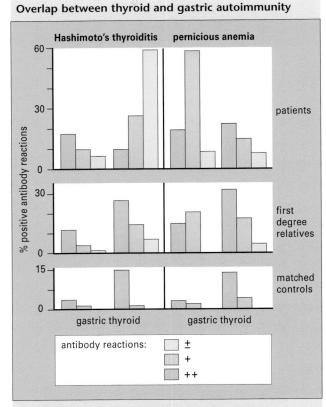

Fig. 20.5 Genetic factors affect the predisposition to autoimmunity and selection of the target organ in the relatives of patients with Hashimoto's thyroiditis and pernicious anemia. (Data adapted from Doniach D, Roitt IM, Taylor KB. Ann NY Acad Sci 1965;124:605)

HLA associations in autoimmune disease

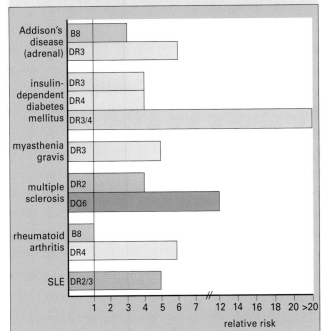

Fig. 20.6 The relative risk is a measure of the increased chance of contracting the disease for individuals bearing the HLA antigen, relative to those lacking it. Virtually all autoimmune diseases studied have shown an association with some HLA specificity. The greater relative risk for Addison's disease associated with HLA-DR3 as compared with HLA-B8 suggests that DR3 is closely linked to or even identical with the 'disease susceptibility gene'. In this case it is not surprising that B8 has a relative risk greater than 1, because it is known to occur with DR3 more often than expected by chance in the general population, a phenomenon termed linkage disequilibrium. Both DQ2 and DQ8 are also associated with type 1 diabetes mellitus, and are usually found in conjunction with the extended haplotype containing the DR3/4 disease-associated alleles. Rheumatoid arthritis is linked to a pentamer sequence in DR1 and certain subtypes of DR4, but not to any HLA-A or HLA-B alleles.

Certain HLA haplotypes predispose to autoimmunity

Further evidence for the operation of genetic factors in autoimmune disease comes from their tendency to be associated with particular HLA specificities (Fig. 20.6).

Rheumatoid arthritis shows no associations with the HLA-A and -B loci haplotypes, but is associated with a nucleotide sequence (encoding amino acids 70–74 in the DRβ chain) that is common to DR1 and major subtypes of DR4. This sequence is also present in the dnaJ **heat-shock proteins** of various bacilli and EBV gp110 proteins, presenting an interesting possibility for the induction of autoimmunity by a microbial cross-reacting epitope (see below).

The plot gets even deeper, though, with the realization that HLA-DR molecules bearing this sequence can bind to another bacterial heat-shock protein, dnaK, and to the human analog, namely hsp73, which targets selected proteins to lysosomes for antigen processing.

The haplotype B8, DR3 is particularly common in the organ-specific diseases, though Hashimoto's thyroiditis tends to be associated more with DR5.

It is notable that for insulin-dependent (type 1) diabetes mellitus, DQ2/8 heterozygotes have a greatly increased risk of developing the disease (see Fig. 20.6).

Usually, a multiplicity of genes underlies susceptibility to autoimmunity

Although HLA risk factors tend to dominate, these disorders are genetically complex and genome-wide searches for mapping the genetic intervals containing genes for predisposition to disease reveal a plethora of genes affecting:

- loss of tolerance;
- sustained inflammatory responses; and
- end-organ targeting.

A notable example is the association of autoimmune disease with a single nucleotide polymorphism (SNP) linked to CTLA-4 (Fig. 20.7), a molecule present on Tregs (see Chapter 19). It should be stressed, however, that this is a single risk factor, one of many that act in concert to provoke autoimmunity, and only rarely have

CTLA-4-linked single nucleotide polymorphism associated with autoimmune disease

signal exon1	B7 bonding domain exon 2	transmembrane domain exon 3	phosphorylation exon 4	CTLA-4 splice variant	mRNA expression of CTLA-4 isoform in:	
					susceptible human genotype	susceptible mouse (NOD) genotype
				full lengh	−	−
				soluble	↓	−
				ligand independent (NOD)	−	↓

Fig. 20.7 The CT60 SNP variant in the non-coding 6.1 kb 3′ region of *CTLA-4* is responsible for the association of autoimmune disease with lower messenger RNA levels of the soluble variant splice isoforms of *CTLA-4*. (Data adapted from Ueda H, et al. Nature 2003;423:506)

single gene mutations leading to autoimmune disease been identified.

Recently it was found that mutations in the transcriptional autoimmune regulator (*Aire*) gene is associated with the multiorgan disorder known as autoimmune polyglandular syndrome type 1, characterized by Addison's disease, hypoparathyroidism, and insulin-dependent diabetes mellitus (IDDM). Deficiency in *Aire* prejudices the establishment of self tolerance to a number of organ-specific antigens such as glutamic acid decarboxylase, GAD65, one of the key autoantigens in IDDM, by preventing its expression in the thymus.

SELF-REACTIVE B AND T CELLS PERSIST EVEN IN NORMAL SUBJECTS

Despite the complex selection mechanisms operating to establish self tolerance during lymphocyte development, the body contains large numbers of lymphocytes, which are potentially autoreactive.

Thus, many autoantigens, when injected with adjuvants, make autoantibodies in normal animals, demonstrating the presence of autoreactive B cells, and it is possible to identify a small number of autoreactive B cells (e.g. anti-thyroglobulin) in the normal population.

Autoreactive T cells are also present in normal individuals, as shown by the fact that it is possible to produce autoimmune lines of T cells by stimulation of normal circulating T cells with the appropriate autoantigen (e.g. myelin basic protein [MBP]) and IL-2.

Autoimmunity results from antigen-driven self-reactive lymphocytes

Given that autoreactive B cells exist, the question remains whether they are stimulated to proliferate and produce autoantibodies by interaction with autoantigens or by some other means, such as non-specific polyclonal activators or idiotypic interactions (see below and Fig. 20.9).

Evidence that B cells are selected by antigen comes from the existence of high-affinity autoantibodies, which arise through somatic mutation, a process that requires both T cells and autoantigen. In addition, patients' serum usually contains autoantibodies directed to epitope clusters occuring on the same autoantigenic molecule. Apart from the presence of autoantigen itself, it is very difficult to envisage a mechanism that could account for the co-existence of antibody responses to different epitopes on the same molecule. A similar argument applies to the induction, in a single individual, of autoantibodies to organelles (e.g. nucleosomes and spliceosomes, which appear as blebs on the surface of apoptotic cells) or antigens linked within the same organ (e.g. thyroglobulin and thyroid peroxidase).

The most direct evidence for autoimmunity being antigen driven comes from studies of the Obese strain chicken, which spontaneously develops thyroid autoimmunity. If the thyroid gland (the source of antigen) is removed at birth, the chickens mature without developing thyroid autoantibodies (Fig. 20.8). Furthermore, once thyroid autoimmunity has developed, later removal of the thyroid leads to a gross decline of thyroid autoantibodies, usually to undetectable levels.

Comparable experiments have been carried out in the non-obese diabetic (NOD) mouse, which models human autoimmune diabetes – chemical destruction of the β cells leads to decline in pancreatic autoantibodies.

DNase treatment of lupus mice ameliorates the disease, presumably by destroying potentially pathogenic immune complexes.

In organ-specific disorders, there is ample evidence for T cells responding to antigens present in the organs under attack. But in non-organ-specific autoimmunity, identification of the antigens recognized by T cells is often inadequate. True, histone-specific T cells are generated in patients with SLE and histone could play a 'piggyback' role in the formation of anti-DNA antibodies by

Effect of neonatal thyroidectomy on Obese chickens

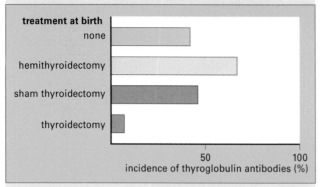

Fig. 20.8 Because removal of the thyroid at birth prevents the development of thyroid autoantibodies, it would appear that the autoimmune process is driven by the autoantigen in the thyroid gland. (Based on data from de Carvalho et al. J Exp Med 1982;155:1255)

substituting for natural antibody in the mechanism outlined in Fig. 20.9.

Another possibility is that the T cells do not see conventional peptide antigen (possibly true of anti-DNA responses), but instead recognize an antibody's idiotype (an antigenic determinant on the V region of antibody).

In this view SLE, for example, might sometimes be initiated as an 'idiotypic disease', like the model presented in Fig. 20.9. In this scheme, autoantibodies are produced normally at low levels by B cells using germline genes. If these then form complexes with the autoantigen, the complexes can be taken up by APCs (including B cells) and components of the complex, including the antibody idiotype, presented to T cells. Idiotype-specific T cells would then help the autoantibody-producing B cells.

Evidence for the induction of anti-DNA and glomerulonephritis by immunization of mice with the idiotype of germline 'natural' anti-DNA autoantibody lends credence to this hypothesis.

CONTROLS ON THE DEVELOPMENT OF AUTOIMMUNITY CAN BE BYPASSED
Molecular mimicry by cross-reactive microbial antigens can stimulate autoreactive B and T cells

Normally, naive autoreactive T cells recognizing cryptic self epitopes are not switched on because the antigen is presented only at low concentrations on 'professional' APCs or it may be presented on 'non-professional' APCs such as pancreatic β-islet cells or thyroid epithelial cells, which lack B7 or other co-stimulator molecules.

However, infection with a microbe bearing antigens that cross-react with the cryptic self epitopes (i.e. have shared epitopes) will load the professional APCs with levels of processed peptides that are sufficient to activate the naive autoreative T cells. Once primed, these T cells

Possible model of T cell help via processing of intermolecular complexes in the induction of autoimmunity

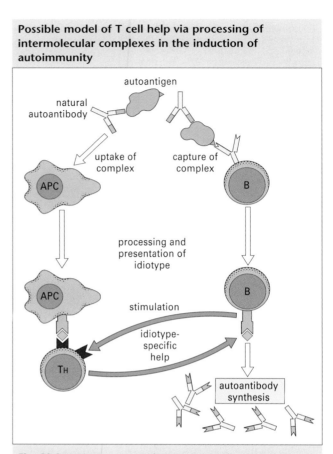

Fig. 20.9 An immune complex consisting of autoantigen (e.g. DNA) and a naturally occurring (germline) autoantibody is taken up by an antigen-presenting cell (APC), and peptides derived by processing of the idiotypic segment of the antibody (Id) are presented to TH cells. B cells that express the 'pathogenic' autoantibody can capture the complex and so can receive T cell help via presentation of the processed Id to the TH cell. Similarly, an anti-DNA-specific B cell that had endocytosed a histone–DNA complex could be stimulated to autoantibody production by histone-specific TH cells.

are able to recognize and react with the self epitope on the non-professional APCs because they:
- no longer require a co-stimulatory signal; and
- have a higher avidity for the target, due to upregulation of accessory adhesion molecules (Fig. 20.10).

Cross-reactive antigens that share B cell epitopes with self molecules can also break tolerance, but by a different mechanism. Many autoreactive B cells cannot be activated because the CD4+ TH cells they need are unresponsive, either because:
- these helper TH cells are tolerized at lower concentrations of autoantigens than the B cells; or
- because they recognize only cryptic epitopes.

However, these 'helpless' B cells can be stimulated if the cross-reacting antigen bears a 'foreign' carrier epitope to which the T cells have not been tolerized (Fig. 20.11). The autoimmune process may persist after clearance of the foreign antigen if the activated B cells now focus

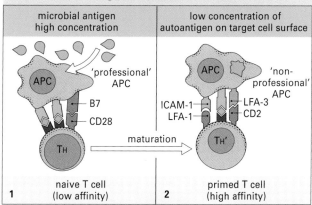

Cross-reactive antigens induce autoimmune TH cells

Fig. 20.10 The inability of naive TH cells to recognize autoantigen on a tissue cell, whether because of low concentration or low affinity, can be circumvented by a cross-reacting microbial antigen at higher concentration or with higher innate affinity, together with a co-stimulator such as B7 on a 'professional' APC; this primes the TH cells (1). Due to increased expression of accessory molecules (e.g. LFA-1 and CD2) the primed TH cells now have high affinity and, because they do not require a co-stimulatory signal, they can interact with autoantigen on 'non-professional' APCs such as organ-specific epithelial cells to produce autoimmune disease (2).

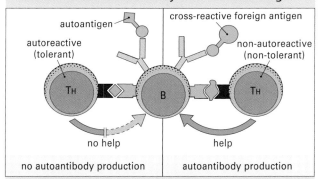

Induction of autoantibodies by cross-reactive antigens

Fig. 20.11 The B cell recognizes an epitope present on autoantigen, but coincidentally present also on a foreign antigen. Normally the B cell presents the autoantigen, but receives no help from autoreactive TH cells, which are functionally deleted. If a cross-reacting foreign antigen is encountered, the B cell can present peptides of this molecule to non-autoreactive T cells and thus be driven to proliferate, differentiate, and secrete autoantibodies.

the autoantigen on their surface receptors and present it to normally resting autoreactive T cells, which will then proliferate and act as helpers for fresh B cell stimulation.

Molecular mimicry operates in rheumatic fever

A disease in which such molecular mimicry operates is rheumatic fever, in which autoantibodies to heart valve antigens can be detected. These develop in a small proportion of individuals several weeks after a streptococcal infection of the throat. Carbohydrate antigens on the streptococci cross-react with an antigen on heart valves, so the infection may bypass T cell self tolerance to heart valve antigens.

Shared B cell epitopes between *Yersinia enterolytica* and the extracellular domain of the thyroid stimulating hormone (TSH) receptor have recently been described.

There may also be cross-reactivity between HLA-B27 and certain strains of *Klebsiella* in connection with ankylosing spondylitis, and cross-reactivity between bacterial heat-shock proteins and DR4 in relationship to rheumatoid arthritis.

In some cases foreign antigen can directly stimulate autoreactive cells

Another mechanism to bypass the tolerant autoreactive TH cell is where antigen or another stimulator directly triggers the autoreactive effector cells.

For example, lipopolysaccharide or Epstein–Barr virus causes direct B cell stimulation and some of the clones of activated cells will produce autoantibodies, though in the absence of T cell help these are normally of low titer and affinity. However, it is conceivable that an activated B cell might pick up and process its cognate autoantigen and present it to a naive autoreactive T cell.

Cytokine dysregulation, inappropriate MHC expression, and failure of suppression may induce autoimmunity

It appears that dysregulation of the cytokine network can also lead to activation of autoreactive T cells.

One experimental demonstration of this is the introduction of a transgene for interferon-γ (IFNγ) into pancreatic β-islet cells. If the transgene for IFNγ is fully expressed in the cells, MHC class II genes are upregulated and autoimmune destruction of the islet cells results. This is not simply a result of a non-specific chaotic IFNγ-induced local inflammatory milieu because normal islets grafted at a separate site are rejected, implying clearly that T cell autoreactivity to the pancreas has been established.

The surface expression of MHC class II in itself is not sufficient to activate the naive autoreactive T cells, but it may be necessary to allow a cell to act as a target for the primed autoreactive TH cells. It was therefore most exciting when cells taken from the glands of patients with Graves' disease were found to be actively synthesizing class II MHC molecules (Fig. 20.12) and so were able to be recognized by CD4⁺ T cells.

In this context it is interesting that isolated cells from several animal strains that are susceptible to autoimmunity are also more readily induced by IFNγ to express MHC class II molecules than cells from non-susceptible strains.

The argument that imbalanced cytokine production may also contribute to autoimmunity receives further support from the unexpected finding that tumor necrosis factor (TNF; introduced by means of a TNF transgene) ameliorates the spontaneous SLE of F₁ (NZB × NZW) mice.

Human thyroid sections stained for MHC class II

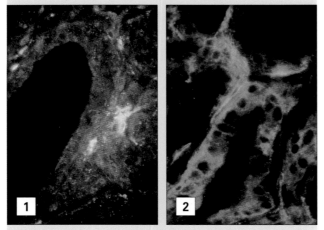

Fig. 20.12 (1) Normal thyroid with unstained follicular cells, and an isolated dendritic cell that is strongly positive for MHC class II. (2) Thyrotoxic (Graves' disease) thyroid with abundant MHC class II molecules in the cytoplasm, indicating that rapid synthesis of MHC class II molecules is occurring.

Defects in the cytokine/hypothalamic–pituitary–adrenal feedback loop in autoimmunity

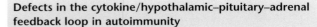
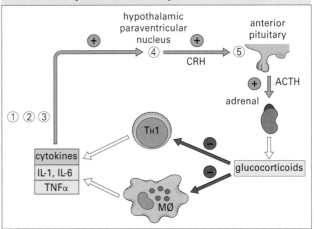

Fig. 20.13 Production of IL-1 is defective in the NOD mouse (1) and diabetes-prone BB rat (2); the disease can be corrected by injection of the cytokine. The same is true for the production of TNFα by the NZB × W lupus mouse (3). Patients with rheumatoid arthritis have a poor hypothalamic response to IL-1 and IL-6 (4). The hypothalamic–pituitary axis is defective in the Obese strain chicken and in the Lewis rat, which is prone to the development of Freund's adjuvant-mediated experimental autoimmune disease (5). (CRH, corticotropin releasing hormone; MØ, macrophage)

Aside from the normal 'ignorance' of cryptic self epitopes, other factors that normally restrain potentially autoreactive cells may include:

- regulatory T cells;
- hormones (e.g. steroids);
- cytokines (e.g. transforming growth factor-β [TGFβ]); and
- products of macrophages.

Deficiencies in any of these factors may increase susceptibility to autoimmunity.

The feedback loop on TH cells and macrophages through the pituitary–adrenal axis is particularly interesting because defects at different stages in the loop turn up in a variety of autoimmune disorders (Fig. 20.13).

For example, patients with rheumatoid arthritis have low circulating corticosteroid levels compared with controls. After surgery, although they produce copious amounts of IL-1 and IL-6, a defect in the hypothalamic paraventricular nucleus prevents the expected increase in adrenocorticotropin (ACTH) and adrenal steroid output.

There is currently intense interest focused on the role of Tregs. Patients with rheumatoid arthritis, for example, reveal a deficiency of Treg function (see below and Fig. 20.24).

A subset of CD4 regulatory cells present in young healthy mice of the NOD strain, which spontaneously develop IDDM, can prevent the transfer of disease provoked by injection of spleen cells from diabetic animals into NOD mice congenic for the severe combined immunodeficiency trait; this regulatory subset is lost in older mice. Prevention of disease in lupus-prone mice by targeting the FcγRIIb inhibitory receptor on B cells points to yet another potential regulatory defect predisposing to immune complex disease.

Pre-existing defects in the target organ may increase susceptibility to autoimmunity

We have already alluded to the undue sensitivity of target cells to upregulation of MHC class II molecules by IFNγ in animals susceptible to certain autoimmune diseases. Other evidence also favors the view that there may be a pre-existing defect in the target organ.

In the Obese strain chicken model of spontaneous thyroid autoimmunity, not only is there a low threshold of IFNγ induction of MHC class II expression by thymocytes, but when endogenous TSH is suppressed by thyroxine treatment, the uptake of iodine into the thyroid glands is far higher in the Obese strain than in a variety of normal strains. Furthermore, this is not due to any stimulating effect of the autoimmunity because immuno-suppressed animals show even higher uptakes of iodine (Fig. 20.14).

Interestingly, the Cornell strain (from which the Obese strain was derived by breeding) shows even higher uptakes of iodine, yet these animals do not develop spontaneous thyroiditis. This could be indicative of a type of abnormal thyroid behavior, which in itself is insufficient to induce autoimmune disease, but does contribute to susceptibility in the Obese strain.

Other situations in which the production of autoantigen is affected are:

- diabetes mellitus, in which one of the genetic risk factors is associated with a microsatellite marker lying

Thyroid ¹³¹I uptake in TSH-suppressed chickens

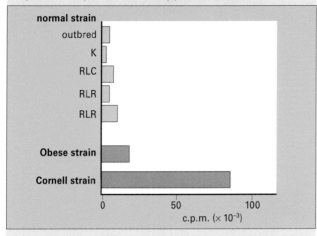

Fig. 20.14 Thyroid ¹³¹I uptake in Obese strain chickens and in the related Cornell strain is abnormally high compared with that in normal strains. Endogenous TSH production was suppressed by administration of thyroxine; therefore the experiment measured TSH-independent ¹³¹I uptake. Values were far higher than normal in Obese strain chickens, which spontaneously develop thyroid autoimmunity, and even higher in the non-autoimmune Cornell strain from which the Obese strain was bred. This abnormality was not due to immune mechanisms because immunosuppression actually increased ¹³¹I uptake into the thyroid gland.

Upregulation of heat-shock protein 60 in endothelial cells at a site of hemodynamic stress

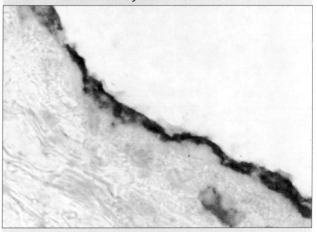

Fig. 20.15 Hsp60 expression (red) co-localized with intercellular adhesion molecule-1 (ICAM-1) expression (black) by endothelial cells and cells in the intima (macrophages) at the bifurcation of the carotid artery of a 5-month-old child. × 240. (Photograph kindly provided by Professor G Wick)

within a transcription factor controlling the rate of insulin production; and
- rheumatoid arthritis, in which the agalacto IgG glycoform is abnormally abundant.

The post-translational modification of arginine to citrulline, producing a new autoantigen in rheumatoid arthritis, represents yet another mechanism by which autoimmunity can be evoked.

Q. What evidence from rheumatoid arthritis supports the view that autoimmune diseases have a multifactorial etiology?

A. Defects in hypothalamic feedback, Tregs and post-translational modification of antigens (glycosylation and citrulline formation) as well as a strong MHC association have all been identified.

The following intriguing observations hint strongly at an autoimmune contribution to the pathology of the atherosclerosis:
- immunization with mycobacterial heat-shock protein 65 (hsp65) elicits atherosclerotic lesions at classical predilection sites subject to major hemodynamic stress; and
- patients with atherosclerosis produce antibodies to human hsp60, which react with heat or TNFα-stressed endothelial cells.

Particularly relevant to the present discussion is the finding of upregulated hsp60 expression at such critical sites even in a 5-month-old child (Fig. 20.15).

Again, one must re-emphasize the considerable importance of multiple factors in the establishment of prolonged autoimmunity.

IN MOST DISEASES ASSOCIATED WITH AUTOIMMUNITY, THE AUTOIMMUNE PROCESS PRODUCES THE LESIONS

Autoimmune processes are often pathogenic. When autoantibodies are found in association with a particular disease there are three possible inferences:
- the autoimmunity is responsible for producing the lesions of the disease;
- there is a disease process that, through the production of tissue damage, leads to the development of auto-antibodies;
- there is a factor that produces both the lesions and the autoimmunity.

Autoantibodies secondary to a lesion (the second possibility) are sometimes found. For example, cardiac autoantibodies may develop after myocardial infarction.

However, sustained production of autoantibodies rarely follows the release of autoantigens by simple trauma. In most diseases associated with autoimmunity, the evidence supports the first possibility, that the autoimmune process produces the lesions.

The pathogenic role of autoimmunity can be demonstrated in experimental models
Examples of induced autoimmunity
The most direct test of whether autoimmunity is responsible for the lesions of disease is to induce autoimmunity deliberately in an experimental animal and see if this leads to the production of the lesions.

Autoimmunity can be induced in experimental animals by injecting autoantigen (self antigen) together with complete Freund's adjuvant, and this does indeed produce organ-specific disease in certain organs. For example:

- thyroglobulin injection can induce an inflammatory disease of the thyroid;
- MBP can cause encephalomyelitis.

In the case of thyroglobulin-injected animals, not only are thyroid autoantibodies produced, but the gland becomes infiltrated with mononuclear cells and the acinar architecture crumbles, closely resembling the histology of Hashimoto's thyroiditis.

THE ABILITY TO INDUCE EXPERIMENTAL AUTOIMMUNE DISEASE DEPENDS ON THE STRAIN OF ANIMAL USED –
For example, it is found that the susceptibility of rats and mice to MBP-induced encephalomyelitis depends on a small number of gene loci, of which the most important are the MHC class II genes.

MBP-induced encephalomyelitis can be induced in susceptible strains by injecting T cells specific for MBP. These pathogenic T cells belong to the CD4/TH1 subset. It has been found that induction of disease can be prevented by treating the recipients with antibody to CD4 just before the expected time of disease onset, blocking the interaction of the TH cells' CD4 with the class II MHC molecules of antigen-presenting target cells (see Chapter 5).

The results indicate the importance of class II-restricted autoreactive TH cells in the development of these conditions, and emphasize the prominent role of the MHC.

Examples of spontaneous autoimmunity
It has proved possible to breed strains of animals that are genetically programmed to develop autoimmune diseases closely resembling their human counterparts.

One well-established example mentioned above is the Obese strain chicken, which parallels human autoimmune thyroid disease in terms of:

- the lesion in the gland;
- the production of antibodies to different components in the thyroid; and
- the overlap with gastric autoimmunity.

So it is of interest that, when the immunological status of Obese strain chickens is altered, quite dramatic effects are seen on the outcome of the disease. For example:

- removal of the thymus at birth appears to exacerbate the thyroiditis, suggesting that the thymus exerts a controlling effect on the disease through Tregs; but
- if the entire T cell population is abrogated by combining thymectomy with massive injections of anti-chick T cell serum, both autoantibody production and the attack on thyroid are completely inhibited.

T cells therefore play a variety of pivotal roles as mediators and regulators of this disease.

More directly, a diabetogenic CD4+ T cell clone can induce the chronic leukocytic infiltrate of T cells and macrophages, which damages the insulin-producing β cells of the pancreatic islets of Langerhans in the NOD murine model of IDDM (Fig. 20.16).

The role of the T cells in mediating this attack is further emphasized by the amelioration and prevention of disease by treatment of the mice with a non-depleting anti-CD4 monoclonal antibody, which in the presence of the pancreatic autoantigens, insulin, and glutamic acid decarboxylase (GAD) induces specific T cell anergy.

The dependence of yet another spontaneous model, the F_1 hybrid of New Zealand Black and White strains, on the operation of immunological processes is aptly revealed by the suppression of the murine SLE, which characterizes this strain, by treatment with anti-CD4 (Fig. 20.17).

Human autoantibodies can be directly pathogenic
When investigating human autoimmunity directly rather than using animal models, it is of course more difficult to carry out experiments. Nevertheless, there is much evidence to suggest that autoantibodies may be important in pathogenesis, and we will discuss the major examples here.

Autoantibodies can give rise to a wide spectrum of clinical thyroid dysfunction
A number of diseases have been recognized in which autoantibodies to hormone receptors may actually mimic the function of the normal hormone concerned and produce disease. Graves' disease (thyrotoxicosis) was the first disorder in which such **anti-receptor antibodies** were clearly recognized.

The phenomenon of neonatal thyrotoxicosis provides us with a natural 'passive transfer' study, because the IgG antibodies from the thyrotoxic mother cross the placenta and react directly with the TSH receptor on the neonatal thyroid. Many babies born to thyrotoxic mothers and showing thyroid hyperactivity have been reported, but the problem spontaneously resolves as the antibodies derived from the mother are catabolized in the baby over several weeks.

Whereas autoantibodies to the TSH receptor may stimulate cell division and/or increase the production of thyroid hormones, others can bring about the opposite effect by inhibiting these functions, a phenomenon frequently observed in receptor responses to ligands that act as agonists or antagonists.

Different combinations of the various manifestations of thyroid autoimmune disease – chronic inflammatory cell destruction, and stimulation or inhibition of growth and thyroid hormone synthesis – can give rise to a wide spectrum of clinical thyroid dysfunction (Fig. 20.18).

A variety of other diseases are associated with autoantibodies
A parallel with neonatal hyperthyroidism has been observed – **antibodies to acetylcholine receptors** from mothers who have myasthenia gravis cross the placenta into the fetus and may cause transient muscle weakness in the newborn baby.

Somewhat rarely, **autoantibodies to insulin receptors and to α-adrenergic receptors** can be found, the latter associated with bronchial asthma.

Destruction of β cells in the pancreatic islets of Langerhans in the non-obese diabetic mouse by a diabetogenic T cell clone

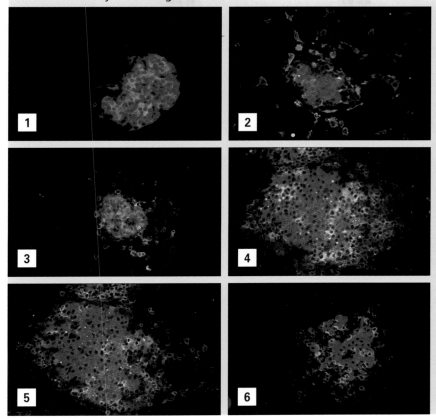

Fig. 20.16 NOD neonates were injected with the diabetogenic CD4+ T cell clone, BDC2.5. The cells infiltrated the pancreas and there was recruitment of other NOD cells. Of the neonates that receive this clone 80% become diabetic within 20 days. Snap-frozen pancreas sections taken from representative neonates killed 10 days after transfer of BDC2.5, before the onset of overt diabetes, were stained for insulin (red fluorescence) and infiltrating cells (green fluorescence). (**1**) Section from a normal NOD neonate showing an islet, but no infiltration of CD3+ T cells. Other sections show islets infiltrated with (**2**) macrophages (F4/80+), (**3**) B cells (B220+), (**4**) CD3+ T cells, (**5**) CD4+ T cells, and (**6**) CD8+ T cells, this section showing serious loss of insulin producing cells. × 400. (Figures generously provided by Drs Jenny Phillips and Anne Cooke)

Neuromuscular defects can be elicited in mice injected with serum containing **antibodies to presynaptic calcium channels** from patients with the Lambert–Eaton syndrome, while **sodium channel autoantibodies** have been identified in the Guillain–Barré syndrome.

Yet another example of autoimmune disease is seen in rare cases of male infertility where **antibodies to spermatozoa** lead to clumping of spermatozoa, either by their heads or by their tails, in the semen.

In pernicious anemia an autoantibody interferes with the normal uptake of vitamin B$_{12}$

Vitamin B$_{12}$ is not absorbed directly, but must first associate with a protein called intrinsic factor; the vitamin–protein complex is then transported across the intestinal mucosa.

Early passive transfer studies demonstrated that serum from a patient with pernicious anemia (PA), if fed to a healthy individual together with intrinsic factor–B$_{12}$ complex, inhibited uptake of the vitamin.

Subsequently, the factor in the serum that blocked vitamin uptake was identified as **antibody against intrinsic factor**. It is now known that plasma cells in the gastric mucosa of patients with PA secrete this antibody into the lumen of the stomach (Fig. 20.19).

Antibodies to the glomerular capillary basement membrane cause Goodpasture's syndrome

In Goodpasture's syndrome, **antibodies to the glomerular capillary basement membrane** bind to the kidney in vivo (see Fig. 25.3). To demonstrate that the antibodies can have a pathological effect, a passive transfer experiment was performed. The antibodies were eluted from the kidney of a patient who had died from this disease, and injected into primates whose kidney antigens were sufficiently similar for the injected antibodies to localize on the glomerular basement membrane. The injected monkeys subsequently died from glomerulonephritis.

Blood and vascular disorders caused by autoantibodies include AHA and ITP

Autoimmune hemolytic anemia (AHA) and idiopathic thrombocytopenic purpura (ITP) result from the synthesis of **autoantibodies to red cells and platelets**, respectively.

The primary antiphospholipid syndrome characterized by recurrent thromboembolic phenomena and fetal loss is triggered by the reaction of **autoantibodies with a complex of β$_2$-glycoprotein 1 and cardiolipin**.

The β$_2$-glycoprotein turns up again as an abundant component of atherosclerotic plaques, and there is

Suppression of autoimmune disease

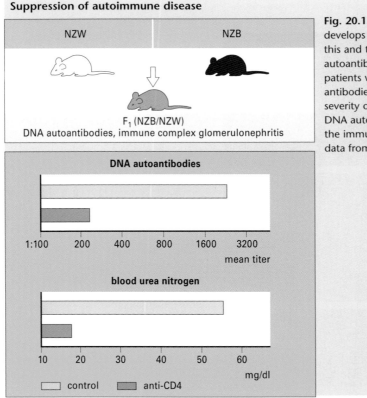

Fig. 20.17 The New Zealand Black (NZB) mouse spontaneously develops autoimmune hemolytic anaemia. The hybrid between this and the New Zealand White (NZW) strain develops DNA autoantibodies and immune complex glomerulonephritis, as in patients with SLE. Immunosuppression with monoclonal antibodies to the TH cell marker CD4 considerably reduced the severity of the glomerulonephritis and the titer of double-stranded DNA autoantibodies at 8 months of age, showing the relevance of the immune processes to the generation of the disease. (Based on data from Wofsy D, Seaman WE. J Exp Med 1985;161:378)

The spectrum of autoimmune thyroid disease

thyroid disease	thyroid destruction	cell division		thyroid hormone synthesis	
		stimulation	inhibition	stimulation	inhibition
Hashimoto's thyroiditis					
Hashimoto's persistent goiter					
autoimmune colloid goiter					
Graves' disease					
non-goitrous hyperthyroidism					
'hashitoxicosis'					
primary myxedema					

Fig. 20.18 Responses involving thyroglobulin and the thyroid peroxidase (microsomal) surface microvillous antigen lead to tissue destruction, whereas autoantibodies to TSH (and other?) receptors can stimulate or block metabolic activity or thyroid cell division. 'Hashitoxicosis' is an unconventional term that describes a gland showing Hashimoto's thyroiditis and Graves' disease simultaneously.

increasing attention to the idea that autoimmunity may initiate or exacerbate the process of lipid deposition and plaque formation in this disease, the two lead candidate antigens being **heat-shock protein 60** (cf. Fig. 20.15) and the low density lipoprotein, **apoprotein B**.

The necrotizing granulomatous vasculitis that characterizes Wegener's granulomatosis is associated with **antibodies to neutrophil cytoplasmic proteinase III (cANCA)**, but their role in the pathogenesis of the vasculitis is ill defined.

Immune complexes appear to be pathogenic in systemic autoimmunity

In the case of SLE, it can be shown that complement-fixing complexes of antibody with DNA and other nucleosome components such as histones are deposited in the

Failure of vitamin B₁₂ absorption in pernicious anemia

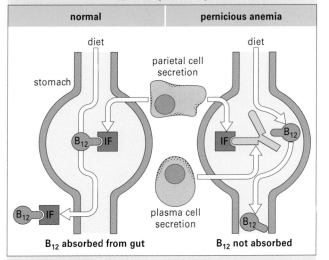

Fig. 20.19 Normally, dietary vitamin B₁₂ is absorbed by the small intestine as a complex with intrinsic factor (IF), which is synthesized by parietal cells in gastric mucosa. In PA, locally synthesized autoantibodies, specific for intrinsic factor, combine with intrinsic factor to inhibit its role as a carrier for vitamin B₁₂.

kidney (see Fig. 25.3), skin, joints, and choroid plexus of patients, and must be presumed to produce type III hypersensitivity reactions as outlined in Chapters 24 and 25.

Cationic anti-DNA antibodies and histones facilitate the binding to heparin sulfate in the connective tissue structures.

Individuals with genetic deficiency of the early classical pathway complement components clear circulating immune complexes very poorly and are unduly susceptible to the development of SLE.

Turning to the experimental models, we have already mentioned the (NZB × NZW) F₁, which spontaneously develops murine SLE associated with immune complex glomerulonephritis and anti-DNA autoantibodies as major features (see Fig. 20.17). Measures that suppress the immune response in these animals (e.g. treatment with azathioprine or anti-CD4) also suppress the disease and prolong survival, adding to the evidence for autoimmune reactions causing such disease.

The erosions of cartilage and bone in rheumatoid arthritis are mediated by macrophages and fibroblasts, which become stimulated by cytokines from activated T cells and immune complexes generated by a vigorous immunological reaction within the synovial tissue (Fig. 20.20).

The complexes can arise through the self-association of IgG rheumatoid factors specific for the Fcγ domains – a process facilitated by the striking deficiency of terminal galactose on the biantennary N-linked Fc oligosaccharides (Fig. 20.21). This agalacto glycoform of IgG in complexes

can exacerbate inflammatory reactions through reaction with mannose-binding lectin and production of TNF.

Evidence for directly pathogenic T cells in human autoimmune disease is hard to obtain

Adoptive transfer studies have shown that TH1 cells are responsible for directly initiating the lesions in experimental models of organ-specific autoimmunity.

In the human, factors that make it abundantly clear that T cells are utterly pivotal for the development of autoimmune disease include:

- the production of high-affinity, somatically mutated IgG autoantibodies characteristic of T-dependent responses;
- the isolation of thyroid-specific T cell clones from the glands of patients with Graves' disease;
- the beneficial effect of ciclosporin in prediabetic individuals; and
- the close associations with certain HLA haplotypes.

However, it is difficult to identify a role for the T cell as a pathogenic agent as distinct from a T helper function in the organ-specific disorders.

Indirect evidence from circumstances showing that antibodies themselves do not cause disease, such as in babies born to mothers with IDDM, may be indicative.

Autoantibodies have diagnostic and prognostic value

Whatever the relationship of autoantibodies to the disease process, they frequently provide valuable markers for diagnostic purposes. A particularly good example is the test for mitochondrial antibodies, used in diagnosing primary biliary cirrhosis (Fig. 20.22). Exploratory laparotomy was previously needed to obtain this diagnosis, and was often hazardous because of the age and condition of the patients concerned.

Autoantibodies often have predictive value. For instance, individuals testing positively for antibodies to both insulin and glutamic acid decarboxylase have a high risk of developing IDDM.

MANY AUTOIMMUNE DISEASES CAN BE TREATED SUCCESSFULLY

Often, in organ-specific autoimmune disorders, the symptoms can be corrected by metabolic control. For example:

- hypothyroidism can be controlled by administration of thyroxine;
- thyrotoxicosis can be controlled by administration of antithyroid drugs;
- in pernicious anemia, metabolic correction is achieved by injection of vitamin B₁₂;
- in myasthenia gravis metabolic correction is achieved by administration of cholinesterase inhibitors.

If the target organ is not completely destroyed, it may be possible to protect the surviving cells by transfection with *FasL* or *TGFβ* genes.

Where function is completely lost and cannot be substituted by hormones, as may occur in lupus nephritis or chronic rheumatoid arthritis, tissue grafts or mechanical

Pathology of rheumatoid arthritis

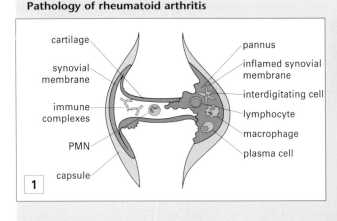

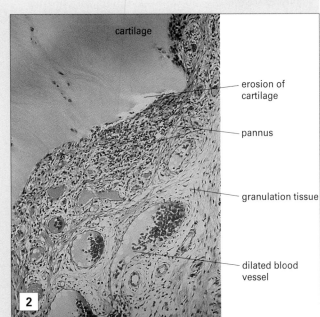

Fig. 20.20 In the rheumatoid arthritis joint an inflammatory infiltrate is found in the synovial membrane, which hypertrophies forming a 'pannus' (**1** and **2**). This covers and eventually erodes the synovial cartilage and bone. Immune complexes and neutrophils (PMNs) are detectable in the joint space and in the extra-articular tissues where they may give rise to vasculitic lesions and subcutaneous nodules. (Histological section reproduced from Woolf N. Pathology: basic and systemic. London: W.B. Saunders; 1998)

Self-associated IgG rheumatoid factors forming immune complexes

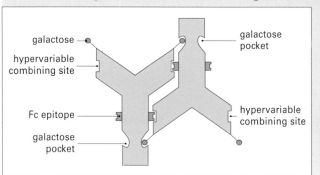

Fig. 20.21 The binding between the Fab on one IgG rheumatoid factor and the Fc of another involves the hypervariable region of the combining site. As it has been established that the Fab oligosaccharides, which occur on approximately one in three different immunoglobulin molecules, are not defective with respect to glycosylation in rheumatoid arthritis, a Fab galactose residue could become inserted in the Fc pocket left vacant by a galactose-deficient $C\gamma2$ oligosaccharide, so increasing the strength of intermolecular binding. The stability and inflammatory potency of these complexes is increased by binding IgM rheumatoid factor and C1q.

substitutes may be appropriate. In the case of tissue grafts, protection from the immunological processes that necessitated the transplant may be required.

Conventional immunosuppressive therapy with antimitotic drugs at high doses can be used to damp down the immune response, but, because of the dangers involved, tends to be used only in life-threatening disorders such as SLE and dermatomyositis.

The potential of ciclosporin and related drugs such as rapamycin has yet to be fully realized, but quite dramatic results have been reported in the treatment of type 1 diabetes mellitus.

Anti-inflammatory drugs are, of course, prescribed for rheumatoid diseases, with the introduction of selective cyclo-oxygenase-2 (COX-2) inhibitors representing a new development.

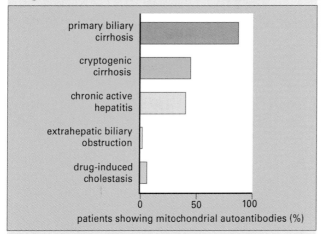

Diagnostic value of anti-mitochondrial antibodies

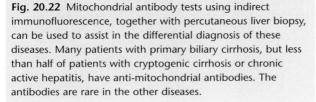

patients showing mitochondrial autoantibodies (%)

Fig. 20.22 Mitochondrial antibody tests using indirect immunofluorescence, together with percutaneous liver biopsy, can be used to assist in the differential diagnosis of these diseases. Many patients with primary biliary cirrhosis, but less than half of patients with cryptogenic cirrhosis or chronic active hepatitis, have anti-mitochondrial antibodies. The antibodies are rare in the other diseases.

Encouraging results are being obtained by the treatment of patients with rheumatoid arthritis with low corticosteroid doses at an early stage to correct the apparently defective production of these corticosteroids by the adrenal feedback loop. For those with more established disease, attention is now focused on the striking remissions achieved by synergistic treatment with anti-

TNFα monoclonal antibody plus methotrexate (Fig. 20.23). It is fascinating to record that the compromised regulatory T cell function in the patients is reversed by such therapy (Fig. 20.24).

Less well-established approaches to treatment may become practicable

As we understand more about the precise defects, and learn how to manipulate the immunological status of the patient, some less well-established approaches may become practicable (Fig. 20.25):

- several centers are trying out autologous stem cell transplantation following hematoimmunoablation with cytotoxic drugs for patients with severe SLE, scleroderma, and rheumatoid arthritis;
- a draconian reduction in the T cells in multiple sclerosis by Campath-1H (anti-CD52) and of the B cell population with anti-CD20 in rheumatoid arthritis and SLE (Fig. 20.26) are giving particularly encouraging results;
- treatment with Campath-1H followed by a non-depleting anti-CD4 has produced excellent remissions in patients with Wegener's granulomatosis who were refractory to normal treatment;
- in an attempt to establish antigen-specific suppression, considerable clinical improvement has been achieved in exacerbating–remitting multiple sclerosis by repeated injection of Cop 1, a random copolymer of alanine, glutamic acid, lysine, and tyrosine meant to simulate the postulated 'guilty' autoantigen, MBP.

Some experimental autoimmune diseases have been treated successfully by:
- feeding antigen to induce oral tolerance;
- the inhalation of autoantigenic peptides and their analogs; and

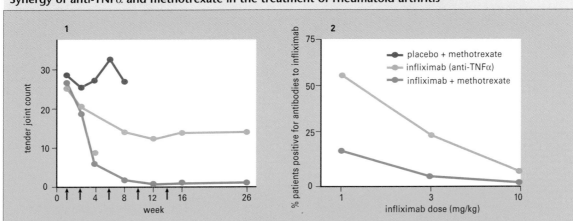

Synergy of anti-TNFα and methotrexate in the treatment of rheumatoid arthritis

Fig. 20.23 (1) Infusions were given at times indicated by the arrows. Median joint scores were more effectively reduced by a combination of anti-TNFα with methotrexate, which (2) eliminated the anti-idiotypic response to infliximab (a humanized anti-TNFα monoclonal antibody). (Data reproduced from Maini RN, et al. Arthritis Rheum 1998;41:1552, with permission of the authors and publishers)

Reversal of compromised regulatory T cell function in rheumatoid arthritis by anti-TNFα therapy

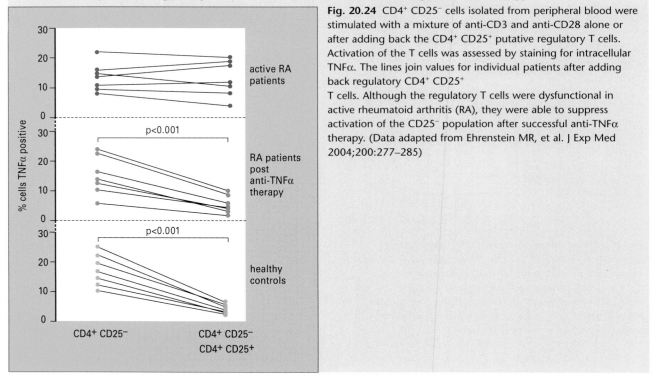

Fig. 20.24 CD4⁺ CD25⁻ cells isolated from peripheral blood were stimulated with a mixture of anti-CD3 and anti-CD28 alone or after adding back the CD4⁺ CD25⁺ putative regulatory T cells. Activation of the T cells was assessed by staining for intracellular TNFα. The lines join values for individual patients after adding back regulatory CD4⁺ CD25⁺ T cells. Although the regulatory T cells were dysfunctional in active rheumatoid arthritis (RA), they were able to suppress activation of the CD25⁻ population after successful anti-TNFα therapy. (Data adapted from Ehrenstein MR, et al. J Exp Med 2004;200:277–285)

Current and potential treatment of autoimmune disease

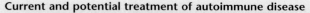
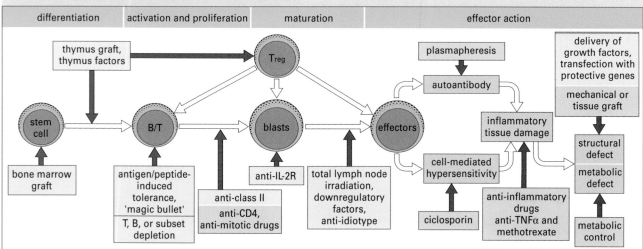

Fig. 20.25 Current treatments for arresting the pathological developments in autoimmune disease are given in blue boxes, and those that may become practicable in green boxes. Anti-mitotic drugs are given in severe cases of SLE or chronic active hepatitis, and anti-inflammatory drugs are widely prescribed in rheumatoid arthritis. Organ-specific disorders (e.g. primary myxedema) can be treated by supplying the defective component (e.g. thyroid hormone). When a live graft is necessary, immunosuppressive therapy can protect the tissue from damage.

Efficacy of B cell depletion in systemic lupus erythematosus

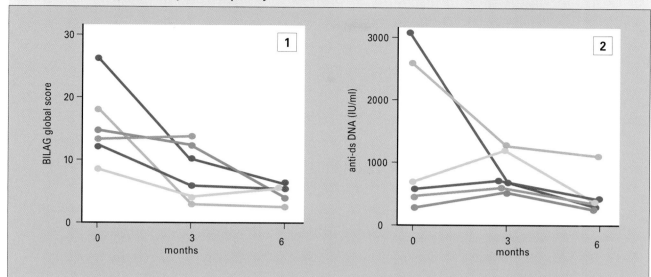

Fig. 20.26 Six female patients with active SLE resistant to standard immunosuppressive therapy were treated on an open-label basis with two infusions of monoclonal anti-CD20 to deplete the B cells, cyclophosphamide, and corticosteroids. Five of the six showed marked clinical improvement as evidenced by reduction of the British Isles Lupus Assessment Group (BILAG) global score (**1**) and significant falls in anti-dsDNA in two patients (**2**). (Data reproduced from Leandro MJ, et al. Arthritis Rheum 2002:46;2673. Copyright 2002 with permission from John Wiley & Sons Inc)

- 'vaccination' with peptides from heat-shock protein 70 or the antigen-specific receptor of autoreactive T cells. This suggests that stimulating normally suppressive functions, including the idiotype network, could be promising.

FURTHER READING

Alt F, Marrack P, eds. Curr Opin Immunol 2003;15(6) and 2004;16 (several critical essays in each annual volume).

Arbuckle MR, McClain MT, Rubertone MV, et al. Development of autoantibodies before the clinical onset of systemic lupus erythematosus. N Engl J Med 2003;349:1526–1533.

Betterle C, Greggio NA, Volpato M. Clinical Review 93: Autoimmune polyglandular syndrome type 1. J Clin Endocrinol Metab 1998;83:1049–1055.

Chapel H, Haeney M, Misbah S, Snowden N. Essentials of clinical immunology, 4th edn. Oxford: Blackwell Science; 1999.

Edwards JC, Szczepanski L, Szechinski J, et al. Efficacy of the novel B cell targeted therapy, rituximab, in patients with active rheumatoid arthritis. N Engl J Med 2004;350:2572–2581.

Keymeulen B, Vandemeulebroucke E, Ziegler AG, et al. Insulin needs after CD3-antibody therapy in new-onset type 1 diabetes. N Engl J Med 2005;352:2598–2608.

McGaha TL, Sorrentino B, Ravetch JV. Restoration of tolerance in lupus targeted inhibiting receptor expression. Science 2005;307:590–593.

Peter JB, Shoenfeld Y, eds. Autoantibodies. Amsterdam: Elsevier; 1996.

Wraith DC, Nicolson KS, Whitely NT. Regulatory CD4+ T cells and the control of autoimmune disease. Curr Opin Immunol 2004;16:695–708.

Critical thinking: Autoimmunity and autoimmune disease (see p. 499 for explanations)

Miss Jacob, a 30-year-old Caribbean woman, was seen in a rheumatology clinic with stiff painful joints in her hands, which were worse first thing in the morning. Other symptoms included fatigue, a low-grade fever, a weight loss of 2 kg, and some mild chest pain. Miss Jacob had recently returned to the UK from a holiday in Jamaica and was also noted to be taking the combined oral contraceptive pill. Past medical history of note was a mild autoimmune hemolytic anemia 2 years previously.

On examination Miss Jacob had a non-specific maculo-papular rash on her face and chest, and patchy alopecia (hair loss) over her scalp. Her mouth was tender and examination revealed an ulcer on the soft palate. She had moderately swollen and tender proximal interphalangeal joints. Her other joints were unaffected, but she had generalized muscle aches. The results of investigations are shown in the table.

investigation	result
radiograph of hands	soft tissue swelling, but no bone erosions
chest radiograph	a small pleural effusion at the right lung base
full blood count	a mild normocytic, normochromic anemia and mild lymphocytopenia
C-reactive protein levels	normal
erythrocyte sedimentation rate	raised
rheumatoid factor	negative
serum IgG levels	raised
anti-nuclear antibodies (ANA)	positive by immunofluorescence
anti-double-stranded DNA, anti-RNA, and anti-histone	positive by ELISA antibodies
complement (C3 and C4) levels	low
skin biopsy from an area unaffected by the rash	deposition of IgG and complement components at the junction between dermis and epidermis (lupus 'band' test)

A diagnosis of systemic lupus erythematosus (SLE) was made. Miss Jacob was treated with chloroquine, an anti-malarial, for the rash on her face and chest.

At a follow-up appointment urinalysis showed protein and red cells. Serum creatinine was mildly elevated as was her blood pressure. A renal biopsy showed membranous lupus nephritis. She was prescribed oral corticosteroids and an antihypertensive agent, which improved her renal function. Her physician also gave advice regarding birth control and pregnancy, and regular check-ups were arranged.

1 What is the immunological mechanism leading to the glomerulonephritis?
2 Are immune complexes the main mediator of systemic damage?
3 What is the mechanism for the vasculitis seen in SLE?
4 Are anti-double-stranded DNA (anti-dsDNA) antibodies pathognomonic of SLE?

Transplantation and Rejection

CHAPTER 21

SUMMARY

- **Transplantation is the only form of treatment** for most end-stage organ failure.

- **The barrier to transplantation** is the genetic disparity between donor and recipient.

- **The immune response in transplantation depends on a variety of factors.** Host versus graft responses cause transplant rejection. Histocompatibility antigens are the targets for rejection. Minor antigens can be targets of rejection even when donor and recipient MHC are identical. Graft versus host reactions result when donor lymphocytes attack the graft recipient.

- **Rejection results from a variety of different immune effector mechanisms.** Hyperacute rejection is immediate and caused by antibody. Acute rejection occurs days to weeks after transplantation. Chronic rejection is seen months or years after transplantation.

- **HLA matching is one of two major methods for preventing rejection of allografts.** The better the HLA matching of donor and recipient, the less the strength of rejection.

- **Successful organ transplantation depends on the use of immunosuppressive drugs.** 6-MP, azathioprine, and MPA are antiproliferative drugs. Ciclosporin, tacrolimus, and sirolimus are inhibitors of T cell activation. Corticosteroids are the anti-inflammatory drugs used for transplant immunosuppression. FTY 720 is a novel immunosuppressive agent under investigation.

- **The ultimate goal in transplantation is to induce donor-specific tolerance.** There is evidence for the induction of tolerance in humans and novel methods for inducing tolerance are being developed. Alloreactive cells can be made anergic. Immune privilege can be a property of the tissue or site of transplant.

- **Shortage of donor organs and chronic rejection limit the success of transplantation.** Living donation is one way to overcome the shortage of donor organs. Alternative approaches are being investigated. The favored animal for xenotransplantation is the pig.

TRANSPLANTATION IS THE ONLY FORM OF TREATMENT FOR MOST END-STAGE ORGAN FAILURE

Transplantation is a central topic for immunologists for two reasons:
- the first is that transplantation is an important clinical procedure;
- the second is that transplantation has proved an important tool for understanding immunological mechanisms – for example, the major histocompatibility complex (MHC; see Chapter 5) was first described in the context of transplantation, and transplantation models continue to be widely used as tools in basic as well as applied immunology.

As a clinical procedure, transplantation is used to replace tissues or organs that have failed. The first successful transplants were those of the cornea, first described in 1906.

Q. Why in retrospect was corneal transplantation more likely to be successful than transplantation of other tissues?
A. The cornea is an immunologically privileged site (see Figs 12.3–12.5).

World War II provided an important impetus, with the problems of skin grafting airmen who had extensive burns motivating a number of scientists, most notably Peter Medawar, to investigate the immunological basis of graft rejection.

The subsequent demonstration by the Medawar group that it was possible to manipulate a recipient animal so that it accepted grafts from an unrelated donor animal encouraged the subsequent clinical development of transplantation. The discovery (by Calne and others) of immunosuppressive drugs and agents then allowed the

Clinical transplantation

organ transplanted	examples of disease
cornea	keratoconus, dystrophies, keratitis
kidney	end-stage renal disease
heart	heart failure
lung/heart–lung	pulmonary hypertension, cystic fibrosis
liver	cancer, cirrhosis, biliary atresia
stem cells (bone marrow/peripheral blood)	leukemia, immunodeficiency
skin (autografts)	burns
pancreas	diabetes mellitus
pancreatic islets	diabetes mellitus
small bowel	cancer, intestinal failure
neuronal cells	Parkinson's disease

Fig. 21.1 Organs and tissues shown in blue are routinely transplanted to treat various conditions. Transplantation of other organs (shown in yellow) is being developed, but has yet to be routinely applied in most centers.

widespread practice of transplantation in the last three to four decades of the 20th century.

In modern practice many transplants are performed routinely (Fig. 21.1). In addition to routine transplantation of the cornea, kidney, heart, lungs, and liver there is increasing interest in transplanting other organs, such as whole pancreas or islet cells for diabetes mellitus and also small bowel.

In general most transplants use organs from dead donors (**cadaveric transplants**), though there is an increasing number of living donors (usually related to the recipients) for kidney transplantation.

In addition to transplantation of organs, there is a large program of transplanting hematopoietic stem cells (cells capable of regenerating blood cells), for example in patients with leukemia or with primary immune deficiencies. These stem cells were previously normally harvested from the bone marrow of (living) donors, though increasingly peripheral stem cells obtained from the blood are used. As discussed below, stem cell transplantation has its own particular problems.

THE BARRIER TO TRANSPLANTATION IS THE GENETIC DISPARITY BETWEEN DONOR AND RECIPIENT

The main immunological problem with transplantation is that the grafted organ or tissue is seen by the immune system as 'foreign' and is recognized and attacked – leading to rejection of the organ.

Transplantation is normally performed between individuals of the same species who are not genetically identical, and the antigenic differences are known as **allogeneic differences**, and result in an **allospecific immune response** (Fig. 21.2).

However, it is also possible in experimental circumstances (and possibly in the future in the clinical setting) to perform grafting between different species. This is termed **xenotransplantation**, and the antigenic differences between donor and recipient form the **xenogeneic barrier**.

Transplantation can also be performed within an individual (e.g. skin grafting), when it is known as an **autograft**.

Syngeneic or **isografts** can be performed between genetically identical individuals. This can occur clinically for identical twins, but is more commonly seen in experimental settings with inbred strains of animals.

In the case of autografts and isografts there should be no antigenic differences between donor and recipient, and so no immune response. This can be readily illustrated using transplantation of skin or organs between inbred strains of animals (Fig. 21.3).

Genetic barriers to transplantation

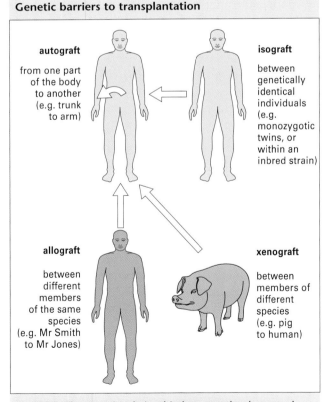

autograft
from one part of the body to another (e.g. trunk to arm)

isograft
between genetically identical individuals (e.g. monozygotic twins, or within an inbred strain)

allograft
between different members of the same species (e.g. Mr Smith to Mr Jones)

xenograft
between members of different species (e.g. pig to human)

Fig. 21.2 The genetic relationship between the donor and recipient determines whether or not rejection will occur. Autografts or isografts are usually accepted, whereas allografts and xenografts are not.

Host versus graft reactions

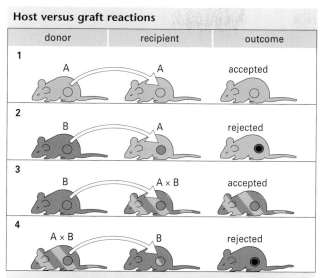

Fig. 21.3 Grafts between genetically identical animals are accepted. Grafts between genetically non-identical animals are rejected with a speed that is dependent on where the genetic differences lie. For example, syngeneic animals that are identical at the MHC locus accept grafts from each other (**1**). Animals that differ at the MHC locus reject grafts from each other (**2**). The ability to accept a graft is dependent on the recipient sharing all the donor's histocompatibility genes; this is illustrated by the difference between grafting from parental to (A × B) F$_1$ animals (**3**) and vice versa (**4**). Animals that differ at loci other than the MHC reject graft from each other, but much more slowly.

THE IMMUNE RESPONSE RESULTS IN GRAFT REJECTION
Host versus graft responses cause transplant rejection

Immune recognition of the antigenic differences between the donor organ and the recipient will, unless treated, lead to an immune response in which the host immune system responds to, and attacks, the donor tissue.

Q. What are the main genetic differences that are recognized by the host, and why should this be so?
A. Differences in MHC molecule allotypes are most important. The reason is that all nucleated cells express MHC molecules, and the T cell receptor on host T cells has a basic structure that interacts with and recognizes MHC molecules. Also the MHC class I and class II molecules have an extremely high level of genetic variability (see Chapter 5).

The nature of the host versus graft response is discussed in more detail below.

Similar to any other adaptive immune response, the immune response against a graft shows memory of previous encounters with an antigen. Therefore, once an animal has rejected an organ graft for the first time, if a second graft is performed from the same species or donor then it is rejected more rapidly (**second set rejection**).

There is a high frequency of T cells recognizing the graft

One of the main features of the immune response against a transplanted organ is that it is much more vigorous and strong than the response seen against a pathogen, such as a virus. This is largely reflected by the frequency of T cells that recognize the graft as foreign and react against it.

Thus, in a naive or unimmunized individual fewer than 1/100 000 T cells respond upon exposure to a virus or a protein immunization; however, 1/100–1/1000 T cells respond to allogeneic antigen-presenting cells (APCs).

This difference can be seen using a mixed lymphocyte reaction, in which T cells are taken from one individual and mixed with APCs from another. The proliferation of the T cells can then be measured (usually by measuring the incorporation of radioactive ^{3}H-thymidine) (Fig. 21.4). This will usually result in a strong proliferation of the T cells.

Measuring the strength of the alloresponse

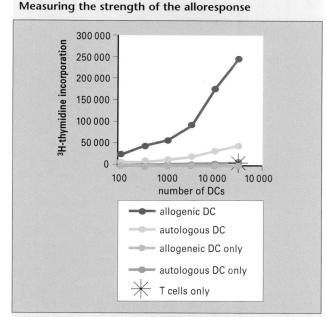

Fig. 21.4 The strength of the alloresponse can be measured in a mixed lymphocyte response. In this assay T cells from an individual were mixed with varying numbers of dendritic cells (DCs) (the most potent form of APCs) from either the same (autologous dendritic cells) or a different (allogeneic dendritic cells) donor. The dendritic cells were irradiated to prevent their proliferation. As a control cultures were included that contained just the dendritic cells or just the T cells. Five days later the cultures were pulsed with ^{3}H-thymidine, which is incorporated into the DNA of dividing cells. After 16 hours the amount of radioactive thymidine in the cells, a measure of the amount they have proliferated, is determined. As can be seen there is strong proliferation of T cells exposed to allogeneic dendritic cells, even though these T cells have not been exposed to the allogeneic cells, so this represents a primary immune response.

However, if the same experiment is performed using APCs and T cells from the same individual, and if a virus or a protein antigen is added, then no or little T cell proliferation is seen unless that person has been previously exposed to the antigen and so has a higher frequency of (memory) T cells capable of recognizing it.

Histocompatibility antigens are the targets for rejection

Early experiments showed that the bulk of the allospecific response is against molecules of the MHC. We now know that these molecules are the MHC class I or class II molecules (see Chapter 5), which are responsible for presenting antigen (in the form of peptides) to either:

- CD8 T cells (MHC class I); or
- CD4 cells (MHC class II).

As discussed in Chapter 7, MHC molecules are highly polymorphic, and it is these polymorphic differences that are seen by alloreactive T cells.

Why is there such a high frequency of allospecific T cells?

Several models seek to explain why there is such a high frequency of allospecific cells in the T cell repertoire.

The first model (**high determinant density model**) (Fig. 21.5) suggests that allospecific T cells recognize the foreign MHC molecules directly, with a low affinity, in a peptide-independent manner. The affinity of the interaction would normally be too low to activate the T cells; however, because the T cells see the MHC molecules directly, and are not recognizing the peptide, this low affinity is compensated for by the high concentration of MHC molecules on allogeneic cells.

The second model (**multiple determinant model**) states that what the allospecific T cells are recognizing are peptides derived from normal, non-polymorphic, host proteins that bind to and are presented by the foreign MHC molecules, but are not presented by self MHC. Due to lack of presentation by self MHC, the T cell repertoire is not tolerant to such peptides. The high frequency of the response is due to the large number of such antigens that can be presented by the graft.

Indirect recognition is important in chronic rejection

In a primary alloresponse, as detected by the mixed lymphocyte reaction, most of the alloreactive T cells recognize the MHC antigens by the direct pathway, as described above. In this interaction the T cell receptors on recipient T cells directly recognize the donor MHC molecules.

However, there are other forms of alloresponse, including:

- those against **minor MHC antigens** (see below); or
- the **indirect response** in which the recipient T cells recognize donor MHC molecules that have been processed by recipient donor APCs and are presented as peptides in the context of recipient MHC class II molecules (Fig. 21.6).

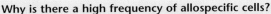

Why is there a high frequency of allospecific cells?

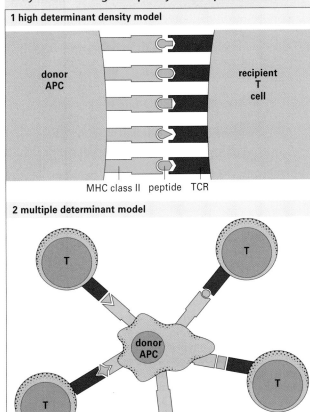

1 high determinant density model

donor APC

recipient T cell

MHC class II   peptide   TCR

2 multiple determinant model

T

T

T

donor APC

T

T

Fig. 21.5 The high precursor frequency of alloreactive T cells can be explained by one of two models. In the first (high determinant density model) the T cell receptor recognizes the MHC molecules on the surface of the APC with a moderate to low affinity. However, this recognition is largely independent of the type of peptide present in the groove of the MHC molecule. The low affinity of the interaction is compensated for by the multiple interactions that form, which provide an avidity advantage. In the multiple determinant model the T cells recognize, with a high affinity, peptide and MHC molecule complexes. The peptides are derived from normal self proteins. As the T cells have not been tolerized in the thymus to those antigens in the context of the donor MHC (though any T cells reactive with the same antigens in the context of self MHC would have been deleted), there is a high frequency of alloreactivity. Which form of allorecognition is most important will depend on the MHC combination of the donor and recipient.

Direct and indirect allorecognition

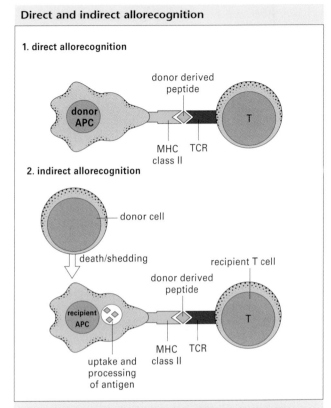

1. direct allorecognition

donor derived peptide

donor APC

MHC class II

TCR

T

2. indirect allorecognition

donor cell

death/shedding

recipient APC

uptake and processing of antigen

donor derived peptide

MHC class II

TCR

recipient T cell

T

Fig. 21.6 **(1)** In direct allorecognition the T cell directly recognizes the donor APC, with the T cell receptor (TCR) binding donor MHC molecules bearing donor peptide. **(2)** Indirect allorecognition is more similar to conventional T cell recognition, in that the recipient T cells recognize foreign (donor derived) antigen that has been taken up and processed by recipient APCs. The TCR therefore recognizes recipient MHC bearing donor peptide. Although the frequency of the direct pathway allorecognition is high, that for the indirect pathway is no higher than that seen for normal antigens.

The indirect response is very similar to conventional T cell recognition of normal antigens, such as those from a pathogen, which are processed by host APCs and presented in the context of host MHC molecules.

Q. **How frequent do you expect the T cells that recognize graft allogeneic molecules encoded outside the MHC to be?**
A. The frequency of allospecific T cells in an unimmunized individual capable of recognizing donor tissue by the indirect pathway is low, equivalent to the frequency of reactivity to any normal antigen.

Nevertheless, the indirect pathway of recognition is important during chronic rejection, when the number of donor-derived professional APCs is no longer high enough to stimulate a direct immune response. It is also important in the rejection of corneal grafts because the cornea lacks large numbers of APCs.

Minor antigens can be targets of rejection even when donor and recipient MHC are identical

Although the MHC is the major target of the alloimmune response, there are also minor histocompatibility antigens. These can serve as targets of rejection even when the MHC is identical between donor and recipient.

The nature of most minor histocompatibility antigens is unknown, though they are assumed to be normal polymorphic molecules, peptides from which bind to host MHC and induce an immune response. In some cases they are expressed in a tissue-specific manner.

Perhaps the best studied minor histocompatibility antigen system is the H-Y system. These are antigens encoded by the Y chromosome, and so are expressed only on male cells. Thus, following immunization, it is possible to demonstrate immune responses and rejection of male organs or skin following transplantation mediated by female animals (2X chromosomes) against male cells (X and Y chromosome).

It is not possible to show responses against female antigens by male animals because the male animals carry one X chromosome in addition to their Y chromosome, and so are tolerant to all antigens encoded for by the X chromosome (Fig. 21.7).

Graft versus host reactions result when donor lymphocytes attack the graft recipient

Although it is usual to think of the immune response recognizing and destroying the transplanted organ, the situation is different when competent immune cells are transplanted into a recipient. This can happen during bone marrow transplantation, when normal donor T cells may be infused into the recipient. In such circumstances the T cells can recognize the MHC molecules and/or minor histocompatibility antigens of the recipient as foreign, and produce an immune response against the recipient. This is known as **graft versus host disease (GvHD)**.

GvHD can be lethal, causing damage in particular to the skin and gut. It can be demonstrated in animal models by transfer of bone marrow to irradiated recipient animals (Fig. 21.8). It can be avoided by:
*   careful matching of the donor and recipient;
*   removal of all T cells from the graft; and
*   immunosuppression.

REJECTION RESULTS FROM A VARIETY OF DIFFERENT IMMUNE EFFECTOR MECHANISMS
The time of rejection is important

Rejection of organs or tissues can occur at various times, each of which is associated with different immune effector mechanisms (Fig. 21.9). These are:
*   hyperacute rejection, which occurs within minutes to hours and is principally mediated by antibody;
*   acute rejection, which usually occurs in days to weeks in animal models and is initiated by alloreactive T cells; and

H-Y minor histocompatibility antigens

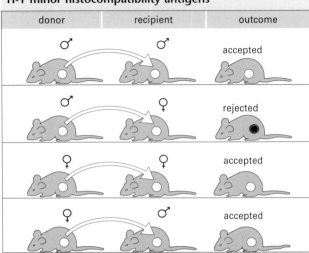

Fig. 21.7 The H-Y antigens are minor histocompatibility antigens expressed on male animals and not on females. Their existence can be demonstrated by skin grafting between animals of the same strain. As would be expected grafts from female mice are always accepted, while those from male mice are accepted on male recipients, but not female recipients.

Graft versus host disease

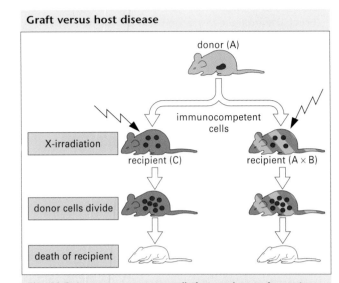

Fig. 21.8 Immunocompetent cells from a donor of type A are injected into an immunosuppressed (X-irradiated) host of type C, or a normal (A × B) F$_1$ recipient. The immunosuppressed individual is unable to reject the cells and the F$_1$ animal is fully tolerant to parental type A cells. In both cases the donor cells recognize the foreign tissue types B or C of the recipient. They divide and react against the recipient tissue cells and recruit large numbers of host cells to inflammatory sites. Very often the process leads to the death of the recipient.

• chronic rejection, which is seen months to years following transplantation.

Hyperacute rejection is immediate and mediated by antibody

Hyperacute rejection is seen when the recipient animal has pre-existing antibodies that are reactive with the donor tissue. This may be because:
• the individual has been sensitized to the donor MHC, for example by previous transplants, multiple blood transfusions, or pregnancy;
• the animal may have natural pre-existing antibodies (e.g. as a result of ABO blood group incompatibility).
A special case is seen in xenotransplantation, where humans and Old World monkeys and apes all have pre-existing antibodies to a carbohydrate antigen α-galactosyl. This carbohydrate is expressed on cell surface proteins of all other donors. Therefore, a xenotransplant of a cellular organ from a pig (or most other species) into a primate is at risk of hyperacute rejection.

Hyperacute rejection is seen within minutes of connecting the circulation into the transplanted organ. It is caused by the pre-existing antibodies binding to the endothelial cells lining the blood vessels and by initiating immune effector functions.

Q. Which immune effector functions would be activated following binding of antibody to the endothelium?
A. Complement will be activated, by the classical pathway (see Chapter 4).

Complement activation can lead to death of the endothelium, or, when the damage is sub-lethal, activation of the endothelial cells. This not only causes an inflammatory response, increasing vascular leakage, but can also cause blood coagulation (Fig. 21.10). The result is rapid destruction of the graft.

Tempo of rejection response

type of rejection	time taken	mechanisms of rejection
hyperacute rejection	minutes to hours	preformed anti-donor antibodies
acute rejection	days to weeks	activation of alloreactive T cells
chronic rejection	months to years	slow cellular response, response of organ to injury, unknown causes

Fig. 21.9 Rejection of organs or tissues can occur at various times, each of which is associated with different immune effector mechanisms, ranging from antibody mediated to acute and chronic cellular responses.

Renal histology showing hyperacute graft rejection

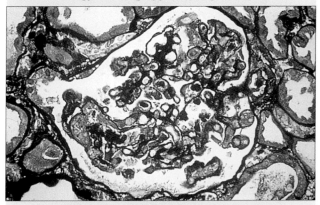

Fig. 21.10 There is extensive necrosis of the glomerular capillary associated with massive interstitial hemorrhage. This extensive necrosis is preceded by an intense polymorphonuclear infiltration, which occurs within the first hour of the graft's revascularization. The changes shown here occurred 24–48 hours after this. H&E stain. × 200.

Prevention of hyperacute rejection is performed by carefully avoiding transplanting an organ into an individual with pre-existing antibodies to that tissue. This is done by:
- ABO matching individuals; and
- cross-matching the donor and recipient.

This involves incubating donor leukocytes with recipient serum in the presence of complement; cell death indicates the presence of anti-donor antibody and is a contraindication to proceeding with transplantation. Such cross-matching is normally performed immediately before surgery.

In the case of xenotransplantation, one solution being developed is the generation of pigs that lack the α-galactosyl carbohydrate epitopes. This is done by knocking out the gene encoding the enzyme (α-galactosyl transferase) that generates this carbohydrate. In preclinical models in which pig organs are transplanted into primates, this approach has led to prolonged graft survival with no evidence of hyperacute rejection.

Acute rejection occurs days to weeks after transplantation

Acute rejection is normally seen days to weeks after transplantation, and is caused by activation of allospecific T cells capable of damaging the graft.

Donor dendritic cells (sometimes called passenger leukocytes) play an important role in triggering acute rejection. Dendritic cells that are present in the organ, following transplantation into the recipient, migrate to the lymph nodes draining the organ and stimulate a primary alloimmune response.

The importance of these dendritic cells can be shown by 'parking experiments' in which:
- a kidney is transplanted from one strain of rat to another under cover of immunosuppression (to prevent rejection) (Fig. 21.11);

- the kidney is kept in that animal long enough to ensure that all the resident dendritic cells have migrated out of the organ;
- the kidney is then transplanted into a third animal, of the same strain as the original recipient, where it shows prolonged graft survival.

However, if the third animal is injected with donor-derived dendritic cells there is rapid graft rejection. These data highlight the contribution of donor dendritic cells in initiating the alloresponse.

Although the direct pathway is thought to predominate in acute rejection, the indirect alloresponse, though significantly weaker, can also cause acute rejection in some animal models.

Once activated the T cells migrate to the organ and lead to tissue damage by standard immunological effector mechanisms (Fig. 21.12). These include:
- the generation of cytotoxic T cells; and
- the induction of delayed-type hypersensitivity reactions.

The role of the T cells in graft rejection can be demonstrated by depletion studies in which antibodies against T cell subsets are administered in vivo. Both of the major T cell subsets, CD4+ and CD8+, can cause graft rejection.

If the animal or patient has already been exposed to the alloantigens expressed by the graft, and as a consequence has been immunized, there will be alloreactive memory cells. This will lead to a much more rapid (accelerated) rejection of the graft (Fig. 21.13).

Chronic rejection is seen months or years after transplantation

In vascularized organs chronic rejection presents as occlusion of blood vessels, which on histological analysis show a thickening of the intima similar in some respects to the thickening seen as a result of atherosclerosis (Fig. 21.14). Smooth muscle cell proliferation is often seen, together with a macrophage infiltrate (together with some lymphocytes). This eventually leads to blockage of the blood vessels and subsequent ischemia of the organ.

A number of mechanisms can lead to chronic rejection. They include:
- a low-grade T cell response (mainly of the indirect allospecific pathway as a result of the loss of passenger leukocytes that activate T cells with direct pathway specificity, see p. 385);
- antibody can also be involved in chronic rejection, as indicated by the deposition of complement components (C4d) in tissues.

Non-immunological processes are also important, such as:
- the response of the graft to injury caused at the time of transplantation or by acute rejection episodes;
- recurrence of the original underlying disease; and
- drug-related toxicities (e.g. the immunosuppressive drug ciclosporin A is nephrotoxic and can damage the kidneys).

In some cases, initiation of chronic rejection may be immunological in nature, but its progression is due to non-immunological mechanisms.

Chronic rejection responds poorly to current immunosuppressive therapy. Therefore, although there has been

Importance of passenger leukocytes in graft sensitization

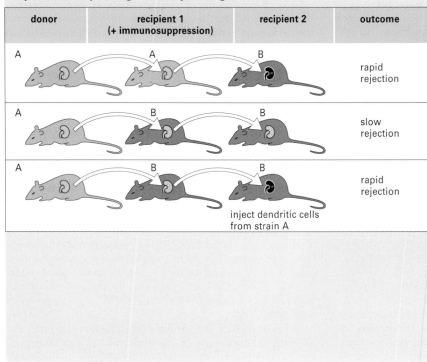

Fig. 21.11 The role of passenger leukocytes (dendritic cells) can be shown by 'parking' experiments in which kidneys are grafted from a rat of strain A into a recipient of strain B. Immunosuppression is used to prevent the animal from rejecting the graft. After a period the grafts are then retransplanted into a fresh strain B rat. There is very slow rejection of the graft (when compared to the rapid rejection seen when the kidney is transferred first into a strain A rat), which is thought to be due to the inability of the kidney from the strain A rat to immunize the strain B recipient due to the loss of dendritic cells during the period when the graft was 'parked' in the first strain A animal. The slow rejection probably occurs via the indirect pathway. The rejection occurs at the normal rapid tempo if strain A dendritic cells are injected into the recipient animal at the same time as the graft, suggesting that dendritic cells are capable of sensitizing the animal to the graft.

Renal histology showing acute graft rejection

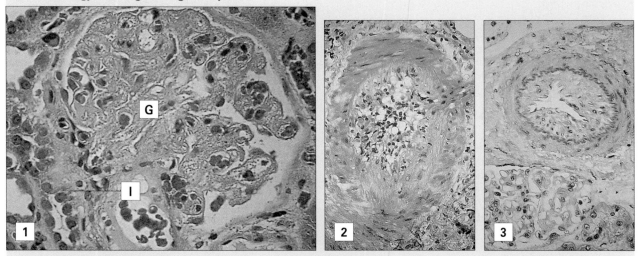

Fig. 21.12 (1) Small lymphocytes and other cells are accumulating in the interstitium of the graft. Such infiltration (I) is characteristic of acute rejection and occurs before the appearance of any clinical signs. H&E stain. (2) H&E stain of acutely rejecting kidney showing vascular obstruction. (3) van Gieson's stain of acutely rejecting kidney showing the end stage of this process. (G, glomerulus)

considerable improvement in overall graft survival over the past decades, this improvement is mostly seen in the first year following transplantation – the subsequent survival of grafts has hardly altered over the past 20 to 30 years (Fig. 21.15). This indicates the need to improve the treatment of chronic rejection.

HLA MATCHING IS IMPORTANT FOR PREVENTING REJECTION

The two major methods for preventing rejection of allografts are:

- to match the donor and recipient to minimize the antigenic differences;

Graft rejection displays immunological memory

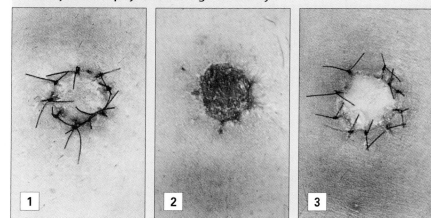

Fig. 21.13 A human skin allograft at day 5 (1) is fully vascularized and the cells are dividing, but by day 12 (2) is totally destroyed. A second graft ('second-set' graft) from the same donor shown here on day 7 (3) does not become vascularized and is destroyed rapidly. This indicates that sensitization to the first graft produces immunological memory.

Chronic rejection

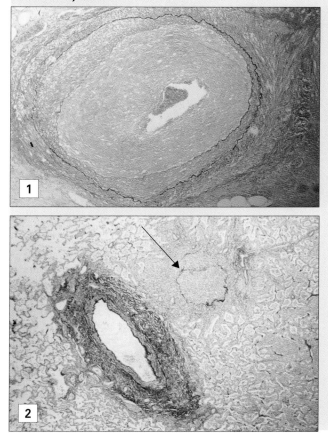

Fig. 21.14 Grafts that survive acute rejection are still capable of undergoing chronic rejection. (1) Section taken from a patient with chronic rejection of their heart graft. The lumen of the blood vessel in the heart has been narrowed as a result of thickening of the wall of the vessel, limiting the blood supply to the heart. (2) Section taken from a patient with chronic rejection of the lung, showing obliterative bronchiolitis (arrow) blocking the airways. (Kindly supplied by Professor Marlene Rose, Imperial College London, Harefield Hospital, and Dr Margaret Burke, Pathology Department, Royal Brompton Hospital and Harefield Hospital)

• to use immunosuppressive regimens that block the immune response against the organ.

However, in animal models (and hopefully in the clinic) there are techniques that can induce tolerance to an organ such that the immune system of the recipient 'learns' to treat the donor organ as 'self' and not destroy it. As discussed below, the ability to induce donor-specific tolerance is the Holy Grail of transplantation immunology (see p. 394).

The better the HLA matching of donor and recipient, the less the strength of rejection

The major antigenic differences recognized by the alloimmune response are found on the MHC molecules

Long-term survival of kidney grafts

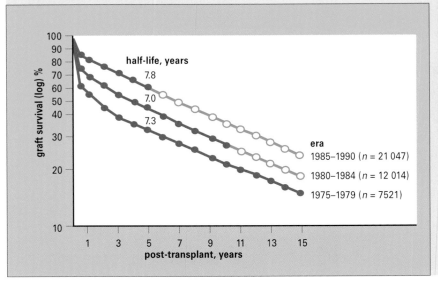

Fig. 21.15 This graph shows the survival of kidney grafts in patients transplanted in three periods: 1975–1979, 1980–1984, and 1985–1990 (with the projections for graft survival shown for later periods). There has been a considerable improvement in graft survival since 1975, but most of the improvement is seen in the first year. After that time the half-life of graft survival is similar for all patient groups. (With permission from UK Transplant, Bristol)

(known as HLA in humans, see Chapter 5). These highly polymorphic molecules have a vital role in presenting antigens to T cells.

There are many different alleles of the MHC molecules, and one way to reduce the strength of a rejection response is to match the donor and recipient so that they share as many alleles as possible. In general matching is now performed using molecular techniques, with polymerase chain reactions (PCR) that are specific for the different alleles.

In humans HLA matching is rarely perfect between unrelated donors because of the difficulty in matching all MHC class I and class II gene loci and the high level of polymorphism at each locus.

Q. How many MHC loci would need to be matched to obtain a perfect match in a human population?

A. There are three HLA class I loci (HLA-A, HLA-B, and HLA-C), and one individual can express up to six different HLA class I molecules (for each antigen there will be a maternally derived and a paternally derived version). Similarly, there are three class II loci (HLA-DR, HLA-DP, and HLA-DQ), and again the maternal and paternal chromosomes would normally be different. In other words there are 12 potentially different loci.

The extensive polymorphism means that there can be more than 600 possible versions (alleles) of each antigen (there are at least 626 different alleles for HLA-B, other antigens are less polymorphic, with 470 DRB and 349 HLA-A alleles, see Appendix 1).

Therefore, even before one considers other polymorphic molecules associated with the HLA locus, there is considerable complexity, which makes it highly unlikely for there to be a complete match.

In cases where the transplant is between living related donors (such as brothers and sisters) there is a greater opportunity for a match because in general the HLA locus

is inherited en bloc as a single set (or haplotype) from each parent.

Loci outside the MHC can also lead to rejection (the minor histocompatibility antigens, see above). However, there is no attempt to match for these antigens because there is little possibility of getting a good match and the effect of matching any single minor antigen is too small to be significant.

It should be noted that even when siblings are perfectly matched at the MHC locus they will not be matched (unless they are identical twins) for the minor histocompatibility antigens.

The importance of HLA matching is not always crucial

HLA matching is very important in bone marrow transplantation (where a large potential donor pool can reduce the risk of GvHD) and has a significant influence on the outcome in kidney transplantation. For other organs the importance is less clear, for example:

- in corneal transplantation there is no benefit of HLA matching;
- for those organs where transplantation is essential to maintain life (such as heart and liver) there is no possibility of waiting for a well-matched organ to become available.

SUCCESSFUL ORGAN TRANSPLANTATION DEPENDS ON THE USE OF IMMUNOSUPPRESSIVE DRUGS

The success of organ transplantation is entirely dependent on the use of immunosuppressive drugs that control the alloimmune response. Although rejection episodes still occur, they are usually kept in check by the drugs so that lasting damage is minimized.

Over recent decades there has been a marked improvement in short-term success rates, such that over 90% of kidney transplants are functioning 1 year after transplantation. The major reason for these improved success rates is the advent of more powerful immunosuppressive agents.

Q. What problems would you expect to result from long-term immunosuppression?

A. These drugs cause blanket suppression of the immune system so transplant recipients are more prone to opportunistic infections and have a raised incidence of malignancy. This is the reason for continuing interest in strategies to promote specific immunological tolerance (see below).

Despite the continuing interest in strategies to promote specific immunological tolerance, clinical transplantation is likely to require non-specific immunosuppression for some years to come. The present challenge is to use the currently available agents intelligently to minimize side effects while preserving graft function.

The commonest cocktail of drugs used for kidney transplant patients involves three agents, each of which has a distinct mode of action:

• a drug that inhibits T cell activation;
• an antiproliferative; and
• an anti-inflammatory agent.

Usually three agents are used in the early post-transplant period while the anti-donor immune response is at its peak.

Numerous clinical trials are addressing the safety of withdrawing one of these three agents within weeks or months of transplantation. It appears that maintenance immunosuppression with two drugs is safe and has an improved side effect profile.

6-MP, azathioprine, and MPA are antiproliferative drugs

The first antiproliferative drug to be used in patients was **6-mercaptopurine (6-MP)**. This was followed by the introduction of **azathioprine**, the parent compound that is converted in vivo to 6-MP. Azathioprine was given to all patients until a more potent alternative arrived on the scene, **mycophenolic acid (MPA)**.

These antiproliferative drugs have related modes of action, namely inhibition of the synthesis of purines that are required for cell division:

• azathioprine is a purine antagonist and competes with inosine monophosphate;
• MPA inhibits an enzyme, inosine monophosphate dehydrogenase, which is essential in the de-novo synthesis of purines.

Clearly purine synthesis is needed in all cell types. Consequently, the risk of such agents is inhibition of other populations of rapidly dividing cell systems, such as the bone marrow. Indeed, close monitoring of white cell and platelet numbers is necessary in patients on antiproliferative drugs.

T cells are particularly sensitive to antiproliferative agents, partly because they are largely dependent on the de-novo synthesis of purines, whereas other cell types have a more efficient salvage pathway. Consequently, at conventional doses there is selective inhibition of T cell-dependent immunity.

Ciclosporin, tacrolimus, and sirolimus are inhibitors of T cell activation
Ciclosporin inhibits the production of IL-2

Drugs that inhibit T cell activation are the mainstay of immunosuppressive regimens. The first such drug to be discovered was **ciclosporin**, a fungal metabolite (Fig. 21.16).

The introduction of ciclosporin revolutionized clinical transplantation in that it led to a marked improvement in early success rates, which rose from approximately 70% to over 90%. Furthermore, the doses of other drugs that were required were substantially lower, so drug side effects were less troublesome.

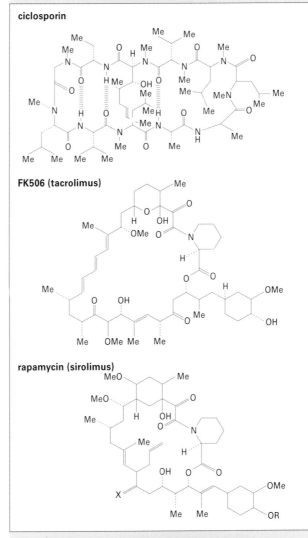

Structure of immunosuppressive fungal macrolides

ciclosporin

FK506 (tacrolimus)

rapamycin (sirolimus)

Fig. 21.16 The immunosuppressive fungal macrolides, ciclosporin, FK506 (tacrolimus), and rapamycin (sirolimus), have quite different structures. They act on lymphocytes in different ways – ciclosporin and FK506 affect cytokine production and rapamycin interferes with signaling through the IL-2 receptor (IL-2R).

Because of the much greater potency of ciclosporin, and its ability to prevent early acute rejection, transplantation of organs other than kidney became routine. Programs of heart, liver, and more recently lung transplantation were established in major transplant centers around the world.

The key effect of ciclosporin is to inhibit the production of the major growth factor for T cells, interleukin-2 (IL-2).

The intracellular mechanism of action of ciclosporin involves binding to **cyclophilin**, and the consequent inhibition of the calcium-dependent phosphatase, **calcineurin**, which would otherwise activate the **NFAT complex**, and lead to IL-2 gene transcription.

Tacrolimus binds to an intracellular protein, FK-binding protein 12

A few years after the introduction of ciclosporin, a Japanese company discovered another fungal metabolite with a similar mode of action and greater molar potency, tacrolimus (**FK506**).

Tacrolimus binds to another intracellular protein, FK-binding protein 12 (FKBP12). The resulting complex then inhibits calcineurin, and the consequences of calcium-dependent signaling, in the same manner as ciclosporin.

Ciclosporin and tacrolimus are used almost interchangeably, and each has its advocates. Perhaps the major factor that is in favor of tacrolimus is that is less nephrotoxic than ciclosporin. On the other hand, tacrolimus is diabetogenic in some patients. As is usually the case, no drug is perfect, and the choice is one of balancing potency against toxicity.

Sirolimus inhibits signals transmitted by IL-2 binding to IL-2R

The third drug in the 'inhibitors of T cell activation' category is **sirolimus** (**rapamycin**).

Sirolimus is a fungal metabolite that was discovered on the Easter Island, Rapa ui, and its mechanism of action is quite distinct. Rather than inhibiting the production of IL-2, it inhibits the response to IL-2, by inhibiting some of the signals transmitted as a result of IL-2 binding to its receptor.

Indeed, sirolimus inhibits signaling through several growth factor receptors – consequently it has quite widespread antiproliferative effects, and was written off as being too non-specific when first studied in vitro.

Sirolimus has attracted much attention recently, for two reasons:
- first, because it appears to be a tolerance-permissive drug – that is, if T cells are exposed to antigen in tolerance promoting conditions, such as co-stimulatory blockade, sirolimus allows tolerance to occur, though in contrast there are some data to suggest that the calcineurin inhibitors may inhibit the development of tolerance under similar circumstances;
- second, the broader antiproliferative effects of sirolimus that almost confined it to the waste basket at the outset are now being claimed as beneficial because they reduce the incidence of some malignancies.

Corticosteroids are anti-inflammatory drugs used for transplant immunosuppression

Corticosteroids, given in combination with azathioprine, were the mainstay of immunosuppression for several decades. Only now is the possibility of rapid corticosteroid withdrawal, after 1 or 2 weeks, being explored.

Corticosteroids are pharmacological derivatives of the glucocorticoid family of steroid hormones, and act through intracellular receptors that are almost ubiquitously expressed.

The anti-inflammatory effects of steroids are highly complex, reflecting the fact that as many as 1% of genes may be regulated by glucocorticoids. Some of the most important effects are:
- inhibition of proinflammatory cytokine secretion (IL-1, IL-3, IL-4, IL-5, IL-8 (CXCL8), TNFα);
- inhibition of nitric oxide synthase;
- inhibition of adhesion molecule expression leading to reduced inflammatory cell migration;
- induction of endonucleases leading to apoptosis in lymphocytes and eosinophils.

The problem of side effects is a major issue with the use of corticosteroids, particularly at high doses. Central weight gain, fluid retention, diabetes mellitus, bone mineral loss, and thinning of the skin, all result from protracted corticosteroid use. It is for this reason that much attention is being devoted to protocols that allow steroid minimization.

FTY 720 is a novel immunosuppressive agent under investigation

Some newer immunosuppressives are under investigation and are the subject of clinical trials. One is FTY 720, which has a dramatic effect on lymphocyte migration, leading to marked sequestration of lymphocytes in lymphoid tissues, and a sharp fall in the circulating numbers of these cells. It remains to be seen whether this will find its way into the armamentarium of clinical immunosuppression.

In light of the continuing pursuit of donor-specific transplant tolerance, an interesting question is whether FTY 720 will favor or impede the development of tolerance.

THE ULTIMATE GOAL IN TRANSPLANTATION IS TO INDUCE DONOR-SPECIFIC TOLERANCE

Although generalized immunosuppression has been highly successful in preventing graft rejection, it comes at a price. This includes:
- the non-specific toxicity of the drugs;
- the need to stay indefinitely on medication; and
- the consequences of generalized immunosuppression such as the increased incidence of cancer and infection.

It would therefore be desirable to induce tolerance to the graft whereby the immune system specifically becomes non-responsive to the donor antigens, yet is still capable of responding normally to other antigens.

Tolerance to grafts was first demonstrated by Peter Medawar's group. They showed that, if allogeneic cells were injected into a neonatal animal, when the animal became adult it would be tolerant to tissue from the donor and would accept grafts without the need for immuno-suppression. There have been numerous examples of inducing tolerance to grafts in animal models since, but this has yet to translate into the clinical setting.

One of the difficulties in the clinical setting is to demonstrate that tolerance really exists. In an animal model it is relatively easy to demonstrate tolerance by:

- performing a second graft (so showing that the immune system will no longer respond to the antigen); or
- demonstrating that an irrelevant third party graft is still rejected (demonstrating that graft survival is not due to a generalized immunosuppression).

However, this is more difficult in humans.

There is evidence for the induction of tolerance in humans

There are two sources of evidence for the induction of tolerance in humans.

First there are patients who have received grafts, but are no longer on immunosuppressive regimens because they cannot tolerate the drugs. They can show long-term graft survival. This is not formal evidence of tolerance, but it is highly suggestive that some people can have an operational tolerance whereby they fail to destroy their organ graft.

Second, it is possible to look at the frequency of alloreactive T cells in patients with grafts. In some groups there is a reduced frequency of these cells, but the response to other antigens remains normal (Fig. 21.17). Again, this is not a formal proof of tolerance because it is not yet known how the in-vitro assays relate to the response in patients. However, it does indicate that it might be possible to develop tests that will allow us to monitor the development of tolerance in patients, and so know how to tailor treatment to the individual (e.g. removing them from immunosuppression when indicated).

Novel methods for inducing tolerance are being developed

There are various ways in which tolerance (or the appearance of tolerance) can occur. Most of these are discussed in more detail in Chapters 11 and 19. An understanding of the mechanisms by which tolerance is induced and maintained allows the development of novel methods for inducing tolerance.

Central tolerance results from deletion of T cells in the thymus and is the most important form of tolerance induction for preventing autoimmunity. It has been harnessed for the induction of tolerance in experimental systems by transplanting the thymus from the donor into the recipient. This approach may be particularly useful in the context of xenotransplantation, where there is an opportunity to manipulate the donor and/or recipient before grafting of the organ. Limited clinical trials of inducing central tolerance using donor bone marrow in kidney transplant recipients are also under way.

Alloreactive cells can be made anergic

In the peripheral organs tolerance induction can result from deletion. However, it is also possible for alloreactive cells to be energized. Anergy describes a state in which the cell is not deleted, but has been rendered unresponsive to further stimulation by the same antigen.

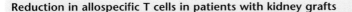

Q. What mechanism causes T cells to become anergic in the presence of an antigen presented on an appropriate MHC molecule?

A. Presentation of the antigen by a non-professional APC that lacks the ability to provide co-stimulatory signals (see Fig. 7.18).

Blockade of co-stimulatory molecules such as CD80 and CD86 with agents like CTLA-4–Ig (a fusion protein between CTLA-4, a ligand for CD80 and CD86, and the Fc part of an antibody molecule) can be used to induce anergy in alloreactive cells (Fig. 21.18). However, it

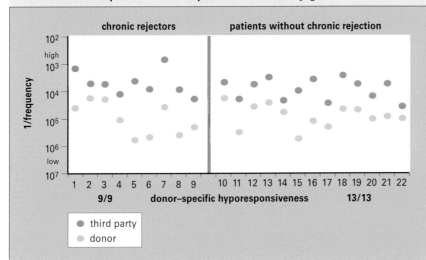

Reduction in allospecific T cells in patients with kidney grafts

chronic rejectors   patients without chronic rejection

1/frequency

10^2
high
10^3
10^4
10^5
10^6
low
10^7

1 2 3 4 5 6 7 8 9   10 11 12 13 14 15 16 17 18 19 20 21 22

9/9   donor–specific hyporesponsiveness   13/13

- ● third party
- ● donor

Fig. 21.17 The graph shows the frequency of T cells capable of producing IL-2 from patients with long-term kidney grafts that react with cells bearing the donor alloantigen or control (third party) alloantigens. The data show two groups of patients – those with evidence of chronic rejection and those without. Both groups of patient show a reduced frequency of T cells capable of recognizing alloantigen from the donor of the organ when compared to the frequency against third party alloantigen. This indicates that the patients show a degree of reduced reactivity to alloantigens.

Co-stimulation blockade

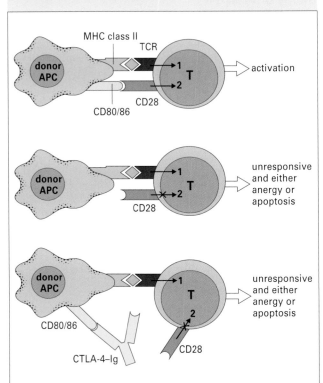

Fig. 21.18 For full T cell activation to occur the T cell needs to receive two signals – signal 1 through the T cell receptor binding the appropriate peptide–MHC complex (which provides antigenic specificity) and signal 2 through co-stimulatory molecules (the most important of which for naive T cells is CD28 on the T cell binding CD80, or CD86 on the APC). Interaction of a T cell with an APC that lacks CD80 or CD86, so that signal 1 only is received, fails to activate the T cell and can result in apoptosis or anergy of the lymphocyte. In experimental or clinical settings it is possible to block the CD28 interaction with CD80/86 by addition of a soluble molecule, CTLA-4–Ig, which consists of the extracellular part of CTLA-4 (an alternative ligand for CD80/86) fused to the Fc of immunoglobulin. This molecule prevents the interaction of CD28 with CD80/86. It can also result in upregulation of immunoregulatory enzyme, indoleamine 2,3-dioxygenase (IDO), as described in the text.

should be noted that the situation can be more complex than this. In many APCs cross-linking of CD80 and CD86 with CTLA-4–Ig results in upregulation of an immuno-modulatory enzyme indoleamine 2,3-dioxygenase (IDO). This enzyme catabolizes tryptophan, and as a result prevents T cell activation both as a result of:

- depriving T cells of this essential amino acid; and
- the products of tryptophan breakdown acting directly on the T cells.

The role of IDO in immune regulation was first recognized in the placenta, where it protects the fetus from immunological rejection – inhibition of IDO causes rejection of histoincompatible fetuses.

Another alternative is to induce a regulatory response to the alloantigen. The phenomenon of T cell regulation has long been recognized (Fig. 21.19), and can be shown in experimental models by transferring T cells from a tolerant animal to a naive recipient, and showing that this results in a transfer of the tolerance. Several types of T cell are capable of regulating the immune response, and strategies that seek to expand these cells may be one method to induce tolerance in vivo.

Immune privilege can be a property of the tissue or site of transplant

Although a failure to reject a graft could be the result of tolerance (or immunosuppression), an alternative is that the graft is immune privileged and protected from the immune response against it:

- when corneal transplantation is performed in an animal model the rejection response is weaker than for other forms of transplantation, indicating the immune privileged nature of the graft;
- skin transplanted onto the anterior chamber (where the cornea is) shows a lower rate of rejection than skin transplanted into other sites.

These data indicate that the anterior chamber is an immune privileged site, and any tissue transplanted into it is protected from the immune response.

Other immune privileged sites include the posterior chamber of the eye, the testes, the brain, and the hamster cheek pouch (see Chapter 12).

It is important to note that immune privilege is not an absolute term. Corneal grafts are rejected, albeit less vigorously than other grafts. It is probably best to think of immune privilege as a spectrum ranging from grafts that show a high degree of privilege (cornea) to those where the immune response against them is very strong (skin), with other grafts somewhere inbetween.

Several mechanisms can be responsible for immune privilege. These include 'ignorance' – the immune system does not see the graft. The cornea is not vascularized, and has a poor lymphatic drainage. It also has a very low concentration of dendritic cells in the center. These features reduce the ability of the graft to stimulate an immune response against it. If this ignorance is disrupted (e.g. by inducing vascularization in the graft bed) then the cornea is more rapidly rejected.

In addition the tissue can deviate the immune response. In the anterior chamber of the eye there is a cytokine environment (high in TGFβ and α-melanocyte stimulating hormone) that deviates the immune response away from a tissue destructive to a non-inflammatory response.

Finally, the tissue being transplanted can itself be privileged. This is also seen in the cornea, which expresses high levels of Fas ligand.

Q. What is the significance of the expression of Fas ligand in the cornea?

A. It results in apoptosis of inflammatory cells expressing Fas that enter the graft (see Chapter 12).

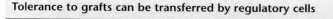

Tolerance to grafts can be transferred by regulatory cells

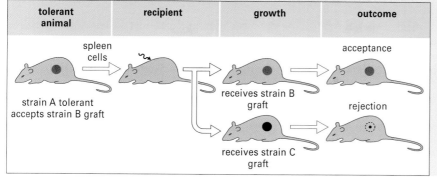

tolerant animal	recipient	growth	outcome

Fig. **21.19** An animal of strain A that has been made tolerant to a graft B can contain regulatory cells. If these cells are removed from the animal and transferred to a lightly irradiated strain A recipient, and this animal is then given a skin graft from strain B, then that graft may be accepted. In most cases this tolerance is specific, so if the second mouse received a graft of strain C it would be rejected.

SHORTAGE OF DONOR ORGANS AND CHRONIC REJECTION LIMIT THE SUCCESS OF TRANSPLANTATION

Two major issues limit success of transplantation:

- the first is the shortage of donor organs – this means that not everyone who would benefit from a transplant receives one, and, given the high success rate of transplantation, an increasing number of patients would benefit;
- the second problem is chronic rejection, which results in a continual loss of transplanted organs and necessitates patients remaining on immunosuppression, with the consequences of drug toxicity, systemic immunosuppression, increased incidence of malignancy, and infection.

The second of these problems, chronic rejection, would be solved if we were able to induce tolerance to grafts in patients. To do this it is necessary that:

- we develop assays that will allow us to determine when tolerance has been induced; and
- translate the therapies developed in animal models to the clinic.

These assays may involve measuring the frequency of alloreactive and/or regulatory T cells in patients. At present it is not clear which tolerance induction procedure is most likely to work in clinical transplantation, and further work in primate models is needed to address this issue.

Living donation is one way to overcome the shortage of donor organs

The shortage of donor organs can be addressed to some extent by increasing the number of potential donors, by increased advertising or changing the legislation. In addition more use could be made of living donations.

Living donation is possible for:

- kidney transplantation because the donor can survive with the one remaining kidney; and
- stem cell transplantation (either bone marrow or peripheral blood) because the donor can replace cells taken for donation.

Although some groups have performed other forms of living donation (e.g. with lung and liver lobes), this is not routine.

In most cases living donation is performed between relatives. When transplants from unrelated subjects are performed it is necessary to ensure that the donation is not coerced and that the necessary ethical standards are upheld.

Alternative approaches to overcoming the shortage of donor organs are being investigated

Although it is very important to increase the donor pool, the approaches discussed above will never provide all the organs needed. Alternatives include:

- the development of artificial mechanical organs;
- in the longer term, use of cloning and/or tissue engineering strategies to make artificial biological organs;
- xenotransplantation (the use of animal organs).

The favored animal for xenotransplantation is the pig

The reasons for the pig being the most suitable animal include the physiological and anatomical compatibility between pigs and humans and the ability to breed large numbers of animals rapidly.

There are several barriers to xenotransplantation, including public acceptability, safety, and scientific issues.

The main safety concern is the risk of transmission of viruses from the pig to the human. It should be noted that acellular xenografts have been performed for many years and are highly successful (e.g. in the case of pig heart valves, which can be used to replace diseased valves). These are not subject to immunological rejection, nor are they potential sources of viral infection.

The scientific issues revolve around preventing graft rejection. As indicated above, a pig organ transplanted into a human would undergo hyperacute rejection as a result of preformed anti-α-galactosyl antibodies in the recipient's circulation. One solution to this has been to engineer pigs (by nuclear cloning from cell lines) that lack the galactosyl transferase enzyme responsible for creating α-galactosyl residues. Organs from these pigs show reasonably long-term survival in primates.

As well as offering scientific challenges, there are also opportunities for using pig organs. The ability to genetically engineer the pig should make it easier to develop tolerance to the organ. This, as well as the ability to carry out transplants in a pre-planned manner, offers considerable advantages over conventional transplantation.

Critical thinking: Kidney transplantation (see p. 500 for explanations)

Mrs X has diabetes mellitus, and this caused severe damage to her kidneys. This complication is called diabetic nephropathy, and is one of the major indications for kidney transplantation. Mrs X was on dialysis treatment, but this was not working well for her and she was advised that she would benefit from renal transplantation. However, it proved very difficult to find a suitable cadaveric donor for Mrs X and it was suggested that a family member might donate an organ. All her immediate family – her husband, five children, and two brothers – agreed to be considered as donors.

The HLA types and blood groups of the family members are shown in the table. On the basis of these tests a donor was selected and the transplant was performed. Despite successful surgery, the kidney soon turned dark and swelled. This started to happen within a few minutes of the restoration of blood flow through the transplant, and necessitated the immediate removal of the graft.

Four years later Mrs X was still very ill on dialysis, no cadaveric donor was available, and it was decided to try again with a living related transplant. Another member of the family

person	age	relationship to patient	HLA genotypes			blood group genes phenotype
			A	B	DR	
Mrs X	46	the patient	1 2	8 44	3 4	BODd BRh⁺
Mr X	52	husband	2 3	14 7	8 2	AOdd ARh⁻
Anne	25	daughter	2 3	44 7	4 2	AOdd ARh⁻
Bert	24	son	1 2	8 14	3 8	ABDd ABRh⁺
Chas	21	son	1 3	8 7	3 2	BOdd BRh⁻
Dave	15	son	2 1	44 60	4 9	BODd BRh⁺
Edna	13	daughter	1 2	8 14	3 8	AODd ARh⁺
Fred	48	brother	1 2	8 44	3 4	ABDd ABRh⁺
Gary	56	brother	2 2	44 14	4 15	BODD BRH⁺

was selected to donate a kidney and it functioned well from the onset. Mrs X was given triple immunosuppression. She had only one rejection episode at about 3 weeks after grafting, and this was treated successfully with anti-rejection therapy. There were no other problems.

The kidney continued to work for 8 years, but its function gradually declined from the fourth year onwards. It seemed there was little the doctors could do to prevent this worsening situation, and Mrs X eventually had to return to dialysis.

1 What are the difficulties in finding a donor organ?
2 Comment on the HLA relationships between Mrs X and her brothers.
3 Comment on the relationships between the children of Mrs X.
4 Classify each member of the family in terms of their HLA relationship to Mrs X (HLA identical, HLA haplotype match, complete HLA mismatch).

5 In terms of HLA matching alone, who was the best donor for Mrs X?
6 Consider what effect the blood group antigens had on the choice of donor. From whom could kidneys have been transplanted, and who would not have been suitable?
7 Of those who had a compatible blood group, who would you have chosen as the best donor? Explain your reasoning.
8 The outcome of the transplantation was a disaster! By what mechanism was the graft attacked?
9 Why was Mrs X at a greater risk of this untoward reaction?
10 What laboratory tests are used to avoid this rejection reaction, and what seems to have gone wrong on this occasion?
11 Four years after the first transplant it was decided to try again with a living related donor. Of all the family members, who would you have chosen as the donor and whose kidney was most likely to survive in Mrs X?

Critical thinking: Kidney transplantation *(Continued)*

12 What is triple therapy immunosuppression?
13 What type of rejection occurred at 3 weeks after transplantation, and what immunological mechanisms were involved?
14 What is anti-rejection therapy?
15 There were no other problems with Mrs X. Can you think of some of the problems that might arise in a transplant recipient?
16 Why did the function of the transplant gradually decline, and why could the doctors not stop this process?

Discussion points

1 What are the ethical issues involved in this form of transplantation?
2 What novel forms of immunotherapy might be available in the future to prevent rejection of grafts?

Immunity to Cancers

SUMMARY

- **Can the immune system protect the host from cancer?** The immune surveillance hypothesis has profound implications in cancer immunology.

- **Tumors can induce immunity.** Mice, rats, hamsters, and frogs can be immunized against tumors. In most tumors of animals, tumor immunity elicited by immunization is specific (or strongest) to the individual tumor that was used to immunize.

- **Tumor antigens have been characterized by three means – immunization-challenge experiments, T cell reactivity, and antibody reactivity.** Immunization-challenge experiments have uncovered the immunogenicity of heat-shock protein-chaperoned antigenic peptides. Antigens identified by reactivity to T cells and antibodies include individual tumor-specific mutated antigens, cancer testes antigens, differentiation antigens, and viral tumor antigens.

- **Vigorous anti-tumor immune responses are compromised by regulatory mechanisms.** Tumors elicit immunity in their primary host, and such immunity is downregulated. Regulatory cells such as $CD25^+$ $CD4^+$ T cells and inhibition of activated anti-tumor T cells through T cell molecules such as CTLA-4 are involved in downregulation of tumor immunity.

- **Three major categories of experimental immunotherapy are used for human cancer.** Vaccination with the idiotypes of B lymphomas, irradiated intact tumor cells, tumor lysate, or HSP–peptide complexes has been used. Vaccination with dendritic cells pulsed with peptides and adoptive immunotherapy using T cells is also being tested.

CAN THE IMMUNE SYSTEM PROTECT THE HOST FROM CANCER?
The immune surveillance hypothesis has profound implications for cancer immunology

Cancer appears to have engaged the minds of immunologists almost since the beginning of immunology itself.

Ehrlich, who opined on all things immunological, believed that the immune system could protect the host from cancer.

Burnet and Thomas refined that idea into the immune surveillance hypothesis of cancer. The hypothesis lived in limbo for several decades, failing to thrive and failing to die, until very recently when the work of Old, Schreiber, and their colleagues demonstrated that mice with a compromised immune status were more prone than immunocompetent mice to developing an array of cancers.

The immune surveillance hypothesis is often regarded as the intellectual underpinning of cancer immunology. Although the hypothesis itself has contributed little to our attempts to treat cancer through immunological means, it has profound implications for understanding the functions of the immune system.

Does infection have an anti-cancer effect?

This idea is an even more ancient stream of thought and effort in cancer immunity, and one that may be relevant to the immune surveillance hypothesis.

German physicians in the 19th century noted dramatic regressions of cancer in occasional patients who developed streptococcal infections. These anecdotes led to a systematic exploration of infections/fever as an immunotherapeutic modality by William Coley, a New York city surgeon.

The idea that a non-specific stimulation of the immune system, such as by an infection, can have an anti-cancer effect, has its origins in Coley's clinical studies. Never entirely applicable, and never to be ignored, the work of Coley and his predecessors continues to remain the permanent Rorscharch's inkblot in cancer immunology. It is only a small exaggeration to say that every idea in cancer immunity has been interpreted at some time or another, in terms of Coley's observations.

TUMORS ELICIT IMMUNITY IN THE PRIMARY HOST

Entirely unrelated to these two lines of enquiry, the study of cancer immunity saw a revival at the hands of those who were transplanting chemically induced tumors into the many inbred mice that began to be available in the 1950s. These investigators 'showed "highly successful" immunization against the "transplantable tumors" and expressed great hopes about cancer vaccination'.

In hindsight, these successful immunizations were simply a result of allogeneic differences between tumors and the host strain of mouse, a theme that played a seminal role in definition of the MHC, but had no relevance for cancer immunity.

Q. What will happen when a tumor from a mouse of one MHC haplotype is transplanted into a recipient with a different haplotype on the first occasion or the second?
A. A transplantation rejection reaction will ensue, and these reactions display specificity and memory (see Chapter 21).

Nonetheless, amidst the barrage of experiments where MHC-mismatched tumors were transplanted into mice, were the experiments of Ludwik Gross, and later those of Prehn and Main, and of George and Eva Klein, who showed that, even when MHC-matched tumors were used to immunize mice, protection against subsequent tumor growth could be achieved (Fig. 22.1). These studies led to two principles, which have informed much of cancer immunology since and are discussed below.

Cancers elicit protective immunity in the primary and syngeneic host

Mice and rats of a given haplotype can be immunized with irradiated cancer cells that arose in animals of the same haplotype. When they are challenged with live cancer cells, they are able to resist the tumor challenge. The following further observations and deductions have been derived from these results.

- The immunogenicity of tumors has provided the foundation stone for the idea of **tumor-specific antigens**. If one could immunize, then antigens must exist.
- Tumor immunity depends on many factors. The degree of tumor immunity depends upon the type of cancer and the method of its induction, or lack of induction. UV-induced cancers are highly immunogenic, methylcholanthrene-induced tumors less so, and spontaneous tumors even less so. Nonetheless, immunogenicity of tumors has been demonstrated in all model systems tested.

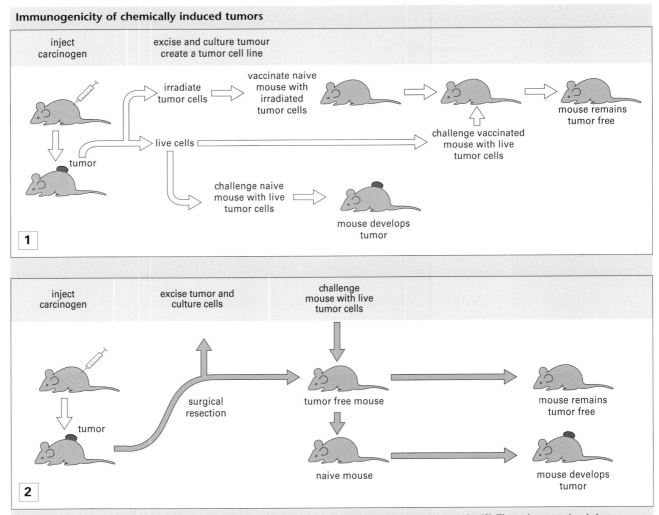

Fig. 22.1 **(1)** Mice immunized with tumor cells are protected against subsequent tumor growth. **(2)** The primary animal that develops the tumor is also immune to subsequent challenges with the same tumor.

- The primary animal develops immunity to subsequent tumor challenge. The Kleins made the seminal observation that not only can the syngeneic animals be immunized, but that the primary animal that develops the tumor is also immune to subsequent challenges with the same tumor (see Fig. 22.1).
- Protective immunity is only seen in prophylactic immunization and not therapeutic immunization – once a mouse has been implanted with a tumor, immunization with irradiated cancer cells (derived from the growing tumor) does nothing to mitigate tumor growth (Fig. 22.2). Exploration of differences between prophylaxis and therapy has led to fundamental insights into tumor immunity (see p. 413).
- It is not possible to test immunogenicity of tumors in humans. The transplantation-challenge experimental paradigm is not applicable to humans and no clearer method of determination of immunogenicity exists. It is therefore impossible to comment on the immunogenicity of human tumors, though references to such immunogenicity are often made. Much of the work in human cancer immunity has been done with melanomas leading to suggestions that, among human tumors, melanomas are particularly immunogenic. This is an erroneous belief – melanomas are simply the easiest human tumors to culture in vitro and hence the easiest to study.

Immunity to a fibrosarcoma is specific to the individual tumor

When mice are immunized against a given fibrosarcoma, they are rendered immune to that fibrosarcoma, but only to that individual fibrosarcoma or lines derived from it. If the mice are challenged with another fibrosarcoma, even one induced by the same carcinogen, tumor growth is unaffected by the prior immunization (Fig. 22.3).

Q. What can you infer about the nature of the immune response to tumors from this observation?
A. It must involve the adaptive immune system.

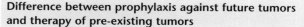

Difference between prophylaxis against future tumors and therapy of pre-existing tumors

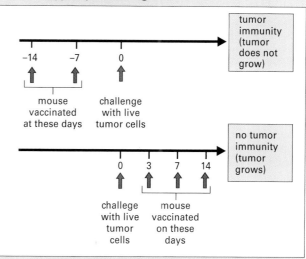

Fig. 22.2 Protective immunity is only seen in prophylactic immunization and not therapeutic immunization – once a mouse has been implanted with a tumor, immunization with irradiated cancer cells (derived from the growing tumor) does nothing to mitigate tumor growth.

Chemically induced tumors are individually distinct. The most extensive interrogation of the individually distinct antigenicity of chemically induced tumors was carried out by Basombrio and Prehn. They induced fibrosarcomas in 25 syngeneic BALB/c mice using methylcholanthrene and tested the immunogenicity of each one against all other tumors in an immunization-challenge model. They concluded that, even though all tumors were induced at the same time, in the same strain of mice of the same age by the same carcinogen and were histologically all fibrosarcomas, they were antigenically individually distinct. Independent tumors induced by the same carcinogen in the same mouse are also antigenically distinct.

Individually distinct antigenicity of chemically induced tumors

tumor used to challenge	tumor used to immunize			
	A	B	C	D
A	+	–	–	–
B	–	+	–	–
C	–	–	+	–
D	–	–	–	+

+ denotes tumor immunity or lack of tumor growth; – denotes lack of tumor immunity or tumor growth

Fig. 22.3 When mice are immunized against a given fibrosarcoma they are rendered immune to that fibrosarcoma, but only to that individual fibrosarcoma or lines derived from it. If the mice are challenged with another fibrosarcoma, even one induced by the same carcinogen, they are sensitive to it.

Spontaneous tumors are also antigenically distinct.

Cross-reactivity among tumors does occur occasionally. Typically, such cross-reactive immunity has been observed to be significantly weaker than the individually specific antigenicity. Efforts at characterization of such cross-reactive tumor-protective antigens have not made much headway, except in the case of virally induced tumors (see p. 409). In contrast, there has been considerable success in identification of individually distinct antigens.

In addition to these experimental studies, several clinical observations point to the existence of tumor-protective immunity in humans. These include the increased relative risk of cancers in patients who are immunosuppressed because they are kidney transplant recipients (Fig. 22.4) or for a variety of other reasons (Fig. 22.5).

Q. The observation that immunosuppressed individuals are more susceptible to tumors can be explained in at least two different ways. Suggest what these explanations might be.
A. The individual may be unable to control virus infections that lead to cancer (oncogenic viruses), or they may be unable to survey and control primary tumors that arise by mutation. The explanations are not mutually exclusive.

TUMOR ANTIGENS HAVE BEEN CHARACTERIZED BY THREE MEANS

The two broad approaches to the identification of tumor antigens are shown in Fig. 22.6 and discussed individually below. Not surprisingly, the approaches have yielded results that are not fully concordant with each other. These differences have helped highlight a fascinating interplay between immunity and tolerance to tumors, as discussed in a later section (see p. 413).

Tumor-specific antigens defined by immunization and challenge all belong to the family of HSPs

When tumors were biochemically fractionated and individual protein fractions tested for their ability to elicit protective tumor immunity, a number of tumor-protective antigens were identified in diverse tumor models, such as mouse sarcomas, melanomas, colon and lung carcinomas, and rat hepatomas.

Interestingly, regardless of the tumor models used, all antigens were found to belong to the family of proteins known as the **heat-shock proteins** (HSPs), which:
- constitute a very large family of intracellular soluble proteins that are organized into HSP families based on molecular size (Fig. 22.7);
- were shown to elicit protective immunity;
- were of the HSP90 (gp96 and HSP90), HSP70 (HSP110 and HSP/c70), calreticulin, and HSP170 (also known as grp170) families.

HSPs have to be isolated directly from tumors to be immunologically active

Two aspects of HSP-elicited tumor immunity are notable.
- First, HSPs are present in normal tissues as well as tumors, and normal tissue-derived HSPs do not elicit

---

Relative risk of tumors in immunosuppressed kidney transplant

tumor type	approximate relative risk
Kaposi's sarcoma	50–100
non-Hodgkin's lymphoma	25–45
carcinoma of the liver	20–35
carcinoma of the skin	20–50
carcinoma of the cervix	2.5–10
melanoma	2.5–10
lung	1–2

Fig. 22.4 In all forms of immunodeficiency the relative risk of developing tumors in which viruses are known to play a role is greatly increased. This is the case for all those listed except cancer of the lung. The relative risks vary in different studies according to the duration of follow-up and the presence of co-factors such as sunlight for skin cancer.

Tumor viruses and immunodeficiency

cause of immunodeficiency	common tumor types	viruses involved
inherited immunodeficiency	lymphoma	EBV
immunosuppression for organ transplants or due to AIDS	lymphoma cervical cancer skin cancer liver cancer Kaposi's sarcoma	EBV papilloma viruses probably papilloma viruses hepatitis B and C viruses human herpes virus 8
malaria	Burkitt's lymphoma	EBV
autoimmunity	lymphoma	EBV

Fig. 22.5 Skin cancer is the most common form of tumor in absolute numbers in organ transplant recipients. In other forms of immunodeficiency, tumors of the immune system dominate. Most normal adults carry both Epstein–Barr virus (EBV) and many papilloma viruses throughout life with no ill effects because they have antiviral immunity.

Comprehensive list of major types of tumor antigen

	category of antigen	individual antigens	tumors in which identified	activity in mouse models	human vaccine trials
tumor transplantation (mouse models)	heat-shock protein–peptide complexes	Gp96	fibrosarcoma, lung carcinoma, lymphoma, prostate carcinoma, etc.	+	phase III trials in renal carcinoma, melanoma underway
		Hsp70	fibrosarcoma, colon carcinoma	+	phase II trials in CML underway
		Hsp90, CRT Hsp110, 170	fibrosarcoma colon carcinoma	+	none yet
T cell/antibody (SEREX) reactivity (mostly human studies, some mouse models)	cancer/testes antigens	NY-ESO-1 MAGE, etc.	melanomas other tumors	N/A**	a number of phase I, II trials completed and underway
	differentiation antigens (lineage-specific)	melan A tyrosinase Gp100 PSA, etc.	melanomas (except PSA) (prostate carcinoma)		
	antigens with broader expression	human – CEA, MUC, HER2, G250	many tumors, except G250 (renal carcinoma only)		
		murine – P1A, gp70	many tumors	–	N/A
	common tumor-specific antigens	mutated p53, mutated ras, BCR-ABL, etc. papilloma virus?	many tumors	N/T*** exc. a single positive study with p53	no significant ongoing clinical effort
	unique tumor-specific antigens (mutations)	human – MUM-1, 2, β-catenin, HLA-A2-R170I, ELF2m, myosin-m, caspase-8, KIAA0205, HSP70-2m CDK4*, TRP2*, NA17A*	melanoma	N/A	N/A
		murine – Erk2, RNA helicase ribosomal proteins L9, L11	fibrosarcomas squamous cell carcinomas	+	none
	viral antigens	(see Fig. 22.5)			

CML, chronic myeloid leukemia; SEREX, serological analysis of recombinant cDNA expression libraries; *expressed on >1 melanoma, but not on any normal tissues; N/A**, not applicable; N/T***, not tested

Fig. 22.6 A comprehensive list of the major types of tumor antigen.

tumor rejection. They have to be isolated from tumors to be immunologically active.

• Second, HSPs elicit immunity specifically against the individual tumors from which they are isolated.

These two observations suggested that HSPs in tumors differ from those in normal tissues and that HSPs in each tumor differ from the same molecules in other tumors.

This conundrum was resolved by the demonstration that the HSP molecules chaperone peptides in a peptide-binding pocket, much as the MHC molecules do (though the structural details of the pockets in HSP and MHC differ) (Fig. 22.8). The specificity of immunogenicity derives from the peptides rather than the HSP itself – dissociation of HSP-associated peptides from HSPs abrogate the tumor rejection activity.

What are the HSP-chaperoned tumor antigenic peptides?

HSPs chaperone a large repertoire of peptides generated within the cells from which they are isolated.

Major heat-shock proteins*

HSP family	members	intracellular location
small HSPs	HSP10, GROES, HSP16, α-crystallin, HSP25, HSP26, HSP27	cytosol
HSP40	HSP40, DNAJ, SIS1	cytosol
HSP47	HSP47	endoplasmic reticulum
calreticulin	calreticulin, calnexin	endoplasmic reticulum
HSP60	HSP60, HSP65, GROEL	cytosol and mitochondria
HSP70	HSP72, HSP/c70/(HSP73), HSP110/SSE, DNAK, SSC1, SSQ1, ECM10, GRP78(BiP), grp170	cytosol / mitochondria / endoplasmic reticulum
HSP 90	HSC84, HSP86, HTPG gp96 (grp94, Erp99, endoplasmin)	cytosol / endoplasmic reticulum
HSP100	HSP104, HSP110** CLP proteins HSP78	cytosol / cytosol / mitochondria

*the list is not all-inclusive; **distinct from the HSP member with the same name; HSP, heat-shock protein

Fig. 22.7 HSPs constitute a very large family of intracellular soluble proteins, which are organized into HSP families based on molecular size. (Redrawn from Srivastava P. Nat Rev Immunol 2002;2:185–194. Copyright 2002, Nature Reviews Immunology www.nature.com/reviews)

HSP-chaperoned peptide pools contain cytotoxic T lymphocyte (CTL) epitopes and CTL epitope precursors for any antigens that the cell expresses (Fig. 22.9). This evidence comes from mouse and human tumors, normal tissues, and virus-infected cells. Hence, the HSP-chaperoned peptides contain among them any tumor-specific antigenic epitopes present in the tumor cell or the antigenic fingerprint of the tumor from which the HSPs are isolated.

HSP molecules bind to APCs and target peptides with high efficiency

The HSP molecule itself plays at least two crucial roles other than chaperoning peptides:

- HSPs bind antigen-presenting cells (APCs) such as macrophages and dendritic cells (DCs) through HSP receptors such as CD91 and thus target the peptides chaperoned by them into the APCs with high efficiency;
- further, the HSP-chaperoned peptides, once introduced into the APC, follow the endogenous as well as the exogenous pathway of antigen presentation and are processed and re-presented by the MHC I and MHC II molecules of the APCs (Fig. 22.10).

Q. How can an APC present internalized antigen via MHC class I molecules?

A. It can do this via the mechanism of cross-presentation (see Fig. 7.15).

It is by this mechanism that immunization with tumor-derived HSPs elicits a CD8 as well as CD4 response against the tumors. In addition, the HSP molecules stimulate the APCs to mediate maturation of DCs and secretion of an array of cytokines that provide the innate milieu for the adaptive response.

Unique immunogenicity of HSP–peptide complexes

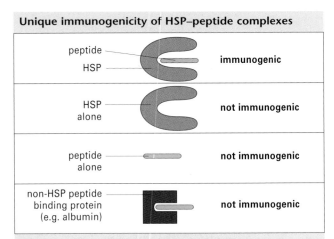

peptide / HSP	**immunogenic**
HSP alone	**not immunogenic**
peptide alone	**not immunogenic**
non-HSP peptide binding protein (e.g. albumin)	**not immunogenic**

Fig. 22.8 HSP molecules chaperone peptides in a peptide-binding pocket. The specificity of immunogenicity derives from the peptides rather than the HSP itself – dissociation of HSP-associated peptides from HSPs abrogated the tumor rejection activity.

CTL epitopes isolated from HSP–peptide complexes

antigen source	HSP with which associated	MHC class I molecule that presents epitope
tumor antigens		
PRL1e mouse leukemia	HSP70, HSP90, gp96	H-2L^d
human melanoma MART-1	HSP70	HLA-A2
human melanoma tyrosinase	HSP70	HLA-A2
human melanoma gp100	HSP70	HLA-A2
viral antigens		
vesicular stomatitis	gp96	H-2K^b
herpes simplex 2	gp96	H-2^d
influenza	gp96, HSP70	H-2K^b
simian virus 40	gp96	H-2D^b, H-2K^b
hepatitis B	gp96	
intracellular bacterial antigens		
Mycobacterium tuberculosis	gp96	H-2^d
Listeria monocytogenes	gp96	H-2^d
model antigens		
β-galactosidase	gp96	H-2L^d
ovalbumin	gp96	H-2K^b
normal cellular antigens		
minor histocompatibility antigens	gp96	H-2K^b, H-2K^b

Fig. 22.9 HSP-chaperoned peptide pools contain CTL epitopes and CTL epitope precursors for any antigens that the cell expresses. (Redrawn from Srivastava P. Nat Rev Immunol 2002;2:185–194. Copyright 2002, Nature Reviews Immunology www.nature.com/reviews)

The immunization-challenge model has led to identification of antigen carriers (i.e. HSPs), but not of the antigens themselves. As a result of exogenous administration, immunization with antigens themselves would generally be expected to elicit CD4 response, which in and of itself is not sufficient to elicit tumor immunity. The HSP-chaperoned antigens were picked up in this assay because they have the ability to elicit CD8 as well as CD4 responses despite being exogenously introduced. As discussed above, this response is derived from the ability of HSPs to interact with APCs through receptors such as CD91.

The status of clinical trials using tumor-derived HSP–peptide complexes for immunotherapy of human cancer is discussed below (see p. 417).

'Tumor-specific antigens' defined by T cells show a wide spectrum of specificity

Many studies have identified tumor-reactive T cells in blood or within a tumor, and these findings have thus supported the idea of tumor antigens.

The work of Thierry Boon and his colleagues first made it technically possible to identify the CTL epitopes of cancer cells being recognized by the tumor-reactive T cells.

Although the idea of tumor-specific antigens in mouse models of cancer was based on tumor rejection in vivo and thus had connotations of tumor specificity, the tumor antigens defined by tumor-reactive T cells show a wider spectrum of specificity, and their connection with tumor immunity in vivo, has been tenuous thus far.

The T cell-defined tumor antigens of murine tumors have been defined in a mastocytoma, two fibrosarcomas, a squamous cell carcinoma, and a colon carcinoma because these tumor lines are in popular use.

Similarly, much of the corresponding work in human tumors has been carried out in melanomas because melanoma cell lines are easier to establish in culture, rather than because of any unique immunogenicity of human melanomas.

The source of T cells is critically different in human and mouse studies

The murine T cells used for definition of tumor antigens have been obtained typically from splenocytes of mice that have been immunized against the tumor and are tumor-immune.

The human T cells have been obtained typically from patient's blood or from the tumor tissue itself.

These differences in the sources of T cells used may lie at the root of some of the differences in the nature of tumor antigens defined in the murine and human systems, as discussed below. The tumor antigens identified as T cell epitopes fall into the following categories (see Fig. 22.6).

Cancer/testes antigens are expressed only in testes

Cancer/testes (CT) antigens, as the name suggests, are expressed on cancer cells and in testes, but not in other normal adult tissues. MAGE, BAGE, GAGE, and NY-ESO1 are examples of this class of antigen. Individual epitopes within CT antigens have been defined for CD8 as well as CD4 lymphocytes. Most CT antigens have been identified in humans, although murine examples such as PEM exist as well.

Differentiation antigens are lineage specific and not tumor specific

Differentiation antigens, which are lineage specific, but not tumor specific, are expressed on normal tissues (melanocytes) as well as tumors (melanomas). Examples of such antigens include MART-1/Melan-A, tyrosinase, gp100, Trp1, and Trp2. Individual epitopes within

Mechanism of specific immunogenicity of HSP–peptide complexes

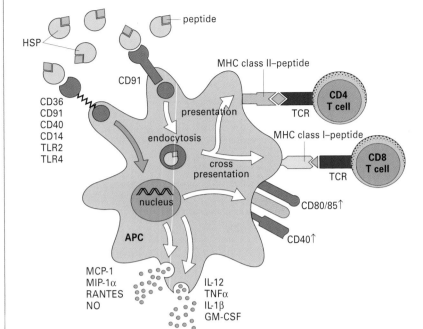

Fig. 22.10 Once introduced into the APC, the HSP-chaperoned peptides follow the endogenous class I as well as the exogenous class II pathway of antigen presentation and are processed and re-presented by the MHC class I and MHC II molecules of the APCs. HSP ligation induces production of chemokines and cytokines, and upregulation of CD40 and CD80/85. (MCP-1, monocyte chemotactic protein-1; MIP-1α, macrophage inflammatory protein-1α) (Redrawn from Srivastava P. Nat Rev Immunol 2002;2:185–194. Copyright 2002, Nature Reviews Immunology www.nature.com/reviews)

differentiation antigens have been defined for CD8 as well as CD4 lymphocytes. Most differentiation antigens have been identified in human melanomas.

Widely expressed antigens are expressed in cancers and normal tissue

These antigens are expressed on normal tissues as well as a wide array of tumors; in some instances differences in glycosylation may confer source specificity. Examples include:

- carcinoembryonic antigen (CEA), HER2/Neu, and Mucin (MUC) in humans; and
- AH1 in a mouse colon carcinoma.

Also in this category is a hypoxia-inducible carbonic anhydrase (MN/CA IX), which has been reported to be expressed in a majority of renal carcinomas, but in very few normal tissues tested.

Common tumor-specific antigens are not expressed on normal tissue

Common tumor-specific antigens can be expressed on tumors, but not on normal tissue. Such antigens, which have only been reported from the human system thus far, include antigenic epitopes generated by apparently tumor-specific alternate splicing such as TRP-2 and NA17-A (both in melanomas). This category also includes the mutated oncogenes, which are discussed in a separate category (see p. 410), because they were not identified on the basis of T cell reactivity.

Unique tumor-specific antigens have been characterized in melanomas

Individually tumor-specific or unique antigens presented by MHC class I or class II molecules have been characterized in:

- human melanomas (CDK-4, MUM-1, MUM-2, β-catenin, HLA-A2-R170I, ELF2m, myosin-m, caspase-8, KIAA0205, HSP70-2m); and
- murine tumors (Erk2, RNA helicase, ribosomal proteins L9, L11) alike (see Fig. 22.6).

In terms of their specificity, these antigens are the most similar to the individually tumor-specific antigens of murine tumors defined by tumor transplantation studies. Immunization with these antigens renders the mice resistant to tumor challenge. These are the only tumor antigens that have been shown to possess this essential property. The defined unique antigens of human tumors have not been tested for clinical activity.

T cell epitopes of viral antigens have been identified

T cell epitopes of viral antigens of virus-induced tumors have been identified such as:

- the T antigen of SV40 and the polyoma viruses;
- the E6 and E7 antigens of the human papilloma viruses that cause cervical cancer; and
- a number of antigens of the EBV (Fig. 22.11).

Some of these, such as the HPV antigens, are being tested for clinical activity against human tumors.

Microorganisms and human tumors

tumor	organism
adult T cell leukemia	human T leukemia virus-I (HTLV-I)
Burkitt's lymphoma and lymphoma in immunosuppression	EBV
cervical cancer	human papilloma viruses (HPV 16 and 18, and others)
liver cancer	hepatitis B and C
nasopharyngeal cancer	EBV
skin cancer	probably human papilloma viruses
stomach cancer	*Helicobacter pylori*

Fig. 22.11 EBV causes Burkitt's lymphoma in endemic malaria areas of Africa and nasopharyngeal carcinoma in China, suggesting that co-factors, either genetic or environmental, are required for tumor development. *Helicobacter pylori* is the only bacterium so far known to be involved in the etiology of human cancer.

'Tumor-specific antigens' defined by antibodies are rarely tumor specific

The search for antibodies that discriminate between cancer cells and normal cells has a long pedigree and has been carried out with the whole range of tools starting from antisera to panning antibody libraries.

This search has helped identify a whole range of molecules central to modern immunology, such as thymus leukemia antigen, CD8, and the T cell receptor (TCR), but, with very rare exceptions, has been largely unable to identify what it set out to do (i.e. identify cancer-specific antigens). The search has been largely unsuccessful and rarely have tumor-specific antibodies been generated.

Most anti-tumor antibodies, like anti-tumor T cells, happen to recognize CT antigens, differentiation antigens, and even more broadly distributed common antigens (see Fig. 22.6).

A recent development in this approach has focused attention on the fact that the tumor-bearing host develops antibodies to a repertoire of antigens that is distinct from the corresponding repertoire of antibodies seen in a non-tumor-bearing host. In this approach (known as SEREX for serological analysis of recombinant cDNA expression libraries), sera of cancer patients or tumor-bearing animals are used to screen expression libraries of tumors and an antibody repertoire is characterized. Although the individual antibodies are not tumor specific, the total repertoire shows relative specificity for cancer. The physiological meaning of this repertoire is unclear, but it appears to be a potent tool for diagnostic as well as monitoring purposes.

Antibodies used in the diagnosis of cancer may not be tumor specific

It is worthwhile at this point to comment on two types of antibodies that are used in diagnosis or treatment of cancers (Fig. 22.12).

As serum antibodies are technically easy to measure, they have always attracted the attention of diagnosticians. Thus:

- antibody to carcinoembryonic antigen (CEA) is often used as a marker for progression or status of certain carcinomas;
- similarly, a SEREX protein array may be used some day to monitor progression of a given cancer.

However, CEA or SEREX antigens are not tumor-specific antigens and diagnostic markers need not necessarily have the specificity required of a 'tumor-specific antigen'.

Antibodies to a B cell surface antigen, CD20, epidermal growth factor receptor, and HER2/Neu have now been approved for treatments, respectively, of B lymphoma, colorectal cancers, and breast cancers. Although these antibodies have shown some efficacy in the treatment of certain cancers at certain stages, they:

- do not recognize tumor-specific antigens;
- are actually used as pharmacological rather than immunological reagents.

This distinction does not diminish their utility and is highlighted only to draw attention to the fact that the term 'tumor-specific antigen' is used here to illustrate primarily the idea of host immune response to cancer, how it is elicited, how it is successful, and how it is not.

Tumor-specific antigens generated by mutated oncogenes may not be tumor protective

The discussion thus far has dealt with tumor antigens defined by experimental tools. Several additional antigens have been tested as tumor antigens because of their restricted or relatively restricted expression on cancer cells, with the reasonable assumption that they would elicit tumor-specific and perhaps tumor-protective immune responses. Antigenic epitopes generated by mutated oncogenes such as *ras* and *p53* as well as gene

(1) Markers for detection of cancers

marker	cancer
carcinoembryonic antigen (CEA)	adenocarcinomas of colon, breast, lung, breast, ovary
Ca 19-9	colon, pancreatic, and breast cancers
Ca 125	ovarian cancer
prostate-specific antigen (PSA)	prostate cancer
prostatic acid phosphatase (PAP)	prostate cancer
alpha-fetoprotein (AFP)	hepatocarcinoma, gonadal germ cell tumor
lactate dehydrogenase (LDH)	lymphoma, Ewing's sarcoma, melanoma
human chorionic gonadotropin (hCG)	gonadal germ cell tumor
calcitonin	medullary cancer of thyroid
catecholamines	pheochromocytoma
common acute lymphoblastic leukemia antigen (CALLA)	acute lymphoblastic leukemia
monoclonal immunoglobulin	myeloma
CD25	hairy cell leukemia, adult T cell lymphoma/leukemia
CD30	Hodgkin's lymphoma

(2) Antibodies used for therapy of selected cancers

antibody	antigen	conjugated to radioactivity/toxin	cancer
Herceptin®	HER2/Neu receptor	none	breast cancers
Rituxan®	CD20	none	non-Hodgkin's B cell lymphoma
Erbitux®	EGFR	none	metastatic colorectal cancers
Campath®	CD52	none	CLL
Zevalin®	CD20	indium-111, yttrium-90	refractory B cell lymphoma
Bexaar®	CD20	iodine-131	refractory B cell lymphoma
Mylotarg®	CD33	calicheamicin toxin	AML

Fig. 22.12 Neither the 'antigens' used as diagnostic cancer markers (1) nor the antibodies used for therapy of selected cancers (2) are tumor specific. CLL, chronic lymphatic leukemia; AML, acute myeloid leukemia.

fusion-generated oncogenes such as *bcr-abl*, which are, by definition, tumor specific, come into this category. These antigens could, in principle, be broadly applicable tumor antigens.

The idea that mutant proteins are recognized by the immune system has been explored to a degree in murine and human systems, and immune reactivity to peptides derived from such mutated oncogenes has been detected. However, no evidence of their general tumor-protective immunogenicity has emerged.

It is conceivable that the immune response to these alterations is tolerized early in tumorigenesis and, indeed, such tolerization may be a pre-condition for tumorigenesis.

The same may be said for telomerase, expression of which in cancer cells allows them to circumvent the rules of cellular mortality, and which too has been conceived of and tested as a tumor antigen with tantalizing but not compelling results.

The non-mutated oncogene HER2/Neu as an immunizing agent has been the subject of extensive studies in HER2/Neu-transgenic mouse models, which develop spontaneous mammary carcinomas. These experiments have shown that immunization with the oncogene inhibits spontaneous mammary carcinogenesis in these mice and may also promote regression of pre-existing lesions. The reasons for the differences between tumor-protective immunogenicities of these various antigens are unclear at present.

VIGOROUS ANTI-TUMOR IMMUNE RESPONSES ARE COMPROMISED BY REGULATORY MECHANISMS
Successful tumor immunity is rare in patients who have cancer

Mechanisms of tumor immunity have been examined mostly in mouse models, partly because successful tumor immunity is rare in patients who have cancer.

Further, as successful tumor immunity is rare in the tumor-bearing setting in mouse models as well, much of the work has been done in a prophylactic setting, which is not applicable to the human situation.

Not surprisingly, the pathways to elicitation of immune response to tumors are straightforward (Fig. 22.13). The tumor inoculum (with its antigenic load) is taken up by the APCs at the site of immunization and is cross-presented by them to the naive CD8 cells in the draining lymph nodes. Both responses are generally necessary in the mouse models tested and both responses have been shown to be present in the cancer patients studied.

Antibodies have not generally been shown to be protective in the natural setting.

NK cell activity has been demonstrated most commonly, but its necessity has been rarely examined critically. In the few studies where it has been examined, it appears that NK cells play a crucial role in the immune response to cancers. Clearly, the cytokines necessary for the effector functions of CD4, CD8, and NK cells, such as IL-2, IFNγ, IL-12, and others, are necessary as well.

In selected models, significant roles for innate components such as neutrophils and eosinophils in tumor rejection have been shown.

Despite an immune response, tumors continue to grow

Despite clear evidence for the existence of tumor-specific antigens and the immune response elicited by them,

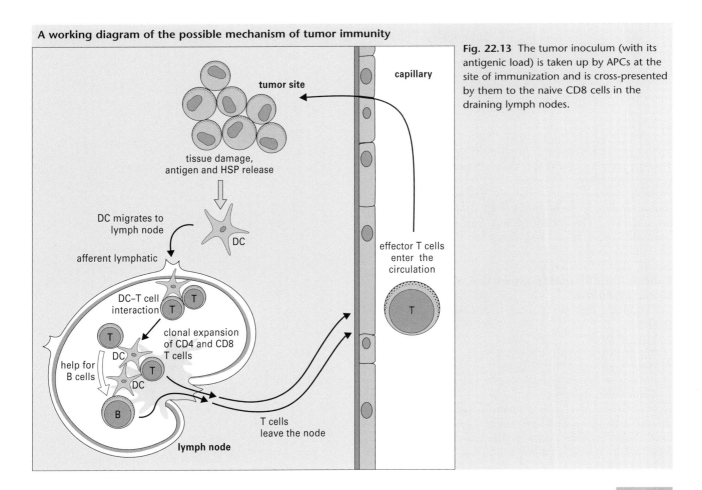

A working diagram of the possible mechanism of tumor immunity

tumor site

tissue damage, antigen and HSP release

DC migrates to lymph node

afferent lymphatic

DC

DC–T cell interaction

clonal expansion of CD4 and CD8 T cells

help for B cells

DC

DC

B

T cells leave the node

lymph node

capillary

effector T cells enter the circulation

Fig. 22.13 The tumor inoculum (with its antigenic load) is taken up by APCs at the site of immunization and is cross-presented by them to the naive CD8 cells in the draining lymph nodes.

Concomitant immunity

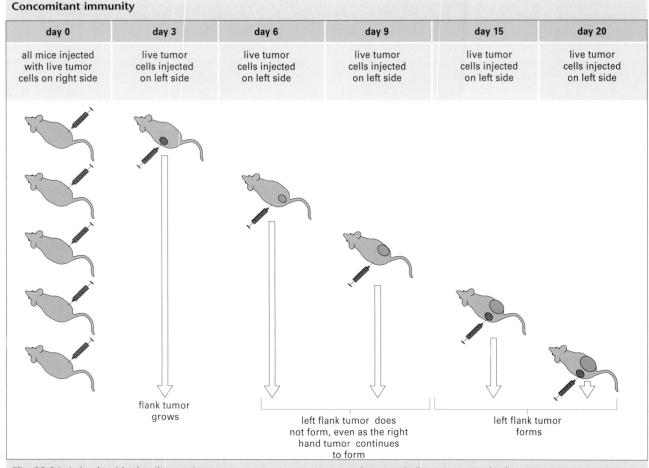

day 0	day 3	day 6	day 9	day 15	day 20
all mice injected with live tumor cells on right side	live tumor cells injected on left side	live tumor cells injected on left side	live tumor cells injected on left side	live tumor cells injected on left side	live tumor cells injected on left side

flank tumor grows

left flank tumor does not form, even as the right hand tumor continues to form

left flank tumor forms

Fig. 22.14 Animals with already growing tumors are resistant to a second tumor challenge even as the first tumor continues to grow.

tumors generally continue to grow. In this regard, Ehrlich made a curious observation that remains at the center of cancer immunity. He noted that animals with already growing tumors were strangely resistant to a second tumor challenge even as the first tumor kept growing (Fig. 22.14). This phenomenon, termed **concomitant immunity** as early as 1908, remained relatively unexamined until recently.

Concomitant immunity shows two aspects of tumor immunity

Concomitant immunity shows two aspects of tumor immunity:
- first, a growing tumor elicits in the primary host a tumor-protective immune response;
- second, although this response is sufficient to eliminate a nascent tumor, it fails to eliminate the tumor that elicited the response.

It was shown that concomitant immunity was tumor specific and operational only within a narrow window of 7–10 days after tumor implantation; if the second tumor was implanted beyond this time, it was not rejected. The lack of immunity beyond the narrow window was attributable to a new population of suppressor T cells that appeared at that time (Fig. 22.15). Similar to the phenomenon of concomitant immunity, it was also noted that mice in the process of rejecting an allograft were unable to concomitantly reject a growing tumor bearing the same alloantigens as the allograft.

Q. How do you interpret the observation above?
A. One would expect an allograft to be rejected in these circumstances, therefore there is something about the tumor that allows it to evade a normal allospecific rejection reaction.

Immunization is effective prophylactically but rarely as therapy

The findings discussed above fit in well with the observations that, although naive mice can be immunized successfully using irradiated tumor cell vaccines in almost any tumor model, the same irradiated cell vaccine is ineffective at treating established tumors.

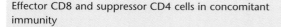

Effector CD8 and suppressor CD4 cells in concomitant immunity

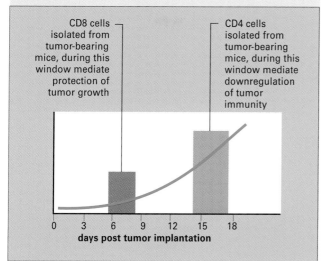

CD8 cells isolated from tumor-bearing mice, during this window mediate protection of tumor growth

CD4 cells isolated from tumor-bearing mice, during this window mediate downregulation of tumor immunity

days post tumor implantation

Fig. 22.15 Concomitant immunity is tumor specific and operational only within a narrow window of 7–10 days after tumor implantation. If the second tumor is implanted beyond this time, it is not rejected. The lack of immunity beyond the narrow window is attributable to a new population of suppressor T cells that appear at that time.

Prophylaxis is relatively effective, even if begun as late as 3 days before tumor implantation, but therapy is ineffective even if begun as early as 2 days after tumor implantation (see Fig. 22.2).

It is easy, and incorrect, to infer from these observations that the tumor-bearing mice or cancer patients are generally immunosuppressed. Tumor-bearing mice generally mount a vigorous immune response to model antigens and even unrelated tumors, almost until the very end of their lives. Similarly, patients with cancer do not generally succumb to the opportunistic infections that are the hallmark of general immunosuppression.

What are the mechanisms behind the change from naive to tumor-bearing states?

Collectively, these and similar other observations have shaped the thinking that, immunologically speaking, the tumor-bearing host is in a radically different state compared with the naive host.

What are the mechanisms behind this change of status? They are exactly the same as envisaged for the mechanisms for the initiation and maintenance of peripheral tolerance. None of the explanations is fully satisfactory by itself, but each perhaps contributes to the final state of tolerance in some measure. Immune unresponsiveness per se is addressed in detail in Chapters 12 and 19. Only some aspects that are of specific relevance to tumor immunity are discussed here (Fig. 22.16).

Downregulation of MHC I molecule expression may result in resistance to recognition and lysis

Loss of MHC class I molecules by tumor cells has often been suggested to be one such mechanism.

A number of studies have shown:
- downregulation of expression of one or more MHC class I alleles;
- loss of β_2-microglobulin; or
- loss or downregulation of any of the several components of the antigen processing machinery.

Although these alterations are clearly likely to inhibit recognition of tumor cells by T cells, they are also more likely to make tumors more susceptible to become targets of NK cells.

On the whole, it is not clear what effect, if any, these alterations have on the net ability of a tumor to escape the immune response in vivo.

Generation of antigen-loss variants is another mechanism that no doubt plays a role to some degree in the immunological escape of tumor cells. However, because we do not yet have a significant knowledge of the identity of truly tumor-protective antigens, the role of antigen-loss variants cannot be critically examined.

Inhibitory cytokines such as TGFβ and IL-10, and others, have often been proposed to downregulate anti-tumor immune responses.

Major mechanisms of suppression of anti-tumor immune response

at the level of generation of response
inhibitory cytokines such as transforming growth factor-β (TGFβ) and interleukin-10 (IL-10)
attenuation of response
general mechanisms of peripheral tolerance inhibition of T cell activity through CTLA-4 downregulation of immune response through CD25⁺ and other suppressor cells
at the effector level
resistance to recognition and lysis by downregulation of MHC class I molecules generation of antigen-loss variants

Fig. 22.16 Only mechanisms of suppression of specific relevance to tumor immunity are listed here.

T cell activity is inhibited through CTLA-4

An exciting explanation for unresponsiveness is the role of inhibition of T cell activity through CTLA-4. CTLA-4 and CD28 belong to the same family of molecules and both are expressed on CD8 T cells.

Q. What are the functions of CD28 and CTLA-4 (CD152) on T cells?

A. CD28 transduces co-stimulatory signals to the T cell, while CTLA-4 also ligates B7, but is inhibitory (see Fig. 22.17).

CTLA-4 inhibits the T cell by raising the stimulatory threshold or by inhibiting the proliferative drive of T cells (Fig. 22.17). The biological role of CTLA-4 appears to lie in limiting the T cell response to foreign antigens as well as to autoantigens.

Administering antibodies to CTLA-4 (that inhibit CTLA-4:B7 interactions) to mice bearing a broad array of tumors inhibited tumor growth, even when the antibody was administered after the tumors were visible and palpable (Fig. 22.18). Such activity was generally seen only against the more immunogenic tumors and not against a poorly immunogenic melanoma (e.g. B16). In that instance, combination of anti-CTLA-4 antibody with a vaccine consisting of irradiated melanoma cells that were also transfected with the cytokine granulocyte–macrophage colony stimulating factor (GM-CSF), resulted in a stronger anti-tumor response than by anti-CTLA-4 antibody or the vaccine alone. Clinical development of this idea is discussed below.

Similar results have been observed in other tumor models. These results support the notion derived from studies on concomitant immunity that progressive tumor

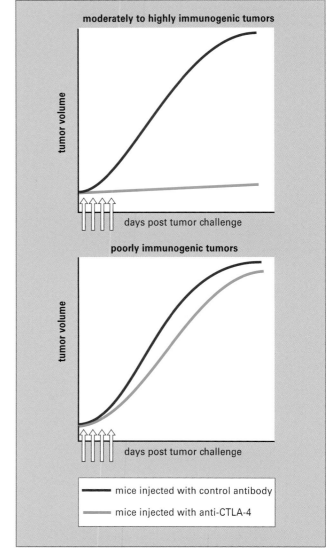

Mouse tumor rejection using anti-CTLA-4 antibody

Fig. 22.18 Administering anti-CTLA-4 to mice bearing a broad array of tumors inhibited tumor growth. Such activity was generally seen only against the more immunogenic tumors and not against poorly immunogenic tumors. The arrows denote the administration of antibodies.

growth results in the generation of inhibitory influences on the anti-tumor immune response.

Abrogation of CD25⁺ cells leads to protective tumor immunity

The notion that progressive tumor growth results in the generation of inhibitory influences on the anti-tumor immune response is further supported by the recent work on the CD25⁺ CD4⁺ Treg cells (see Chapter 19). These cells have been shown to play a regulatory (i.e. suppressive) role in CD8 T cell responses in general, including autoimmune responses.

Mechanism of action of anti-CTLA-4 antibody

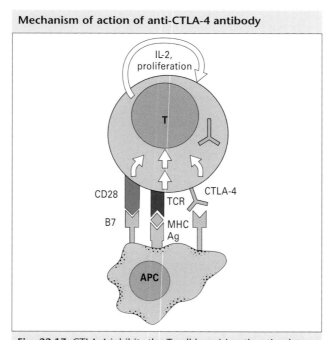

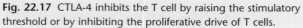

Fig. 22.17 CTLA-4 inhibits the T cell by raising the stimulatory threshold or by inhibiting the proliferative drive of T cells.

Recent studies have shown that abrogation of the CD25+ subpopulation (through anti-CD25 antibodies or through genetic manipulation) in tumor-bearing mice leads to a robust T cell response and protective tumor immunity even in an aggressive tumor model such as the B16 melanoma. Conversely, re-addition of these cells can suppress the anti-tumor immune response.

Results consistent with these have been observed in patients with melanoma whose regulatory CD4+ T cells specifically inhibit the CD8+ activity against autologous melanoma cells, but not against other targets.

More recent studies have examined this paradigm through the prism of the CD25+ T cells. In a study of patients with ovarian cancer, such cells were shown to be associated with a higher risk of death and reduced survival. Interestingly, the CD25+ T cells were shown to migrate preferentially to the solid tumors and the ascites, but rarely to the draining lymph nodes.

Such results have begun to point inexorably to the general theme that, despite the poor clinical outcomes in advanced cancer, the host does mount a vigorous anti-tumor immune response, which is compromised by regulatory mechanisms. Manipulation of such regulatory mechanisms for enhancing cancer immunity is bound to influence the fine balance between tolerance and auto-immunity. In certain contexts, that may be a reasonable price to pay.

IMMUNOTHERAPY FOR HUMAN CANCER
Animal models are limited in the translation of therapy

There exists a 'common wisdom' that treatment of cancers of mice is easy and has no bearing on treatment of human cancers. This belief is as common as it is incorrect. Mouse tumors are hard to cure – there does not exist a single publication that reports curing a mouse with stage IV disseminated disease.

Most approaches study prophylactic vaccination in mice, a smaller number begin treatment on the day of tumor challenge, and only a handful of studies begin treatment more than 10 days after tumor challenge. In most mouse tumor models, mice die within 4–6 weeks of tumor challenge, and thus the window of treatment is extremely narrow.

Most approaches to immunotherapy of human cancer have either never been tested in appropriate mouse models or have failed to show anti-tumor activity when tested. It is important to bear this in mind while examining the three major categories of approaches to immunotherapy of human cancer, discussed below.

Antibodies have been used successfully

As antibodies are the oldest known immunological reagents, it is only to be expected that the first, and thus far among the most successful, approaches to human cancer immunotherapy has been made using these reagents.

Nearly 20 years ago, Ronald Levy and colleagues treated patients with B cell lymphomas using individual patient's tumor-specific anti-idiotypic antibodies on the premise that the antibodies will recognize and help eliminate their targets – the surface immunoglobulin on the monoclonal lymphomas. The treatment was successful clinically, leading to significant objective tumor regressions, but was limited by the re-emergence of escape variants that did not express the idiotype. This approach has not been pursued further, but remains a powerful reminder of what true tumor-specific antibodies can do to real-life tumors. The transformation of this approach to vaccination is discussed below.

Selected antibodies are now approved for clinical use, but these represent pharmacological rather than immunological use of antibodies (see Fig. 22.12) and include antibodies to:
- CD20 – rituximab – against B cell lymphoma;
- HER2/Neu – trastuzumab (Herceptin®) – against breast cancer;
- epidermal growth factor receptor – cetuximab (Erbitux®) – against colon cancer.

It is ironic that the anti-tumor antibodies that may recognize truly or relatively tumor-specific molecules, and that were the earliest hopes of much of the efforts in this area, have yet to enter the phase of randomized clinical testing. Such antibodies are difficult to characterize and therefore have been slow in development. Nonetheless, they exist and may be expected to be tested by themselves or with radioactive or toxic tags in the near future. Unfortunately, a number of antibodies that were thus tagged and already tested in clinical trials were not very specific and did not show compelling clinical results.

Vaccination can be used to treat cancer

Although the term vaccination is typically used to indicate prophylactic vaccination, cancer researchers use it to indicate the treatment of someone who already has cancer, with agents that stimulate anti-cancer immune response. Several vaccination approaches are currently being pursued (Fig. 22.19).

The idiotypes of B lymphomas have been used as vaccines

Following the use of anti-idiotypic antibodies and the attendant limitations discussed above, the idiotypes of B lymphomas have been used as vaccines. In this approach, a patient's idiotype is determined by polymerase chain reactions from the tumor tissues, and a synthetic idiotype, conjugated to a carrier such as keyhole limpet hemocyanin, is administered along with GM-CSF. Phase I and II trials with this approach have yielded promising results and phase III trials in patients with follicular B lymphoma are now in progress. For obvious reasons, this approach is limited to B lymphoma and related hematological malignancies.

Q. Which other group of cells is (theoretically) susceptible to anti-idiotypic targeting of tumor therapy?

A. The recombined T cell receptor is also expressed on specific clones of cells. The limitations that apply to the therapy of B cell lymphomas (mutation escape) also apply here, and it is in any case more difficult to generate antibodies to the T cell receptor.

Vaccination approaches to immunotherapy of human cancer currently being tested

vaccine	cancer
unique antigen (individually patient-specific) approaches	
idiotypes + KLH + GM-CSF	B lymphoma
intact autologous irradiated tumor cells + BCG	colon cancer
intact autologous haptenated irradiated tumor cells	melanoma
intact autologous GM-CSF transfected tumor cells	melanoma, renal cancer, lung cancer
autologous tumor lysates	renal cancer
HSP–peptide complexes	melanoma, renal cancer, colon cancer, chronic myeloid leukemia
shared tumor antigen approaches	
allogeneic irradiated cell lines	melanoma
differentiation antigens	melanoma
cancer/testes antigens	melanoma

Fig. 22.19 Several vaccination approaches are currently being pursued.

Immunization with irradiated intact tumor cells has been tested against many cancers

The first randomized trials of immunizing cancer patients with irradiated intact tumor cells were carried out in patients with colorectal cancer, where each patient in the treatment arm received autologous irradiated tumor cells mixed with BCG. The trials showed detectable clinical activity in the vaccine arm, but the activity failed to achieve statistical significance.

Autologous haptenated tumor cells and autologous GM-CSF transfected tumor cells have also been used as vaccines in patients with melanoma, renal carcinoma, pancreatic cancer, and non-small cell lung cancer. Some of the early trials with these approaches have been suggestive of clinical activity.

A non-autologous whole cell strategy has been pursued in stage III and IV melanoma where the vaccines were not made from autologous tumors, but from a collection of irradiated allogeneic lines. The rationale offered for this approach was that melanomas may be expected to contain a number of shared immunogenic antigens and immunization with a collection of melanoma lines increases the odds of immunizing against the antigens expressed by the melanoma of any given patient. However, analysis of the phase III trial indicated lack of any clinical benefit to

immunized patients and the trial has now been discontinued.

Q. What evidence is there that this approach to therapy is unlikely to be successful?
A. The result is consistent with the earliest observations in the history of cancer immunity that showed that the immuno-protective antigens of tumors are individually unique and not shared among tumors (see Fig. 22.3).

Tumor lysate immunization is still being tested

Immunization with whole tumor lysates (as opposed to intact irradiated cells) also has a long pedigree and is still being tested.

An allogeneic melanoma lysate named Melacine® was initially tested without significant success.

Autologous tumor lysates have been tested in patients with renal carcinoma in the post-nephrectomy adjuvant setting and a randomized trial using such lysates has shown statistically significant benefit for the immunized patients. The manufacturers of this vaccine have presently applied for it to be approved as standard treatment for patients with renal carcinoma. In principle, this method would be applicable to any cancer.

Defined MHC I epitope immunotherapy does not lead to clinical benefit

The antigenic epitopes of differentiation antigens and cancer/testes antigens have been used extensively and several hundred patients with melanoma have been treated with these. Although anti-peptide CD8 responses have been detected in most studies, these have not generally translated into clinical benefit even for those patients who have shown good CD8 responses. Attempts to understand this anomaly and to build upon these studies are in progress.

Particularly interesting are efforts to vaccinate with altered peptide epitopes with higher affinity for the cognate T cell receptors. Immunization with such altered peptides is able to break tolerance against these self antigens where immunization with native peptides is not.

Q. What problem is intrinsic to this type of tumor therapy?
A. Immunization with differentiation antigens is premised on breaking tolerance and hence carries the near certainty of generating autoimmune responses (see Chapter 19).

This approach relies on the existence of a therapeutic window, which will permit anti-cancer immunity without debilitating autoimmunity.

Immunization with HSP–peptide complexes demonstrates clinical benefit

The role of HSP–peptide complexes in eliciting tumor immunity has been discussed earlier.

The highly successful murine studies have been translated into a series of phase I and II trials involving patients with pancreatic, gastric, stomach, and renal cancers, and with melanoma, B lymphoma, and chronic myelogenous leukemia.

In these trials, surgically obtained tumor specimens (or leukemia cells obtained by leukopheresis) from a given patient are used as the starting material for preparation of gp96–peptide or hsp70–peptide complexes specifically for that patient (Fig. 22.20).

The early trials have shown suggestions of clinical activity in immunized patients and have led to randomized phase III trials in renal carcinoma and melanoma. Interim results from a randomized trial in patients with stage IV melanoma have shown that patients with early stage IV disease, who were treated with gp96, survived longer than those in the control arm. The final results of this trial, and of the phase III renal cancer trial, are expected in early 2006.

Adoptive immunotherapy using T cells: the clinical benefits

Adoptive immunotherapy using T cells has a successful pedigree in murine models of cancer (Fig. 22.21). Clinical experience with bone marrow transplant recipients also provides a strong rationale for the approach.

Patients undergoing high-dose chemotherapy lose their bone marrow and are re-constituted with allogeneic stem cells, which engraft in the recipient. However, the T cells from the donor may see the normal tissues of the host as foreign, thus causing graft versus host disease (GVHD).

Interestingly, patients who develop GVHD also have a lower cancer relapse or graft versus tumor (GVT) incidence. The clinical experience with GVHD and GVT has long remained a compelling piece of evidence for the premise that T cells can eliminate human cancers in vivo (Fig. 22.22).

A number of studies have isolated tumor-infiltrating T cells from cancer patients, expanded them in vitro and infused the expanded cells back into the patients. Such studies have occasionally shown remarkable shrinkage of tumors. However, the fact that such responses are seen only occasionally points to the fact that there remain inherent hurdles that need to be identified and rectified.

Adoptive immunotherapy with T cells

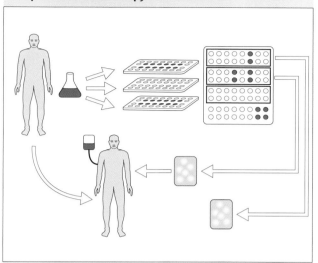

Fig. 22.21 Lymphocytes removed from a patient with a tumor are expanded in vitro. Cells that recognise the tumor are selected and reinfused into the original patient. Adoptive therapy with allogeneic lymphocytes may also be carried out. (Redrawn from Dudley ME, Rosenberg SA. Adoptive-cell-transfer therapy for the treatment of patients with cancer. Nat Rev Cancer 2003;3:666–675. Copyright 2002, Nature Reviews Cancer, Macmillan Magazines Ltd)

In a variation of this approach, cloned T cells with defined specificity have been expanded to very large numbers and infused into patients with melanoma, also to show dramatic tumor shrinkage.

However, hurdles to expansion of T cells as well as their effector functions in vivo remain, and there is considerable ongoing experimental effort to engineer T cells that will retain specificity and autonomy of growth and will be relatively refractory to downregulatory influences of the host.

Immunotherapy with peptide pulsed DCs has shown early promise

In such studies, DCs are isolated from a cancer patient, expanded in vitro, pulsed with antigenic peptides, whole proteins, or tumor lysates and infused back into the patient.

The most advanced randomized phase III clinical trials with this approach have been carried out in patients with prostate cancer who have received autologous DCs pulsed with prostatic acid phosphatase. Patients in the control arm received a placebo. Patients who received acid phosphatase pulsed DCs survived measurably longer than patients who received placebo. This trial may form the basis of approval of this treatment for patients with prostate cancer.

Inhibition of downregulation of immune modulation may be clinically valuable

The role of downregulation of tumor immunity in progressive tumor growth in mouse models has been discussed earlier. Inhibition of such downregulation is an

Treatment of cancer patients with HSP–peptide complexes

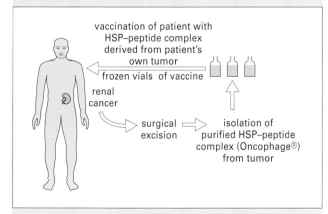

Fig. 22.20 Surgically obtained tumor specimens from a given patient are used as the starting material for preparation of gp96–peptide or HSP70–peptide complexes specifically for that patient.

Graft versus host disease and graft versus tumor

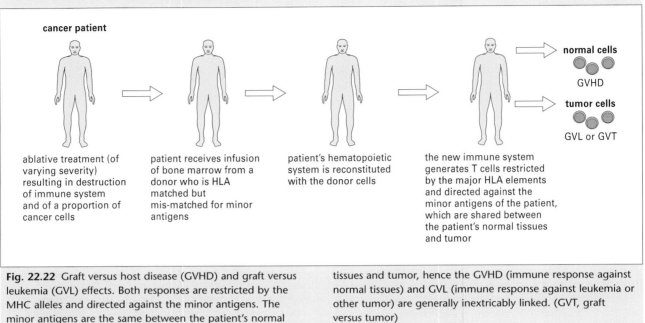

Fig. 22.22 Graft versus host disease (GVHD) and graft versus leukemia (GVL) effects. Both responses are restricted by the MHC alleles and directed against the minor antigens. The minor antigens are the same between the patient's normal tissues and tumor, hence the GVHD (immune response against normal tissues) and GVL (immune response against leukemia or other tumor) are generally inextricably linked. (GVT, graft versus tumor)

attractive target of translation and antibodies to CTLA-4 are under clinical testing in this regard.

A number of phase I and II clinical trials using antibodies to CTLA-4 have been completed in patients with melanoma and ovarian and renal cancer.

The most dramatic results have been obtained in patients who had previously been vaccinated with autologous GM-CSF transfected tumor cells as part of another study and had not shown significant response to that vaccination. When these patients were treated with anti-CTLA-4 antibody, they showed dramatic tumor shrinkage and infiltration of the tumors with lymphocytes and granulocytes.

Interestingly, patients previously immunized with differentiation antigen vaccines and who received the same anti-CTLA-4 antibody did not show clinical responses.

The synergy between vaccination with GM-CSF transfected tumor cells and administration of anti-CTLA-4 antibody was also previously seen in a mouse model of melanoma. Further clinical exploration of this attractive strategy is now in progress.

Most successful treatment approaches are based on individually distinct tumor antigens

A perusal of the various approaches discussed above will show that some approaches are based on the premise that immunoprotective antigens of tumors are individually distinct, whereas others pursue the idea of immunoprotective antigens shared among individual tumors (see Fig. 22.19).

The most successful clinical data obtained thus far have been seen in trials with:

- autologous cancer cells plus BCG (colon cancers);
- idiotype vaccines (follicular B lymphoma);
- autologous tumor lysates (renal carcinoma);
- autologous tumor vaccines plus anti-CTLA-4 antibody (melanoma, ovarian cancers);
- acid phosphatase pulsed DCs; and
- gp96–peptide complexes from autologous tumors.

Of these, all approaches except the acid phosphatase pulsed DCs are based on individually distinct rather than shared immunoprotective tumor antigens. That bias is certainly consistent with the individually unique antigenicity seen in mouse tumors, as discussed at the beginning of this chapter.

FURTHER READING

Belli F, Testori A, Rivoltini L, et al. Vaccination of metastatic melanoma patients with autologous tumor-derived heat shock protein gp96–peptide complexes: clinical and immunologic findings. J Clin Oncol 2002;20:4169–4180.

Coulie PG, Karanikas V, Lurquin C, et al. Cytolytic T-cell responses of cancer patients vaccinated with a MAGE antigen. Immunol Rev 2002;188:33–42.

Egen JG, Kuhns MS, Allison JP. CTLA-4: new insights into its biological function and use in tumor immunotherapy. Nat Immunol 2002;3:611–618.

Fehervari Z, Sakaguchi S. CD4+ Tregs and immune control. J Clin Invest 2004;114:1209–1217.

Ho WY, Blattman JN, Dossett ML, et al. Adoptive immunotherapy:

engineering T cell responses as biologic weapons for tumor mass destruction. Cancer Cell 2003;3:431–437.

Klein G. The strange road to the tumor-specific transplantation antigens (TSTAs). Cancer Immun 2001;1:6.

North RJ. Down-regulation of the antitumor immune response. Adv Cancer Res 1985;45:1–43.

Scanlan MJ, Gure AO, Jungbluth AA, et al. Cancer/testis antigens: an expanding family of targets for cancer immunotherapy. Immunol Rev 2002;188:22–32.

Srivastava PK. Do human cancers express shared protective antigens? or the necessity of remembrance of things past. Semin Immunol 1996;8:295–302.

Srivastava PK. Interaction of heat shock proteins with peptides and antigen presenting cells: chaperoning of the innate and adaptive immune responses. Annu Rev Immunol 2002;20:395–425.

Van Der Bruggen P, Zhang Y, Chaux P, et al. Tumor-specific shared antigenic peptides recognized by human T cells. Immunol Rev 2002;188:51–64.

Wick M, Dubey P, Koeppen H, et al. Antigenic cancer cells grow progressively in immune hosts without evidence for T cell exhaustion or systemic anergy. J Exp Med 1997;186:229–238.

Critical thinking: Immunity to cancers (see p. 501 for explanations)

1 Animals can be easily immunized against cancers. Why then do the same cancers grow progressively and kill their hosts?

2 Heat-shock proteins do not differ between tumors and normal tissues. Yet, HSP preparations isolated from tumors elicit tumor immunity, whereas similar preparations from normal tissues do not. Explain the mechanistic basis of this phenomenon.

3 How have tumor antigens been defined? How many classes of tumor antigen have been defined thus far?

4 Explain the phenomenon of concomitant immunity.

5 Discuss the evidence that the immune response to tumors is downregulated in tumor-bearing mice and in patients with cancer.

Hypersensitivity

Immediate Hypersensitivity (Type I)

SUMMARY

- **Hypersensitivity reactions are based on the classification of Coombs and Gell.**

- **Historical observations have shaped our understanding of immediate hypersensitivity.** The severity of symptoms depends on IgE antibodies, the quantity of allergen, and also a variety of factors that can enhance the response including viral infections and environmental pollutants.

- **Most allergens are proteins.**

- **IgE is distinct from the other dimeric immunoglobulins.** Production of IgE in genetically predisposed (i.e. atopic) individuals occurs in response to repeated low-dose exposure to inhaled allergens such as dust mite, cat dander, or grass pollen.

- **Allergens are the antigens that give rise to immediate hypersensitivity and contribute to asthma.**

- **Mast cells and basophils contain histamine.** IgE antibodies bind to a specific receptor, FcεRI, on mast cells and basophils. When bound IgE is cross-linked by specific allergen, mediators including histamine, leukotrienes, and cytokines are released.

- **Multiple genes have been associated with asthma in different populations.** Multiple genetic loci influence the production of IgE, the inflammatory response to allergen exposure, and the response to treatment. Polymorphisms have been identified in the genes, in promoter regions, and in the receptors for IgE, cytokines, leukotrienes, and the β_2-receptors.

- **Skin tests are used for diagnosis and investigation.**

- **Several different pathways contribute to the chronic symptoms of allergy.**

- **Allergens contribute to asthma.**

- **Immunotherapy can be used for hayfever and anaphylactic sensitivity.**

- **New approaches are being investigated for treating allergic disease.**

- **IgE antibodies play a critical role in defense against helminths.** The biological role of immediate hypersensitivity is to control helminth infections such as schistosomiasis, hookworm, or ascariasis. However, it is likely to be a combination of effector TH2 cells, basophils, and eosinophils, as well as IgE antibodies on mast cells, that control these worms.

HYPERSENSITIVITY REACTIONS ARE BASED ON THE CLASSIFICATION OF COOMBS AND GELL

The adaptive immune response provides specific protection against infection with bacteria, viruses, parasites, and fungi. In particular, it is able to provide rapid protection against a repeated challenge with the same or a similar foreign organism or toxin. Some immune responses, however, give rise to an excessive or inappropriate reaction – this is usually referred to as **hypersensitivity**.

The term hypersensitivity evolved from the observations of Richet and Portier one hundred years ago, who described the catastrophic result of exposing a pre-sensitized animal to systemic antigen. The resulting outcome, termed **anaphylaxis**, became the prototype of immediate hypersensitivity responses.

Coombs and Gell in 1963 proposed a classification scheme in which allergic hypersensitivity of the type described by Portier and Richet was termed type I, and broadened the definition of hypersensitivity to include:
- reactions that resulted from antibody–antigen reactions, including cytotoxic reactions which they termed type II (see Chapter 24);
- immune complex reactions of the Arthus type, which were termed type III reactions (see Chapter 25);
- delayed-type hypersensitivity responses were given the classification type IV to describe reactions typified by cutaneous contact reactions upon exposure to certain agents such as nickel (see Chapter 26).

The original Coombs and Gell classification is shown in Fig. 23.1.

The Coombs and Gell classification of the four types of hypersensitivity reaction

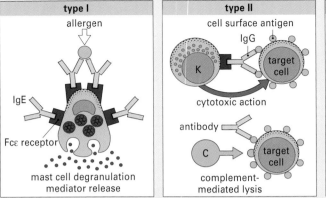
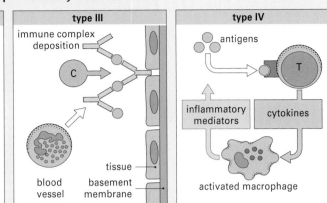

Fig. 23.1 In type I, mast cells bind IgE via their Fc receptors. On encountering allergen the IgE becomes cross-linked, inducing degranulation and release of mediators that produce allergic reactions. In type II, antibody is directed against antigen on an individual's own cells (target cell) or foreign antigen, such as transfused red blood cells. This may lead to cytotoxic action by K cells, or complement-mediated lysis. In type III, immune complexes are deposited in the tissue.

Complement is activated and polymorphs are attracted to the site of deposition, causing local tissue damage and inflammation. In type IV, antigen-sensitized T cells release lymphokines following a secondary contact with the same antigen. Cytokines induce inflammatory reactions and activate and attract macrophages, which release inflammatory mediators.

In the past several years it has become apparent that the Combs and Gell classification artificially divided mechanistically related antibody reactions (such as types I, II, and III), which contribute to the pathophysiology of many common immune-mediated diseases, while including the T cell-mediated reactions of delayed-type hypersensitivity (DTH) in a common classification (termed type IV).

Based on our current understanding of the underlying pathways of inflammation triggered by antigen exposure and the disease conditions observed, common mechanisms appear to operate in types I, II, and III hypersensitivity. These common mechanisms involve the engagement by antibody–antigen complexes with cellular receptors for the Fc region of antibodies (termed **Fc receptors**).

Understanding the mechanisms underlying these categories has resulted in the development of novel therapeutics based on the common pathways activated by these reactions and may result in the broader applicability of such therapeutics to multiple disease states.

Immediate hypersensitivity responses:
- have traditionally been referred to as type I hypersensitivity; and
- are characterized by the production of IgE antibodies against foreign proteins that are commonly present in the environment (e.g. pollens, animal danders, or house dust mites).

Antibody-mediated reactions:
- were previously referred to as type II;
- occur when IgG or IgM antibodies are produced against surface antigens on cells of the body.

These antibodies can trigger either by activating complement (e.g. autoimmune hemolytic anemia) or by facilitating the binding of natural killer cells (NK).

Type III hypersensitivity:
- involves the formation of immune complexes in the circulation that are not adequately cleared by macrophages or other cells of the reticuloendothelial system.

The formation of immune complexes requires significant quantities of antibody and antigen (typically microgram quantities of each). The classical diseases in which immune complexes are thought to be involved are systemic lupus erythematosus (SLE), chronic glomerulonephritis, and serum sickness.

Cell-mediated reactions:
- were previously referred to as type IV;
- are those in which specific T cells are the primary effector cells.

Examples of T cells causing unwanted responses are:
- contact sensitivity (e.g. to nickel or plants such as poison ivy);
- graft rejection;
- the hypersensitivity skin responses of leprosy or tuberculosis;
- the exaggerated response to viral infections such as measles; and
- the persistent symptoms of allergic disease.

HISTORICAL OBSERVATIONS HAVE SHAPED OUR UNDERSTANDING OF IMMEDIATE HYPERSENSITIVITY

The classical allergic disease is seasonal hayfever caused by pollen grains entering the nose (rhinitis) and eyes (conjunctivitis). In severe cases patients also get seasonal asthma and seasonal dermatitis.

Charles Blackley in 1873 demonstrated that pollen grains placed into the nose could induce symptoms of rhinitis. He also demonstrated that pollen extract could produce a wheal and flare skin response in patients with hayfever.

The **wheal and flare skin response** is an extremely sensitive method of detecting specific IgE antibodies. The timing and form of the skin response is indistinguishable from the local reaction to injected histamine. Furthermore, the immediate skin response can be effectively blocked with antihistamines.

In 1903 Portier and Richet discovered that immunization of guinea pigs with a toxin from the jellyfish *Physalia* could sensitize them so that a subsequent injection of the same protein would cause rapid onset of breathing difficulty, influx of fluid into the lungs, and death. They coined the term **anaphylaxis** (from the Greek *ana*, non, and *phylaxos*, protection) and speculated about the relationship to other hypersensitivity diseases. They noted that:

- human anaphylaxis had no familial characteristics (unlike most of the other allergic diseases); and
- natural exposure to inhaled allergens did not cause anaphylaxis or urticaria.

Subsequently, it became clear that injection of any protein into an individual with immediate hypersensitivity to that protein can induce anaphylaxis. Thus, anaphylaxis occurs when a patient with immediate hypersensitivity is exposed to a relevant allergen in such a way that antigen enters the circulation rapidly.

Q. In what circumstances can large amounts of allergen enter the circulation rapidly?

A. Following direct injection of the antigen into the tissue, such as a bee sting, a therapeutic injection for hyposensitization, or injection of a drug.

Anaphylaxis may also occur as a result of eating an allergen such as peanut or shellfish, or following the rupture of hydatid cysts with the rapid release of parasite antigens (Fig. 23.2).

The term **allergen** was first used by von Pirquet to cover all foreign substances that could produce an immune response. Subsequently, the word 'allergen' came to be used selectively for the proteins that cause 'supersensitivity'. Thus, **an allergen is an antigen that gives rise to immediate hypersensitivity**.

MOST ALLERGENS ARE PROTEINS

Substances that can give rise to wheal and flare responses in the skin and to the symptoms of allergic disease are derived from many different sources (see www.allergen.org). When purified they are almost all found to be proteins and their size ranges in molecular weight from 10 000–40 000 Da. These proteins are all freely soluble in aqueous solution, but have many different biological functions including digestive enzymes, carrier proteins, calycins, and pollen recognition proteins.

Any allergen can be described or classified by its source, route of exposure, and nature of the specific protein (Fig. 23.3).

Anaphylaxis and urticaria

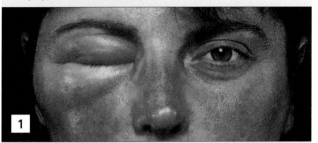

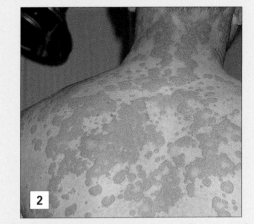

Fig. 23.2 (1) The anaphylactic response to bee venom in a patient who has IgE antibodies to the venom protein, phospholipase A. The immediate reaction occurs within 20 minutes and is mediated by the release of histamine and other mediators from mast cells. The patient shown had been stung on the face, but the reaction can become generalized, leading to a fall in blood pressure, generalized urticaria, and/or bronchospasm (i.e. anaphylaxis). **(2)** Diffuse urticaria on a patient with severe chronic urticaria. The lesions have a raised edge and come up within minutes or hours. The lesions almost always resolve within 12 hours leaving no trace on the skin.

Extracts used for skin testing or in-vitro measurement of IgE antibodies are made from the whole material, which contains multiple different proteins, any of which can be an allergen. Indeed, it is clear that individual patients can react selectively to one or more different proteins within an extract.

Q. Name one genetic factor that determines whether an individual can make an immune response to a specific allergen.

A. The individual's MHC haplotypes determine which antigens and antigen fragments are presented.

Estimates of exposure can be made either by visual identification of particles (e.g. pollen grains or fungal spores) or by immunoassay of the major allergens (e.g. Fel d 1 or Der p 1).

Properties of allergens

source	airborne particles	dimension of airborne particle (μm)	allergen		
			name	MW (kDa)	function/homologies
dust mite – *Dermatophagoides pteronyssinus*	feces	10–40	Der p 1 Der p 2	25 13	cysteine protease (epididymal protein)
cats – *Felis domesticus*	dander particles	2–15	Fel d 1	36	uteroglobin
German cockroach – *Blattella germanica*	frass saliva	≥ 5	Bla g 2 Bla g 4 Bla g 5	36 21 23	aspartic protease calycin glutathione-*S*-transferase
rat – *Rattus norvegicus*	urine on bedding ?	2–20	Rat n 1	19	pheromone binding protein
grass	pollen	30	Lol p 1	29	not known
fungi – *Alternaria alternata,* *Aspergillus fumigatus*	spores spores	14 × 10 2	Alt a 1 Asp f 1	28 18	not known mitogillin

Fig. 23.3 Patients who become 'allergic' to one of the well-recognized sources of allergens have actually produced an IgE antibody response to one or more of the proteins produced by mites, trees, grass, cats, or fungi. The proteins are predominantly water soluble with a molecular weight (MW) ranging from 10 000 to 40 000 kDa. In many cases the function of the proteins is known, but it is not clear whether function such as enzymic activity alters the ability of these proteins to induce an allergic response. The properties of the particles carrying these allergens are very important because they influence both how much becomes airborne, and also where the allergen is deposited in the respiratory tract. The dimensions of the particles airborne vary from ≤ 2 μm for *Aspergillus* or *Penicillium* spores to ≥ 20 μm for mite fecal pellets and some pollen grains. (Sizes are given as diameter in μm)

IgE IS DISTINCT FROM THE OTHER DIMERIC IMMUNOGLOBULINS

In 1921 Küstner, who was allergic to fish, injected his own serum into the skin of Prausnitz, who was allergic to grass pollen but not fish, and demonstrated that it was possible to passively transfer immediate hypersensitivity (the Prausnitz–Küstner or P–K test). Prausnitz would also notice that an immediate wheal and flare occurred at the site of passive sensitization when he ate fish. This showed that intact fish allergen can be absorbed into the circulation.

Over the next 30 years it was established that P–K activity was a general property of the serum of patients with immediate hypersensitivity and that it was allergen specific (i.e. behaved like an antibody).

In 1967 Ishizaka and his colleagues purified the P–K activity from a patient with ragweed hayfever and proved that this was a novel isotype of immunoglobulin – IgE. However, it was obvious that the concentration of this immunoglobulin isotype in serum was very low.

The initial antisera to IgE made it possible to identify a patient with multiple myeloma whose serum contained a very high concentration of IgE (~10 mg/ml). Purification of this myeloma protein by Johansson and Bennich led to the full structure of IgE and also to the production of potent antisera.

Antisera to IgE are used in the radioallergosorbent test (RAST) to measure IgE antibodies in serum, as well as for measuring total serum IgE.

IgE is distinct from the other dimeric immunoglobulins (see Fig. 3.8) because it has:

- an extra constant region domain;
- a different structure to the hinge region; and
- binding sites for both **high-** and **low-affinity IgE receptors**, **FcεRI** and **FcεRII**, respectively (Fig. 23.4).

The primary cells that bear FcεRI are **mast cells** and **basophils**, which are the only cells in the human that contain significant amounts of histamine.

Low-affinity receptors for IgE – FcεRII or CD23 – are also present on B cells and may play a role in antigen presentation.

In addition in atopic dermatitis dendritic cells in skin can express a high-affinity receptor for IgE, but this receptor lacks the β chain of FcεRI.

The properties of IgE can be separated into three areas:

- the characteristics of the molecule including its half-life and binding to IgE receptors;
- the control of IgE and IgG antibody production by T cells; and
- the consequences of allergen cross-linking IgE on the surface of mast cells or basophils.

IgE molecules

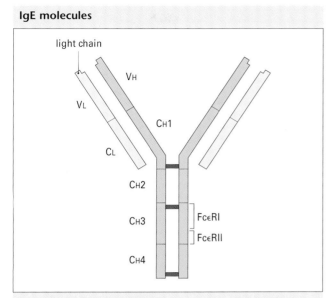

Fig. 23.4 The IgE molecule has four heavy chain constant regions. The binding sites for the high-affinity IgE receptor FcεRI and for the low-affinity receptor FcεRII, or CD23, are shown. Monoclonal antibodies to the binding site for FcεRI also block FcεRII.

The half-life of IgE is short compared with that of other immunoglobulins

The concentration of IgE in the serum of normal individuals is very low compared to all the other immunoglobulin isotypes. Values range from < 10 to 10 000 IU/ml, and the international unit (IU) is equivalent to 2.4 ng. Most sera contain < 400 IU/ml (i.e. < 1 µg/ml). The reasons why serum IgE is so low include:

• serum IgE has a much shorter half-life than other isotypes (≈ 2 days compared with 21–23 days for IgG);

• IgE is produced in small quantities and is only produced in response to a select group of antigens (allergens and parasites); and

• IgE antibodies are sequestered on the high-affinity receptor on mast cells and basophils.

Q. What fundamental reason explains the low production of IgE?
A. The class switch from IgM to IgE happens infrequently and is controlled by T cells. The position of the IgE constant region gene is towards the distal end of the Ig gene stack (see Fig. 8.19), but the position alone cannot explain the infrequency of the switch to IgE.

The half-life of IgE in the serum has been measured both by injecting radiolabeled IgE and by infusing plasma from allergic patients into normal and immune-deficient patients.

The half-life of IgE in serum is less than 2 days; by contrast, IgE bound to mast cells in the skin has a half-life of approximately 10 days.

The low quantities of IgE in the serum must reflect a more rapid breakdown of IgE, as well as removal from the circulation by binding onto mast cells.

The most important site of breakdown of IgE is thought to be within **endosomes** where the low pH facilitates breakdown of free immunoglobulin by cathepsin.

Serum is constantly being taken up by endocytosis. Most macromolecules including IgE degrade in the endosome. One major exception is IgG, which is protected by binding to the neonatal Fc gamma receptor, FcγRn (Fig. 23.5).

IgG4 is transferred across the placenta, but IgE is not

In cord blood the concentration of IgE is very low indeed, generally < 1 IU/ml (i.e. < 2 ng/ml). Thus, there appears to be almost no transfer across the placenta.

Endocytosis of plasma

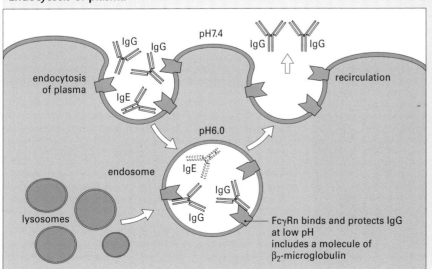

Fig. 23.5 Endocytosis of plasma contributes to the short half-life of IgE as plasma proteins are taken up and the pH falls because of lysosomes combining with the endosome. At low pH IgG including IgG4 molecules bind to the neonatal Fc γ receptor (FcγRn). By contrast, IgE molecules do not bind to FcγRn so are not protected and are digested by cathepsin. As the endosomes recirculate, the pH rises to 7.4 and the undamaged IgG molecules are released into the circulation. The FcγRn includes a molecule of β2-microglobulin. In keeping with this model the half-life of IgG is shorter than normal in mice that have had the gene for β2-microglobulin removed (or knocked out).

By contrast, IgG, including IgG4 antibodies to allergens such as those from dust mite or cat, are very efficiently transferred across the placenta. This process also involves endocytosis and receptor-mediated transport.

Passive transfer of IgE to the fetus may be blocked because IgE is broken down in the endosomes, or because an Fc receptor that is essential for transport is absent on the cells that comprise the placental tissues. In prenatal transfer IgG is protected in endosomes by binding to FcγRn. Although IgE can be seen on fetal villous stroma, this is not through FcεRI or FcγRn, but may be through FcγRI on fetal macrophages.

ROLE OF T CELLS IN THE IMMUNE RESPONSE TO INHALANT ALLERGENS
IgE production is dependent on TH2 cells

Experiments in animals have established that the production of IgE is completely dependent on T cells. It is also clear that T cells can suppress IgE production.

T cells that suppress IgE production:
- act predominantly by producing interferon-γ (IFNγ); and
- are produced when the animal (e.g. mouse, rat, or rabbit) is primed in the presence of Freund's complete adjuvant.

This adjuvant, which includes bacterial cell walls and probably bacterial DNA, is a very potent activator of macrophages.

With the discovery of TH1 and TH2 cells, it became clear that IgE production is dependent on TH2 cells and that any priming that generates a TH1 response will inhibit IgE production.

The main cytokines that are specifically relevant to a TH1 response include:
- interleukin-12 (IL-12) produced by macrophages; and
- IFNγ produced by T cells.

By contrast, the primary cytokines relevant to a TH2 response are:
- IL-4 (IL13);
- IL-5; and
- IL-10 (Fig. 23.6).

It is clear from experiments in mice and humans that the expression of the gene for IgE is dependent on IL-4. Thus, if immature human B cells are cultured with anti-CD40 and IL-4, they will produce IgE antibodies.

Cytokines regulate the production of IgE

In humans IgE antibodies are the dominant feature of the response to a select group of antigens and most other immune responses do not include IgE.

T cell differentiation during human immune responses

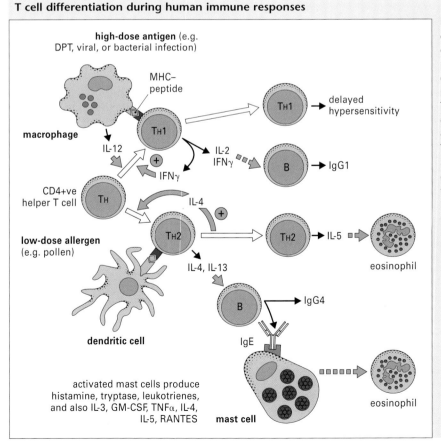

Fig. 23.6 The differentiation of TH cells depends on the antigen source, the quantity of allergen, and the cytokines produced. Bacterial antigens or a high dose of antigen will induce IL-12 from macrophages. In addition, the developing TH1 cells produce IFNγ, which further enhances the production of TH1 cells. Low-dose antigen without adjuvant will induce TH2 cells, which produce both IL-4 and IL-5. IL-4 plays a role in (i) enhancing the growth of TH2 cells; (ii) the expression of the gene for IgE. In turn IgE binds to the high-affinity receptor for IgE (FcεRI) on mast cells.

The classical allergens are inhaled in very small quantities (5–20 ng/day) either perennially indoors or over a period of weeks or months outdoors. Immunization of mice with repeated low-dose antigen is a very effective method of inducing IgE responses.

By contrast, the routine immunization of children with diphtheria and tetanus toxoid does not induce persistent production of IgE antibodies. This is clear because we do not routinely take precautions against anaphylaxis when administering a booster injection of tetanus.

Q. Which cytokines promote the production of IgE, and which inhibit production?

A. TH2 cytokines, including IL-4, promote production of IgE, whereas TH1 cytokines (e.g. IL-12) inhibit production.

As T cells differentiate, TH1 cells express the functional IL-12 receptor with the IL-12 β2 chain. By contrast, TH2 cells express only part of the IL-12 receptor and this part is non-functional.

IL-4 is important in the differentiation of TH2 cells and is also a growth factor for these cells. Because it is produced by TH2 cells, it is at least in part acting on the cell that produced it (i.e. in an autocrine fashion). The interaction of IL-4 with T cells can be blocked either with:

- an antibody to IL-4; or
- a soluble form of the IL-4 receptor (IL-4R).

The release of soluble IL-4R from T cells may be a natural mechanism for controlling T cell differentiation.

It follows that inhaling recombinant soluble IL-4R is a potential therapeutic strategy to control allergic responses in the lung. However, recent evidence suggests that in-vivo responses are controlled by T cells producing either IL-10 or transforming growth factor-β (TGFβ).

Both IgE and IgG4 are dependent on IL-4

The genes for immunoglobulin heavy chains are in sequence on chromosome 14. The gene for ε occurs directly following the gene for γ4. Both of these isotypes are dependent on IL-4 and they may be expressed sequentially (Fig. 23.7).

The mechanisms by which IgG4 is controlled separately from IgE are not well understood, but this may include a role for IL-10. Thus, immunotherapy for patients with anaphylactic sensitivity to honey bee venom will induce IL-10 production by T cells, decreased IgE, and increased IgG4 antibodies to venom antigens.

Recently, it has been shown that children raised in a house with a cat can produce an IgG response, including IgG4 antibody, without becoming allergic. A modified TH2 response (increased IgG4 and decreased IgE) therefore represents an important mechanism of tolerance to allergens (Fig. 23.8). IgG4 antibody responses without IgE antibody are a feature of immunity/tolerance to insect venom, rat urinary allergens, and food antigens as well as cat allergens.

ALLERGENS ARE THE ANTIGENS THAT GIVE RISE TO IMMEDIATE HYPERSENSITIVITY
Allergens have similar physical properties

In mice a wide range of proteins can be used to induce an IgE antibody response. The primary factors that influence the response are:

- the strain of mouse;
- the dose; and
- adjuvants used.

Thus, repeated low-dose immunization with alum or pertussis (but not complete Freund's adjuvant) will produce IgE responses. However, the dose necessary to induce a optimal response varies greatly from one strain to another.

The allergens that have been defined have similar physical properties (i.e. freely soluble in aqueous solution with a molecular weight between 10 000 and 40 000 Da), but are very diverse biologically.

Cloning has revealed sequence homology between allergens and diverse proteins including calycins, pheromone binding proteins, enzymes, and pollen recognition proteins.

Although many of the allergens have homology with known enzymes, this is not surprising because enzymic activity is an important property of proteins in general.

Some important allergens, for example Der p 2 from mites, Fel d 1 from cats, and Amb a 5 from ragweed pollen, have neither enzymic activity nor homology with known enzymes. Thus, enzymic activity is not essential for immunogenicity.

Nevertheless, the group I allergens of dust mites are cysteine proteases and in several model situations it has been shown that this enzymic activity influences the immunogenicity of the protein. Thus cleavage of CD23 or CD25 on lymphocytes by Der p 1 can enhance immune responses.

Chromosome 14

Fig. 23.7 Switch regions and heavy chain genes for immunoglobulin are arranged sequentially on chromosome 14. Both Cγ4 and Cε expression are dependent on IL-4 produced by T cells. The switch region of IgE often includes elements from Sγ4 indicating that the switching occurs sequentially. However, IgG4 responses can occur without IgE antibody responses.

429

Modified TH2 response

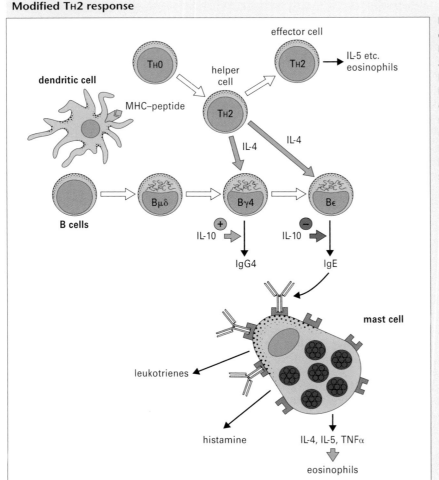

Fig. 23.8 The TH2 response includes T effector cells as well as help for IgE and IgG4 antibody production. In turn IgE plays a major role in triggering mast cells. However, increasing evidence shows that higher doses of allergen (e.g. bee venom, cat dander, or rat urine) can induce a modified or tolerant TH2 response. This response includes IgG4 antibodies, but not IgE. The cytokine IL-10 may well play a role in enhancing IgG4 antibody while suppressing production of IgE.

Alternatively, it has been shown that Der p 1 can disrupt epithelial junctions and alter the entry of proteins through the epithelial layer. The interest in this property is increased because many different mite allergens are inhaled together in the fecal particle so the enzymic activity of one protein (i.e. Der p 1) could facilitate either the physical entry or the immune response to other mite proteins. However, the lungs contain many different naturally occurring proteinases (as well as anti-proteases), which are just as potent as these allergens.

The primary characterization of allergens relates to their route of exposure. The routes includes:
- inhaled allergens;
- foods;
- drugs;
- antigens from fungi growing on the body (e.g. *Aspergillus* spp.); and
- venoms.

The routes are important because they define the ways in which the antigens are presented to the immune system. Because antigen presentation may well be the site at which genetic influences play the biggest role, the properties of the different groups of allergen need to be considered separately.

The inhalant allergens cause hayfever, chronic rhinitis, and asthma

The inhalant allergens are:
- the primary causal agents in hayfever, chronic rhinitis, and asthma among school-aged children and young adults;
- play an important role in atopic dermatitis.

Almost all evidence about the genetics of allergic disease relates to inhalant allergens.

Allergens can only become airborne in sufficient quantity to cause an immune response or symptoms when they are carried on particles. Pollen grains, mite fecal particles, particles of fungal hyphae or spores, and animal skin flakes (or dander) are the best defined forms in which allergens are inhaled (Fig. 23.9).

In each case it is possible to define the approximate particle size and the quantity of protein on the particle as well as the speed with which the proteins in the particle dissolve in aqueous solution (see Fig. 23.3).

Thus, for grass pollen, mite fecal pellets, and cat dander:
- the relevant allergens are present in high concentrations (up to 10 mg/cm^3);
- the particles are 'large' (i.e. 3–30 μm diameter); and
- the allergens elute rapidly in aqueous solution.

Particles carrying airborne allergens – mite fecal pellets and pollen grains

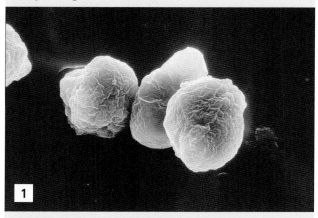

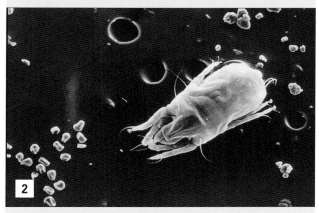

Fig. 23.9 The dust mite is the most important source of allergen in house dust, largely as fecal particles (**1**). A mite is shown in (**2**) with pollen grains lower left and fecal particles upper right. The mite is approximately 300 µm in length (i.e. just visible but not small enough to become airborne). Mite fecal particles are approximately 10–40 µm in diameter and become airborne during domestic disturbance. Pollen grains are similar in size to mite fecal particles (i.e. approximately 30 µm in diameter). The important allergic sources of pollen (i.e. grass, ragweed, and trees) are wind pollinated and the grains are designed to travel in the air for long distances.

The allergens within these particles will be delivered to the nasal epithelium because a large proportion of particles of this size will impact on the mucous membrane during passage of inhaled air through the nose.

Small quantities of inhalant allergen cause immediate hypersensitivity

Estimates of the quantity of mite or pollen-derived proteins inhaled vary from 5 to 50 ng/day. Thus exposure to some allergens may be as little as 1 µg/year. This is very important because it probably explains:

- why the immune response is consistently of this one kind (i.e. immediate hypersensitivity); and
- why no respiratory diseases, other than asthma, have been associated with these allergens.

The quantities inhaled also seriously restrict the models about how allergens contribute to asthma. Inhaling between 10 and 100 particles per day will produce localized areas of inflammation in the lungs, but would not be expected to induce acute bronchospasm. Inhaling a small number of 'large' particles (10–30 µm in diameter) could produce local areas of inflammation but could not give rise to alveolitis, acute bronchospasm, or progressive lung fibrosis. Equally, the quantities inhaled severely restrict the quantity that enters the blood stream and make it extremely unlikely that the fetus is sensitized or primed to inhalant allergens in utero.

Only a small number of food proteins are common causes of allergic responses

Although many food proteins can occasionally give rise to IgE responses, only a small number are common causes of allergic responses. These include egg, milk, wheat, soy, tree nuts, peanut, fish, and shellfish. In contrast to inhaled allergens, these proteins are often eaten in very large quantities (i.e. ≈10–100 g/day).

In general only a small fraction of the food proteins are absorbed. However, small peptides can be freely absorbed and may be recognized by T cells and even by IgE antibodies in a minority of individuals. Nevertheless, the bulk of the allergic and anaphylactic responses to foods are thought to be related to food proteins that have not been digested, either triggering mast cells in the intestine or entering the circulation.

Q. Recent evidence from Dr Sampson and his colleagues has shown that some children produce IgE antibodies against linear epitopes on food allergens. What implication does this have for induction of allergy in cooked food?
A. Denaturation of a protein by heat will not destroy linear epitopes, consequently cooking will not alter the allergenicity.

IgE binding sites can be identified on the tertiary structure of allergens

Many different allergens have been cloned, and for a few the tertiary structure is now known either from X-ray crystallography (e.g. Bet v 1), by nuclear magnetic resonance (e.g. Der p 2), or by modeling relationships to known homologs (Fig. 23.10).

Knowledge of the tertiary structure makes it possible to predict surface residues and to define IgE binding sites using site-directed mutagenesis. This approach provides the potential to design molecules that have decreased IgE binding properties, but with preserved T cell epitopes.

Given the importance of T cells to the control of IgE antibody production and their potential role in the recruitment of inflammatory cells, it is logical to try to use molecules that will directly 'desensitize' T cells. The approaches used include:

- allergen molecules modified by glutaraldehyde (allergoids);
- site-directed mutagenesis;
- allergens combined with two to four molecules of CpG;
- peptides.

Tertiary structure of two important allergens – Der p 2 and Bla g 2

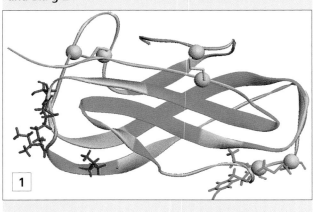

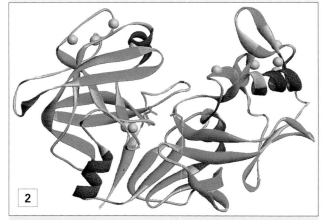

Fig. 23.10 The tertiary structure of the dust mite allergen, Der p 2 (**1**), was derived by nuclear magnetic resonance. This protein has no known function, and the structure shows no enzymic sites. On this structure the amino acids that are part of the binding sites for two monoclonal antibodies are shown (DPX green and 7A1 red). Knowledge of the structure makes it possible to alter the antibody binding sites using site-directed mutagenesis. (Courtesy of Drs Alisa Smith and Geoffrey Mueller) (**2**) The tertiary structure of a cockroach allergen, Bla g 2, shows the enzymic cleft and three residues that are considered to form the active site of an aspartic protease. However, the molecule has no enzymic activity due to other changes in the primary amino acid sequence. Some allergens (e.g. Der p 1 and Bla g 5) are active enzymes, but it remains an open question whether this activity contributes to their activity as allergens. (Courtesy of Drs A Pomes and M Chapman) On each structure the β sheets are shown as green bands, the α-helical structures in Bla g 2 are shown in red. In addition, cysteines are shown as yellow spheres.

The approach with peptides has been to test overlapping peptides of different lengths of between 12 and 35 amino acids.

Therapeutic trials have been carried out with peptides from ragweed pollen antigens and the cat allergen Fel d 1. The results show that peptide recognition is restricted by the HLA-DR type of the patient, which means that a wide range of peptides are necessary for treatment. In addition, there is clear evidence that peptides can produce a significant response in the lungs (Fig. 23.11). This is the clearest evidence yet that T cells in the lung can contribute to an asthmatic response.

MAST CELLS AND BASOPHILS CONTAIN HISTAMINE

The only human cell types that contain histamine are mast cells and basophils. In addition, these are the only cells that express the high-affinity receptor for IgE (FcεRI) under resting conditions.

Under most circumstances the primary and most rapid consequence of allergen exposure in an allergic individual is cross-linking of IgE receptors on mast cells and basophils:

- basophils are circulating polymorphs that are not present in normal tissue, but can be recruited to a local site by cytokines released from either T cells or mast cells;

Late asthmatic response to peptides from cat allergen

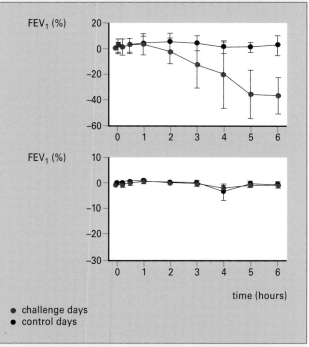

- challenge days
- control days

Fig. 23.11 Late asthmatic reactions induced in cat allergic patients by the intradermal injection of peptides derived from the cat allergen, Fel d 1. The nine responders show a mean fall in forced expiratory volume in 1 second (FEV_1) of approximately 30%. The response to the peptides is MHC-restricted and correlated with the ability of the patients' T cells to respond to these peptides in vitro. On challenge days (red filled circle) injection of peptides was associated with a fall in FEV_1 which did not occur on the control days (black filled circle). Data are shown for nine responders (upper graph) and 31 non-responders (lower graph). (Courtesy of Dr M Larché from J Exp Med 1999;189:1885)

Rat peritoneal mast cells

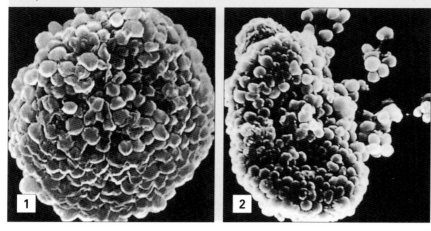

Fig. 23.12 Scanning electron micrograph (SEM) of rat peritoneal mast cells. (**1**) An intact mast cell with the cell membrane shrunk onto the granules (see Fig. 2.11). (**2**) A rat peritoneal mast cell degranulating following incubation with anti-IgE for 30 seconds. SEM. × 1500. (Courtesy of Dr TSC Orr)

- mast cells cannot be identified in the circulation, but are present in connective tissue and at mucosal surfaces throughout the body (Fig. 23.12).

Mast cells in different tissues are morphologically and cytogenetically distinct.

Both the cells that contain histamine and the biology of these cells may be very different in other species. For example:

- in the rabbit the histamine content of the peripheral blood is almost all in platelets;
- in the mouse there are few if any circulating basophils; and
- in rats the degranulation of mast cells appears to be one granule at a time (see Fig. 23.12).

By contrast, human granules tend to fuse and release their contents together (Fig. 23.13).

MMCs and CTMCs have distinct granule proteases

Mast cells were originally identified by Ehrlich who named them based on the distinctive, tightly packed granules. (*Mast* means well fed, or fattening, in German.)

Mast cells in different tissues can be distinguished by staining for proteases, and the content of these enzymes may be relevant to their role in allergic diseases.

The granule proteases of mast cells have been cloned and sequenced and are distinct for two types of mast cell (Fig. 23.14):

- mucosal mast cells (MMCs) are characterized by the presence of tryptase without chymase;
- by contrast, connective tissue mast cells (CTMCs) contain both chymase and tryptase.

These enzymes may play a direct role in the lung inflammation of asthma, either by breaking down mediators or, in the case of tryptase, by acting as a fibroblast growth factor. Basophils contain very little of either of these proteases.

Staining of basophils in tissue sections requires special fixation and staining. Without this staining the granules in basophils cannot be identified and the cells appear as neutrophils (i.e. polymorphs without special granules).

In allergic individuals mast cells can be recruited to the skin and to the nose

Although mast cells are present in normal non-inflamed tissue, their numbers are increased in response to inflammation. It is assumed that this accumulation is T cell dependent because in rats infected with *Nippostrongylus brasiliensis* accumulation of mast cells in the gut is dependent on T cells and can be suppressed by corticosteroids.

In guinea pigs the immune response to tick bites includes a large local accumulation of basophils. Indeed, the tick is thought to be killed by basophils that it ingests.

In allergic individuals mast cell recruitment has been demonstrated both:

- in the skin in response to repeated allergen exposure; and
- in the nose during the pollen season.

In both situations basophils are also recruited.

In the nose the recruitment of cells represents a shift so that mast cells move from the subepithelium into the epithelium while basophils appear in the nasal mucus. This process, which brings histamine-containing cells closer to the site of entry of allergen, is one of the ways in which allergic individuals become more sensitive. It is likely but less well established that equivalent processes occur in the human lung and gut.

Cross-linking of two FcεRI receptors results in degranulation

The process of degranulation in human mast cells and basophils involves fusing of the membrane of the granules containing histamine with the exterior cell membrane (see Fig. 23.13). The granule membrane becomes part of the cell membrane. The granule contents rapidly dissolve and are secreted, leaving behind a viable degranulated or partially degranulated cell. This process is initiated in most cases by cross-linking of two specific IgE molecules by their relevant allergen.

When two IgE receptors (FcεRI) are cross-linked, signal transduction through the γ chains of the receptor

Human basophils

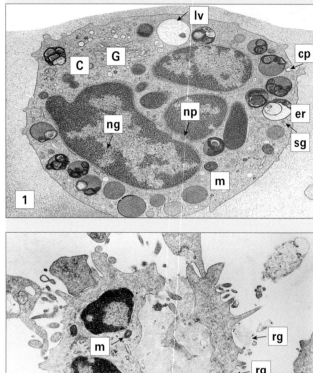

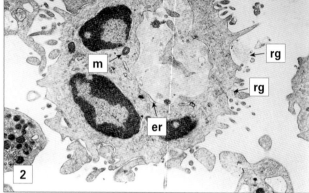

Fig. 23.13 Basophils are circulating mononuclear cells that have multilobed nuclei and distinctive granules that stain with metachromatic stains (1). Basophils can be recruited into local tissues such as the skin, nose, lungs, or gut by allergic and other immune responses. (2) A basophil degranulating 4 minutes after adding allergen. The degranulation that releases histamine occurs by fusion of the granule membrane with the external membrane of the cell. The arrows show connections between granule and the exterior of the cell. (Courtesy of Robin Hastie) (C, centriole; cp, coated pit; er, endoplasmic reticulum; np, nuclear pore; G, Golgi apparatus; lv, lucent vesicle; m, mitochondria; ng, nuclear granule; rg, residual material from granules; sg, small granules)

1 Differences between mast cell populations

	MMC	CTMC
location in vivo	gut and lung	ubiquitous
life span	< 40 days (?)	> 40 days (?)
T cell dependent	+	−
number of Fcε receptors	25×10^5	3×10^4
histamine content	+	++
cytoplasmic IgE	+	−
major AA metabolite LTC$_4$: PGD$_2$ ratio	25:1	1:40
DSGG/theophylline inhibits histamine release	−	+
major proteoglycan	chondroitin sulfate	heparin

Fig. 23.14 (1) There are at least two subpopulations of mast cell, the mucosal mast cells (MMCs) and the connective tissue mast cells (CTMCs). The differences in their morphology and pharmacology suggest different functional roles in vivo. MMCs are associated with parasitic worm infections and, possibly, allergic reactions. In contrast to the CTMC, the MMC is smaller, shorter lived, T cell dependent, has more Fcε receptors, and contains intracytoplasmic IgE. Both cells contain histamine and serotonin in their granules; the higher histamine content of the CTMC may be accounted for by the greater number of granules. Major arachidonic acid (AA) metabolites (prostaglandins [PGs] and leukotrienes [LTs]) are produced by both mast cell types, but in different amounts. For example, the ratios of production of the leukotriene LTC$_4$ to the prostaglandin PGD$_2$ are 25:1 in the MMC and 1:40 in the CTMC. The effect of drugs on degranulation is different between the two cell types. Sodium cromoglycate (DSCG) and theophylline both inhibit histamine release from the CTMC, but not from the MMC. (This may have important implications in the treatment of asthma.) Note that some of these data come from rodent studies and may not apply to humans.

(see Fig. 3.22) leads to influx of calcium, which initiates both degranulation and the synthesis of newly formed mediators (Fig. 23.15).

Cross-linking of IgE antibodies on FcεRI by allergens is the primary method by which mediators are released from basophils and mast cells; however, other mechanisms can be involved. Experimentally, degranulation can be triggered through FcεRI by using:

- lectins such as phytohemagglutinin (PHA) or concanavalin A (Con A); or
- antibodies to the α chain of the receptor.

Histamine release can also be triggered by agents that act on other receptors on the cell surface.

Q. Give an example of a mediator that can cause mast cell degranulation without cross-linking FcεRI.

A. Typical examples include the complement components C5a and C3a (see Fig. 6.21).

2 Differences between mast cell populations

cell type	location	amount per cell (pg)	
		tryptase	chymase
MC$_T$ (MMC)	lung and nasal cavity, intestinal mucosa	10	< 0.04
MC$_{TC}$ (CTMC)	skin, blood vessels, intestinal submucosa	35	4.5
basophil	circulation	0.04	< 0.04

Fig. 23.14 Cont'd (2) Tryptase is a tetramer of 134 kDa that may comprise as much as 25% of the mast cell protein. Chymase is a monomer of 30 kDa. The relative proportions of these proteases in mast cells define MC$_T$ and MC$_{TC}$ populations, which have different distributions in human tissues. Basophils have very low amounts of both proteases. (The suffixes T and TC represent tryptase and chymase present in the respective cells.)

Drugs such as codeine or morphine, the antibiotic vancomycin, and contrast media used for imaging the kidneys also degranulate mast cells. Acute reactions to these agents, which are not thought to involve IgE antibodies, are referred to as **anaphylactoid**.

Mast cell mediator release

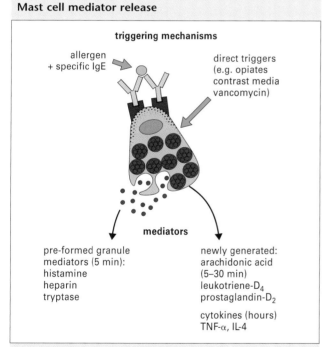

Fig. 23.15 Mast cells release mediators after cross-linking of the IgE receptors on their surface. Pre-formed mediators are released rapidly while arachidonic acid metabolites such as leukotriene D$_4$ and prostaglandin D$_2$ are released more slowly. Mast cells can also be triggered by opiates, contrast media, vancomycin, and the complement components C3a and C5a. The mediators, which are also released by basophils, include histamine, TNFα, and IL-4. Histamine released by mast cells can be measured in serum following anaphylaxis or extensive urticaria, but it has a half-life in minutes. By contrast, tryptase can be measured in serum for many hours after an anaphylactic reaction.

MULTIPLE GENES HAVE BEEN ASSOCIATED WITH ASTHMA IN DIFFERENT POPULATIONS

Children with one allergic parent have a 30% chance of developing allergic disease; those who have two allergic parents have as high as a 50% chance.

Systematic studies of allergic diseases are difficult because the phenotypes for diseases, such as hayfever and asthma, are not well defined and depend on the approach used to make the diagnosis (Fig. 23.16).

Asthma defined by a patient questionnaire is therefore less specific than asthma defined by testing of specific or non-specific bronchial hyperreactivity. Furthermore, studies on asthma are complicated because both IgE antibody responses and bronchial reactivity are genetically controlled.

Indeed, it is important not to confuse simple genetic diseases like cystic fibrosis or hemophilia with complex traits such as asthma or type II diabetes mellitus.

It is therefore not surprising that multiple genes have been associated with asthma in different populations.

A further major problem in genetic analyses of allergic disease comes from the progressive increase in the incidence of asthma between 1960 and 2000. Clearly this increase cannot be attributed to genetic change and implies that some of the genes identified would influence asthma only in the presence of other changes either in the environment or in lifestyle. This is referred to as a gene–environment interaction.

Multiple genes or genetic regions are associated with asthma. Analyses of the genetics of immediate hypersensitivity have identified both allergen-specific and non-specific influences. There are therefore HLA associations with atopy in general and also with sensitization to specific allergens. These genetic studies have given the clearest associations when purified allergens are used to test sensitization (Fig. 23.17).

The genetics of asthma has been studied both by genomic screening and by using candidate genes. Genomic screening identifies regions of the genome that link to asthma so that this region can be examined to identify specific genes.

If a candidate gene is identified, it is possible to examine the gene for polymorphisms that link to asthma. However, a brief consideration of the possible targets (Fig. 23.18)

IgE levels and atopic disease

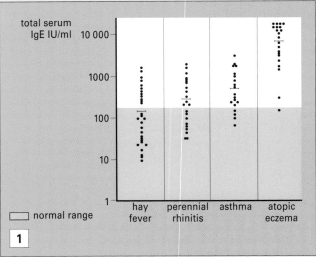

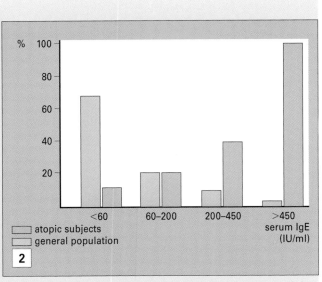

Fig. 23.16 **(1)** The serum concentration of IgE (which is around 100 IU/ml) is only approximately 0.001% that of IgG (around 10 mg/ml) and comprises less than 0.001% of the total immunoglobulin. Levels in atopic patients tend to be raised, and this is especially so in atopic eczema (1 IU = 2.4 ng).

(2) The higher the level of IgE the smaller the percentage of the population affected, but the greater the likelihood of atopy. Where the level is greater than 450 IU/ml the majority of subjects are atopic.

Allergens and HLA associations

Fig. 23.17 HLA association of IgE responses to allergens from ragweed and ryegrass. (Courtesy of Dr D Marsh)

systematic name	old name	mol. wt (Da)	primary association	p value
Ambrosia (ragweed) spp.				
Amb a I	AgE	37 800	none	–
Amb a III	Ra3	12 300	A2	0.01
Amb a VI	Ra6	11 500	DR5	$< 10^{-7}$
Amb a V	Ra5	5000	DR2/Dw2	$< 10^{-9}$
Amb t V	Ra5G	4400	DR2/Dw2	$< 10^{-3}$
Lolium (ryegrass) spp.				
Lol p I	rye I	27 000	DR3/Dw3	$< 10^{-3}$
Lol p II	rye II	11 000	DR3/Dw3	$< 10^{-3}$
Lol p III	rye III	11 000	DR3/Dw3	$< 10^{-4}$

makes it clear how complex the analysis of asthma is likely to be, and indeed is proving to be. Typical examples include polymorphisms of the promoter region for IL-4 and polymorphisms of the gene for IL-5.

Q. What effect might polymorphism in these genes have?
A. The level of production of IL-4, and the activity of IL-5, will vary between individuals, each of which will affect the type of immune response that develops – TH1 versus TH2 – either of which could directly influence the inflammatory response that occurs as a result of exposure to allergens.

Alternatively, a series of polymorphisms have been identified that influence the response of asthma to treatment. These include:

- variants of the β_2-adrenergic receptor α chain; and
- genetic differences that influence the therapeutic response to leukotriene antagonists.

In the past 10 years multiple 'genes' or genetic regions associated with asthma have been identified. At present, it appears that the overall effects are too complex to be of any practical significance. Certainly it is most unlikely that gene transfer will ever be of significance. However, as genetic screening becomes easier, pharmacogenetics may

Genetic influences over asthma and allergic disease

allergen specific	HLA related
IgE	total production
	FcεRI
	FcεRII
cytokines	IL-4 promoter and receptor
	IL-5
	IL-10
	IFNγ
	TGFβ promoter
	IL-11
	IL-13 and receptor
leukotriene pathway	five lipoxygenase activating protein (FLAP)
	lipoxygenase
	LTC$_4$ synthase
β$_2$-adrenergic receptor	leukotriene receptors – LTRI, LTRII
chemokines	polymorphisms
	CCR3 receptor

Fig. 23.18 Allergic diseases run in families, but the inheritance is not simple. Population-based studies have established that the inheritance of allergic diseases is influenced by multiple genes. Some of these, such as HLA-linked control of the response to pollen antigens or genes controlling total IgE, are related to the immune response. However, many others are related to the mechanisms of inflammation (e.g. IL-4 and IL-5 gene polymorphisms) or to the response to treatment (e.g. leukotriene receptor genes or polymorphisms of the β$_2$-adrenergic receptor).

well become an important method for identifying the best drugs for individual patients.

SKIN TESTS ARE USED FOR DIAGNOSIS AND INVESTIGATION

The primary method for diagnosing immediate hypersensitivity is skin testing. The characteristic response is a **wheal and flare** (Fig. 23.19):

- the wheal is caused by extravasation of serum from capillaries in the skin, which occurs as a direct effect of histamine and is accompanied by pruritus (also a direct effect of histamine);
- the larger erythematous flare is mediated by an axon reflex.

This skin response takes 5–15 minutes to develop and may persist for 30 minutes or more. Techniques for skin testing include:

- a prick test, in which a 25-gauge needle or a lancet is used to introduce 0.1 μl of extract into the dermis;
- alternatively, an intradermal injection of 0.02–0.03 ml is used.

All allergen injections have the potential to cause anaphylaxis and for safety reasons the intradermal test, which introduces approximately 100 times more extract, should always be preceded by a prick test.

Skin tests are evaluated by the size of the wheal compared to a positive (histamine) and negative (saline) control. In general, a 3×3 mm wheal in children and a 4×4 mm wheal in adults can be considered a positive response to a prick test.

A positive skin test indicates that the patient has specific IgE antibodies on the mast cells in their skin. In turn this implies that bronchial or nasal challenge would also be positive if sufficient antigen were administered.

In most cases (i.e. ≈ 80%) where the skin prick test is positive, IgE antibody will be detectable in the serum. However, blood tests for IgE antibody are generally less sensitive than intradermal skin tests.

Q. Suggest explanations for the higher sensitivity of the skin test.

A. Most IgE is located on the high-affinity receptor on mast cells. Its half-life is 10 days on the mast cell as opposed to 2 days in blood. The skin test has intrinsic amplification steps caused by mast cell degranulation and mediator release.

Positive skin tests are common

Epidemiologically, sensitization to a relevant inhalant allergen is a 'risk factor' for allergic disease. An individual with a positive skin test to grass pollen is therefore up to ten times more likely to have hayfever during the grass pollen season (odds ratio ≥ 10) than a skin test-negative individual.

Equally an individual with a positive skin test to dust mite or cat allergen is more likely to have asthma (odds ratios 2–6).

It is assumed that allergen exposure contributes to the risk, but that relationship is not simple.

Positive skin tests are common, and in individual cases may not be relevant, perhaps because the patient is not exposed to the allergen, for example:

- skin tests to grass pollen are not relevant to understanding symptoms occurring during autumn;
- equally skin tests to cat dander or cockroach allergens may not be relevant if the patient has moved to an area or house where those allergens are not present.

In addition up to one-third of skin test-positive individuals do not experience symptoms when they are exposed to the relevant allergen.

Late skin reactions probably include several different events

Late reactions can occur following an immediate response to allergen, in either the skin or the lungs.

Skin tests

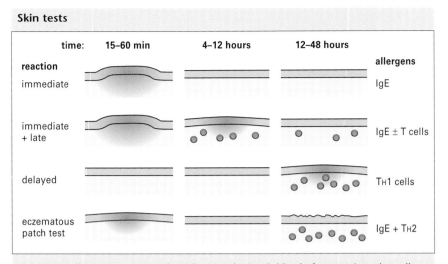

Fig. 23.19 Skin tests are carried out by introducing 0.02 ml of extract intradermally. With allergens such as pollen, cat, or dust mite, the positive reaction is an immediate (i.e. within 20 min) wheal, which in some cases is followed by an indurated response occurring late (i.e. at 4–12 hours). Non-allergic individuals make no discernible reaction to testing with these allergens. A delayed skin response is the commonest form of positive response to tuberculin, tetanus, and mumps, or to fungi such as *Trichophyton* and *Candida* spp. The skin typically shows no reaction up to 12 hours and then gradually develops an erythematous, indurated, delayed hypersensitivity response, which is maximal at 24–48 hours. Patch tests are performed by applying a gauze pad with allergen to a patch of skin that has been mildly abraded. This procedure may give an immediate wheal response, but this is followed at 24–48 hours by an indurated, erythematous response, which has many of the features of eczema. The patch test is not a diagnostic test, but has provided extensive information about the role of allergens in atopic dermatitis.

A late skin response is only common following a large immediate response (i.e. wheal size 10×10 mm). The late response, which is diffuse, erythematous, and indurated, generally starts 2–3 hours after the wheal and may last for up to 24 hours. The late reaction is considered to be a model of the events that lead to persistent inflammation in the nose, lungs, or skin.

Late reactions probably include several different events:
- the direct effects of prostaglandins, leukotrienes, and cytokines released by mast cells following the initial release of histamine;
- infiltration of lymphocytes, eosinophils, basophils, and neutrophils into the local site mediated by chemokines and other cytokines released from mast cells;
- release of products from the infiltrating cells.

In general, these events are occurring in parallel over a period of hours.

True delayed skin test responses (i.e. without an immediate response) are:
- characteristic of the response to tuberculin; and
- common with fungal antigens, particularly to the yeast *Candida albicans* or the dermatophyte fungus *Trichophyton* spp.

By contrast true delayed responses are very rare following skin testing with pollen, animal dander, or dust mites.

Epidermal spongiosis and a dermal infiltrate are features of a positive patch (atopy) test

The infiltration of cells into the skin that occurs in the 24 hours after an allergen is applied can be studied in several ways:
- by local intradermal injections;
- by applying a patch of allergen on gauze that stays on the skin for 2 days; or
- by fixing a chamber containing allergen over a denuded area of skin.

The skin chamber allows repeated sampling whereas the other two techniques require biopsy of the skin.

In the **patch test** 10 μg allergen is applied on a gauze pad 2.5 cm², and the biopsy is carried out at 24 or 48 hours. A positive patch response induces:
- macroscopic eczema;
- spongiosis of the epidermis (a hallmark of eczema); and
- an infiltrate of cells into the dermis (Fig. 23.20).

The cellular infiltrate includes eosinophils, basophils, and lymphocytes.

With persistent allergen at a site (i.e. 6 days), the eosinophils degranulate locally. This is in keeping with the

Eczema induced by patch test with mite allergen

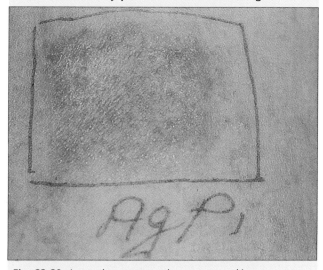

Fig. 23.20 An erythematous and eczematous skin response 48 hours after the application of 5 μg of the mite allergen Der p 1 to the skin of a patient with atopic dermatitis who had 56 IU/ml of IgE antibody to the dust mite *Dermatophagoides pteronyssinus*. Biopsy of the patch site revealed an infiltrate of eosinophils, basophils, and lymphocytes.

evidence that the skin of patients with eczema contains large quantities of the eosinophil granule major basic protein (MBP), even though very few whole eosinophilic cells are visible (Fig. 23.21).

Biopsy of patch tests also yields T cells that are specific for the allergen used, which in most cases has been dust mite, thus establishing that antigen-specific T cells are present in the skin after antigen challenge.

Some groups have succeeded in cloning allergen-specific T cells from the skin of patients with eczema without a preceding patch. This is never possible with skin from normal individuals or allergic patients without eczema.

Answering whether allergen-specific T cells are present at local sites is important because T cells could play a role both as effector cells and in the recruitment of other cells.

Establishing whether T cells play an effector role is also relevant to the nose in rhinitis, the lungs in asthma, the conjunctiva in hayfever, as well as the skin in atopic dermatitis.

Biopsy of patch test sites has also established that the Langerhans' cells in the skin of patients with eczema express FcεRI. Thus, these antigen-presenting cells use IgE antibodies to help capture allergens and to increase the efficiency of antigen presentation.

Part of the patch test response can be passively transferred by serum

Following injection of serum from a patient with atopic dermatitis into the skin of a non-allergic individual, a patch test can be carried out. Biopsy of this passively transferred response reveals large numbers of eosinophils. At least part of the eczematous response can therefore be passively transferred. The mechanisms for this response are thought to be:

- passive sensitization of IgE antibodies onto mast cells in the dermis;
- triggering of the local mast cells with allergen to release histamine, leukotrienes, and cytokines;
- recruitment of eosinophils by IL-5 as well as by chemokines such as CCL5 and CCL11 (eotaxin).

Eosinophil major basic protein in the skin of atopic dermatitis

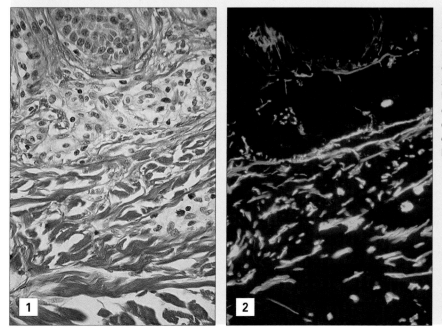

Fig. 23.21 Skin biopsy from a patient with severe atopic dermatitis. The hematoxylin and eosin (H&E) stain (1) shows an inflammatory infiltrate, but very few intact eosinophils are present. The same section stained with antibodies to eosinophil major basic protein (MBP) (2) shows extensive deposition of MBP in the dermis, demonstrating that eosinophils had degranulated in the skin. (Courtesy of Dr K Lieferman)

SEVERAL DIFFERENT PATHWAYS CAN CONTRIBUTE TO THE CHRONICITY OF SYMPTOMS OF ALLERGY

The diagnosis of allergy is made by:
- skin tests; or
- serum assays of IgE antibodies.

These antibodies form part of an immune response, which also includes antibodies of other isotypes (IgG1, IgG4, and IgA), as well as T cells, which are characteristically TH2.

The release of histamine within 15 minutes after allergen exposure can only explain a small proportion of allergic disease. In particular, the chronic inflammation in the lungs of patients with asthma and/or in the skin of patients with atopic dermatitis has many features that cannot be explained by histamine:
- first, the time course is too long;
- second, there is a cellular infiltrate in these tissues; and
- third, there are major differences in disease between patients who have apparently similar IgE antibodies in their serum and skin (Fig. 23.22).

Several different pathways contribute to chronic symptoms and can alter the severity of allergic disease as follows:
- local recruitment of mast cells and basophils, combined with increased 'releasability' of these cells, allows an increased response to the same allergen challenge – this mechanism plays a major role in the increased symptoms in the nose during the pollen season;
- release of leukotrienes, chemokines, and cytokines from mast cells or basophils – the mediators can have direct effects on blood vessels and smooth muscles – IL-5, tumor necrosis factor (TNF), and chemokines are each thought to contribute to the recruitment of inflammatory cells;
- the local actions of T effector cells – T cells release a wide range of cytokines, which can have direct inflammatory effects.

Inflammatory response in asthmatic bronchi

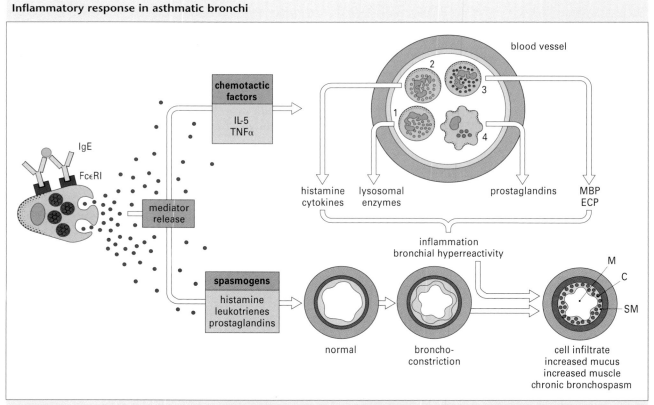

Fig. 23.22 Mast cells release factors that can induce immediate bronchospasm (e.g. histamine and LTD_4), but also release chemotactic factors such as LTB_4, IL-5, and TNFα. The spasmogens can induce edema, increased mucus, and smooth muscle constriction, resulting in an immediate decrease in airway conductance and a fall in FEV_1. By contrast, chemotactic factors recruit cells out of the circulation including eosinophils, neutrophils, lymphocytes, and macrophages. These cells can chronically modify the lung with goblet cell hyperplasia, collagen deposition below the basement membrane, and possibly smooth muscle hyperplasia. In addition, these cells and their products produce non-specific bronchial hyperreactivity. Thus, chronic bronchospasm includes elements of hypersecretion, inflammatory infiltrate thickening the walls of the small bronchi, and bronchial smooth muscle spasm. Evidence for this inflammatory response can be obtained from increased exhaled nitric oxide; increased eosinophils or eosinophil cationic protein (ECP) in induced sputum; and experimentally from biopsies of the lung. (1, neutrophils; 2, basophils; 3, eosinophils; 4, monocytes; C, cells; M, mucus; SM, smooth muscle)

Separating out the different factors influencing chronic allergic symptoms is difficult. Information may be obtained from:

- the effects of different drugs, particularly disodium cromoglycate, leukotriene antagonists, and anti-IgE; and
- passive transfer experiments.

The fact that cromoglycate can inhibit both the immediate and the late response of the lung to allergen challenge has been taken as evidence that the late reaction is also dependent on mast cell triggering. However, cromoglycate can control only part of the chronic inflammation.

By contrast, corticosteroids, which are an effective treatment for most of the inflammation in asthma, act selectively on the late response. The response to corticosteroid treatment cannot be used to distinguish the delayed effects of mast cell triggering from the direct effects of T cells because corticosteroids can inhibit both of these mechanisms (Fig. 23.23).

Local or systemic injection of IgE antibodies can passively transfer the wheal and flare skin response. Passive transfer of serum from an allergic patient (i.e. containing IgE antibodies) into the skin of a non-allergic individual can also transfer some aspects of the delayed or cellular response.

Both late reactions following an intradermal injection of allergen and the patch test response at 48 hours can be passively transferred. This experiment demonstrates that cross-linking of IgE antibody on mast cells in the tissue of a non-allergic individual can lead to local recruitment of eosinophils in the absence of antigen-specific T cells.

Therefore, in any analysis of the factors influencing the severity of allergic disease (e.g. response to pharmacological treatment or response to immunotherapy), it is necessary to consider the relevance of both mast cells and effector T cells.

ALLERGENS CONTRIBUTE TO ASTHMA

The causal role of bee venom in anaphylaxis or grass pollen in seasonal hayfever is obvious because:

- these diseases occur in individuals who have positive skin tests; and
- the symptoms are directly related to increased exposure.

By contrast, the role of inhaled allergens in chronic asthma is less obvious because exposure is perennial, the patients are often not aware of the relationship, and only a proportion of skin test-positive individuals develop asthma.

The evidence that allergens derived from dust mites, cats, dogs, the German cockroach, or the fungus *Alternaria* spp. contribute to asthma comes from several different lines of evidence:

- the epidemiological evidence that positive skin tests or serum IgE antibodies are a major risk factor for asthma;
- bronchial challenge with nebulized extracts can produce both rapid bronchospasm, within 20 minutes, and a late reaction, in 4–8 hours, which is characterized by renewed mediator production and a cellular infiltrate;
- reduced exposure to allergens can lead to decreased symptoms and decreased non-specific bronchial reactivity – this avoidance can be achieved either by moving patients to an allergen-free unit or by controlling exposure in the home.

Bronchi in the lungs of patients with asthma are characterized by increased mast cells, lymphocytes of the TH2 type, eosinophils, and products of eosinophils. In addition, there is increased mucus production secondary to goblet cell hyperplasia, epithelial desquamation, and collagen deposition below the basement membrane. These changes are a reflection of chronic inflammation, and it is generally considered that eosinophils play a major role in these events (see Fig. 23.22).

Q. Some recent evidence has shown that anti-IL-5 treatment has limited effects on asthma, though it decreases circulating eosinophils. How do you interpret this result?
A. Other cells, including basophils, mast cells, effector T cells, and macrophages, all contribute to the non-specific bronchial reactivity.

BAL analysis after allergen challenge demonstrates mast cell and eosinophil products

Analysis of bronchoalveolar lavage (BAL) after an allergen challenge demonstrates the presence of products derived from mast cells and eosinophils.

Actions of corticosteroids in allergic disease

- act primarily on the delayed or chronic effects of allergen exposure and are seen as anti-inflammatory
- in allergen challenge situations, block the delayed or late response in the lungs and inhibit the influx of eosinophils, basophils, and lymphocytes into local sites
- following systemic administration, circulating eosinophils decrease rapidly because of margination
- prevent eosinophil production in the bone marrow
- bind to a receptor that leads to inhibition of the transcription of the genes for many cytokines, including IL-5, TNFα, and also some chemokines
- are thought to have limited effects on leukotriene production and do not inhibit histamine release
- downregulate T cell activity as shown by the result of their clinical effect on contact sensitivity and blockade of delayed hypersensitivity skin tests

Fig. 23.23 Locally active corticosteroids are widely used in seasonal rhinitis, perennial rhinitis, asthma, and atopic dermatitis. In addition, courses of systemic corticosteroid are used for the treatment of exacerbations of asthma.

Q. What products would you expect to detect in BAL following challenge?
A. Histamine, prostaglandins, and leukotrienes from mast cells; major basic protein (MBP) and eosinophil cationic protein (ECP) from eosinophils (see Chapter 2).

Furthermore, MBP is present in biopsies of the lungs and can produce epithelial change typical of asthma in vitro (Fig. 23.24).

The subepithelial collagen deposition present in many patients with asthma is probably a reflection of fibroblast responses to local inflammation.

Although it has been suggested that these changes, which are referred to as 'remodeling', can lead to progressive decreases in lung function, the evidence for this view is not clear. In particular, progressive loss of lung function is unusual in asthma and there are no studies showing a correlation between the extent of collagen deposition and changes in lung function. Nonetheless, inhaled corticosteroids, which can block many different aspects of inflammation, are an effective long-term treatment that can control asthma.

Bronchial hyperreactivity is a major feature of asthma

Non-specific bronchial hyperreactivity (BHR) is present in patients with asthma and is a major feature of the disease. Thus, airway obstruction, induced by cold air or exercise, and nocturnal asthma all correlate with non-specific bronchial reactivity.

BHR can be demonstrated by challenging the lungs with histamine, methacholine, or cold air.

The mechanism by which exercise or cold air induces a bronchial response is thought to be evaporation of water with associated cooling of the epithelium. However, it is unclear whether this process triggers nerve endings directly or by causing local mediator release.

Evidence for inflammation of the lungs of patients with asthma is indirect

Bronchoscopy is not possible in patients with asthma except as a research procedure. Therefore the only evidence for inflammation of the lungs that can be obtained routinely is indirect:

- peripheral blood or nasal smear eosinophils are increased in most patients presenting with an acute episode of asthma (Fig. 23.25);
- nasal secretions may contain increased ECP and CXCL8.

Additional evidence about inflammation in the lungs can be obtained either from exhaled air or from condensates of exhaled air. Nitric oxide (NO$^{\bullet}$) gas is increased in patients with asthma, and this decreases following systemic or local corticosteroid treatment.

Q. Why should NO$^{\bullet}$ be increased in the lungs of asthmatic patients?
A. Macrophage activation causes synthesis of inducible nitric oxide synthase (iNOS) and consequent NO$^{\bullet}$ production in the lungs (see Fig. 9.31).

Localization of MBP in the lung of a severe asthmatic

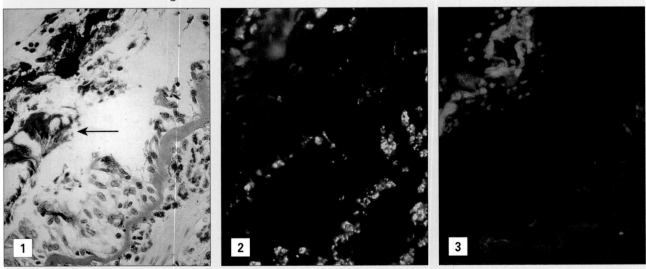

Fig. 23.24 (1) Respiratory epithelium showing striking submucosal eosinophil infiltration and a cluster of desquamated epithelial cells in the bronchial lumen (arrowed) next to a 'stringy' deposit of soot. H&E stain. (2) The same section stained for major basic protein (MBP) showing immunofluorescent localization in infiltrating eosinophils. MBP deposits are also seen on desquamated epithelial cells on the luminal surface. (3) A control section stained with normal rabbit serum does not stain eosinophils or bronchial tissue, but does show some non-specific staining of the sooty deposit. (Courtesy of Dr G Gleich, reprinted from J Allergy Clin Immunol 1982;70:160–169, with permission from American Academy of Allergy Asthma and Immunology)

Nasal eosinophils

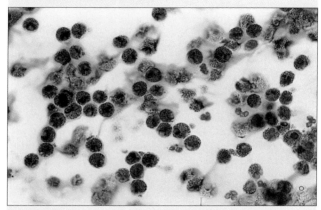

Fig. 23.25 Nasal smear from an 8-year-old boy presenting with acute asthma. Most of the cells are eosinophils – polymorphonuclear cells with a cytoplasm that stains red using H&E stain. He was known to be allergic to dust mites and had recently had a rhinovirus infection as judged by polymerase chain reaction on nasal secretions.

In addition, the pH of the condensate decreases during acute episodes. The increased exhaled NO˙ may reflect upregulation of the enzyme NOS. Alternatively, the release of NO˙ gas could also increase acutely as a consequence of airway acidification.

In adults further information about the inflammation in the 'respiratory tract' can be obtained from computed tomography (CT) of the nasal sinuses. Extensive opacification of the sinuses is present in approximately one-third of patients presenting with acute asthma. This reflects both:

- chronic sinusitis, which is a major feature of late-onset asthma; and
- sinus inflammation secondary to acute rhinovirus infection.

Whether the changes in the sinuses are a reflection of similar effects occurring in the lungs, or a source of mediators, or T cells that contribute to lung inflammation, is not clear.

IMMUNOTHERAPY IS AN EFFECTIVE TREATMENT FOR HAYFEVER AND ANAPHYLACTIC SENSITIVITY TO VENOM

Immunotherapy (or hyposensitization) with allergen extracts was introduced in 1911 by Noon and Freeman. At that time they were trying to establish immunity against pollen toxin.

Immunotherapy requires regular injections of allergen over a period of months. It is an established treatment for:

- seasonal hayfever; and
- anaphylactic sensitivity to bees, wasps, and hornets.

In addition, immunotherapy is an effective treatment for selected cases of other allergic diseases including asthma.

The dose is increased progressively, starting with between 1 and 10 ng and increasing up to approximately 10 µg allergen per dose.

The response to treatment includes:

- an increase in serum IgG antibodies;
- a striking decrease in the response of peripheral blood T cells to antigen in vitro; and
- a marked decrease in late reactions in the skin.

Over a longer period of time there is a progressive decrease in IgE antibodies in the serum (Fig. 23.26).

The change in antibodies, lymphocyte responses, and symptoms could all be secondary to changes in T cells. Given the known mechanisms of allergic inflammation, a response of T cells to allergen injections could influence symptoms in several ways as follows:

- decreased local recruitment of mast cells and basophils;
- decreased recruitment of eosinophils to the nose or lungs;
- increased IgG including IgG4 antibodies with progressive decreases in IgE – the IgG antibodies may act as blocking antibodies by binding allergen before it cross-links IgE on mast cells.

Some studies of cytokine RNA have suggested that immunotherapy produces a shift in T cells from a TH2 profile (i.e. IL-4 and IL-5) towards a profile that is more typical of TH1 (i.e. IFNγ). Although this could explain decreased help for IgE, and decreased eosinophil recruit-

Effects of immunotherapy on allergic rhinitis

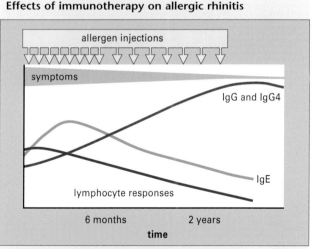

Fig. 23.26 During desensitization or immunotherapy the allergic patient receives regular subcutaneous injections of the relevant allergen. The immunological changes that occur include an initial increase in IgE antibodies followed by a gradual decline, which in pollen-allergic patients is largely due to a blunting of the seasonal increase. Antibodies of the IgG and specifically IgG4 isotype increase progressively and may reach concentrations of ten times those present before treatment. Symptoms decline, starting as early as 3 months, but generally not maximally until 2 years. Changes in T cells are less well defined, but include decreased in-vitro response to allergens and increased production of IL-10.

443

ment, this would not explain the production of IgG4. The expression of the gene for IgG4 is dependent on IL-4, and may also require the cytokine IL-10. The response to immunotherapy is therefore better seen as a modification of the TH2 response.

NEW APPROACHES FOR TREATING ALLERGIC DISEASE
Modified forms of allergen-specific immunotherapy
Peptides from the primary sequence of an allergen that can stimulate T cells in vitro

Peptides from the primary sequence of an allergen, usually approximately 20 amino acids in length, stimulate T cells in vitro.

In theory, peptides provide a mechanism for stimulating or desensitizing T cells without the risk of anaphylaxis, which is always present with traditional allergens.

Whether incomplete stimulation of T cells by peptides can lead to 'tolerance' or a change in the cytokine profile is not clear. Problems include:
- significant reactions in the lung with a fall in FEV_1; and
- the fact that multiple peptides are necessary to allow presentation of antigen in patients with different HLA types.

MODIFIED RECOMBINANT ALLERGENS HAVE DECREASED BINDING – Genetically modified recombinant allergens that have decreased binding to IgE antibodies can be produced. Their advantage is that the primary sequence with the T cell epitopes is preserved. Even if the molecule is extensively modified, any full-length protein has the potential to induce anaphylaxis in allergic individuals. Thus, the use of genetically modified molecules would always require precautions similar to those for traditional immunotherapy. A potential but unlikely problem is that patients would develop IgE antibodies against new epitopes.

ADJUVANTS CAN SHIFT THE IMMUNE RESPONSE TO TH1 – Adjuvants 'attached' to allergen molecules have been designed to shift the immune response from TH2 towards TH1. Possible co-molecules that act like an adjuvant include:
- the cytokine IL-12; or
- immunostimulatory sequences (ISSs).

ISSs are DNA sequences such as cytosine phosphoguanidine (CpG) that are common in bacterial DNA and have a profound effect on the mammalian immune system.

In mice combining an antigen with two or three molecules of CpG can induce a TH1 response or downregulate IgE responses.

Combining CpG with allergen not only influences the response, but also reduces the reactivity of the allergen with IgE.

Thus immunization with allergen and CpG may produce a greater immune response with less potential for an acute allergic reaction.

Preliminary trials in allergic individuals using ragweed antigen linked to CpG have been successful.

DNA vaccines are being designed to change the immune response

The concept of immunizing with the gene for an antigen is well established (i.e. DNA vaccines).

This approach has potential for the treatment of allergy because the DNA vector can be designed to change the immune response.

Prokaryotic DNA includes CpG motifs so that, as the antigen is expressed, it will induce a TH1 response.

Experiments with DNA vaccines have been very successful in mice, both in inducing a TH1 response initially and in controlling an existing IgE antibody response. However, the consequences of expressing an allergen within the tissue of an allergic individual are not known. Equally, it is not clear whether inducing a TH1 response to a ubiquitous allergen such as cat dander would give rise to other forms of inflammatory disease.

New forms of non-specific therapy
Humanized monoclonal anti-IgE

Humanized monoclonal anti-IgE treatment can reduce sensitivity and significantly decrease the number of acute episodes of asthma per year.

Antibodies directed against the binding site for FcεRI on IgE can bind to IgE in the circulation, but not when it is attached to mast cells or basophils. An antibody of this kind can therefore remove IgE from the circulation but will not induce anaphylaxis. It also downregulates IgE production by simultaneously binding to the B cell IgE surface receptor and the FcγRIIb receptor.

A mouse monoclonal antibody to IgE has been progressively humanized so that the molecule can be safely injected into patients and will bind IgE with very high affinity.

Treatment with anti-IgE antibodies has reduced the symptoms of both asthma and hayfever. In addition, continued treatment that controls free IgE below 10 ng/ml leads to a progressive decrease in the number of IgE receptors on mast cells. Thus, the treatment may achieve a secondary effect, further decreasing the sensitivity of histamine-containing cells to allergen.

The role of anti-IgE in treating food allergy, atopic dermatitis, and drug allergy remains to be established.

Recombinant soluble IL-4R can block the biological activity of IL-4

Given the central role of IL-4 in the TH2 response, it is not surprising that several efforts have been made to block its action. These include:
- a mutated IL-4 (Y124D);
- antibodies to IL-4; and
- recombinant soluble IL-4 receptor (sIL-4R).

Treatment with sIL-4R has proved moderately effective in clinical trials of allergic asthma. The mechanism is that sIL-4R binds to IL-4 before it can react with the receptor on T cells or B cells, and thus blocks its biological activity. However, it is less clear which of the many actions of IL-4 is relevant to the clinical effects:
- blocking the action of IL-4 on B cells may reduce IgE production, but would probably require several weeks to produce a clinical effect;

- the autocrine effect of IL-4 on TH2 cells may be an essential growth factor.

The efficacy of sIL-4R provides indirect evidence for the role of T cells in allergic disease.

Humanized monoclonal anti-IL-5 decreases circulating eosinophils

Anti-IL-5 (like anti-IgE) is a humanized mouse monoclonal antibody.

Following successful studies in baboons, anti-IL-5 has been shown to decrease circulating eosinophils in patients. It is therefore assumed that binding IL-5 produced by T cells (or mast cells) can decrease the production of eosinophils in the bone marrow. However, the results do not answer whether the treatment acts on IL-5 in the circulation or on IL-5 produced by T cells (or mast cells) locally in the bone marrow and/or the respiratory tract.

To the surprise of most investigators in the field, treatment with anti-IL-5 was not effective as a treatment for asthma despite an approximately 90% decrease in circulating eosinophils.

Some new treatment approaches may not be practical

The treatment of allergic disease is based on:
- allergen avoidance;
- pharmacological management including disodium cromoglycate, leukotriene antagonists, and local corticosteroids; and
- immunotherapy.

The treatment approaches using peptides, modified allergens, or allergens linked to CpG may not be practical because each allergen would have to go through clinical trials.

Although specific antagonists to other cytokines appear to be an attractive target for treatment, it is increasingly unlikely that they will be clinically successful in competition with anti-IgE, corticosteroids, and leukotriene antagonists.

IgE ANTIBODIES PLAY A CRITICAL ROLE IN DEFENSE AGAINST HELMINTHS

The biological role of IgE has been studied both in relation to human disease and using animal models. In tropical countries total serum IgE is usually much higher than in the West. Typical mean serum IgE levels among rural populations in tropical countries are 1000– 2000 IU/ml compared to approximately 100–200 IU/ml in the West.

The best established cause of increased IgE is infection with helminths (e.g. ascaris, hookworm, or schistosomiasis). Elevated serum IgE is not a feature of protozoal infections such as malaria and trypanosomiasis, or of bacterial infections such as tuberculosis or leprosy.

The hypothesis is that IgE antibodies play a critical role in the defense against helminths, primarily by acting as a gate-keeper.

A good example is to consider the possible role of immediate skin sensitivity in the protection against schistosomiasis. As the schistosomules enter through the skin of a sensitized individual, they trigger mast cell degranulation with release of histamine, leukotrienes, and

cytokines. These mediators lead to the local accumulation of serum (which contains IgG antibodies) and eosinophils. IgG antibodies bound to schistosomules interact with FcγR on eosinophils leading to degranulation on the surface of the worm, which kills it (Fig. 23.27).

Another important protective mechanism against helminths is the expulsion of worms from the gut. This involves increased mucus production and activated peristalsis, as well as a role for eosinophils and mast cells.

Eosinophil adhesion and degranulation

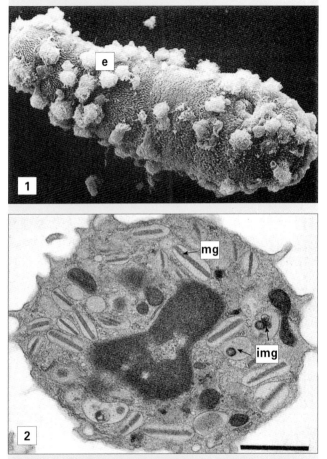

Fig. 23.27 (1) A schistosomule being killed by eosinophils that had been cultured from mouse bone marrow in the presence of IL-5. The larval helminth had first been treated with IgG antibodies and the eosinophils adhere by means of their Fcγ receptors. (Courtesy of Dr C Sanderson) (2) Transmission electron micrograph of an eosinophil. Degranulation of eosinophils usually leads to death of the cells. The mediators released include major basic protein (MBP), eosinophil cationic protein (ECP), eosinophil peroxidase (EPO), and eosinophil derived neurotoxin (EDN). In addition, eosinophils can produce leukotrienes and the cytokines IL-5, granulocyte–macrophage colony stimulating factor (GM-CSF) and TGFα. Scale bar 1 µm. (img, immature granules; mg, mature granules with crystalline core) (Courtesy of Dr C Sanderson)

Whether IgE and IgE antibodies are essential for this expulsion is not clear. However, the best analysis is that protection against worm infection is a primary role of the TH2 system. This includes roles for effector T cells, mast cells, basophils, and IgE antibodies. Furthermore, the primary mechanisms are focused on preventing entry of new worms.

Given that one third of the world's population is infested with helminths, it is clear that a protective system could have sufficient survival advantage to explain the presence of an effective TH2 system.

Perhaps as a consequence of living in the West without helminth infection, a large proportion of the population generates a TH2-based allergic response against irrelevant antigens such as those on pollen grains, cat dander, or mite fecal particles.

FURTHER READING

Akdis CA, Blaser K. IL-10-induced anergy in peripheral T cell and reactivation by microenvironmental cytokines: two key steps in specific immunotherapy. FASEB J 1999;13:603–609.

Beaven MA, Metzger H. Signal transduction by Fc receptors: the FcεRI case. Immunol Today 1993;14:222–226.

Borish L, Rosenwasser L. TH1/TH2 lymphocytes: doubt some more. J Allergy Clin Immunol 1997;99:161–164.

Bruynzeel-Koomen C, Wichen D, Toonstra J, et al. The presence of IgE molecules on epidermal Langerhans' cells in patients with atopic dermatitis. Arch Dermatol Res 1986;278:199–205.

Coca AF, Cooke RA. On the classification of the phenomenon of hypersensitiveness. J Immunol 1923;8:163.

Coyle AJ, Wagner K, Bertrand C, et al. Central role of immunoglobulin (Ig) E in the induction of lung eosinophil infiltration and T helper 2 cell cytokine production: inhibition by a non-anaphylactogenic anti-IgE antibody. J Exp Med 1996;183:1303–1310.

Galli SJ. New concepts about the mast cell. N Engl J Med 1993;328:257–265.

Geha RF. Regulation of IgE synthesis in humans. J Allergy Clin Immunol 1992;90:143–150.

Haselden BM, Kay AB, Larch M. Immunoglobulin E-independent major histocompatibility complex-restricted T cell peptide epitope-induced late asthmatic reactions. J Exp Med 1999;189:1885–1894.

Marsh DG, Neely JD, Breezeale DR, et al. Linkage analysis of IL-4 and other chromosome 5q31.1 markers and total serum immunoglobulin E concentrations. Science 1994;264:1152–1156.

Miller JS, Schwartz LB. Human mast cell proteases and mast cell heterogeneity. Curr Opin Immunol 1989;1:637–642.

Montford S, Robinson HC, Holgate ST. The bronchial epithelium as a target for inflammatory attack in asthma. Clin Exp Immunol 1992;22:511–520.

Platts-Mills TAE, Vervloet D, Thomas WR, et al. Indoor allergens and asthma: report of the Third International Workshop. J Allergy Clin Immunol 1997;100:S2–S24.

Platts-Mills TAE, Vaughan JW, Squillace S, Woodfolk JA, Sporik RB. Sensitisation, asthma and a modified TH2 response in children exposed to cat allergen. Lancet 2001;357:752–756.

Prausnitz C, Kustner H. In: Gell PGH, Coombes RRA, eds. Clinical aspects of immunology. Oxford: Blackwell Scientific Publications; 1962:808–816.

Sporik R, Holgate ST, Platts-Mills TAE, Cogswell JJ. Exposure to house-dust mite allergen (Der p I) and the development of asthma in childhood. A prospective study. N Engl J Med 1990;323:502–507.

Spry CJF, Kay AB, Gleich GJ. Eosinophils 1992. Immunol Today 1992;13:384–387.

Wan H, Winton HL, Soeller C, et al. Der p 1 facilitates transepithelial allergen delivery by disruption of tight junctions. J Clin Invest 1999;104:123–133.

Wide L, Bennich H, Johansson SGO. Diagnosis of allergy by an in vitro test for allergen antibodies. Lancet 1967;ii:1105.

Critical thinking: Severe anaphylactic shock (see p. 501 for explanations)

Sixty-two-year-old Mrs Young was stung by a bee from a hive in her back garden. Harvesting the honey had left her with several stings during the course of the summer. Several minutes after the recent sting she complained of an itching sensation in her hands, feet, and groin accompanied by cramping abdominal pain. Shortly afterwards she felt faint and acutely short of breath. Moments later she collapsed and lost consciousness. Her husband, a doctor, noticed that her breathing was rapid and wheezy and that she had swollen eyelids and lips. She was pale and had patchy erythema across her neck and arms.

On examination her apex beat could be felt, but her radial pulse was weak. Her husband immediately administered 0.5 ml of 1/1000 epinephrine (adrenaline) intramuscularly and 10 mg of chlorpheniramine (chlorphenamine) (an H_1-receptor antihistamine) intravenously with 100 mg of hydrocortisone. She regained consciousness and her respiratory rate dropped. By the following day she had recovered completely. Results of investigations at this time are shown in the table.

Mrs Young had no previous history of adverse reactions to

investigation	result (normal range)
hemoglobin (g/dl)	14.2 (11.5–16.0)
white cell count ($\times 10^9$/l)	7.5 (4.0–11.0)
neutrophils ($\times 10^9$/l)	4.4 (2.0–7.5)
eosinophils ($\times 10^9$/l)	0.40 (0.04–0.44)
total lymphocytes (($\times 10^9$/l)	2.4 (1.6–3.5)
platelet count ($\times 10^9$/l)	296 (150–400)
serum immunoglobulins 　IgG (g/l) 　IgM (g/l) 　IgA (g/l) 　IgE (IU/ml)	10.2 (5.4–16.1) 0.9 (0.5–1.9) 2.1 (0.8–2.8) 320 (3–150)
RAST 　bee venom 　wasp venom	class 4 class 0
skin prick tests	grade (0–5)
bee venom (10 µg/ml)	3+

bee venom, foods, or antibiotics. In addition there was no history of asthma, allergic rhinitis, food allergy, or atopic dermatitis. A diagnosis of anaphylactic shock due to bee venom sensitivity was made based on the history and investigations, and a decision taken to commence desensitization therapy.

Mrs Young was made aware of the possible risk of the procedure and consented to it. She was injected subcutaneously with gradually increasing doses of bee venom, the procedures being performed in hospital with access to

resuscitation apparatus. No further allergic reactions occurred and she was maintained on a dose of bee venom at 1-month intervals for the next 2 years. She was stung by a bee the following summer and had no adverse reaction.

1 What mechanisms are involved in anaphylaxis?
2 What are the clinical features and management of acute anaphylaxis?
3 How may such sensitivity be detected and what can be done to desensitize patients?

Hypersensitivity (Type II)

SUMMARY

- **Type II hypersensitivity is mediated by antibodies binding to specific cells.** Type II hypersensitivity reactions are caused by IgG or IgM antibodies against cell surface and extracellular matrix antigens. The antibodies damage cells and tissues by activating complement, and by binding and activating effector cells carrying Fcγ receptors.

- **Type II hypersensitivity reactions may target cells.** Transfusion reactions to erythrocytes are produced by antibodies to blood group antigens, which may occur naturally or may have been induced by previous contact with incompatible tissue or blood following transplantation, transfusion or during pregnancy.

- **Hemolytic disease of the newborn** occurs when maternal antibodies to fetal blood group antigens cross the placenta and destroy the fetal erythrocytes.

- **Type II hypersensitivity reactions may target tissues.** Damage to tissues may be produced by antibody to functional cell surface receptors through Fab regions. In doing so, they may enhance or inhibit the normal activity of the receptor. Examples include myasthenia gravis, pemphigus, and Goodpasture's syndrome.

- **The role of autoantibodies in disease is not always clear.** Antibodies to intracellular components are not normally pathogenetic, but they may be diagnostically useful.

- **Cytotoxic antibodies are increasingly being used for therapeutic indications.**

TYPE II HYPERSENSITIVITY REACTIONS ARE CAUSED BY IgG OR IgM ANTIBODIES AGAINST CELL SURFACE AND EXTRACELLULAR MATRIX ANTIGENS

Type II hypersensitivity reactions are mediated by IgG and IgM antibodies binding to specific cells or tissues. The damage caused is therefore restricted to the specific cells or tissues bearing the antigens. In general:

- antibodies directed against cell surface antigens are usually pathogenic;
- antibodies directed against internal antigens are usually not pathogenic.

Type II reactions therefore differ from type III reactions, which involve antibodies directed against soluble antigens in the serum, leading to the formation of circulating antigen–antibody complexes. Damage occurs when the complexes are deposited non-specifically onto tissues and/or organs (see Chapter 25).

Cells engage their targets using Fc and C3 receptors

In type II hypersensitivity, antibody directed against cell surface or tissue antigens interacts with the **Fc receptors (FcR)** on a variety of effector cells and can activate complement to bring about damage to the target cells (Fig. 24.1).

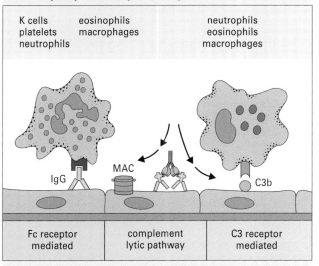

Antibody-dependent cytotoxicity

K cells eosinophils		neutrophils
platelets macrophages		eosinophils
neutrophils		macrophages

| Fc receptor mediated | complement lytic pathway | C3 receptor mediated |

Fig. 24.1 Effector cells – K cells, platelets, neutrophils, eosinophils, and cells of the mononuclear phagocyte series – all have receptors for Fc, which they use to engage antibody bound to target tissues. Activation of complement C3 can generate complement-mediated lytic damage to target cells directly, and also allows phagocytic cells to bind to their targets via C3b, C3bi, or C3d, which also activate the cells. (MAC, membrane attack complex)

Once the antibody has attached itself to the surface of the cell or tissue, it can bind and activate complement component C1, with the following consequences:

- complement fragments (C3a and C5a) generated by activation of complement attract macrophages and polymorphs to the site, and also stimulate mast cells and basophils to produce chemokines that attract and activate other effector cells;
- the classical complement pathway and activation loop lead to the deposition of C3b, C3bi, and C3d on the target cell membrane;
- the classical complement pathway and lytic pathway result in the production of the C5b–9 membrane attack complex (MAC) and insertion of the complex into the target cell membrane.

Effector cells – in this case macrophages, neutrophils, eosinophils, and NK cells – bind to either:

- the complexed antibody via their Fc receptors; or
- the membrane-bound C3b, C3bi, and C3d, via their C3 receptors (CR1, CR3, CR4).

The mechanisms by which these antibodies trigger cytotoxic reactions in vivo have been investigated in FcR-deficient mice. Anti-red blood cell antibodies trigger erythrophagocytosis of IgG-opsonized red blood cells in an FcR-dependent manner. Fc receptor γ chain-deficient mice were protected from the pathogenic effect of these antibodies whereas complement-deficient mice were indistinguishable from wild-type animals in their ability to clear the targeted red cells.

Q. How do you interpret this observation?

A. These experiments indicate that phagocytosis of antibody-sensitized red cells depends on FcR-mediated binding to the phagocytes and is not dependent on opsonization by C3b deposited via the classical pathway.

Cells damage targets by exocytosis of their normal immune effector molecules

The mechanisms by which neutrophils and macrophages damage target cells in type II hypersensitivity reactions reflect their normal methods of dealing with infectious pathogens (Fig. 24.2).

Normally pathogens would be internalized and then subjected to a barrage of microbicidal systems including defensins, reactive oxygen and nitrogen metabolites, hypohalites, enzymes, altered pH, and other agents that interfere with metabolism (see Chapters 9 and 14).

If the target is too large to be phagocytosed, the granule and lysosome contents are released in apposition to the sensitized target in a process referred to as **exocytosis**. Cross-linking of the Fc and C3 receptors during this process causes activation of the phagocyte with production of reactive oxygen intermediates, as well as activation of phospholipase A2 with consequent release of arachidonic acid from membrane phospholipids.

Q. What inflammatory mediators are synthesized from arachidonic acid?

A. This metabolite is the precursor of eicosanoids – prostaglandins and leukotrienes (see Fig. 6.21).

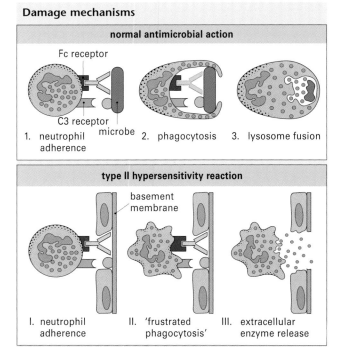

Damage mechanisms

normal antimicrobial action

Fc receptor

C3 receptor

1. neutrophil adherence   microbe   2. phagocytosis   3. lysosome fusion

type II hypersensitivity reaction

basement membrane

I. neutrophil adherence   II. 'frustrated phagocytosis'   III. extracellular enzyme release

Fig. 24.2 Neutrophil-mediated damage is a reflection of normal antibacterial action. (**1**) Neutrophils engage microbes with their Fc and C3 receptors. (**2**) The microbe is then phagocytosed and destroyed as lysosomes fuse to form the phagolysosome (**3**). In type II hypersensitivity reactions, individual host cells coated with antibody may be similarly phagocytosed, but where the target is large, for example a basement membrane (**I**), the neutrophils are frustrated in their attempt at phagocytosis (**II**). They exocytose their lysosomal contents, causing damage to cells in the vicinity (**III**).

In some situations, such as the eosinophil reaction against schistosomes (see Chapter 15), exocytosis of granule contents is normal and beneficial. However, when the target is host tissue that has been sensitized by antibody, the result is damaging (Fig. 24.3).

Antibodies may also mediate hypersensitivity by NK cells. In this case, however, the nature of the target, and whether it can inhibit the NK cells' cytotoxic actions, are as important as the presence of the sensitizing antibody.

The resistance of a target cell to damage varies. Susceptibility depends on:

- the amount of antigen expressed on the target cell's surface; and
- the inherent ability of different target cells to sustain damage.

For example, an erythrocyte may be lyzed by a single active C5 convertase site, whereas it takes many such sites to destroy most nucleated cells – their ion-pumping capacity and ability to maintain membrane integrity with anti-complementary defenses is so much greater.

Phagocytes attacking a basement membrane

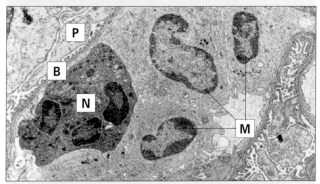

Fig. 24.3 This electron micrograph shows a neutrophil (N) and three monocytes (M) binding to the capillary basement membrane (B) in the kidney of a rabbit containing anti-basement membrane antibody. × 3500. (P, podocyte) (Courtesy of Professor GA Andres)

Q. What molecules protect the surface of nucleated cells from complement-mediated damage?
A. Decay accelerating factor (CD55) and CD59 (see Figs 4.9 and 4.11).

The rest of this chapter examines some of the instances where type II hypersensitivity reactions are thought to be of prime importance in causing target cell destruction or immunopathological damage.

TYPE II HYPERSENSITIVITY REACTIONS MAY TARGET BLOOD CELLS AND PLATELETS

Some of the most clearcut examples of type II reactions are seen in the responses to erythrocytes. Important examples are:

- incompatible blood transfusions, where the recipient becomes sensitized to antigens on the surface of the donor's erythrocytes;
- hemolytic disease of the newborn, where a pregnant woman has become sensitized to the fetal erythrocytes;
- autoimmune hemolytic anemias, where the patient becomes sensitized to his or her own erythrocytes.

Reactions to platelets can cause thrombocytopenia, and reactions to neutrophils and lymphocytes have been associated with systemic lupus erythematosus (SLE).

Transfusion reactions occur when a recipient has antibodies against donor erythrocytes

More than 20 blood group systems, generating over 200 genetic variants of erythrocyte antigens, have been identified in humans.

A blood group system consists of a gene locus that specifies an antigen on the surface of blood cells (usually, but not always, erythrocytes).

Within each system there may be two or more phenotypes. In the ABO system, for example, there are four phenotypes (A, B, AB, and O), and therefore four possible blood groups.

An individual with a particular blood group can recognize erythrocytes carrying allogeneic (non-self) blood group antigens, and will produce antibodies against them. However, for some blood group antigens such antibodies can also be produced 'naturally' (i.e. without previous sensitization by foreign erythrocytes, see below).

Transfusion of allogeneic erythrocytes into an individual who already has antibodies against them may produce erythrocyte destruction and symptoms of a 'transfusion reaction'.

Some blood group systems (e.g. ABO and Rhesus) are characterized by antigens that are relatively strong immunogens; such antigens are more likely to induce antibodies.

When planning a blood transfusion, it is important to ensure that donor and recipient blood types are compatible with respect to these major blood groups, otherwise transfusion reactions will occur.

Some major human blood groups are listed in Fig. 24.4.

The ABO blood group system is of primary importance

The epitopes of the **ABO blood group system** occur on many cell types in addition to erythrocytes and are located on the carbohydrate units of glycoproteins. The structure of these carbohydrates, and of those determining the

Five major blood group systems involved in transfusion reactions

system	gene loci	antigens	phenotype frequency (%)
ABO	1	A, B, or O	A 42 B 8 AB 3 0 47
Rhesus	2 closely linked loci: major antigen=RhD	C or c D or d E or e	RhD+ 85 RhD− 15
Kell	1	K or k	K 9 k 91
Duffy	1	Fyª, Fyᵇ, or Fy	FyªFyᵇ 46 Fyª 20 Fyᵇ 34 Fy 0.1
MN	1	M or N	MM 28 MN 50 NN 22

Fig. 24.4 Not all blood groups are equally antigenic in transfusion reactions – thus RhD evokes a stronger reaction in an incompatible recipient than the other Rhesus antigens; and Fyª is stronger than Fyᵇ. Frequencies stated are for Caucasian populations – other races have different gene frequencies.

ABO blood group antigens

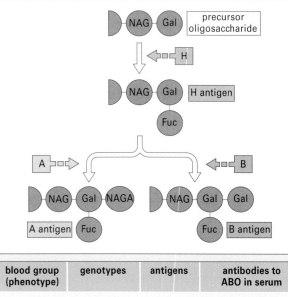

blood group (phenotype)	genotypes	antigens	antibodies to ABO in serum
A	AA, AO	A	anti-B
B	BB, BO	B	anti-A
AB	AB	A and B	none
O	OO	H	anti-A and anti-B

Fig. 24.5 The diagram shows how the ABO blood groups are constructed. The enzyme produced by the H gene attaches a fucose residue (Fuc) to the terminal galactose (Gal) of the precursor oligosaccharide. Individuals possessing the A gene now attach *N*-acetylgalactosamine (NAGA) to this galactose residue, whereas those with the B gene attach another galactose, producing A and B antigens, respectively. People with both genes make some of each. The table indicates the genotypes and antigens of the ABO system. Most people naturally make antibodies to the antigens they lack. (NAG, *N*-acetylglucosamine)

Erythrocyte blood group antigens

erythrocyte surface glycoprotein	blood groups expressed	number of epitopes per cell
anion transport protein	ABO, Ii	10^6
glycophorin A	MN	10^6
glucose transporter	ABO, Ii	5×10^5
Mr 45 000–100 000	ABO	
Mr 30 000	ABO, Rh	1.2×10^5
glycophorin B	N, Ss	2.5×10^5
glycophorins C & D	Gerbich (Ge)	10^5
DAF	Cromer	<10 000
CD44 (80 kDa)	Ina/Inh	3000–6000
zinc endopeptidase	Kell	3000–6000
DARC	Fy	12 000
laminin-binding glycoprotein	lutheran	1500–4000

Fig. 24.6 Note that blood group epitopes based on carbohydrate moieties, such as ABO and Ii (expressed on the precursor of the ABO polysaccharide), can appear on many different proteins, including Rhesus antigens. Antigens such as Rhesus and Duffy are proteins, so the epitope appears on only one type of molecule. In general, the most important blood group antigens are present at high levels on the erythrocytes, thus providing plenty of targets for complement-mediated lysis or Fc receptor-mediated clearance. (DAF, decay accelerating factor; DARC, Duffy antigen receptor for chemokines)

related Lewis blood group system, is determined by genes coding for enzymes that transfer terminal sugars to a carbohydrate backbone (Fig. 24.5).

Most individuals develop antibodies to allogeneic specificities of the ABO system without previous sensitization by foreign erythrocytes. This sensitization occurs through contact with identical epitopes, coincidentally and routinely expressed on a wide variety of microorganisms.

Antibodies to ABO antigens are therefore extremely common, making it particularly important to match donor blood to the recipient for this system. However, all people are tolerant to the O antigen, so O individuals are **universal donors** with respect to the ABO system.

The Rhesus system is a major cause of hemolytic disease of the newborn

The Rhesus system is also of great importance because it is a major cause of **hemolytic disease of the newborn (HDNB)**.

Rhesus antigens are associated with membrane proteins of 30 kDa, which are expressed at moderate levels on the erythrocyte surface. The antigens are encoded by two closely linked loci, RhD and RhCcEe, with 92% homology.

RhD is the most important clinically due to its high immunogenicity, but in RhD⁻ individuals the RhD locus is missing completely. The RhCcEe locus encodes a molecule that expresses the RhC/c and RhE/e epitopes.

Transfusion reactions can be caused by minor blood groups

MN system epitopes are expressed on the *N*-terminal glycosylated region of glycophorin A, a glycoprotein present on the erythrocyte surface. Antigenicity is determined by polymorphisms at amino acids 1 and 5.

The related **Ss system** antigens are carried on glycophorin B.

Proteins expressed on erythrocytes that display allelic variation can also act as blood group antigens. Examples of these include:

- the Kell antigen, a zinc endopeptidase;
- the Duffy antigen receptor for chemokines (DARC); and
- variants of decay accelerating factor (DAF).

The relationship of the blood groups to erythrocyte surface proteins is listed in Fig. 24.6.

Transfusion reactions caused by the minor blood groups are relatively rare unless repeated transfusions are given. The risks are greatly reduced by accurately cross-matching the donor blood to that of the recipient.

Cross-matching ensures that a recipient does not have antibodies against donor erythrocytes

The aim of cross-matching is to ensure that the blood of a recipient does not contain antibodies that will be able to react with and destroy transfused (donor) erythrocytes. For example:
- antibodies to ABO system antigens cause incompatible cells to agglutinate in a clearly visible reaction;
- minor blood group systems cause weaker reactions that may only be detectable by an indirect Coombs' test (see Fig. 24.10).

If the individual is transfused with whole blood, it is also necessary to check that the donor's serum does not contain antibodies against the recipient's erythrocytes. However, transfusion of whole blood is unusual – most blood donations are separated into cellular and serum fractions, to be used individually.

Transfusion reactions involve extensive destruction of donor blood cells

Transfusion of erythrocytes into a recipient who has antibodies to those cells produces an immediate reaction. The symptoms include:
- fever;
- hypotension;
- nausea and vomiting; and
- pain in the back and chest.

The severity of the reaction depends on the class and the amounts of antibodies involved:

Antibodies to ABO system antigens are usually IgM, and cause agglutination, complement activation, and intravascular hemolysis.

Other blood groups induce IgG antibodies, which cause less agglutination than IgM. The IgG-sensitized cells are usually taken up by phagocytes in the liver and spleen, though severe reactions may cause erythrocyte destruction by complement activation. This can cause circulatory shock, and the released contents of the erythrocytes can produce acute tubular necrosis of the kidneys.

These transfusion reactions are often seen in previously unsensitized individuals and develop over days or weeks as antibodies to the foreign cells are produced. This can result in anemia or jaundice.

Q. Why do antibodies to the ABO blood group that are normally present in a mother not damage the erythrocytes that are present in a fetus she is carrying when the fetus has a different blood group?
A. Antibodies to the ABO blood group are usually IgM, which is not transported across the placenta (see Fig. 3.19).

Transfusion reactions to other components of blood may also occur, but their consequences are not usually as severe as reactions to erythrocytes.

Hyperacute graft rejection is related to the transfusion reaction

Hyperacute graft rejection occurs when a graft recipient has preformed antibodies against the graft tissue. It is only seen in tissue that is revascularized directly after transplantation, in kidney grafts for example.

The most severe reactions in this type of rejection are due to the ABO group antigens expressed on kidney cells. The damage is produced by antibody and complement activation in the blood vessels, with consequent recruitment and activation of neutrophils and platelets.

Donors and recipients are now always cross-matched for ABO antigens, and this reaction has become extremely rare. Antibodies to other graft antigens (e.g. MHC molecules) induced by previous grafting can also produce this type of reaction.

HDNB is due to maternal IgG reacting against the child's erythrocytes in utero

Hemolytic disease of the newborn (HDNB) occurs when the mother has been sensitized to antigens on the infant's erythrocytes and makes IgG antibodies to these antigens. These antibodies cross the placenta and react with the fetal erythrocytes, causing their destruction (Figs 24.7 and 24.8). Rhesus D (RhD) is the most commonly involved antigen.

A risk of HDNB arises when a Rh^+-sensitized Rh^- mother carries a second Rh^+ infant. Sensitization of the

Hemolytic disease of the newborn

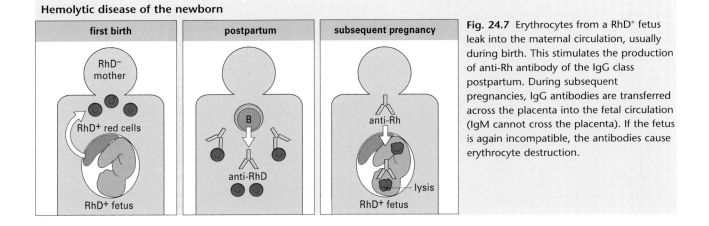

first birth	postpartum	subsequent pregnancy

RhD⁻ mother
RhD⁺ red cells
RhD⁺ fetus
B
anti-RhD
anti-Rh
lysis
RhD⁺ fetus

Fig. 24.7 Erythrocytes from a RhD⁺ fetus leak into the maternal circulation, usually during birth. This stimulates the production of anti-Rh antibody of the IgG class postpartum. During subsequent pregnancies, IgG antibodies are transferred across the placenta into the fetal circulation (IgM cannot cross the placenta). If the fetus is again incompatible, the antibodies cause erythrocyte destruction.

A child with hemolytic disease of the newborn

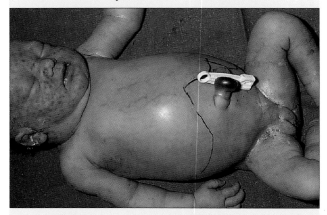

Fig. 24.8 There is considerable enlargement of the liver and spleen associated with erythrocyte destruction caused by maternal anti-erythrocyte antibody in the fetal circulation. The child had elevated bilirubin (breakdown product of hemoglobin). The facial petechial hemorrhaging was due to impaired platelet function. The most commonly involved antigen is RhD. (Courtesy of Dr K Sloper)

Rh⁻ mother to the Rh⁺ erythrocytes usually occurs during the birth of the first Rh⁺ infant, when some fetal erythrocytes leak back across the placenta into the maternal circulation and are recognized by the maternal immune system. The first incompatible child is therefore usually unaffected, whereas subsequent children have an increasing risk of being affected, as the mother is resensitized with each successive pregnancy.

Reactions to other blood groups may also cause HDNB, the second most common being the Kell system K antigen. Reactions due to anti-K are much less common than reactions due to RhD because of the relatively low frequency (9%) and weaker antigenicity of the K antigen.

The risk of HDNB due to Rhesus incompatibility is known to be reduced if the father is of a different ABO group to the mother. This observation led to the idea that

these Rh⁻ mothers were destroying Rh⁺ cells more rapidly because they were also ABO incompatible. Consequently, fetal Rh⁺ erythrocytes would not be available to sensitize the maternal immune system to RhD antigen.

This notion led to the development of **Rhesus prophylaxis** – preformed anti-RhD antibodies are given to Rh⁻ mothers immediately after delivery of Rh⁺ infants, with the aim of destroying fetal Rh⁺ erythrocytes before they can cause Rh⁻ sensitization. This practice has successfully reduced the incidence of HDNB due to Rhesus incompatibility (Fig. 24.9). Although the number of cases of HDNB has fallen dramatically and progressively, the proportion of cases caused by other blood groups, including Kell and the ABO system, has increased.

Autoimmune hemolytic anemias arise spontaneously or may be induced by drugs

Reactions to **blood group antigens** also occur spontaneously in the autoimmune hemolytic anemias, in which patients produce antibodies to their own erythrocytes.

Autoimmune hemolytic anemia is suspected if a patient gives a positive result on a **direct antiglobulin test** (Fig. 24.10), which identifies antibodies present on the patient's erythrocytes. These are usually antibodies directed towards erythrocyte antigens, or immune complexes adsorbed onto the erythrocyte surface.

The direct antiglobulin test is also used to detect antibodies on red cells in mismatched transfusions, and in HDNB (see above).

Autoimmune hemolytic anemias can be divided into three types, depending upon whether they are caused by:
- warm-reactive autoantibodies, which react with the antigen at 37°C;
- cold-reactive autoantibodies, which can only react with antigen at below 37°C;
- antibodies provoked by allergic reactions to drugs.

Warm-reactive autoantibodies cause accelerated clearance of erythrocytes

Warm-reactive autoantibodies are frequently found against Rhesus system antigens, including determinants of the RhC and RhE loci as well as RhD. They differ from

Rhesus prophylaxis

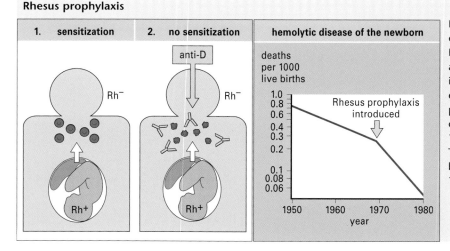

Fig. 24.9 **(1)** Without prophylaxis, Rh⁺ erythrocytes leak into the circulation of a Rh⁻ mother and sensitize her to the Rh antigen(s). **(2)** If anti-Rh antibody (anti-D) is injected immediately postpartum it eliminates the Rh⁺ erythrocytes and prevents sensitization. The incidence of deaths due to HDNB fell during the period 1950–1966 with improved patient care. The decline in the disease was accelerated by the advent of Rhesus prophylaxis in 1969.

Direct antiglobulin test

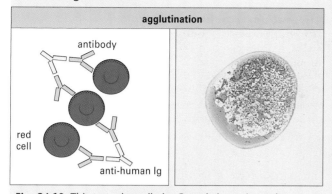

Fig. 24.10 This test, also called a Coombs' test, is used to detect antibody on a patient's erythrocytes. If antibody is present the erythrocytes can be agglutinated by anti-human immunoglobulin. If no antibody is present on the red cells, they are not agglutinated by anti-human immunoglobulin.

the antibodies responsible for transfusion reactions in that they appear to react with different epitopes.

Warm-reactive autoantibodies to other blood group antigens exist, but are relatively rare.

Most of these hemolytic anemias are of unknown cause, but some are associated with other autoimmune diseases.

Q. What mechanisms could lead to the anemia associated with these autoantibodies?
A. Fc receptor-mediated erythrophagocytosis or complement-dependent lysis.

The anemia appears to be a result of accelerated clearance of the sensitized erythrocytes by spleen macrophages more often than being caused by complement-mediated lysis.

Cold-reactive autoantibodies cause erythrocyte lysis by complement fixation

Cold-reactive autoantibodies are often present in higher titers than the warm-reactive autoantibodies. The antibodies are primarily IgM and fix complement strongly. In most cases they are specific for the Ii blood group system. The I and i epitopes are expressed on the precursor polysaccharides that produce the ABO system epitopes, and are the result of incomplete glycosylation of the core polysaccharide.

The reaction of the antibody with the erythrocytes takes place in the peripheral circulation (particularly in winter), where the temperature in the capillary loops of exposed skin may fall below 30°C. In severe cases, peripheral necrosis may occur due to aggregation and microthrombosis of small vessels caused by complement-mediated destruction in the periphery.

The severity of the anemia is therefore directly related to the complement-fixing ability of the patient's serum. (Fc-mediated removal of sensitized cells in the spleen and liver is not involved because these organs are too warm for the antibodies to bind.)

Most cold-reactive autoimmune hemolytic anemias occur in older people. Their cause is unknown, but it is notable that the autoantibodies produced are usually of very limited clonality.

Q. Why would you expect the autoimmune response to Ii antigens to be of limited clonality? There are two reasonable explanations, which are not mutually exclusive.
A. The numbers of autoreactive clones may have been curtailed by negative selection during B cell development. In addition, the antigens are carbohydrate and induce an IgM response (T independent) which has not been subject to diversification.

However, some cases may follow infection with *Mycoplasma pneumoniae*, and these are acute-onset diseases of short duration with polyclonal autoantibodies. Such cases are thought to be due to cross-reacting antigens on the bacteria and the erythrocytes, producing a bypass of normal tolerance mechanisms (see Chapter 19).

Drug-induced reactions to blood components occur in three different ways

Drugs (or their metabolites) can provoke hypersensitivity reactions against blood cells, including erythrocytes and platelets. This can occur in three different ways (Fig. 24.11).

- The drug binds to the blood cells and antibodies are produced against the drug – In this case it is necessary for both the drug and the antibody to be present to produce the reaction. This phenomenon was first recorded by Ackroyd, who noted thrombocytopenic purpura (destruction of platelets leading to purpuric rash) following administration of the drug Sedormid.

  Hemolytic anemias have been reported following the administration of a wide variety of drugs, including:
  – penicillin;
  – quinine; and
  – sulfonamides.

  All these conditions are rare.

Drug-induced reactions to blood cells

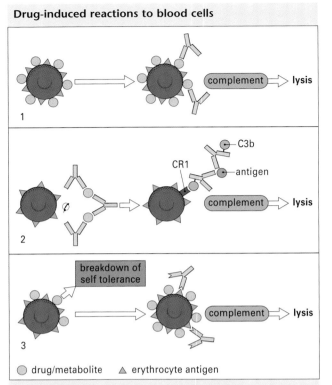

Fig. 24.11 Three ways that drug treatment can cause damage are illustrated. **(1)** The drug adsorbs to cell membranes. Antibodies to the drug bind to the cell and complement-mediated lysis occurs. **(2)** Immune complexes of drugs and antibody become adsorbed to the red cell. This could be mediated by an Fc receptor, but is more probably via the C3b receptor CR1. Damage occurs by complement-mediated lysis. **(3)** Drugs, presumably adsorbed onto cell membranes, induce a breakdown of self tolerance, possibly by stimulating TH cells. This leads to the formation of antibodies to other blood group antigens on the cell surface. Note that in examples 1 and 2 the drug must be present for cell damage to occur, whereas in 3 the cells are destroyed whether they carry adsorbed drug or not.

- Drug–antibody immune complexes are adsorbed onto the erythrocyte cell membrane – When drug–antibody immune complexes are adsorbed on to the erythrocyte cell membrane damage occurs by complement-mediated lysis.
- The drug induces an allergic reaction – The drug induces an allergic reaction and autoantibodies are directed against the erythrocyte antigens themselves, as occurs in 0.3% of patients given a-methyldopa. The antibodies produced are similar to those in patients with warm-reactive antibody. However, the condition remits shortly after the cessation of drug treatment.

Reactions against other blood cells have been associated with SLE and with thrombocytopenia

Autoantibodies to neutrophil cytoplasmic antigens (ANCAs) are associated with a number of diseases. For example:

- antibody to proteinase-3, a cytoplasmic antigen (c-ANCA), is associated with Wegener's granulomatosis;
- antibodies to myeloperoxidase are seen more commonly in systemic lupus erythematosus (SLE), and are located in perinuclear granules (p-ANCA).

Other granule components may also act as antigens in SLE, but less commonly than myeloperoxidase. Such autoantigens are generally neutrophil specific and antibodies can be detected by immunofluorescent staining (Fig. 24.12).

By contrast, antibodies to MHC antigens, which are also seen in SLE, are highly non-tissue specific.

p-ANCAs are particularly characteristic of vasculitis and glomerulonephritis. Their contribution to disease pathogenesis appears to be relatively small, although they have some diagnostic use.

Autoantibodies to platelets are seen in ITP

Autoantibodies to platelets are seen in up to 70% of cases of **idiopathic thrombocytopenic purpura** (ITP), a disorder in which there is accelerated removal of platelets from the circulation, mediated primarily by splenic macrophages. The mechanism of removal is via the immune adherence receptors on these cells.

ITP most often develops after bacterial or viral infections, but may also be associated with autoimmune diseases including SLE.

Antibodies to neutrophils

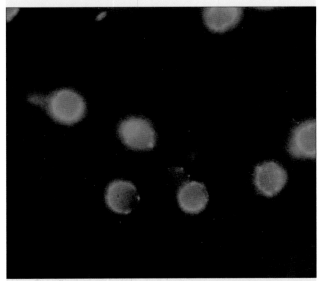

Fig. 24.12 Antibodies to neutrophils are demonstrated by immunofluorescence. In this instance, normal neutrophils were stained with antibodies from a neonate suffering from alloimmune neonatal neutropenia.

In SLE, antibodies to cardiolipin, which is present on platelets, can sometimes be detected. Autoantibodies to cardiolipin and other phospholipids can inhibit one aspect of blood clotting (**lupus anticoagulant**) and can be associated, in some cases, with venous thrombosis and recurrent abortions.

Thrombocytopenia may also be induced by drugs by similar mechanisms to those outlined in Fig. 24.11.

TYPE II HYPERSENSITIVITY REACTIONS TARGET TISSUES

A number of autoimmune conditions occur in which antibodies to tissue antigens cause immunopathological damage by activation of type II hypersensitivity mechanisms. The antigens are extracellular, and may be expressed on structural proteins or on the surface of cells. The resulting diseases are discussed here and include:

- Goodpasture's syndrome;
- pemphigus;
- myasthenia gravis.

It is often possible to demonstrate autoantibodies to particular cell types, but in these cases the antigens are intracellular, and the importance of the type II mechanisms is less well established. In these cases, recognition of autoantigen by T cells is probably more important pathologically, and the autoantibodies are of secondary importance.

Antibodies against basement membranes produce nephritis in Goodpasture's syndrome

A number of patients with nephritis are found to have **antibodies to collagen type IV**, which is a major component of basement membranes (see Fig. 25.3).

Collagen type IV undergoes alternate RNA splicing, which produces a number of variant proteins (**Goodpasture antigen**), but the antibodies appear to bind just those forms that retain the characteristic N terminus. The antibody is usually IgG and, in at least 50% of patients, it appears to fix complement.

Goodpasture's syndrome usually results in severe necrosis of the glomerulus, with fibrin deposition. The association of this type of nephritis with lung hemorrhage was originally noticed by Goodpasture (hence Goodpasture's syndrome). Although the lung symptoms do not occur in all patients, the association of lung and kidney damage is due to cross-reactive autoantigens in the basement membranes of the two tissues.

Animal models for Goodpasture's syndrome have been developed

In nephrotoxic serum nephritis (Masugi glomerulonephritis), heterologous antibodies to glomerular basement membrane are injected into rats or rabbits. The injected antibody is deposited onto the basement membranes, and this is followed by further deposition of host antibodies to the injected antibody – this precipitates acute nephritis. Development of nephritis and proteinuria depends on the accumulation of neutrophils, which bind via complement-dependent and complement-independent mechanisms. Similar lesions can be induced by immunization with heterologous basement membrane (Steblay model).

Another animal model (Heymann nephritis), caused by raising autoantibodies to a protein present in the brush border of glomerular epithelial cells, resembles human membranous glomerulonephritis. In this model, the damage is mostly complement mediated – complement depletion of the animals alleviates the condition.

Pemphigus is caused by autoantibodies to an intercellular adhesion molecule

Pemphigus is a serious blistering disease of the skin and mucous membranes. Patients have **autoantibodies against desmoglein-1 and desmoglein-3**, components of desmosomes, which form junctions between epidermal cells (Fig. 24.13). The antibodies disrupt cellular adhesion, leading to breakdown of the epidermis.

Clinical disease profiles can be related to the specificity of the antibodies. For example:

- patients with only anti-desmoglein-3 tend to show mucosal disease;
- those with anti-desmoglein-1 and anti-desmoglein-3 have skin and mucosal involvement.

Disease has been correlated with the incidence of IgG4 antibodies against a different part of the molecule.

Pemphigus is strongly linked to a rare haplotype of HLA-DR4 (DRB1*0402), and this molecule has been shown to present a peptide of desmoglein-3, which other DR4 subtypes cannot. This is therefore a clear example of an autoimmune disease producing pathology by type II mechanisms.

Autoantibodies in pemphigus

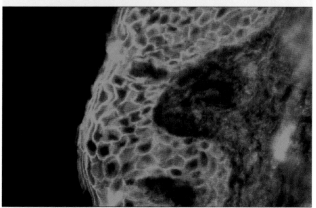

Fig. 24.13 The antibodies in pemphigus bind to components of the desmosome involved in cell adhesion. Desmoglein-1 and desmoglein-3 are most commonly involved, but other molecules, including the plakins and desmocollin, may also act as autoantigens. Immunofluorescence of human skin stained with anti-IgA. (Courtesy of Dr R Mirakian and Mr P Collins)

In myasthenia gravis and Lambert–Eaton syndrome autoantibodies to acetylcholine receptors cause muscle weakness

Myasthenia gravis, a condition in which there is extreme muscular weakness, is associated with **antibodies to the acetylcholine receptors** on the surface of muscle membranes. The acetylcholine receptors are located at the motor endplate where the neuron contacts the muscle. Transmission of impulses from the nerve to the muscle takes place by the release of acetylcholine from the nerve terminal and its diffusion across the gap to the muscle fiber.

It was noticed that immunization of experimental animals with purified acetylcholine receptors produced a condition of muscular weakness that closely resembled human myasthenia. This suggested a role for antibody to the acetylcholine receptor in the human disease.

Analysis of the lesion in myasthenic muscles indicated that the disease was not due to an inability to synthesize acetylcholine, nor was there any problem in secreting it in response to a nerve impulse – the released acetylcholine was less effective at triggering depolarization of the muscle (Fig. 24.14).

Examination of neuromuscular endplates by immunochemical techniques has demonstrated IgG and the complement proteins, C3 and C9, on the postsynaptic folds of the muscle (Fig. 24.15).

Further evidence for a pathogenetic role for IgG in this disease was furnished by the discovery of transient muscle weakness in babies born to mothers with myasthenia gravis. This is significant because it is known that IgG can and does cross the placenta, entering the blood stream of the fetus.

IgG and complement are thought to act in two ways:
- by increasing the rate of turnover of the acetylcholine receptors; and
- by partial blocking of acetylcholine binding.

Cellular infiltration of myasthenic endplates is rarely seen, so it is assumed that damage does not involve effector cells.

Lambert–Eaton syndrome is caused by defective release of acetylcholine

In a Lambert–Eaton syndrome, a condition related to myasthenia gravis, muscular weakness is caused by defective release of acetylcholine from the neuron. If serum or

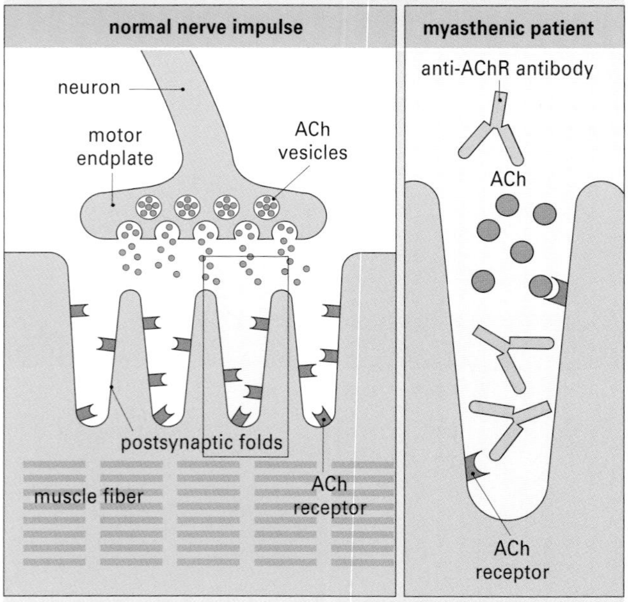

Fig. 24.14 Normally a nerve impulse passing down a neuron arrives at a motor endplate and causes the release of acetylcholine (ACh). This diffuses across the neuromuscular junction, binds ACh receptors (AChR) on the muscle, and causes ion channels in the muscle membrane to open, which in turn triggers muscular contraction. In myasthenia gravis, antibodies to the receptor block binding of the ACh transmitter. The effect of the released vesicle is therefore reduced, and the muscle can become very weak. Antibody blocking receptors are only one of the factors operating in the disease.

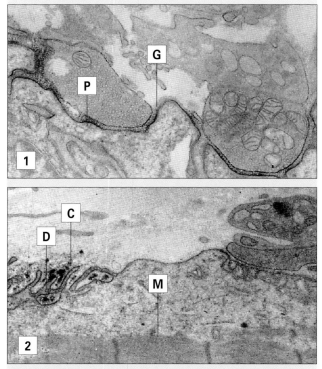

Fig. 24.15 (1) Electron micrograph showing IgG deposits (G) in discrete patches on the postsynaptic membrane (P). × 13 000. (2) Electron micrograph illustrating C9 (C) shows the postsynaptic region denuded of its nerve terminal – it consists of debris and degenerating folds (D). There is a strong reaction for C9 on this debris. × 9000. (M, muscle fiber) (Courtesy of Dr AG Engel)

IgG from patients with Lambert–Eaton syndrome is transfused into mice, the condition is also transferred, indicating the presence of autoantibody. The autoantibodies are directed against components of **voltage-gated calcium channels or the synaptic vesicle protein synaptotagmin**.

The different forms of Lambert–Eaton syndrome are thought to relate to the target antigen and the class and titer of antibodies involved.

Q. Predict whether inhibitors of acetylcholinesterase will have any value in alleviating the symptoms of myasthenia gravis or Lambert–Eaton syndrome.

A. These drugs are often useful in myasthenia gravis because acetylcholine is present and an inhibitor of acetylcholinesterase will prolong its activity. They are less useful in Lambert–Eaton syndrome because acetylcholine is not released in the first place.

Autoantibodies may block receptors or mimic receptors agonists

Myasthenia gravis and Lambert–Eaton syndrome exemplify conditions where autoantibodies to receptors block the normal function of the receptor. There are other diseases, however, where the autoantibody has an opposite effect, for example in some forms of autoimmune thyroid disease antibodies to the thyroid-stimulating hormone (TSH) receptor mimic TSH, thereby stimulating thyroid function (see Chapter 21).

AUTOANTIBODIES MAY BE PRESENT IN THE ABSENCE OF DISEASE

Although many autoantibodies react with tissue antigens, their significance in causing tissue damage and pathology in vivo is not always clear. For example, although autoantibodies to pancreatic islet cells can be detected in vitro using sera from some diabetic patients (Fig. 24.16), most

Islet cell autoantibodies

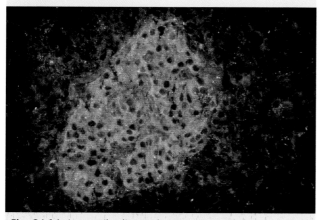

Fig. 24.16 Autoantibodies to the pancreas in diabetes mellitus may be demonstrated by immunofluorescence. The antibodies are diagnostically useful, and may contribute to the pathology. (Courtesy of Dr B Dean)

of the immunopathological damage in autoimmune diabetes is thought to be caused by autoreactive T cells.

Until recently it was thought that autoantibodies against intracellular antigens would not usually cause immunopathology because they could not reach their antigen within a living cell. However, it now appears that antibodies such as anti-ribonucleoprotein (anti-RNP) and anti-DNA can reach the cell nucleus and modulate cell function – in some cases, they can induce apoptosis.

Although the relative importance of antibody in causing cell damage is still debated, autoantibodies against internal antigens of cells often make excellent disease markers because they are frequently detectable before immunopathological damage occurs.

CYTOTOXIC ANTIBODIES ARE INCREASINGLY USED FOR THERAPEUTIC INDICATIONS

It is now realized that high-specificity monoclonal antibodies can be used to induce cell death as a therapeutic procedure mediated via type II hypersensitivity mechanisms.

Some of antibodies increasingly being used for therapeutic indications work by blocking signaling pathways important in disease pathophysiology, for example:

* the **antihuman epidermal growth factor receptor 2 (anti-HER2) antibody, trastuzumab,** used in breast cancer; and
* the **anti-TNF antibody, infliximab,** used in Crohn's disease.

However, of relevance to type II hypersensitivity reactions, other monoclonal antibodies work by inducing antibody-dependent cell-mediated cytotoxicity (ADCC) and/or activation of complement pathways. The most widely used of these is the **anti-CD20 antibody, rituximab.** CD20 is expressed on normal B cells as well as most B cell malignancies and rituximab is now an established part of the treatment of B lineage non-Hodgkin's lymphomas.

Anti-CD20 therapy is also proving useful for treatment of autoimmune disease resistant to standard therapies including immune thrombocytopenia, rheumatoid arthritis, and SLE, where its activity is due to elimination of host autoreactive B cells.

Other antibodies in clinical use include the **anti-CD52 antibody, alemtuzumab,** which targets an antigen found on immune cells (both B and T cells). Alemtuzumab is used for the treatment of chronic B and T cell leukemias as well as for immune suppression in patients undergoing allogeneic hematopoietic stem cell transplantation.

FURTHER READING

Alarçon-Segovia D, Ruiz-Argüelles A, Llorente L. Broken dogma: penetration of autoantibodies into living cells. Immunol Today 1996;17:163–164.

Amagai M. Autoantibodies against desmosomal cadherins in pemphigus. J Dermatol Sci 1999;20:92–102.

Anstee DJ. Blood group active substances of the human red blood cell. Vox Sang 1990;58:1.

Bhol K, Natarajan K, Nagarwalla N, et al. Correlation of peptide specificity and IgG subclass with pathogenic and non-pathogenic auto-antibodies in pemphigus vulgaris: a model for autoimmunity. Proc Natl Acad Sci USA 1995;92:5239–5243.

Black M, Mignogna MD, Scully C. Pemphigus vulgaris. Oral Dis 2005;11:119–130.

Bloy C, Blanchard D, Lambin P, et al. Characterization of the D, C, E and G antigens of the Rh blood group system with human monoclonal antibodies. Mol Immunol 1988;25:926–930.

Dean FG, Wilson GR, Li M, Edgtton KL, et al. Experimental autoimmune Goodpasture's disease: a pathogenetic role for both effector cells and antibody injury. Kidney Int 2005;67:566–575.

Druet P, Glotz D. Experimental autoimmune nephropathies: induction and regulation. Adv Nephrol 1984;13:115.

Engelfriet CP, Reesink HW, Judd WJ, et al. Current status of immunoprophylaxis with anti-D immunoglobulin. Vox Sang 2003;85:328–337.

Le van Kim C, Mouro I, Cherif-Zahar B, et al. Molecular cloning and primary structure of the human blood group RhD polypeptide. Proc Natl Acad Sci USA 1992;89:10925–10929.

King MJ. Blood group antigens on human erythrocytes – distribution, structure and possible functions. Biochim Biophys Acta 1994;1197:14–44.

Lang B, Newsom-Davis J. Immunopathology of the Lambert–Eaton myasthenic syndrome. Springer Semin Immunopathol 1995;17:3–15.

Lindstrom J. Immunobiology of myasthenia gravis, experimental autoimmune myasthenia gravis and Lambert–Eaton syndrome. Annu Rev Immunol 1985;3:109–131.

Mauro I, Colin Y, Chenif-Zahar B, et al. Molecular genetic basis of the human Rhesus blood group system. Nature Genet 1993;5:62–65.

Naparstek Y, Plotz PH. The role of autoantibodies in autoimmune disease. Annu Rev Immunol 1993;11:79–104.

Race R, Sanger R. Blood groups in man. 6th edn. Oxford: Blackwell Scientific Publications; 1975.

Russo D, Redman C, Lee S. Association of XK and Kell blood group proteins. J Biol Chem 1998;273:13950–13956.

Schulz DR, Tozman EC. Anti-neutrophil cytoplasmic antibodies: major autoantigens, pathophysiology, and disease associations. Semin Arthritis Rheum 1995;25:143–159.

Vincent A. Antibody-mediated disorders of neuro-muscular transmission. Clin Neurophysiol Suppl 2004;57:147–158.

Yamamoto F-I, Clausen H, White T, et al. Molecular genetic basis of the histo-blood group ABO system. Nature 1990;345:229.

Critical thinking: Blood groups and hemolytic disease of the newborn (see p. 502 for explanations)

Mrs Chareston has the blood group O, Rhesus negative, and her husband Mr Chareston is A, Rhesus positive. They have had four children, of which two have been affected by hemolytic disease of the newborn (HDNB), as follows:

- first child born 1968 – unaffected;
- second child born 1974 – mildly affected;
- third child born 1976 – seriously affected, required intrauterine blood transfusion;
- fourth child born 1980 – unaffected.

In both affected cases (second and third), the cause of the hemolytic disease was identified as antibodies to Rhesus D binding to the child's red cells. Following the second, third, and fourth deliveries, Mrs Chareston was given antibodies to the Rhesus D blood group (Rhesus prophylaxis was introduced in the UK in 1972).

1. From this information, what can you deduce about the blood group of the first child?
2. Why does HDNB usually become more serious with successive pregnancies?

3. What is the reason for giving anti-Rhesus D antibodies to the mother?
4. Why are the antibodies given postpartum and not earlier?
5. Give an explanation of why the Rhesus prophylaxis after the second delivery failed to prevent HDNB in the third child.
6. What explanation can be given to account for the fact that the fourth child is unaffected?

When the blood groups of the children are examined it is found that they are:

- first child – O, Rh$^+$;
- second child – B, Rh$^+$;
- third child – A, Rh$^+$;
- fourth child – A, Rh$^-$.

7. As Mrs Chareston has antibodies to blood group A, why was the fourth child not affected by HDNB caused by these antibodies?
8. One of these children was definitely not fathered by Mr Chareston – which child?

Hypersensitivity (Type III)

SUMMARY

- **Diseases caused by immune complexes can be divided into three groups.** Immune complexes are formed every time antibody meets antigen and are removed by the mononuclear phagocyte system following complement activation. Persistence of antigen from continued infection or in autoimmune disease can lead to immune complex disease.

- **Immune complexes can trigger a variety of inflammatory processes.** Fc–FcR interactions are the key mediators of inflammation. Most importantly, Fc regions within immune deposits within tissues engage Fc receptors on activated neutrophils, lymphocytes, and platelets to induce inflammation. During chronic inflammation B cells and macrophages are the predominant infiltrating cell type, and activation of endogenous cells within the organ participates in fibrosis and disease progression.

- **Experimental models demonstrate the main immune complex diseases.** Serum sickness can be induced with large injections of foreign antigen. Autoimmunity causes immune complex disease in the NZB/NZW mouse. Injection of antigen into the skin of presensitized animals produces the Arthus reaction.

- **Immune complexes are normally removed by the mononuclear phagocyte system.** Complement helps to disrupt antigen–antibody bonds and keeps immune complexes soluble. Primate erythrocytes bear a receptor for C3b and are important for transporting complement-containing immune complexes to the spleen for removal. Complement deficiencies lead to the formation of large, relatively insoluble complexes, which deposit in tissues.

- **The size of immune complexes affects their deposition.** Deposition of circulating, soluble immune complexes is limited by physical factors, such as the size and charge of the complexes. Small, positively charged complexes have the greatest propensity for deposition within vessels. Large immune complexes are rapidly removed in the liver and spleen.

- **Immune complex deposition in the tissues results in tissue damage.** Immune complexes can form both in the circulation, leading to systemic disease, and at local sites such as the lung. Charged cationic antigens have tissue-binding properties, particularly for the glomerulus, and help to localize complexes to the kidney. Factors that tend to increase blood vessel permeability enhance the deposition of immune complexes in tissues.

- **Deposited immune complexes can be visualized using immunofluorescence.**

DISEASES CAUSED BY IMMUNE COMPLEXES CAN BE DIVIDED INTO THREE GROUPS

Immune complexes are formed every time antibody meets antigen, and generally they are removed effectively by the mononuclear phagocyte system.

Occasionally, however, immune complexes persist and eventually deposit in a range of tissues and organs. The complement and effector cell-mediated damage that follows is known as a type III hypersensitivity reaction or immune complex disease.

The sites of immune complex deposition are partly determined by the localization of the antigen in the tissues and partly by how circulating complexes become deposited.

Diseases resulting from immune complex formation can be divided broadly into three groups:
- those due to persistent infection;
- those due to autoimmune disease; and
- those caused by inhalation of antigenic material (Fig. 25.1).

Persistent infection with a weak antibody response can lead to immune complex disease

The combined effects of a low-grade persistent infection and a weak antibody response lead to chronic immune complex formation, and eventual deposition of complexes in the tissues (Fig. 25.2). Diseases with this etiology include:
- leprosy;
- malaria;
- dengue hemorrhagic fever;
- viral hepatitis; and
- staphylococcal infective endocarditis.

Three categories of immune complex disease

cause	antigen	site of complex deposition
persistent infection	microbial antigen	infected organ(s), kidney
autoimmunity	self antigen	kidney, joint, arteries, skin
inhaled antigen	mold, plant, or animal antigen	lung

Fig. 25.1 This table indicates the source of the antigen and the organs most frequently affected.

Immunofluorescence study of immune complexes in infectious disease

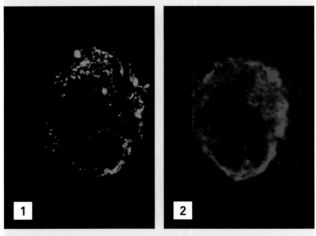

Fig. 25.2 These serial sections of the renal artery of a patient with chronic hepatitis B infection are stained with fluoresceinated anti-hepatitis B antigen (**1**) and rhodaminated anti-IgM (**2**). The presence of both antigen and antibody in the intima and media of the arterial wall indicates the deposition of complexes at this site. IgG and C3 deposits are also detectable with the same distribution. (Courtesy of Dr A Nowoslawski)

Immune complex disease is a frequent complication of autoimmune disease

Immune complex disease is common in autoimmune disease, where the continued production of autoantibody to a self antigen leads to prolonged immune complex formation. As the number of complexes in the blood increases, the systems responsible for the removal of complexes (mononuclear phagocyte, erythrocyte, and complement) become overloaded, and complexes are deposited in the tissues (Fig. 25.3). Diseases with this etiology include:
- rheumatoid arthritis;
- systemic lupus erythematosus (SLE); and
- polymyositis.

Immunofluorescence study of immune complexes in autoimmune disease

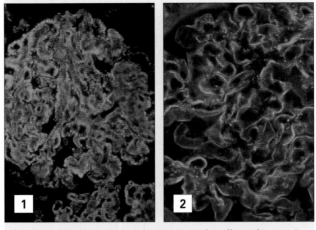

Fig. 25.3 These renal sections compare the effect of systemic lupus erythematosus (type III hypersensitivity) (**1**) and Goodpasture's syndrome (type II hypersensitivity) (**2**). In each case the antibody is detected with fluorescent anti-IgG. Complexes, formed in the blood and deposited in the kidney, form characteristic 'lumpy bumpy' deposits (**1**). The anti-basement membrane antibody in Goodpasture's syndrome forms an even layer on the glomerular basement membrane (**2**). (Courtesy of Dr S Thiru)

Immune complex following inhalation of antigen

Immune complexes may be formed at body surfaces following exposure to extrinsic antigens.

Such reactions are seen in the lungs following repeated inhalation of antigenic materials from molds, plants, or animals. This is exemplified in:
- farmer's lung, where there are circulating antibodies to actinomycete fungi (found in moldy hay); and
- pigeon fancier's lung, where there are circulating antibodies to pigeon antigens.

Both diseases are forms of **extrinsic allergic alveolitis**, and occur only after repeated exposure to the antigen. Note that the antibodies induced by these antigens are primarily IgG, rather than the IgE seen in type I hypersensitivity reactions. When antigen again enters the body by inhalation, local immune complexes are formed in the alveoli leading to inflammation and fibrosis (Fig. 25.4).

Precipitating antibodies to actinomycete antigens are found in the sera of 90% of patients with farmer's lung. However, they are also found in some people with no disease, and are absent from some patients, so it seems that other factors are also involved in the disease process, including type IV hypersensitivity reactions.

IMMUNE COMPLEXES CAN TRIGGER A VARIETY OF INFLAMMATORY PROCESSES

Immune complexes are capable of triggering a wide variety of inflammatory processes:

Extrinsic allergic alveolitis

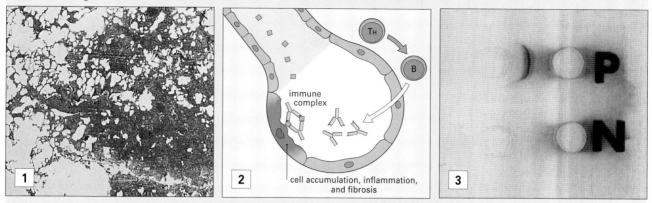

Fig. 25.4 The histological appearance of the lung in extrinsic allergic alveolitis (**1**) shows consolidated areas due to cell accumulation. When fungal antigen is inhaled into the lung of a sensitized individual, immune complexes are formed in the alveoli (**2**). Complement fixation leads to cell accumulation, inflammation, and fibrosis. Precipitin antibody (P) present in the serum of a patient with pigeon fancier's lung (**3**) is directed against the fungal antigen *Micropolyspora faeni*. Normal serum (N) lacks antibodies to this fungus.

- they interact directly with basophils and platelets (via Fc receptors) to induce the release of vasoactive amines (Fig. 25.5);
- macrophages are stimulated to release cytokines, particularly tumor necrosis factor-α (TNFα) and interleukin-1 (IL-1), which have important roles in inflammation;
- they interact with the complement system to generate **C3a and C5a (anaphylatoxins)** – these complement fragments stimulate the release of vasoactive amines (including histamine and 5-hydroxytryptamine) and chemotactic factors from mast cells and basophils; and C5a is also chemotactic for basophils, eosinophils, and neutrophils.

Recent work with knockout mice indicates that complement has a less proinflammatory role than previously thought, whereas cells bearing Fc receptors for IgG and IgE appear to be critical for developing inflammation, with complement having a protective effect.

The vasoactive amines released by platelets, basophils, and mast cells cause endothelial cell retraction and thus increase vascular permeability, allowing the deposition of immune complexes on the blood vessel wall (Fig. 25.6). The deposited complexes continue to generate C3a and C5a.

Platelets also aggregate on the exposed collagen of the vessel basement membrane to form microthrombi.

Q. Aggregation may be directly enhanced by the presence of immune complexes on the basement membrane. How can platelets recognize immune complexes?
A. They have an Fc receptor, FcγRIIa (see Fig. 3.18).

The aggregated platelets continue to produce vasoactive amines and to stimulate the production of C3a and

C5a. (Platelets are also a rich source of growth factors – these may be involved in the cellular proliferation seen in immune complex diseases such as **glomerulonephritis** and **rheumatoid arthritis**.)

Polymorphs are chemotactically attracted to the site by C5a. They attempt to engulf the deposited immune complexes, but are unable to do so because the complexes are bound to the vessel wall. They therefore exocytose their lysosomal enzymes onto the site of deposition (see Fig. 25.6). If simply released into the blood or tissue fluids these lysosomal enzymes are unlikely to cause much inflammation, because they are rapidly neutralized by serum enzyme inhibitors. But if the phagocyte applies itself closely to the tissue-trapped complexes through Fc binding, then serum inhibitors are excluded and the enzymes may damage the underlying tissue.

Type II and type III hypersensitivity cause damage by similar mechanisms

It is important to understand that the inflammatory pathways involved in type II and type III reactions are identical. The distinction is based on where the antigens are derived from and how the immune complexes form:
- in type II hypersensitivity reactions, the autoantibodies bind to autoantigens where they normally reside;
- by contrast, in type III hypersensitivity reactions, the antigens may be either self (i.e. auto) or foreign and the immune deposits may form by either deposition of soluble immune complexes or in situ by initial deposition of unbound circulating antigen followed by binding of circulating antibody.

Nevertheless, the effector mechanisms leading to inflammation and tissue injury are similar in type II and type III reactions and dependent on the capacity of deposited antibodies to engage FcRs and activate complement.

Immune complexes as a trigger for increasing vascular permeability

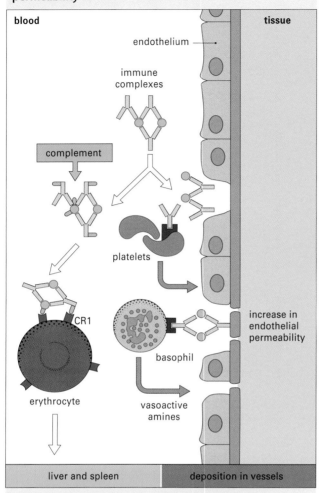

Fig. 25.5 Immune complexes normally bind complement and are removed to the liver and spleen after binding to CR1 on erythrocytes. In inflammation, immune complexes act on basophils and platelets (in humans) to produce vasoactive amine release. The amines released (e.g. histamine, 5-hydroxytryptamine) cause endothelial cell retraction and thus increase vascular permeability.

Complement is an important mediator of type III hypersensitivity

In many diseases, complement activation is triggered inappropriately and drives a vicious cycle, causing:
- further tissue damage;
- increased inflammation; and
- perpetuation of the disease.

This scenario is particularly evident in autoimmune diseases where immune complexes deposit in tissues and there activate complement, causing damage and destruction of host cells. Examples include:
- the kidney in various autoimmune glomerular diseases; and
- the joint in rheumatoid arthritis.

Deposition of immune complexes in blood vessel walls

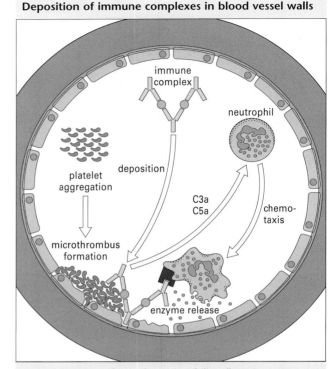

Fig. 25.6 Increased vascular permeability allows immune complexes to be deposited in the blood vessel wall. This induces platelet aggregation and complement activation. The aggregated platelets form microthrombi on the exposed collagen of the basement membrane of the endothelium. Neutrophils are attracted to the site by complement products, but cannot ingest the complexes. They therefore exocytose their lysosomal enzymes, causing further damage to the vessel wall.

Staining of these tissues for complement deposits reveals the full extent of involvement. The tissues are often packed with C3 fragments and other complement proteins. Complement activation is also evident in the blood in these diseases:
- complement activity and the plasma concentrations of the major components C3 and C4 are reduced due to consumption in the tissues; and
- levels of complement activation fragments are increased.

In SLE, autoantibodies are generated against cell contents including DNA, cytoplasmic proteins, and mitochondria. Immune complexes form whenever cell contents are released and these deposit in capillary beds in organs such as skin, kidney, joint, and brain where they activate complement causing further tissue damage. Here complement is playing dual roles:
- the important immune complex solubilizing roles will prevent immune complex deposition until the capacity of the system is exceeded;
- beyond this threshold complexes deposit and activate complement in the tissues, causing pathology.

Complement changes from hero to villain. Patients with SLE often have markedly decreased plasma levels of complement activity and the components C3 and C4 due to the massive and widespread activation of the system. Levels of these parameters can be used to monitor disease activity.

Autoantibodies to complement components can modulate complement activity

Autoantibodies may also develop that directly target the complement components and complexes.

Autoantibodies against C1q are commonly found in SLE, correlating particularly with renal involvement.

Antibodies against the alternative pathway C3 convertase bind and stabilize the complex, markedly increasing its functional half-life and thus consuming C3.

These autoantibodies were first identified in patients with **membranoproliferative glomerulonephritis (MPGN)** and were therefore termed **C3 nephritic factors (C3NeF)**, but may also be found in SLE.

C3NeF are also associated with a bizarre 'wasting' disorder characterized by loss of adipose tissue, termed **partial lipodystrophy**, which may occur with or without associated MPGN. The syndrome was, until recently, unexplained, but recent evidence suggests that activation of the alternative pathway is a feature of normal lipid handling in adipose tissue. Stabilization of the convertase by C3NeF will then cause local increased complement activation and fat cell destruction.

Rarely, autoantibodies against the classical pathway C3 convertase, termed **C4 nephritic factors (C4NeF)**, are found in association with MPGN or SLE. These too stabilize the convertase and cause increased complement activation to drive disease.

EXPERIMENTAL MODELS DEMONSTRATE THE MAIN IMMUNE COMPLEX DISEASES

Experimental models are available for each of the three main types of immune complex disease described above:
- **serum sickness**, induced by injections of foreign antigen, mimics the effect of a persistent infection;
- the NZB/NZW mouse demonstrates **autoimmunity**;
- the **Arthus reaction** is an example of local damage by extrinsic antigen.

Care must be taken when interpreting animal experiments because the erythrocytes of rodents and rabbits lack the receptor for C3b (known as CR1), which readily binds immune complexes that have fixed complement. This receptor is present on primate erythrocytes.

Serum sickness can be induced with large injections of foreign antigen

In serum sickness, circulating immune complexes deposit in the blood vessel walls and tissues, leading to increased vascular permeability and thus to inflammatory diseases such as glomerulonephritis and arthritis.

In the pre-antibiotic era, serum sickness was a complication of serum therapy, in which massive doses of antibody were given for diseases such as diphtheria. Horse anti-diphtheria serum was usually used, and some individuals made antibodies against the horse proteins.

Serum sickness is now commonly studied in rabbits by giving them an intravenous injection of a foreign soluble protein such as bovine serum albumin (BSA). After about 1 week antibodies are formed, which enter the circulation and complex with antigen. Because the reaction occurs in antigen excess, the immune complexes are small (Fig. 25.7). These small complexes are removed only slowly by the mononuclear phagocyte system and therefore persist in the circulation.

Q. Suggest two reasons why small immune complexes would be cleared more slowly than large complexes.
A. Small complexes activate complement less effectively than large complexes because C1 must bind to several Fc regions before it is activated. The avidity of complexes for binding to phagocytes will also be increased when several Fc regions are available to bind to the Fc receptors on a phagocyte. If this were not so, monomeric antibody would block binding of complexes to Fc receptors.

The formation of complexes is followed by an abrupt fall in total hemolytic complement.

The clinical signs of serum sickness that develop are due to granular deposits of antigen–antibody and C3 forming along the glomerular basement membrane (GBM) and in small vessels elsewhere. As more antibody is formed and the reaction moves into antibody excess, the size of the complexes increases and they are cleared more efficiently, so the animals recover. Chronic disease is induced by daily administration of antigen.

Time course of experimental serum sickness

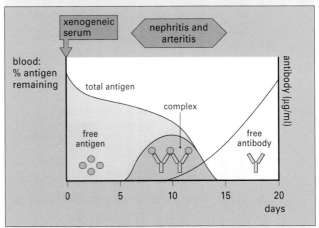

Fig. 25.7 Following an injection of xenogeneic serum there is a lag period of approximately 5 days, in which only free antigen is detectable in serum. After this time, antibodies are produced to the foreign proteins and immune complexes are formed in serum; it is during this period that the symptoms of nephritis and arteritis appear. To begin with, small soluble complexes are found in antigen excess; with increasing antibody titers, larger complexes are formed, which are deposited and subsequently cleared. At this stage the symptoms disappear.

Q. Why would immune complexes deposit in the glomerulus when the complexes are formed outside the kidney?
A. The glomerulus has fenestrated endothelium and is a site of filtration.

Autoimmunity causes immune complex disease in the NZB/NZW mouse

The F_1 hybrid NZB/NZW mouse produces a range of autoantibodies (including anti-erythrocyte, anti-nuclear, anti-DNA, and anti-Sm) and suffers from an immune complex disease similar in many ways to SLE in humans.

A NZB/NZW mouse is born clinically normal, but within 2–3 months shows sign of hemolytic anemia. Tests for anti-erythrocyte antibody (the Coombs' test), anti-nuclear antibodies, lupus cells, and circulating immune complexes are all positive, and there are deposits in the glomeruli and choroid plexus of the brain. The disease is much more marked in the females, who die within a few months of developing symptoms (Fig. 25.8).

The role of Fc receptors in the 'treatment' of immune complex disease

The restoration of 'tolerance' in murine lupus disease has been achieved by the transduction of the inhibitory Fc receptor FcγRIIb. Animals so treated showed:
* a prolonged life span;
* lower levels of kidney disease as measured by reduced proteinuria; and
* lower levels of autoantibody (see Chapter 20).

Injection of antigen into the skin of presensitized animals produces the Arthus reaction

The Arthus reaction takes place at a local site in and around the walls of small blood vessels. It is most frequently demonstrated in the skin.

An animal is immunized repeatedly until it has appreciable levels of serum antibody (mainly IgG). Following

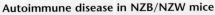

Autoimmune disease in NZB/NZW mice

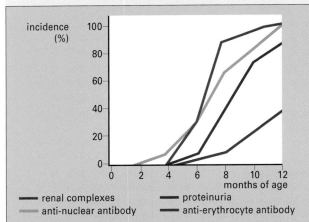

Fig. 25.8 The graph shows the onset of autoimmune disease in female NZB/NZW mice with advancing age. Incidence refers to the percentage of mice with the features identified. Immune complexes were detected by immunofluorescent staining of a kidney section. Anti-nuclear antibodies were detected in serum by indirect immunofluorescence. Proteinuria reflects kidney damage. Autoantibodies to erythrocytes develop later in the disease and so are less likely to relate to kidney pathology. Onset of autoimmune disease is delayed in male mice by approximately 3 months.

subcutaneous or intradermal injection of the antigen a reaction develops at the injection site, sometimes with marked edema and hemorrhage, depending on the amount of antigen injected. The reaction reaches a peak after 4–10 hours, then wanes and is usually minimal by 48 hours (Fig. 25.9).

Immunofluorescence studies have shown that initial deposition of antigen, antibody, and complement in the vessel wall is followed by neutrophil infiltration and

The appearance of the three main skin test reactions

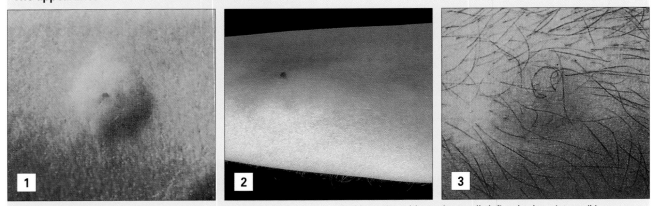

Fig. 25.9 A type I hypersensitivity reaction (**1**) produces a raised wheal, 5–7 mm in diameter and with a well defined edge after about 15 minutes. A type III hypersensitivity Arthus reaction (**2**) produces a reaction after 5–12 hours that is larger (≥ 50 mm) and has a less well defined edge. A type IV (delayed) hypersensitivity reaction shows as a red indurated lesion, about 5 mm in diameter at 24–48 hours (**3**).

intravascular clumping of platelets (Fig. 25.10). This platelet reaction can lead to vascular occlusion and necrosis in severe cases. After 24–48 hours the neutrophils are replaced by mononuclear cells, and eventually some plasma cells appear.

Complement activation via either the classical or alternative pathways was thought to be essential for the Arthus reaction to develop. But C3, C4, or C5 deficient mice were able to mount a normal Arthus reaction. However, when mice were made deficient in FcγRI or FcγRIII they were unable to produce the reaction. Furthermore, when recombinant soluble FcγRII receptors were given they inhibited the development of the Arthus reaction.

TNFα enhances cell-mediated immune responses in various ways (see Chapter 9). Treatment with antibodies to TNF can reduce severity in the Arthus reaction and, interestingly, anti-TNF is useful in treating rheumatoid arthritis.

The ratio of antibody to antigen is directly related to the severity of the ensuing reaction. Complexes formed in either antigen or antibody excess are much less toxic than those formed at equivalence.

IMMUNE COMPLEXES ARE NORMALLY REMOVED BY THE MONONUCLEAR PHAGOCYTE SYSTEM

Immune complexes are opsonized with C3b following complement activation, and removed by the mononuclear phagocyte system, particularly in the liver and spleen. Removal is mediated by the complement C3b receptor, CR1.

In primates, the bulk of CR1 in blood is found on erythrocytes. (Non-primates do not have erythrocyte CR1, and must therefore rely on platelet CR1.) There are about 700 receptors per erythrocyte, and their effectiveness is enhanced by the grouping of receptors in patches, allowing high-avidity binding to the large complexes.

CR1 readily binds immune complexes that have fixed complement, as has been shown by experiments with animals lacking complement (Fig. 25.11).

In normal primates the erythrocytes provide a buffer mechanism, binding complexes that have fixed complement and effectively removing them from the plasma. In small blood vessels 'streamline flow' allows the erythrocytes to travel in the center of the vessel surrounded by the flowing plasma. Thus it is only the plasma that makes contact with the vessel wall. Only in the sinusoids of the liver and spleen, or at sites of turbulence, do the erythrocytes make contact with the lining of the vessels.

The complexes are transported to the liver and spleen, where they are removed by fixed tissue macrophages (Fig. 25.12). Most of the CR1 is also removed in the process, so in situations of continuous immune complex formation the number of active receptors falls rapidly, impairing the efficiency of immune complex handling.

In patients with SLE, for example, the number of receptors may well be halved. With fewer complement receptors the complexes are cleared rapidly to the liver, but these complexes, which arrive directly rather than on red cells, are later released into the circulation again and may then deposit in the tissues elsewhere and lead to inflammation.

The Arthus reaction

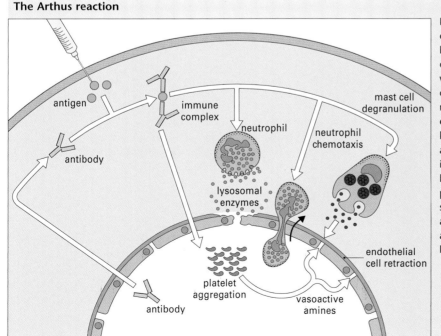

antigen

immune complex

antibody

neutrophil

lysosomal enzymes

mast cell degranulation

neutrophil chemotaxis

endothelial cell retraction

platelet aggregation

antibody

vasoactive amines

Fig. 25.10 Antigen injected intradermally combines with specific antibody from the blood to form immune complexes. The complexes act on platelets and mast cells, which release vasoactive amines. Immune complexes also induce macrophages to release TNF and IL-1 (not shown). Mast cell products, including histamine and leukotrienes, induce increased blood flow and capillary permeability. The inflammatory reaction is potentiated by lysosomal enzymes released from the polymorphs. The Arthus reaction can be seen in patients with precipitating antibodies, such as those with extrinsic allergic alveolitis associated with farmer's lung disease.

Effects of complement depletion on handling of immune complexes

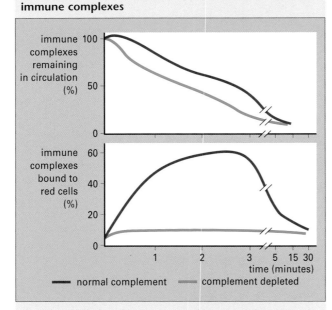

Fig. 25.11 A bolus of immune complexes was infused into the circulation of a primate. In animals with a normal complement system the complexes were bound quickly by the CR1 on erythrocytes. In animals whose complement had been depleted by treatment with cobra venom factor, the erythrocytes hardly bound immune complexes at all. Paradoxically, this results in slightly faster removal of complexes in the depleted animals, with the complexes being deposited in the tissues rather than being removed by the spleen. (Based on data from Waxman FJ, et al. J Clin Invest 1984;74:1329–1340)

Complexes can also be released from erythrocytes in the circulation by the enzymatic action of factor I.

Q. What action does factor I have in the complement system?
A. It cleaves C3b and C4b into fragments (see Figs 4.7–4.9).

This action leaves a small fragment (C3dg) attached to the CR1 on the cell membrane. These soluble complexes are then removed by phagocytic cells, particularly those in the liver, bearing receptors for IgG Fc (Fig. 25.13).

Complement solubilization of immune complexes

It has been known since Heidelberger's work on the precipitin curve in the 1930s that complement delays precipitation of immune complexes, though this information was forgotten for a long time.

The ability to keep immune complexes soluble is a function of the classical complement pathway. The complement components reduce the number of antigen epitopes that the antibodies can bind (i.e. they reduce the valency of the antigen) by intercalating into the lattice of the complex, resulting in smaller, soluble complexes. In

Clearance of immune complexes in the liver

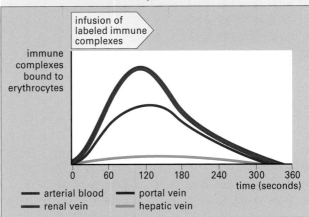

Fig. 25.12 ^{125}I-BSA/anti-BSA complexes were infused into a primate over a period of 120 seconds. Blood was sampled from renal, portal, and hepatic veins, and the level of immune complexes bound to the erythrocytes was measured by radioactive counting. The levels of complexes in the renal and portal veins were similar to that in arterial blood. However, complexes were virtually absent from hepatic venous blood throughout, indicating that complexes bound to erythrocytes are removed during a single transit through the liver. (Based on data from Cornacoff JB, et al. J Clin Invest 1983;71:236–247)

primates these complement-bearing complexes are readily bound by the C3b receptor (CR1) on erythrocytes.

Complement can rapidly resolubilize precipitated complexes through the alternative pathway (Fig. 25.14). The solubilization appears to occur by the insertion of complement C3b and C3d fragments into the complexes.

It may be that complexes are continually being deposited in normal individuals, but are removed by solubilization. If this is the case, then the process will be inadequate in hypocomplementemic patients and lead to prolonged complex deposition.

Solubilization defects have indeed been observed in sera from patients with systemic immune complex disease, but whether the defect is primary or secondary is not known.

Q. What evidence implies that defective solubilization of complexes is a primary cause of immune complex disease?
A. Genetic deficiency of classical pathway components (i.e. primary defects) are associated with SLE and some other immune complex diseases (see Figs 4.16 and 16.11).

Complement deficiency impairs clearance of complexes

In patients with low levels of classical pathway components there is poor binding of immune complexes to erythrocytes. The complement deficiency may result from:
- depletion, caused by immune complex disease; or
- a hereditary disorder, as is the case in C2 deficiency.

Immune complex clearance

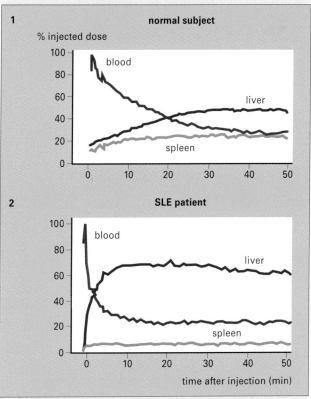

Fig. 25.13 (1) Immune complex clearance in a healthy normal subject. (2) Immune complex clearance in a patient with SLE. Radiolabeled soluble complexes were injected intravenously and immune complex localization monitored by dynamic imaging. In the normal subject complexes remained longer in the blood through binding to CR1 on red cells, followed by clearance to the liver and the spleen, where immune complexes take part in immunoregulation. In the hypocomplementemic patient with SLE there was little binding to red cells, but rapid clearance to organs such as the liver, with little localizing to the spleen, leading to impaired immunoregulation, which may be a factor in the persistence of autoimmunity.

Solubilization of immune complexes by complement

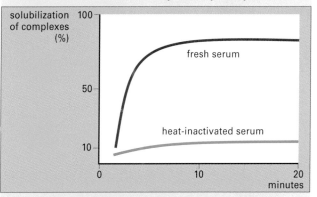

Fig. 25.14 Complement can solubilize precipitable complexes in vitro. Addition of fresh serum containing active complement to insoluble complexes induces solubilization over about 15 minutes at 37°C. Some of the complexes resist resolubilization. Heated serum (56°C for 30 minutes) lacks active complement and cannot resolubilize the complexes. Intercalation of complement components C3b and C3d into the complex causes their solubilization by disrupting antigen–antibody bonds. Complexes that have been artificially connected by covalent bonds cannot be solubilized by complement.

This might be expected to result in persistent immune complexes in the circulation, but in fact the reverse occurs, with the complexes disappearing rapidly from the circulation. These non-erythrocyte-bound complexes are taken up rapidly by the liver (but not the spleen) and are then released to be deposited in tissues such as skin, kidney, and muscle, where they can set up inflammatory reactions (Fig. 25.15).

Infusion of fresh plasma, containing complement, restores the clearance patterns to normal, illustrating the importance of complement in the clearance of immune complexes.

Failure to localize in the spleen not only results in immune complex disease, but may also have important implications for the development of appropriate immune responses. This is because the spleen plays a vital role in antigen processing and the induction of immune responses (see Chapter 2).

The size of immune complexes affects their deposition

In general, larger immune complexes are rapidly removed by the liver within a few minutes, whereas smaller complexes circulate for longer periods (Fig. 25.16). This is because larger complexes are:
- more effective at binding to Fc receptors and at fixing complement, so binding better to erythrocytes;
- released more slowly from the erythrocytes by the action of factor I.

Anything that affects the size of complexes is therefore likely to influence clearance.

It has been suggested that a genetic defect that favors the production of low-affinity antibody could lead to the formation of smaller complexes, and so to immune complex disease.

Antibodies to self antigens may have low affinity and recognize only a few epitopes. This results in small complexes and long clearance times because the formation of large, cross-linked lattices is restricted.

Affinity maturation is dependent on efficient somatic mutation and selection of B cells within germinal centers following binding of antigen. This process is far more effective when B cells are stimulated by antigen or immune complexes coated with complement. Patients with complement deficiencies are particularly prone to develop immune complex disease and recent evidence indicates that another way that this is brought about is through poor targeting of antigen complexes to germinal centers, so preventing affinity maturation.

Immune complex transport and removal

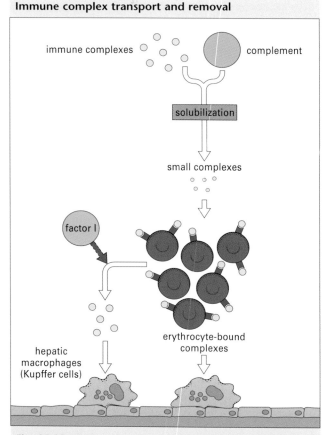

Fig. 25.15 In primates, complexes solubilized by complement are bound by CR1 on erythrocytes and transported to the liver where they are removed by hepatic macrophages. Complexes released from erythrocytes by factor I are taken up by cells (including macrophages) bearing receptors for Fc and complement.

Immunoglobulin classes affect the rate of immune complex clearance

Striking differences have been observed in the clearance of complexes with different immunoglobulin classes:

- IgG complexes are bound by erythrocytes and are gradually removed from the circulation;
- IgA complexes bind poorly to erythrocytes, but disappear rapidly from the circulation, with increased deposition in the kidney, lung, and brain.

Q. Provide an explanation for the different patterns of localization of immune complexes containing IgG and those containing IgA.

A. IgG-containing immune complexes activate the complement classical pathway and can bind to CR1 on erythrocytes. IgA does not activate the classical pathway, but can bind to Fcα receptors on mononuclear phagocytes (see Figs 3.18 and 4.3).

Complex clearance by mononuclear phagocytes

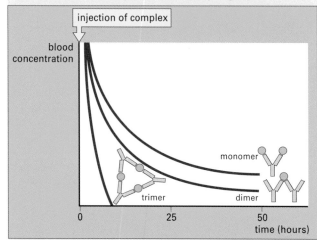

Fig. 25.16 Large immune complexes are cleared most quickly because they present an IgG–Fc lattice to mononuclear phagocyte cells with Fc receptors, permitting higher avidity binding to these cells. They also fix complement better than small complexes.

Phagocyte defects allow complexes to persist

Opsonized immune complexes are normally removed by the mononuclear phagocyte system, mainly in the liver and spleen. However, when large amounts of complex are present, the mononuclear phagocyte system may become overloaded, leading to a rise in the level of circulating complex and increased deposition in the glomerulus and elsewhere.

Defective mononuclear phagocytes have been observed in human immune complex disease, but this may be the result of overload rather than a primary defect.

Carbohydrate on antibodies affects complex clearance

Carbohydrate groups on immunoglobulin molecules have been shown to be important for the efficient removal of immune complexes by phagocytic cells.

Abnormalities of these carbohydrates occur in immune complex diseases such as rheumatoid arthritis, thus aggravating the disease process. IgG Fc oligosaccharides lack the normally terminating galactose residue, enhancing rheumatoid factor binding. Recently, mannan-binding protein has been shown to bind agalactosyl IgG and subsequently activate complement.

IMMUNE COMPLEX DEPOSITION IN TISSUES RESULTS IN TISSUE DAMAGE

Immune complexes may persist in the circulation for prolonged periods of time. However, simple persistence is not usually harmful in itself; the problems start only when complexes are deposited in the tissues.

Two questions are relevant to tissue deposition:
- Why are complexes deposited?
- Why do complexes show affinity for particular tissues in different diseases?

The most important trigger for immune complex deposition is probably an increase in vascular permeability

Animal experiments have shown that inert substances such as colloidal carbon will be deposited in vessel walls following the administration of vasoactive substances, such as histamine or serotonin. Circulating immune complexes are deposited in a similar way following the infusion of agents that cause the liberation of mast cell vasoactive amines (including histamine). Pretreatment with antihistamines blocks this effect.

In studies of experimental immune complex disease in rabbits, long-term administration of vasoactive amine antagonists, such as chlorpheniramine and methysergide, has been shown to reduce immune complex deposition considerably (Fig. 25.17). More importantly (from the point of view of disease prevention), young NZB/NZW mice treated with methysergide show less renal pathology than controls (Fig. 25.18).

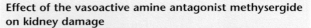

Effect of the vasoactive amine antagonist methysergide on kidney damage

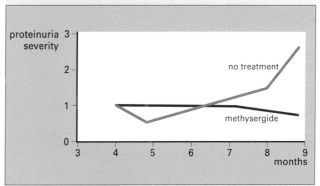

Fig. 25.18 Kidney damage, assessed by proteinuria, was measured in NZB/NZW mice over 5 months. Untreated animals developed severe proteinuria, whereas methysergide-treated animals did not. Methysergide blocks the formation of the vasoactive amine 5-hydroxytryptamine (5-HT), and thus blocks a variety of inflammatory events (e.g. deposition of complexes, neutrophil infiltration of capillary walls, and endothelial proliferation), all of which produce the glomerular pathology.

Effect of a vasoactive amine antagonist on immune complex disease

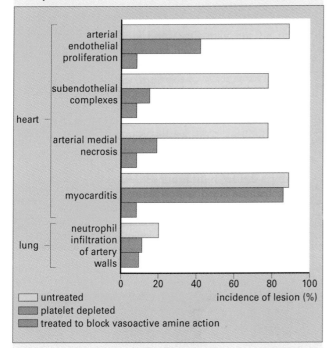

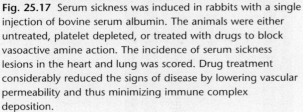

Fig. 25.17 Serum sickness was induced in rabbits with a single injection of bovine serum albumin. The animals were either untreated, platelet depleted, or treated with drugs to block vasoactive amine action. The incidence of serum sickness lesions in the heart and lung was scored. Drug treatment considerably reduced the signs of disease by lowering vascular permeability and thus minimizing immune complex deposition.

Increases in vascular permeability can be initiated by a range of mechanisms, which vary in importance, depending on the diseases and species concerned. This variability makes interpretation of some of the animal models difficult. In general, however, complement, mast cells, basophils, and platelets must all be considered as potential producers of vasoactive amines.

Immune complex deposition is most likely where there is high blood pressure and turbulence

Many macromolecules deposit in the glomerular capillaries, where the blood pressure is approximately four times that of most other capillaries (Fig. 25.19).

If the glomerular blood pressure of a rabbit is reduced by partially constricting the renal artery or by ligating the ureter, deposition is also reduced. If the glomerular blood pressure is increased by experimentally induced hypertension, immune complex deposition is enhanced as shown by the development of serum sickness. Elsewhere, the most severe lesions also occur at sites of turbulence:
- at turns or bifurcations of arteries; and
- in vascular filters such as the choroid plexus and the ciliary body of the eye.

Q. Why should the site of bifurcation in an artery be more susceptible to damage than other sites?

A. This site is subject to high pressure and more erratic shear forces, which may affect the integrity of the endothelium (see Fig. 25.19). In addition blood cells and platelets are not segregated from the vessel wall by laminar flow (see above).

Hemodynamic factors affecting complex deposition

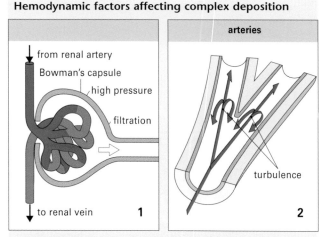

Fig. 25.19 Factors that affect complex deposition include filtration and high blood pressure, both of which occur in the formation of ultrafiltrate in the renal glomerulus (**1**). Turbulence at curves or bifurcations of arteries (**2**) also favors deposition of immune complexes.

Affinity of antigens for specific tissues can direct complexes to particular sites

Local high blood pressure explains the tendency for deposits to form in certain organs, but does not explain why complexes are deposited on specific organs in certain diseases. In SLE, the kidney is a particular target, whereas in rheumatoid arthritis, although circulating complexes are present, the kidney is usually spared and the joints are the principal target.

It is possible that the antigen in the complex provides the organ specificity, and a convincing model has been established to support this hypothesis. In the model, mice are given endotoxin causing cell damage and release of DNA, which then binds to healthy glomerular basement membrane. Anti-DNA is then produced by polyclonal activation of B cells, and is bound by the fixed DNA leading to local immune complex formation (Fig. 25.20). The production of rheumatoid factor (IgM anti-IgG) allows further immune complex formation to occur in situ.

It is possible that in other diseases antigens will be identified with affinity for particular organs.

The charge of the antigen and antibody may be important in some systems. For example, positively charged antigens and antibodies are more likely to be deposited in the negatively charged glomerular basement membrane.

The degree of glycosylation also affects the fate of complexes containing glycoprotein antigens because certain clearance mechanisms are activated by recognition of sugar molecules (e.g. mannan-binding protein).

In certain diseases the antibodies and antigens are both produced within the target organ. The extreme of this is reached in rheumatoid arthritis, where IgG anti-IgG rheumatoid factor is produced by plasma cells within the synovium; these antibodies then combine with each other (self-association), so setting up an inflammatory reaction.

Tissue binding of antigen with local immune complex formation

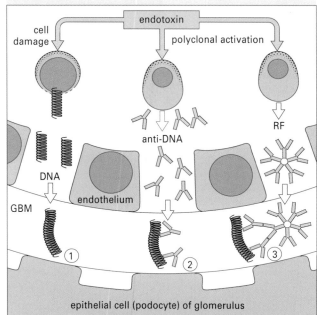

Fig. 25.20 Endotoxin injected into mice increases vascular permeability and induces cell damage and release of DNA. The DNA can then become deposited (**1**) on the collagen of the glomerular basement membrane (GBM) in the kidney. Endotoxin can also induce a polyclonal stimulation of B cells, some of which produce autoantibodies such as anti-DNA and anti-IgG – the latter are known as rheumatoid factors (RFs). Anti-DNA antibody can then bind to the deposited DNA forming a local immune complex (**2**). RFs have a low affinity for monomeric IgG, but bind with high avidity to the assembled DNA–anti-DNA complex (**3**). Thus further immune complex formation occurs in situ.

The site of immune complex deposition depends partly on the size of the complex

The fact that the site of immune complex deposition depends partly on the size of the complex is exemplified in the kidney:

- small immune complexes can pass through the glomerular basement membrane, and end up on the epithelial side of the membrane;
- large complexes are unable to cross the membrane and generally accumulate between the endothelium and the basement membrane or the mesangium (Fig. 25.21).

The size of immune complexes depends on the valency of the antigen, and on the titer and affinity of the antibody.

The class of immunoglobulin in an immune complex can also influence its deposition

There are marked age- and sex-related variations in the class and subclass of anti-DNA antibodies seen in SLE.

Immune complex deposition in the kidney

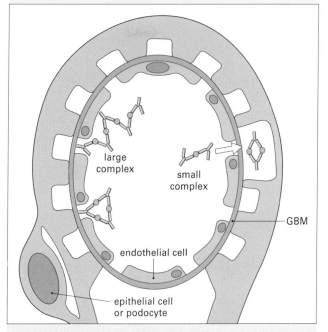

Fig. 25.21 The site of complex deposition in the kidney is dependent on the size of the complexes in the circulation. Large complexes become deposited on the glomerular basement membrane, whereas small complexes pass through the basement membrane and are seen on the epithelial side of the glomerulus.

Antibody classes in immune complex disease

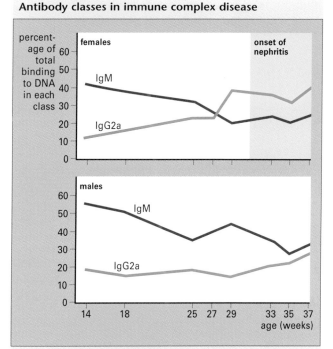

Fig. 25.22 Immune complex disease is automatic in the NZB/NZW mouse and follows a class switch during early development, from IgM to IgG2a. The graphs show the proportions of anti-DNA antibodies of the IgM and IgG2a isotypes in females and males. Both the class switch and fatal renal disease occur earlier in the female mice of this strain.

Similarly, as NZB/NZW mice grow older there is a class switch, from predominantly IgM to IgG2a. This occurs earlier in females than in males and coincides with the onset of renal disease, indicating the importance of antibody class in the tissue deposition of complexes (Fig. 25.22).

DEPOSITED IMMUNE COMPLEXES CAN BE VISUALIZED USING IMMUNOFLUORESCENCE

The ideal place to look for immune complexes is in the affected organ.

Tissue samples may be examined by immunofluorescence for the presence of immunoglobulin and complement. The composition, pattern, and particular area of tissue affected all provide useful information on the severity and prognosis of the disease. For example:

- patients with the continuous, granular, subepithelial deposits of IgG found in membranous glomerulonephritis have a poor prognosis;
- in contrast, those whose complexes are localized in the mesangium have a good prognosis.

Not all tissue-bound complexes give rise to an inflammatory response; for example, in SLE complexes are frequently found in skin biopsies from normal-looking skin, as well as from inflamed skin.

Assays for immune complexes in serum are more readily performed than in-situ immunofluorescence, although the results have to be interpreted carefully (Method box 25.1)

METHOD BOX 25.1
Assays for circulating immune complexes

Circulating complexes are found in two separate compartments:
- bound to erythrocytes; and
- free in plasma.

Erythrocyte-bound complexes are less likely to be damaging, so it is of more interest to determine the level of free complexes. Care is required when collecting the sample – bound complexes can easily be released during clotting by the action of factor I. To obtain accurate assays of free complexes, the erythrocytes should be rapidly separated from the plasma to prevent the release of bound complexes.

Circulating complexes are often identified by their affinity for complement C1q, using either radiolabeled C1q or solid-phase C1q. Complexes can also be detected by their low solubility in polyethylene glycol (Figs 1 and 2).

An assay for soluble immune complexes based on polyethylene glycol (PEG)

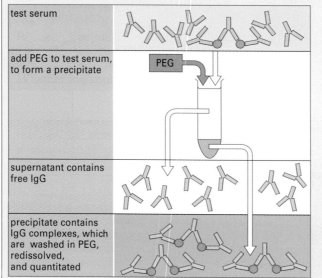

Fig. 1 Polyethylene glycol (PEG) is added to the test serum containing IgG complexes and IgG monomer. When the concentration of PEG reaches 2%, complexes are selectively precipitated; the free antibody remains in solution. The test tube is then centrifuged and the complexes form a pellet at the bottom. The supernatant containing free antibody is removed. The precipitate is washed and redissolved so that the amount of complexed IgG can be measured (e.g. by single radial immunodiffusion, nephelometry, or radioimmunoassay (Fig. 2).

Radioimmunoassay for soluble immune complexes

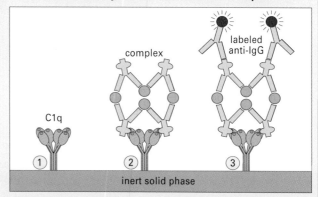

Fig. 2 A three-layer radioimmunoassay for immune complexes based on the use of C1q. (1) C1q is linked to an inert solid-phase support, usually a polystyrene tube or plate. (2) Serum containing complexes is added. The complexes bind to the solid-phase C1q by means of the array of Fc regions presented to the C1q. (3) Radiolabeled anti-IgG antibody is added. The amount of radioactivity remaining on the solid phase after washing is measured in a gamma-counter, and is used to calculate the amount of complex bound to the C1q.

FURTHER READING

Agnello V. Immune complex assays in rheumatic diseases. Hum Pathol 1983;14:343–349.

Arthus M. Injections répétées de sérum de cheval chez le lapin. C R Seances Soc Biol Filiales 1903;55:817.

Birmingham DJ, Herbert LA, Cosio FG, et al. Immune complex erythrocyte complement receptor interactions in vivo during induction of glomerulonephritis in non-human primates. J Lab Clin Med 1990;116:242–252.

Boackle SA, Holer VM, Karp DR. CD21 augments antigen presentation in immune individuals. Eur J Immunol 1997;27:122–129.

Boruchov AM, Heller G, Veri MC, et al. Activating and inhibitory IgG Fc receptors on human DCs mediate opposing functions. J Clin Invest 2005; 115:2914–2923.

Bruhns P, Samuelsson A, Pollard JW, Ravetch JV. Colony-stimulating factor-1-dependent macrophages are responsible for IVIG protection in antibody-induced autoimmune disease. Immunity 2003;18:573–581

Clynes R, Maizes JS, Guinamard R, et al. Modulation of immune complex-induced inflammation in vivo by the co-ordinate expression of activation and inhibitory Fc receptors. J Exp Med 1999;189:179–185.

Cornacoff JB, Hebert LA, Smead WL, et al. Primate erythrocyte immune complex clearing mechanism. J Clin Invest 1983;71:236–247.

Czop J, Nussenzweig V. Studies on the mechanism of solubilization of immune precipitates by serum. J Exp Med 1976;143:615–630.

Davies KA, Hird V, Stewart S, et al. A study of in vivo immune complex formation and clearing in man. J Immunol 1990;144:4613–4620.

Davies KA, Peters AM, Beynon HLC, Walport MJ. Immune complex processing in patients with systemic lupus erythematosus – in vivo imaging and clearance studies. J Clin Invest 1992;90:2075–2083.

Davies KA, Chapman PT, Norsworthy PJ, et al. Clearance pathway of soluble immune complexes in the pig. Insights into the adaptive nature of antigen clearance in humans. J Immunol 1995;155:5760–5768.

Davies KA, Schifferli JA, Walport MJ. Complement deficiency and immune complex diseases. Springer Semin Immunopathol 1994;15:397–416.

Dixon FJ, Joseph D, Feldman JD, et al. Experimental glomerulonephritis: the pathogenesis of a laboratory model resembling the spectrum of human glomerulonephritis. J Exp Med 1961;113:899–919.

Dixon FJ, Vazquez JJ, Weigle WO, et al. Pathogenesis of serum sickness. Arch Pathol 1958;65:18–28.

Emlen W, Carl V, Burdick CG. Mechanism of transfer of immune complexes from red blood cell CR1 to monocytes. Clin Exp Immunol 1992;89:8–17.

Finbloom DS, Magilvary DB, Harford JB, et al. Influence of antigen on immune complex behaviour in mice. J Clin Invest 1981;68:214–224.

Fukuyama H, Nimmerjahn F, Ravetch JV. The inhibitory Fc gamma receptor modulates autoimmunity by limiting the accumulation of immunoglobulin G+ anti-DNA plasma cells. Nat Immunol 2005;6:99–106.

Heidelberger M. Quantitative chemical studies on complement or alexin. J Exp Med 1941;73:681–709.

Inman RD. Immune complexes in SLE. Clin Rheum Dis 1982;8:49–62.

Johnston A, Auda GR, Kerr MA, et al. Dissociation of primary antigen–antibody bonds is essential for complement mediated solubilization of immune complexes. Mol Immunol 1992;29:659–665.

Kijlstrea H, Van Es LA, Daha MR. The role of complement in the binding and degradation of immunoglobulin aggregates by macrophages. J Immunol 1979;123:2488–2493.

Lachmann PJ. Complement deficiency and the pathogenesis of autoimmune complex disease. Chem Immunol 1980;49:245–263.

Lucisano Valim M, Lachmann PJ. The effects of antibody isotype and antigenic epitope density on the complement-fixing activity of immune complexes: a systematic study using chimaeric anti-NIP antibodies with human Fc regions. Clin Exp Immunol 1991;84:1–8.

McGaha TL, Sorrentino B, Ravetch JV. Restoration of tolerance in lupus by targeted inhibitory receptor expression. Science 2005 Jan 28;307:590–593.

McKenzie SE, Taylor SM, Malladi P, et al. The role of the human Fc receptor FcγRIIA in the immune clearance of platelets: a transgene mouse model. J Immunol 1999;162:4311–4318.

Miller GW, Nussenzweig V. A new complement function: solubilization of antigen–antibody aggregates. Proc Natl Acad Sci 1975;72:418–422.

Moll T, Nitschke L, Carroll M, et al. A critical role for Fc gamma RIIB in the induction of rheumatoid factors. J Immunol 2004;173:4724–4728.

Olsson M, Bruhns P, Frazier WA, et al. Platelet homeostasis is regulated by platelet expression of CD47 under normal conditions and in passive immune thrombocytopenia. Blood 2005;105:3577–3582.

Park SY, Ueda S, Ohno H, et al. Resistance of Fc receptor-deficient mice to fatal glomerulonephritis. J Clin Invest 1998;102:1229–1238.

Qiao J-H, Castellani LW, Fishbein MC, et al. Immune complex-mediated vasculitis increases coronary artery lipid accumulation in autoimmune-prone MRL mice. Arterioscler Thromb 1993;13:932–943.

Ravetch JV. Fc receptors. Curr Opin Immunol 1997;9:121–125.

Ravetch JV. A full complement of receptors in immune complex diseases. J Clin Invest 2002;110:1759–1761.

Schifferli JA, Ng YC, Peters DK. The role of complement and its receptor in the elimination of immune complexes. N Engl J Med 1986;315:488–495.

Sylvestre DL, Ravetch JV. A dominant role for mast cell Fc receptors in the Arthus reaction. Immunity 1996;5:387–390.

Takata Y, Tamura N, Fujita T. Interaction of C3 with antigen–antibody complexes in the process of solubilisation of immune precipitates. J Immunol 1984;132:2531–2537.

Terino FL, Powell MS, McKenzie IF, Hogarth PM. Recombinant soluble human FcγRII: production, characterization, and inhibition of the Arthus reaction. J Exp Med 1993;178:1617–1628.

Theofilopoulos AN, Dixon FJ. The biology and detection of immune complexes. Adv Immunol 1979;28:89–220.

Warren JS, Yabroff KR, Remick DG, et al. Tumour necrosis factor participates in the pathogenesis of acute immune complex alveolitis in the rat. J Clin Invest 1989; 84:1873–1882.

Waxman FJ, Hebert LE, Cornacoff JB, et al. Complement depletion accelerates the clearance of immune complexes from the circulation of primates. J Clin Invest 1984;74:1329–1340.

Whaley K. Complement and immune complex diseases. In: Whaley K, ed. Complement in health and disease. Lancaster: MTP Press Ltd; 1987.

Williams RC. Immune complexes in clinical and experimental medicine. Massachusetts: Harvard University Press; 1980.

World Health Organization Scientific Group. Technical report 606. The role of immune complexes in disease. Geneva: WHO; 1977.

Critical thinking: Type III serum sickness after factor IX administration (see p. 503 for explanations)

An 8-year-old boy with factor IX deficiency has had repeated episodes of bleeding into his joints and skin, despite requiring administration of factor IX. Ten days after receiving a dose, he developed fever, swelling of multiple joints, and a skin rash. On physical exam, his temperature was 39°C, he had a diffuse maculopapular skin rash involving his torso and extremities, and both elbows and knees were red, warm, and appeared inflamed. His mother thought the appearance and distribution were very different from the typical appearance after either minor trauma or bleeding into his joints, which he had

sustained on multiple previous occasions. His pediatrician ordered the following tests (results shown in Table 1) and prescribed a short course of corticosteroids.

1 What immunologic mechanisms are involved in this inflammatory reaction after the boy received the factor IX?
2 Why were corticosteroids prescribed?
3 What is the likelihood that this type of reaction will develop again?
4 What measures would you take to prevent this reaction from occurring again?

variable	result	normal
C3 (mg/dl)	38	85–155
C4 (mg/dl)	4	12–45
anti-nuclear antibody	negative	
hemoglobin (g/dl)	11.2	
white cell count (cells/mm^3)	11 000	
eosinophils (%)	1	

Table 1

He responds to treatment and his symptoms resolve, but 1 year later his mother notices that his face is swollen in the morning and his feet are swollen at the end of the day. Otherwise the boy feels well.

On physical exam, his blood pressure is elevated at 140/90 mmHg and his ankles are very edematous. His joints do not appear inflamed and the skin does not show either evidence of recent bleeding or inflammation. Results of tests are shown in Table 2.

5 What immunologic mechanisms are involved in this inflammatory reaction after the boy received the factor IX? How do they differ from the previous episode?
6 What is the likelihood that this type reaction will develop again?
7 What measures would you take to prevent this reaction again?

variable	result	normal
C3 (mg/dl)	142	85–155
C4 (mg/dl)	44	12–45
anti-nuclear antibody	negative	
hemoglobin (g/dl)	11.6	
white cell count (cells/mm^3)	8600	
eosinophils (%)	< 1	
albumin (g/dl)	2.5	3.5–5.5
urine protein (g/24 h)	8	< 0.2

Table 2

Hypersensitivity (Type IV)

SUMMARY

- **DTH reflects the presence of antigen-specific CD4 T cells.**

- **There are three variants of type IV hypersensitivity reaction** – contact, tuberculin, and granulomatous.

- **Contact hypersensitivity occurs at the point of contact with an allergen.** Langerhans' cells internalize and process epicutaneously applied hapten and migrate to the draining lymph nodes where they present it to antigen-specific T cells. Cytokines produced by immune-competent skin cells (e.g. keratinocytes, Langerhans' cells, T cells) recruit antigen-non-specific T cells and macrophages.

- **Tuberculin-type hypersensitivity is induced by soluble antigens from a variety of organisms.** It is useful as a diagnostic test for exposure to a number of infectious agents.

- **Granulomatous hypersensitivity is clinically the most important form of type IV hypersensitivity.** Persistence of antigen leads to differentiation of macrophages to epithelioid cells, and fusion to form giant cells. This pathological response is termed a granulomatous reaction and it results in tissue damage. Granuloma formation is driven by T cell activation of macrophages, and is dependent on TNF. Inhibition of TNF leads to breakdown in granulomas.

- **Many chronic diseases manifest type IV granulomatous hypersensitivity.** These include tuberculosis, leprosy, schistosomiasis, sarcoidosis, and Crohn's disease.

DTH REFLECTS THE PRESENCE OF ANTIGEN-SPECIFIC CD4 T CELLS

Delayed-type hypersensitivity (DTH) is a T cell-mediated inflammatory response in which the stimulation of antigen-specific effector T cells leads to macrophage activation and localized inflammation and edema within tissues. This effector T cell response is:
- a normal component of adaptive immunity; and
- essential for the control of intracellular and other pathogens.

However, if the response is excessive it can damage host tissues.

The T cell response may be made to exogenous agents, such as microbial antigens or sensitizing chemicals, or to self-antigens. Typically T cells are sensitized to the foreign antigen during infection with the pathogen or by absorption of a contact sensitizing agent across the skin.

Q. Where in the body are T cells sensitized and how?

A. Typically, T cells are sensitized in the T cell areas of secondary lymphoid tissues, by dendritic cells.

Subsequent exposure of the sensitized individual to the exogenous antigen, either injected intradermally or applied to the epidermis, results in the recruitment of antigen-specific T cells to the site and the development of a local inflammatory response over 24–72 hours.

If the foreign antigen persists in the tissues, chronic activation of T cells and macrophages may lead to granuloma formation and tissue damage.

If the antigen is an organ-specific self antigen, autoreactive T cells may produce localized cellular inflammation resulting in autoimmune disease, such as type I diabetes mellitus.

According to the Coombs and Gell classification, type IV or DTH reactions take more than 12 hours to develop and involve cell-mediated immune reactions rather than antibody responses to antigens. Some other hypersensitivity reactions may straddle this definition with:
- a rapid antibody-mediated phase; and
- a later cell-mediated phase.

For example, the late-phase IgE-mediated reaction may peak 12–24 hours after contact with an allergen, and cells, such as helper T (TH2) cells and eosinophils, contribute to the inflammation as well as IgE (see Chapter 22).

In contrast to other forms of hypersensitivity, type IV hypersensitivity is transferred from one animal to another by T cells, particularly CD4 TH1 cells in mice, rather than by serum. Therefore it can occur in antibody-deficient humans, but is lost with the decline in CD4 T cells in HIV infection and AIDS.

Type IV hypersensitivity reflects the presence of antigen-specific CD4 T cells and is associated with protective immunity against intracellular and other pathogens.

However, there is not a complete correlation between type IV hypersensitivity and protective immunity, and progressive infections can develop in the presence of strong DTH reactivity.

THERE ARE THREE VARIANTS OF TYPE IV HYPERSENSITIVITY REACTION

Three variants of type IV hypersensitivity reaction are recognized (Fig. 26.1):

- **contact hypersensitivity** and **tuberculin-type hypersensitivity** both occur within 72 hours of antigen challenge;
- **granulomatous hypersensitivity reactions** develop over a period of 21–28 days – the granulomas are formed by the aggregation of macrophages and lymphocytes and may persist for weeks – this is the most important type of type IV hypersensitivity response for producing clinical consequences.

These three types of delayed hypersensitivity were originally distinguished according to the reaction they produced when antigen was applied directly to the skin (epicutaneously) or injected intradermally. The degree of the response is usually assessed in animals by measuring thickening of the skin.

Q. What causes the skin to become thickened during a chronic immune response?

A. The migration of lymphocytes and macrophages into the dermis, the proliferation of cells in the dermis in response to cytokines, and the deposition of new extracellular matrix components can all contribute to skin thickening.

The local response is also accompanied by a variety of systemic immune responses, such as T cell proliferation and synthesis of cytokines including interferon-γ (IFNγ).

CONTACT HYPERSENSITIVITY OCCURS AT THE POINT OF CONTACT WITH AN ALLERGEN

Contact hypersensitivity is characterized by an eczematous reaction in the skin at the point of contact with an allergen (Fig. 26.2). It is often seen following contact with agents such as nickel, chromate, rubber accelerators, and

Clinical and patch test appearances of contact hypersensitivity

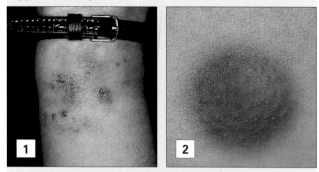

Fig. 26.2 (1) The eczematous area at the wrist is due to sensitivity to nickel in the watch-strap buckle. (2) The suspected allergy may be confirmed by applying potential allergens, in the relevant concentrations and vehicles, to the patient's upper back (patch testing). A positive reaction causes a localized area of eczema at the site of the offending allergen 2–4 days after application.

pentadecacatechol, which is the sensitizing agent in poison ivy. This is distinct from the non-immune-mediated inflammatory response to irritants.

The immunologically active components of sensitizing agents are called **haptens**. Haptens are:

- too small to be antigenic by themselves, having a molecular weight often less than 1 kDa;
- lipophilic and penetrate the epidermis where they conjugate, most often covalently, to self proteins to form **neo-antigens**.

The sensitizing potential of a hapten cannot reliably be predicted from its chemical structure, though there is some correlation with the ability of the molecule to penetrate the skin and the number of haptens attached to the carrier protein.

Some potent haptens, such as dinitrochlorobenzene (DNCB), sensitize nearly all individuals and can be used to assess cell-mediated immunity. DNCB applied to the skin binds to epidermal proteins and to MHC-linked peptides through the -NH$_2$ groups of lysine.

Langerhans' cells and keratinocytes have key roles in contact hypersensitivity
The Langerhans' cell is the principal APC

Contact hypersensitivity is primarily an epidermal reaction, and the dendritic **Langerhans' cell**, located in the suprabasal epidermis, is the principal antigen-presenting cell (APC) involved (Fig. 26.3).

Langerhans' cells (see Chapter 2) are specialized dendritic cells derived from bone marrow and express:

- CD1;
- MHC class II molecules;
- langerin; and
- surface receptors for Fc and complement.

Electron microscopy shows **Birbeck granules**, which are organelles derived from cell membrane and are characteristic of Langerhans' cells (see Fig. 26.3).

The variants of delayed hypersensitivity

delayed reaction	maximal reaction time
contact	48–72 hours
tuberculin	48–72 hours
granulomatous	21–28 days

Fig. 26.1 Contact and tuberculin-type hypersensitivity have a similar time course and are maximal at 48–72 hours. In certain circumstances (e.g. with insoluble antigen) granulomatous reactions also develop at 21–28 days (e.g. skin testing in leprosy).

Langerhans' cells

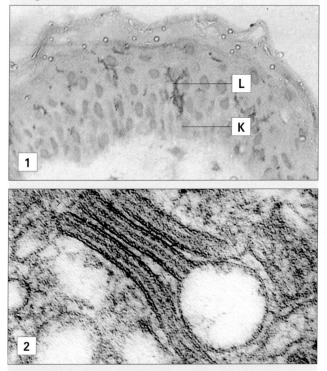

Fig. 26.3 (1) These dendritic cells constitute 3% of all cells in the epidermis. They express a variety of surface markers, which allow them to be visualized. Here they have been revealed in a section of normal skin using a monoclonal antibody that reacts with the CD1 antigen (counterstained with Mayer's hemalum). (L, Langerhans' cell; K, keratinocyte) × 312. (2) Electron micrograph of a Langerhans' cell showing the characteristic 'Birbeck granule'. This organelle is a plate-like structure with a distinct central striation and often has a bleb-like extension at one end. × 132 000.

Langerhans' cells are inactivated by ultraviolet B, which can therefore prevent or alleviate the effects of contact hypersensitivity.

Langerhans' cells take up hapten-modified proteins by micropinocytosis, and under the influence of interleukin-1 (IL-1) and tumor necrosis factor (TNF) from keratinocytes and other cells:
- undergo maturation;
- increase the expression of MHC and co-stimulatory molecules; and
- migrate to draining lymph nodes.

Keratinocytes produce a range of cytokines important to the contact hypersensitivity response
Keratinocytes provide the structural integrity of the epidermis and have a central role in epidermal immunology.

Keratinocytes can be activated by a number of stimuli, including sensitizing agents and irritants. They may express MHC class II molecules and intercellular adhesion molecule-1 (ICAM-1) in the cell membrane.

Activated keratinocytes produce a wide range of cytokines, including:
- TNF, IL-1, and granulocyte–macrophage colony stimulating factor (GM-CSF), which may activate Langerhans' cells;
- IL-3, which can also activate Langerhans' cells, co-stimulate proliferative responses, recruit mast cells, and induce the secretion of immunosuppressive cytokines, such as IL-10 and transforming growth factor-β (TGFβ) – the latter dampen the immune response and may induce clonal anergy or immunological unresponsiveness in TH1 cells.

A contact hypersensitivity reaction has two stages – sensitization and elicitation
Sensitization stimulates a population of memory T cells
Sensitization takes 10–14 days in humans.

Once absorbed, the hapten combines with a protein and is internalized by epidermal Langerhans' cells, which leave the epidermis and migrate as veiled cells through the afferent lymphatics to the paracortical areas of regional lymph nodes. Here they present processed hapten–protein conjugates in association with MHC class II molecules to CD4+ lymphocytes, producing:
- effector/memory CD4+ T cells; and
- regulatory CD4+ T cells (Fig. 26.4).

In addition, MHC class I-restricted CD8+ T cells are important in contact hypersensitivity responses in humans and mice and are the major effector cells for some allergens. For example, lipid-soluble urushiol from poison ivy can enter the cytoplasm of APCs and access the MHC class I processing pathway, leading to the activation of allergen-specific CD8+ T cells. Activated T cells change the pattern of adhesion molecules on their surface by down-regulating the chemokine receptor, CCR7, and CD62L.

Q. What effect will loss of CCR7 and CD62L have on T cell function?

A. CD62L promotes adhesion of lymphocytes to high endothelial venules and CCR7 allows the cells to respond to CCL21 expressed in secondary lymphoid tissues (see Appendix 4). Hence cells lacking these receptors will lose their propensity to traffic into lymph tissues.

The expression of leukocyte functional antigen-1 (LFA-1), very late antigen-4 (VLA-4), and the chemokine receptors CXCR3 and CCR5 is increased. As a result the activated/memory T cells remain within the circulation rather than trafficking through lymphoid tissue, and are able to bind to adhesion molecules on the endothelium of inflamed tissues.

Elicitation involves recruitment of CD4+ lymphocytes and monocytes
The application of a contact allergen leads to:
- rapid expression proinflammatory cytokines; and
- recruitment of effector T cells and monocytes to the site (Fig 26.5).

There is induction of mRNA for TNF, IL-1β, and GM-CSF in Langerhans' cells within 30 minutes of exposure

Sensitization phase of contact hypersensitivity

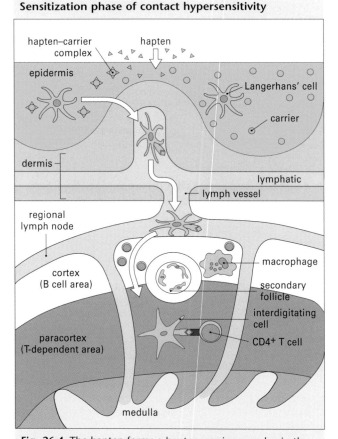

Fig. 26.4 The hapten forms a hapten–carrier complex in the epidermis. Langerhans' cells internalize the antigen, undergo maturation, and migrate via afferent lymphatics to the paracortical area of the regional lymph node where peptide–MHC molecule complexes on the surface of the Langerhans' cell can also be directly haptenated. As interdigitating cells, they present antigen to CD4⁺ T cells.

to allergen, and increased transcription of mRNA for IL-1α, macrophage inflammatory protein-2 (CXCL2), and interferon-induced protein-10 (CXCL10) by keratinocytes.

TNF and IL-1 are potent inducers of endothelial cell adhesion molecules, including:

- E-selectin and vascular cell adhesion molecule-1 (VCAM-1) within 2 hours; and
- ICAM-1 within 8 hours (Fig. 26.6).

VCAM-1 and ICAM-1 are the receptors for VLA-4 and LFA-1, respectively, on the surface of effector/memory T cells and contribute to their recruitment across the endothelium. These locally released cytokines and chemokines also produce a gradient signal for the movement of mononuclear cells towards the dermoepidermal junction and epidermis.

During this initial response to allergen, Langerhans' cells migrate from the epidermis to the dermis, where they may activate any resident memory T cells in the dermis, and to the draining lymph nodes.

The earliest histological change, seen after 4–8 hours, is the appearance of mononuclear cells around blood vessels. Macrophages and lymphocytes invade the dermis and epidermis, peaking at 48–72 hours (Fig. 26.7).

The recruitment of memory T cells is antigen non-specific, with less than 1% of infiltrating lymphocytes bearing hapten-specific αβ T cell receptors. However, these hapten-specific T cells are stimulated by dermal Langerhans' cells expressing hapten–peptide complexes to expand and to increase the expression of adhesion molecules. This leads to the retention of hapten-specific T cells at the inflamed site.

Most infiltrating lymphocytes are CD4⁺ TH1-like T cells secreting IFNγ, with a small proportion of CD8⁺ T cells. The CD8⁺ T cells contribute to inflammation by both a direct cytolytic effect on epidermal cells and the release of IFNγ.

Q. What is the name of this class of cytotoxic cells?
A. They are Tc1 cells (see Chapter 11).

Effector αβ T cells are essential for experimental contact sensitivity in mice, but NK T cells and γδ T cells also contribute to the induction and elicitation of the response.

Interestingly, hapten-specific IgM antibodies from B-1 cells are also important during the elicitation phase in mice by activating complement and recruiting T cells to the challenge site.

Experiments in gene-targeted mice show that selectins, ICAM-1, and the integrins, LFA-1 and VLA-4, are all required for the elicitation of contact and delayed hypersensitivity.

Suppression of the inflammatory reaction is mediated by multiple mechanisms

The reaction to cutaneous application of sensitizer wanes after 48–72 hours. This is due to the removal of antigenic stimulus following degradation of the hapten–conjugate and a variety of inhibitory mechanisms (see Fig. 26.6) including:

- macrophages and keratinocytes produce PGE, which inhibits IL-1 and IL-2 production;
- TGFβ from dermal mast cells, activated keratinocytes, and lymphocytes inhibits inflammation and blocks the proliferative effects of IL-1 and IL-2;
- IL-10 downregulates MHC class II molecule expression, and suppresses cytokine production and antigen-specific proliferation by TH1 cells;
- CD4⁺ regulatory T cells directly inhibit effector T cells;
- external factors may also be involved – in mice UV light induces a specific inhibitor of IL-1 activity.

TUBERCULIN-TYPE HYPERSENSITIVITY

Tuberculin-type hypersensitivity is induced by soluble antigens from a variety of organisms. Tuberculin-type hypersensitivity was originally described by Koch. He observed that if patients with tuberculosis were injected subcutaneously with a tuberculin culture filtrate (antigens

Elicitation phase of contact hypersensitivity

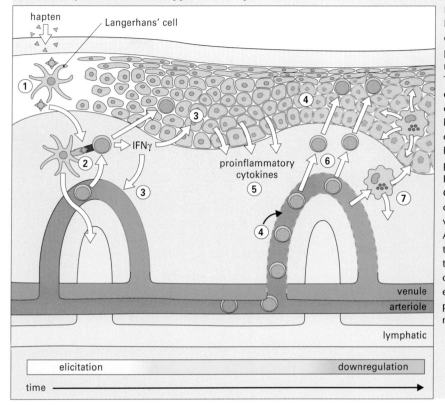

Fig. 26.5 Langerhans' cells carrying the hapten–carrier complex (**1**) move from the epidermis to the dermis, where they present the hapten–carrier complex to memory CD4⁺ T cells (**2**). Activated CD4⁺ T cells release IFNγ, which induces expression of ICAM-1 (**3**) and, later, MHC class II molecules (**4**) on the surface of keratinocytes and on endothelial cells of dermal capillaries, and activates keratinocytes, which release proinflammatory cytokines such as IL-1, IL-6, and GM-CSF (**5**). Non-antigen-specific CD4⁺ T cells are attracted to the site by cytokines (**6**) and may bind to keratinocytes via ICAM-1 and MHC class II molecules. Activated macrophages are also attracted to the skin, but this occurs later. Thereafter the reaction starts to downregulate. This downregulation may be influenced by eicosanoids such as prostaglandin E (PGE) produced by activated keratinocytes and macrophages (**7**).

derived from the causative agent, *Mycobacterium tuberculosis*) they reacted with fever and generalized sickness. An area of hardening and swelling developed at the site of injection.

Soluble antigens from a number of other organisms, including *Mycobacterium leprae* and *Leishmania tropica*, induce similar reactions in sensitized people.

The skin reaction is frequently used to test for T cell-mediated responses to the organisms following previous exposure (Fig. 26.8).

This form of hypersensitivity may also be induced by T cell responses to non-microbial antigens, such as beryllium and zirconium.

The tuberculin skin test reaction involves monocytes and lymphocytes

The tuberculin skin test is an example of the recall response to soluble antigen previously encountered during infection. Dendritic cells infected with *M. tuberculosis* in the lung undergo maturation and migrate to the draining mediastinal lymph nodes where they activate CD4⁺ and CD8⁺ T cells.

Q. How can dendritic cells activate CD8⁺ T cells?
A. This involves the process of cross-presentation (see Fig. 7.15).

Following intradermal tuberculin challenge in a previously infected individual, mycobacteria-specific memory

T cells are recruited and activated to secrete IFNγ, which activates macrophages to produce TNFα and IL-1. These proinflammatory cytokines and chemokines from T cells and macrophages act on endothelial cells in dermal blood vessels to induce the sequential expression of the adhesion molecules E-selectin, ICAM-1, and VCAM-1. These molecules bind receptors on leukocytes and recruit them to the site of the reaction.

The initial influx at 4 hours is of neutrophils, but this is replaced at 12 hours by monocytes and T cells. The infiltrate, which extends outwards and disrupts the collagen bundles of the dermis, increases to a peak at 48 hours. CD4⁺ T cells outnumber CD8⁺ cells by about 2 to 1. CD1⁺ cells (Langerhans'-like cells, but lacking Birbeck granules) are also found in the dermal infiltrate at 24 and 48 hours, and a few CD4⁺ cells infiltrate the epidermis between 24 and 48 hours.

Monocytes constitute 80–90% of the total cellular infiltrate. Both infiltrating lymphocytes and macrophages express MHC class II molecules, and this increases the efficiency of activated macrophages as APCs. Overlying keratinocytes express HLA-DR molecules 48–96 hours after the appearance of the lymphocytic infiltrate. These events are summarized in Fig. 26.9.

Macrophages are probably the main APCs in the tuberculin hypersensitivity reaction. However, there are CD1⁺ cells in the dermal infiltrate, which suggests that Langerhans' cells or other indeterminate dendritic cells may also participate.

Cytokines, prostaglandins, and cellular interactions in contact hypersensitivity

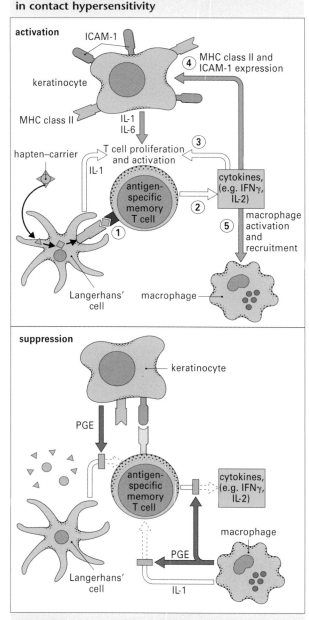

Fig. 26.6 Cytokines and prostaglandins are central to the complex interactions between Langerhans' cells, CD4+ T cells, keratinocytes, macrophages, and endothelial cells in contact hypersensitivity. The act of antigen presentation (**1**) causes the release of a cascade of cytokines (**2**). This cascade initially results in the activation and proliferation of CD4+ T cells (**3**), the induction of expression of ICAM-1 and MHC class II molecules on keratinocytes and endothelial cells (**4**), and the attraction of further T cells and macrophages to the skin (**3, 5**). Subsequent PGE production by keratinocytes and macrophages may have an inhibitory effect on IL-1 and IL-2 production. Production of PGE, binding of activated T cells to keratinocytes, and enzymatic and cellular degradation of the hapten–carrier complex all contribute to the downregulation of the reaction.

Histological appearance of the lesion in contact hypersensitivity

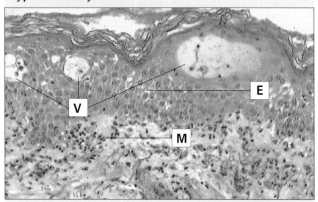

Fig. 26.7 Mononuclear cells (M) infiltrate both dermis and epidermis. The epidermis is pushed outwards and microvesicles (V) form within it due to edema (E). H&E stain. × 130.

Clinical and histological appearances of tuberculin-type sensitivity

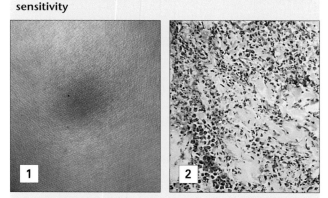

Fig. 26.8 The response to an injection of leprosy bacillus into a sensitized individual is known as the Fernandez reaction. The reaction is characterized by an area of firm red swelling of the skin and is maximal 48–72 hours after challenge (**1**). Histologically (**2**), there is a dense dermal infiltrate of leukocytes. H&E stain. × 80.

Q. What is the function of CD1?
A. It can present lipoprotein and glycolipid antigens to T cells (see Fig. 5.22).

The circulation of immune cells to and from the regional lymph nodes is thought to be similar to that for contact hypersensitivity. The tuberculin lesion normally resolves within 5–7 days, but if there is persistence of antigen in the tissues it may develop into a granulomatous reaction.

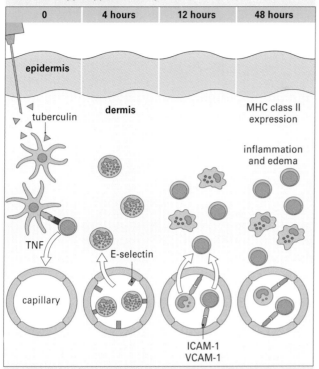

Tuberculin-type hypersensitivity

Fig. 26.9 This diagram illustrates cellular movements following intradermal injection of tuberculin. Within 1–2 hours there is expression of E-selectin on capillary endothelium leading to a brief influx of neutrophil leukocytes. By 12 hours ICAM-1 and VCAM-1 on endothelium bind the integrins LFA-1 and VLA-4 on monocytes and lymphocytes, leading to accumulation of both cell types in the dermis. This peaks at 48 hours and is followed by expression of the MHC class II molecules on keratinocytes. There is no edema of the epidermis.

Tuberculin-like DTH reactions are used practically in two ways

First, reaction to soluble antigens from a pathogen demonstrates past infection with that pathogen. Thus, tuberculin reactivity confirms past or latent infection with *M. tuberculosis*, but not necessarily active disease. However, subjects with latent tuberculosis infection have an increased lifelong risk of 7–10% for the reactivation of active tuberculosis.

Second, DTH responses to frequently encountered microbes are a general measure of cell-mediated immunity. This can be tested with intradermal injection of single antigens from common pathogens or vaccine antigens, such as *Candida albicans* or tetanus toxoid, or a multipuncture device, which delivers multiple common microbial antigens in a standardized fashion. Loss of recall responses to specific antigens occurs in a wide range of diseases and infections, including HIV infection, which impair T cell function, and during therapy with corticosteroids or immunosuppressive agents.

GRANULOMATOUS HYPERSENSITIVITY

Granulomatous hypersensitivity is clinically the most important form of type IV hypersensitivity. Granulomatous hypersensitivity causes many of the pathological effects in diseases that involve T cell-mediated immunity. It usually results from the persistence within macrophages of:
- intracellular microorganisms, which are able to resist macrophage killing; or
- other particles that the cell is unable to destroy.

This leads to chronic stimulation of T cells and the release of cytokines. The process results in the formation of **epithelioid cell granulomas** with a central collection of epithelioid cells and macrophages surrounded by lymphocytes.

The histological appearance of the granuloma reaction is quite different from that of the tuberculin-type reaction. However, both types of reaction may be caused by T cells sensitized to similar microbial antigens, for example the antigens of *M. tuberculosis* and *M. leprae* (Fig. 26.10).

Role of the antigen-specific TH lymphocyte in type IV hypersensitivity

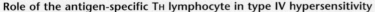

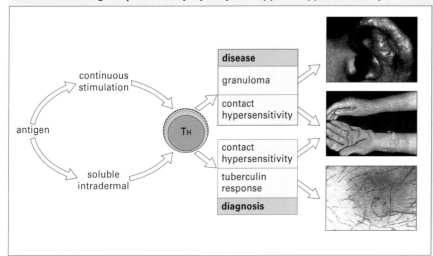

Fig. 26.10 The tuberculin skin reaction (lower photograph, courtesy of Professor JHL Playfair) is the classic diagnostic test for cell-mediated immunity in tuberculosis. If there is continuous antigenic stimulation instead of a single injection of soluble antigen, a granulomatous reaction (upper photograph, courtesy of Dr A du Vivier) or contact hypersensitivity (middle photograph, courtesy of Dr D Sharvill) follows. This granulomatous reaction can also occur if the macrophages cannot destroy the antigen.

Electron micrograph of an epithelioid cell

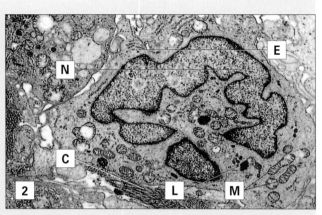

Fig. 26.11 The epithelioid cell is the characteristic cell of granulomatous hypersensitivity. Compare the extent of the endoplasmic reticulum (E) in the epithelioid cell (**1**, × 4800) with that of a tissue macrophage (**2**, × 4800). (C, collagen; L, lysosome; M, mitochondria; N, nucleus; U, nucleolus) (Courtesy of MJ Spencer)

Granulomas occur with chronic infections associated with predominantly TH1-like T cell responses, such as tuberculosis, leprosy, and leishmaniasis, and with TH2-like T cells, as in schistosomiasis.

Immune-mediated granuloma formation also occurs in the absence of infection, as in the sensitivity reactions to zirconium and beryllium, and in sarcoidosis and Crohn's disease where the antigens are unknown.

Foreign body granuloma formation occurs in response to talc, silica, and a variety of other particulate agents, when macrophages are unable to digest the inorganic matter. These non-immunological granulomas may be distinguished by the absence of lymphocytes in the lesion.

Epithelioid cells and giant cells are typical of granulomatous hypersensitivity

Epithelioid cells are large and flattened with increased endoplasmic reticulum (Fig. 26.11). They:
- are derived from activated macrophages under the chronic stimulation of cytokines;
- continue to secrete TNF and thus potentiate continuing inflammation.

Giant cells are formed when epithelioid cells fuse to form multinucleate giant cells (Fig. 26.12), sometimes referred to as **Langhans' giant cells** (not to be confused with the Langerhans' cell discussed earlier). Giant cells have several nuclei, but these are not at the center of the cell. There is little endoplasmic reticulum, and the mitochondria and lysosomes appear to be undergoing degeneration. The giant cell may therefore be a terminal differentiation stage of the monocyte/macrophage line.

The granuloma contains epithelioid cells, macrophages, and lymphocytes

An immunological granuloma typically has a core of epithelioid cells and macrophages, sometimes with giant cells. In some diseases, such as tuberculosis, this central area may have a zone of necrosis, with complete destruction of all cellular architecture.

Clinical and histological appearances of the Mitsuda reaction in leprosy seen at 28 days

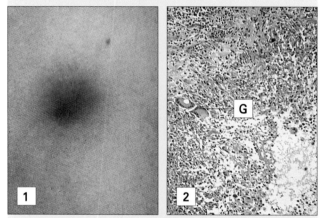

Fig. 26.12 (1) The resultant skin swelling (which may be ulcerated) is much harder and better defined than at 48 hours. (2) Histology shows a typical epithelioid cell granuloma (H&E stain. × 60). Giant cells (G) are visible in the center of the lesion, which is surrounded by a cuff of lymphocytes. This response is more akin to the pathological processes in delayed hypersensitivity diseases than the self-resolving tuberculin-type reaction. The reaction is due to the continued presence of mycobacterial antigen.

The macrophage/epithelioid core is surrounded by a cuff of lymphocytes, and there may also be considerable fibrosis (deposition of collagen fibers) caused by proliferation of fibroblasts and increased collagen synthesis.

Examples of granulomatous reactions are:
- the **Mitsuda reaction** to *M. leprae* antigens (see Fig. 26.12); or

Delayed hypersensitivity reactions

type	reaction time	clinical appearance	histology	antigen
contact	48–72 hours	eczema	lymphocytes, later macrophages; edema of epidermis	epidermal (e.g. antigen, nickel, rubber, poison ivy)
tuberculin	48–72 hours	local induration	lymphocytes, monocytes, macrophages	intradermal (e.g. tuberculin)
granuloma	21–28 days	hardening (e.g. skin of lung)	macrophages, epithelioid cells, giant cells, fibrosis	persistent antigen or antibody complexes or non-immunoglobulin stimuli (e.g. talc)

Fig. 26.13 The characteristics of type IV reactions comparing contact, tuberculin, and granulomatous reactions.

- the **Kveim test**, where patients who have sarcoidosis react to unknown splenic antigens derived from other patients with sarcoidosis.

The three types of delayed hypersensitivity are summarized in Fig. 26.13.

CELLULAR REACTIONS IN TYPE IV HYPERSENSITIVITY
T cells bearing αβ TCRs are essential

Experiments with gene knockout mice have confirmed that T cells bearing αβ TCRs rather than γδ TCRs are essential for initiating delayed hypersensitivity reactions in response to infection with intracellular bacteria.

Sensitized αβ T cells, stimulated with the appropriate antigen and APCs, undergo lymphoblastoid transformation before cell division (Fig. 26.14). This forms the basis of the lymphocyte stimulation test as a measure of T cell function. Lymphocyte stimulation is accompanied by DNA synthesis and this can be measured by assaying the uptake of radiolabeled thymidine, a nucleoside required for DNA synthesis. Lymphocytes from a patient are stimulated in culture with the suspect antigen to determine whether it induces transformation. It is important to stress that this is a test for T cell memory only, and does not necessarily imply the presence of protective immunity.

Following activation by APCs, T cells release a number of proinflammatory cytokines, which attract and activate macrophages. These include IFNγ, lymphotoxin-α, IL-3, and GM-CSF.

Q. How can IFNγ cause the attraction of macrophages to an inflammatory site?
A. It causes the production of chemokines, including CCL2, CCL5, and CXCL10, and induces adhesion molecules ICAM-1 and VCAM-1 on the endothelium (see Chapter 6).

This TH1-like pattern of cytokines is enhanced by activation of the T cells in the presence of IL-12 and IL-23, which are released by dendritic cells on exposure to bacterial products. IL-12 suppresses the cytokine response of TH2 cells.

IFNγ is required for granuloma formation in humans

The role of individual cytokines can be analyzed in gene knockout mice deficient for a single cytokine. For example, IFNγ gene knockout mice are unable to activate macrophages and control infection with *M. tuberculosis* (Fig. 26.15).

The absolute requirement of IFNγ for granuloma formation in humans is confirmed by the syndrome of Mendelian susceptibility to mycobacterial disease. Subjects deficient in the IFNγ receptor have markedly increased susceptibility to environmental mycobacteria and the vaccine strain, BCG, and fail to develop granulomas.

TNF and lymphotoxin-α are essential for granuloma formation during mycobacterial infections

TNF and the related cytokine, lymphotoxin-α, are both essential for the formation of granulomas during mycobacterial infections (Fig. 26.16), and act in part through the regulation of chemokine production.

Transformed lymphocytes

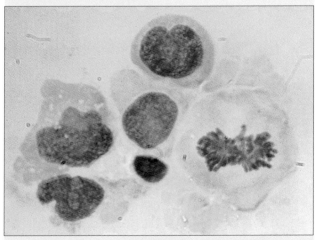

Fig. 26.14 Following stimulation with appropriate antigen, T cells undergo lymphoblastoid transformation before cell division. Blast cells with expanded nuclei and cytoplasm (as well as one lymphocyte in the metaphase of cell division) are shown.

The importance of IFNγ in the activation of macrophages

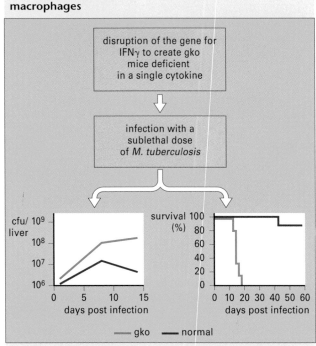

Fig. 26.15 Mice deficient in IFNγ (gene knockout [gko] mice) are unable to activate macrophages in response to infection with an intracellular bacterium. Macrophages initially accumulate at the site of infection, but do not form typical granulomas. Uncontrolled infection (graph, left) causes widespread tissue necrosis and death (graph, right). (cfu, colony forming units of infectious agent in the liver)

Both macrophage- and T cell-derived TNF contribute to this process, but within granulomas activated macrophages become the major source of TNF, driving the differentiation of macrophages into epithelioid cells and the fusion of epithelioid cells to form giant cells (Figs 26.17 and 26.18). The maintenance of granulomas is also dependent on TNF. Consequently, inhibition of TNF activity suppresses the granulomatous inflammation in Crohn's disease and sarcoidosis.

MANY CHRONIC DISEASES MANIFEST TYPE IV GRANULOMATOUS HYPERSENSITIVITY

There are many chronic diseases in humans that manifest type IV hypersensitivity. Most are due to infectious agents such as mycobacteria, protozoa, and fungi, though in other granulomatous diseases such as sarcoidosis and Crohn's disease no infectious agent has been established. Important diseases in this respect include:

- leprosy;
- tuberculosis;
- schistosomiasis;
- sarcoidosis;
- Crohn's disease.

Macrophage differentiation

Fig. 26.16 Bacterial products stimulate macrophages to secrete IL-12. Activation of T cells in the presence of IL-12 leads to the release of IFNγ and other cytokines, lymphotoxin (LT), IL-3, and GM-CSF. These cytokines activate macrophages to kill intracellular parasites. Failure to eradicate the antigenic stimulus causes persistent cytokine release and promotes differentiation of macrophages into epithelioid cells, which secrete large amounts of TNFα. Some fuse to form multinucleate giant cells.

The importance of TNF in the formation of granulomas

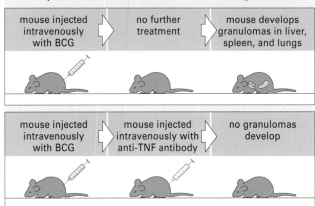

Fig. 26.17 TNF is essential for the development of epithelioid cell granulomas. If BCG-injected mice are injected with anti-TNFα antibodies, they do not develop granulomas.

Epithelioid cells in a granuloma from the lung of a patient with sarcoidosis

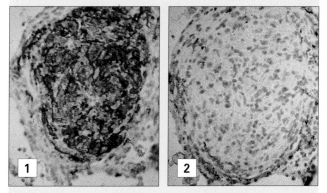

Fig. 26.18 (1) The epithelioid cells and giant cells in the center have been stained with the specific antibody RFD-9. (2) Mature tissue macrophages surrounding the granuloma are stained with the antibody RFD-7; the exact specificity of the antibody is not known. (Courtesy of CS Munro)

The immunological spectrum of leprosy

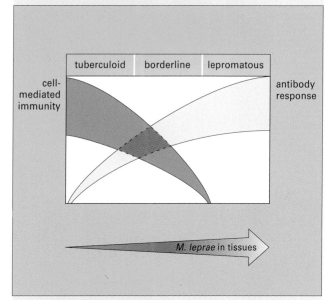

Fig. 26.19 The clinical spectrum of leprosy ranges from tuberculoid disease with few lesions and bacteria to lepromatous leprosy, with multiple lesions and uncontrolled bacterial proliferation. This range reflects host immunity as measured by specific cellular and antibody responses to *M. leprae*, and the tissue expression of cytokines.

A common feature of these infections is that the pathogen presents a persistent, chronic, antigenic stimulus. Activation of macrophages by lymphocytes may limit the infection, but continuing stimulation may lead to tissue damage through the release of macrophage products including reactive oxygen intermediates and hydrolases.

Although delayed hypersensitivity is a measure of T cell activation, the infection is not always controlled, with the result that protective immunity and delayed hypersensitivity do not necessarily coincide. Therefore some subjects showing delayed hypersensitivity may not be protected against disease in the future.

Leprosy is caused by infection with *M. leprae*

Leprosy is a chronic granulomatous disease of skin and nerves caused by infection with *M. leprae*. It is divided clinically into three main types – tuberculoid, borderline, and lepromatous:

- in tuberculoid leprosy, the skin may have a few well-defined hypopigmented patches, which show an intense lymphocytic and epithelioid cell infiltrate and no microorganisms;
- by contrast, the polar reaction of lepromatous leprosy shows multiple confluent skin lesions characterized by numerous bacilli, 'foamy' macrophages, and a paucity of lymphocytes;
- borderline leprosy has characteristics of both tuberculoid and lepromatous leprosy (Fig. 26.19).

In leprosy, protective immunity is usually associated with cell-mediated immunity, but this declines across the leprosy spectrum towards the lepromatous pole with a rise in non-protective anti-*M. leprae* antibodies.

The borderline leprosy reaction is a dramatic example of delayed hypersensitivity. Borderline reactions occur either spontaneously or following drug treatment. In these reactions, hypopigmented skin lesions containing *M. leprae* become swollen and inflamed (Fig. 26.20) because

the patient is now able to mount a T cell response to the mycobacteria resulting in a delayed-type hypersensitivity reaction. The histological appearance shows a more tuberculoid pattern with an infiltrate of IFNγ-secreting lymphocytes. The process may occur in peripheral nerves, where Schwann cells contain *M. leprae*; this is the most important cause of nerve destruction in this disease. The lesion in borderline leprosy is typical of granulomatous hypersensitivity (see Fig. 26.20).

In patients with a tuberculoid-type reaction, T cell sensitization may be assessed in vitro by lymphocyte proliferation or the release of IFNγ following stimulation with *M. leprae* antigens (Fig. 26.21).

Tuberculosis is caused by *M. tuberculosis*

In tuberculosis, the granuloma provides the microenvironment in which lymphocytes stimulate macrophages to kill the intracellular *M. tuberculosis*. The formation and maintenance of granulomas are essential to control the infection.

In most (>90%) subjects with latent tuberculosis infection, the mycobacteria remain dormant within small granulomas in the lung. There is, however, a balance between the effects of activated macrophages:

- controlling the infection on the one hand; and
- causing tissue damage in infected organs on the other.

In those who progress to clinical tuberculosis, granulomatous reactions lead to cavitation in the lung and spread of bacteria. The reactions are frequently accompanied by

Leprosy

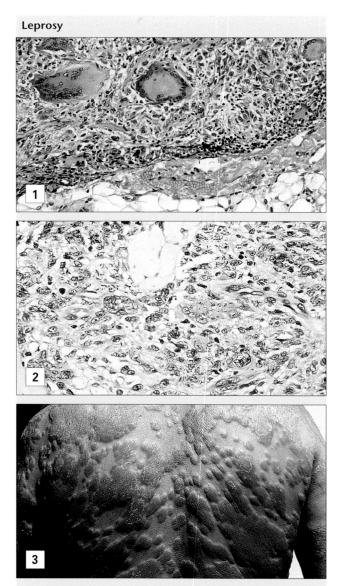

Fig. 26.20 (**1**) A borderline leprosy reaction. This small nerve is almost completely replaced by the granulomatous infiltrate. (**2**) Lepromatous leprosy. Large numbers of bacilli are present. (Courtesy of Dr Phillip McKee) (**3**) Borderline lepromatous leprosy. There are gross infiltrated erythematous plaques with well-defined borders. (Courtesy of Dr S Lucas)

Lymphocyte stimulation test in leprosy

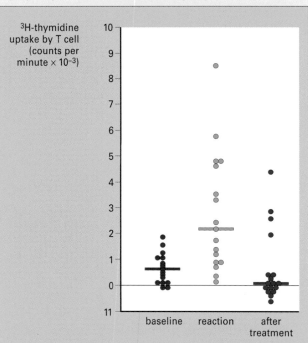

Fig. 26.21 During a borderline leprosy reaction, the lymphocyte stimulation response to *M. leprae* rises. There is a fall in response when the reaction is treated successfully with corticosteroids. The lymphocyte stimulation responses to sonicated *M. leprae* (measured by uptake of ^{3}H-thymidine) are shown for 17 patients who developed such reactions before starting treatment with anti-leprosy drugs (baseline); during the reaction; and following successful treatment with corticosteroids. Medians are indicated by horizontal bars.

Chest radiograph of a patient with pulmonary tuberculosis

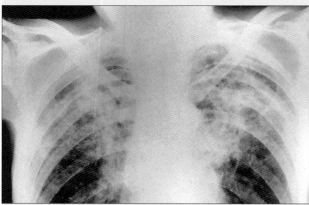

Fig. 26.22 There is extensive parenchymal streaking, predominantly in the upper fields of the lungs. These changes are typical of chronic bilateral pulmonary tuberculosis. Some enlargement of the heart is also evident.

extensive fibrosis and the lesions may be seen in the chest radiographs of affected patients (Fig. 26.22).

Q. What factors might affect the balance that controls a latent infection with tuberculosis?
A. Immunosuppression by drugs or infection (e.g. AIDS) (see Chapter 17) can allow reactivation of infection with tuberculosis.

The histological appearance of the lesion is typical of a granulomatous reaction, with central caseous (cheesy) necrosis (Fig. 26.23). This is surrounded by an area of

Histological appearance of a tuberculous section of lung

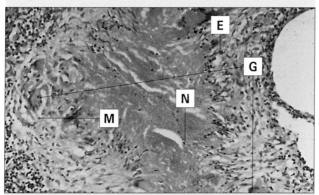

Fig. 26.23 This shows an epithelioid cell granuloma (E) with giant cells (G). Mononuclear cell infiltration can be seen (M). There is also marked caseation and necrosis (N) within the granuloma. H&E stain. × 75.

epithelioid cells, with a few giant cells. Mononuclear cell infiltration occurs around the edge.

Schistosomiasis is caused by parasitic trematode worms

In schistosomiasis, which is caused by parasitic trematode worms (schistosomes), the host becomes sensitized to the ova of the worms, leading to a typical granulomatous reaction in the parasitized tissue mediated essentially by TH2 cells (Fig. 26.24; see also Chapter 15). In this case the cytokines IL-5 and IL-13 are responsible for the recruitment of eosinophils and the formation of the granulomas around the ova. When the eggs have been deposited in the liver, the subsequent IL-13-dependent fibrosis causes hepatic scarring and portal hypertension.

Histological appearance of the liver in schistosomiasis

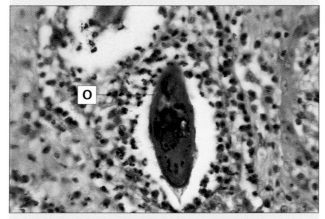

Fig. 26.24 The epithelioid cell granuloma surrounds the schistosome ovum (O) and eosinophils are prominent. H&E stain. × 300. (Courtesy of Dr Phillip McKee)

The cause of sarcoidosis is unknown

Sarcoidosis is a chronic disease of unknown etiology in which activated macrophages and non-caseating granuloma accumulate in many tissues, frequently accompanied by fibrosis (Fig. 26.25). The disease particularly affects lymphoid tissue and the lungs, and enlarged lymph nodes may be detected in chest radiographs of affected patients (Fig. 26.26). No infectious agent has been isolated, though mycobacteria have been implicated because of the similarities in the pathology.

Histological appearance of sarcoidosis in a lymph node biopsy

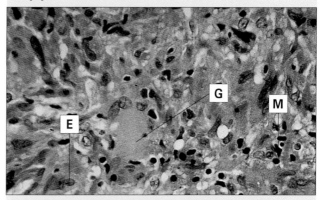

Fig. 26.25 The granuloma of sarcoidosis is typically composed of epithelioid cells (E) and multinucleate giant cells (G), but without caseous necrosis. There is only a sparse mononuclear cell infiltrate (M) evident at the periphery of the granuloma. H&E stain. × 240.

The chest radiograph of a patient with sarcoidosis

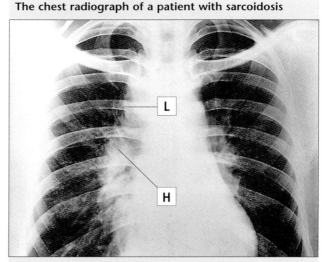

Fig. 26.26 There is enlargement of the lymph nodes adjacent to the hilar (H) and paratracheal (L) areas of the lungs, with diffuse pulmonary infiltration characteristic of the disease.

One of the paradoxes of clinical immunology is that this disease is usually associated with depression of delayed hypersensitivity both in vivo and in vitro. Patients with sarcoidosis are anergic on testing with tuberculin; however, when cortisone is injected with tuberculin antigen the skin tests are positive, suggesting that cortisone-sensitive T inhibitory cells are responsible for the anergy.

Q. What effect does cortisone normally have on an immune response, and why does its effect here appear paradoxical?
A. Cortisone would normally suppress delayed hypersensitivity, principally by its actions on macrophages.

In sarcoidosis, granulomas develop in a variety of organs, most commonly the lungs, lymph nodes, bone, nervous tissue, and skin. Patients may present acutely with fever and malaise, though in the longer term those with pulmonary involvement develop shortness of breath caused by lung fibrosis. The diagnosis is often suggested by the clinical pattern and radiographic changes and confirmed by tissue biopsy. Angiotensin converting enzyme (ACE) and serum calcium levels are sometimes elevated because activated macrophages are a source of both ACE and 1,25-dihydroxy-cholecalciferol (the active metabolite of vitamin D_3).

The cause of Crohn's disease is unknown

Crohn's disease is another non-infectious disease in which granulomas are prominent.

Crohn's disease is a chronic inflammatory disease of the ileum and colon, in which lymphocytes and macrophages accumulate in all layers of the bowel. The granulomatous reaction and fibrosis cause stricture of the bowel and penetrating fistulas into other organs. The natures of the antigens or infectious agents initiating and perpetuating this granulomatous reaction are unknown.

Activated T cells, showing a restricted T cell receptor repertoire and a TH1-like profile of cytokine production are responsible for macrophage activation and the release of inflammatory cytokines, such as TNF, reactive oxygen metabolites, and nitric oxide. These initiate and maintain the transmural intestinal inflammation.

Inhibition of TNF activity with antibody or soluble TNF receptor reduces inflammation in patients with Crohn's disease, but this therapy may be associated with reactivation of tuberculosis in subjects with latent tuberculosis infection and with other granulomatous infectious diseases.

FURTHER READING

American Thoracic Society. Statement on sarcoidosis. Am J Respir Crit Care Med 1999;160:736–755.

Askenase PW. Yes T cells, but three different T cells (αβ, γδ and NK T cells) and also B-1 cells mediate contact sensitivity. Clin Exp Immunol 2001;125:345–350.

Bean AGD, Roach DR, Briscoe H, et al. Structural deficiencies in granuloma formation in tumor necrosis factor gene-targeted mice underlie the heightened susceptibility to aerosol *Mycobacterium tuberculosis* infection which is not compensated for by lymphotoxin. J Immunol 1999;162:3504–3511.

Bjune G, Barnetson RStC, Ridley DS, et al. Lymphocyte transformation test in leprosy; correlation of the response with inflammation of lesions. Clin Exp Immunol 1976;25:85–94.

Britton WJ, Garsia RJ. Mycobacterial infections. In: Bradley J, McCluskey J, eds. Clinical immunology, vol. 38. London: Oxford University Press; 1997:483–498.

Britton WJ, Lockwood DN. Leprosy. Lancet 2004;363:1209–1219.

Casanova J-L, Abel L. Genetic dissection of immunity to mycobacteria: the human model. Annu Rev Immunol 2002;40:581–620.

Daniel H, Present MD, Rutgeerts P, et al. Infliximab for the treatment of fistulas in patients with Crohn's disease. N Engl J Med 1999;18:1398–1405.

Enk AH, Katz SI. Contact hypersensitivity as a model for T-cell activation in skin. J Invest Dermatol 1995;105:805–835.

Flynn JL, Chan J. Immunology of tuberculosis. Annu Rev Immunol 2001;19:93–129.

Flynn JL, Chan J, Triebold KJ, et al. An essential role for interferon-γ in resistance to *Mycobacterium tuberculosis* infection. J Exp Med 1993;178:2249–2254.

Girolomoni G, Sebastiani S, Albanesi C, Cavani A. T cell sub-populations in the development of atopic and contact allergy. Curr Opin Immunol 2001;13:733–737.

Grabbe S, Schwarz, T. Immunoregulatory mechanisms involved in elicitation of allergic contact hypersensitivity. Immunol Today 1998;19:37–43.

Kalish RS, Wood JA, LaPorte A. Processing of urushiol (poison ivy) hapten by both endogenous and exogenous pathways for presentation to T cells in vitro. J Clin Invest 1994;93:2039–2047.

Kindler V, Sappino A-P, Gran GE, et al. The inducing role of tumour necrosis factor in the development of bactericidal granulomas during BCG infection. Cell 1989;56:731–740.

Klimas N. Delayed hypersensitivity skin testing. In: Manual of clinical laboratory immunology, 5th edn. Washington: ASM Press; 1997:276–280.

Roach DR, Briscoe H, Saunders B, et al. Secreted lymphotoxin-alpha is essential for the control of intracellular bacterial infection. J Exp Med 2001;193:239–246.

Roach DR, Bean AGD, Demangel C, et al. Tumor necrosis factor regulates chemokine induction essential for cell recruitment, granuloma formation and clearance of mycobacterial infection. J Immunol 2002;168:4620–4628.

Romagnani P, Annunziato F, Baccari M, et al. T cells and cytokines in Crohn's disease. Curr Opin Immunol 1997;9:793–799.

Salgame P. Host innate and TH1 responses and the bacterial factors that contain *Mycobacterium tuberculosis* infection. Curr Opin Immunol 2005;17:374–380.

Trinchieri G. Interleukin-12: a cytokine at the interface of inflammation and immunity. Adv Immunol 1998;70:133–195.

Von Andrian UH, Mackay CR. T cell function and migration: two sides of the same coin. N Engl J Med 2000;343:1020–1034.

Wallis RS, Broder MS, Wong JY, et al. Granulomatous infectious disease associated with tumor necrosis factor. Clin Infect Dis 2004;38:1261–1265.

Wang B, Eshe C, Mamelak A, et al. Cytokine knockouts in contact hypersensitivity research. Cytokine Growth Factor Rev 2003;14:381–389.

Wynn TA, Thompson RW, Cheever AW, Mentink-Kane MM. Immunopathogenesis of schistosomiasis. Immunol Rev 2004;201:156–167

Yamamura M, Uyemura K, Deans RJ, et al. Defining protective immune responses to pathogens: cytokine profiles in leprosy lesions. Science 1991;254:277–279.

Websites

http://users.path.ox.ac.uk/~cholt/ – a home page describing macrophage biology and the role of macrophages in the host response to infectious disease

http://www.who.int/lep/disease/disease.htm – a home page describing leprosy infection

Critical thinking: A hypersensitivity type IV reaction (see p. 503 for explanations)

An 8-year-old boy with recent weight loss and mild fever is found to have an enlarged lymph node on the right side of the neck. He has no cough and his chest radiograph is normal. Surgical biopsy of the lymph node reveals a granulomatous infiltrate with no evident acid-fast bacilli. The result of micro-biological culture for *Mycobacterium tuberculosis* is awaited. Intradermal skin testing with tuberculin causes swelling and erythema of 20 mm in diameter after 48 hours.

1 What cell types make up the granulomas in the lymph node and what cytokines are involved in their formation?

2 What is the pathology at the site of the skin testing and how does it differ from that in the lymph node?

3 What type of lymphocyte is responsible for the skin test reactivity?

4 What other conditions cause granulomas in lymph nodes and how are they diagnosed?

5 When the family members are tested, the boy's 5-year-old brother is found to have a positive tuberculin reaction (18 mm at 48 hours), but he is well with a normal chest radiograph. What does this result indicate about his immune responses and what is its significance?

491

Critical Thinking: Explanations

1. SPECIFICITY AND MEMORY IN VACCINATION

1.1 The immunological 'memory' induced by vaccination does not depend just on the antibodies. Memory is due to long-lived memory lymphocytes, which persist in the lymphoid tissues for many years. They will be reactivated if the individual encounters the toxin or the vaccine on a later occasion.

1.2 The tetanus toxoid is a stable molecule – it does not change or mutate, so antibodies and lymphocytes that recognize it continue to be effective. By contrast, influenza A mutates every year. Last year's antibodies are marginally effective or ineffective against this year's virus. Researchers must identify newly emerging virus strains and prepare vaccine from those strains they think will produce new epidemics. Often they get it right, but not always.

1.3 Recommendations are based on practicality. It is impossible to prepare sufficient vaccine each year to immunize everyone against influenza. There is not enough time to do it and not enough laboratory resources available. So the highest risk groups are targeted – health workers because they will likely be in contact with the disease and old people because the disease can lead to serious complications.

Discussion point

If we could immunize every person in the world against influenza A in 1 year, do you think that this would lead to total eradication of the disease?

2. DEVELOPMENT OF THE IMMUNE SYSTEM

2.1 The total numbers of blood lymphocytes are drastically reduced, with T cells being virtually absent and B cells significantly reduced – B cells require T cells to complete their own development. The lymph nodes are much reduced in size, and this particularly affects the paracortex (T cell areas). Compare this with diGeorge syndrome. The animals have a reduced ability to fight infections, but this is selective, affecting particularly some viruses and parasites – possibly because there is still good NK cell activity and macrophage-mediated antibacterial defenses.

2.2 Adult thymectomy has very little effect on the individual's ability to fight infection. By adulthood, there is a large pool of peripheral T cells that may to some extent self renew. The thymus progressively involutes and becomes less important as a site of T cell development in the adult.

2.3 Because the lymphocyte precursors fail to make productive rearrangements of their antigen receptor genes, they die by apoptosis during development. This leads to a profound immune deficiency of all lymphocytes, which is analogous to severe combined immunodeficiency (SCID) in humans.

2.4 Interleukin-7 is required for lymphocyte development in primary lymphoid organs. There is a profound reduction in thymocytes and peripheral lymphocytes and a total absence of $\gamma\delta$ T cells.

2.5 The $\alpha_4\beta_7$-integrin is required for binding of cells to adhesion molecules on the high endothelial venule (HEV) of gut-associated lymphoid tissue (GALT), so this knockout results in drastically reduced lymphocyte numbers in these tissues.

3. THE SPECIFICITY OF ANTIBODIES

3.1 In the presence of the antibodies, mutated variants of the virus are selected that do not bind those antibodies. By detecting which of the virus proteins are mutated, one can infer that these are the proteins that normally would bind to the antibody. Neutralizing antibodies against viruses are generally directed against proteins in the capsid of the virus, particularly against the proteins that the virus uses to attach to the surface of its target cell. Antibodies cannot gain access to the inside of the virus, so neutralizing antibodies do not bind the core protein VP4.

3.2 The antibody VP1-a binds to an epitope that includes two closely spaced residues (91 and 95). This is a 'continuous epitope' and is located on a single external loop of polypeptide. By contrast, the epitope recognized by VP1-b is located in at least two distinct areas of the polypeptide chain (83–85 and 138–139). This is a 'discontinuous epitope': examination of the VP1 antigen shows that these residues are located on two adjacent areas of β-pleated sheet.

3.3 A mutation of residue 138 does not affect the epitope recognized by antibody VP1-a, so it continues to bind with high affinity to the antigen. This confirms that the epitopes recognized by VP1-a and VP1-b are physically separate. The mutant with Gly at position 95 still binds the VP1-a antibody weakly. Glycine is a smaller amino acid than aspartate, which is present in the wild type, hence the antibody can still bind to the epitope, although the 'fit' is less good, so the affinity of binding is lower. By contrast, lysine (Lys) is a larger residue than aspartate. It protrudes further out into the antibody's binding site and completely disrupts the antigen–antibody bond.

4. COMPLEMENT DEFICIENCY

4.1 Deficiencies of components of the classical or alternative pathways, particularly of C3, produce a reduced ability to opsonize bacteria, resulting in impaired phagocytosis by macrophages and neutrophils. Patients suffer from repeated bacterial infections from Gram-positive bacteria (e.g. staphylococci, streptococci). These children are unable to clear bacterial infections because their phagocytes do not take up bacteria efficiently. Deficiencies in the lytic pathway components (C5–C9) can render patients more susceptible to neisserial infections because the lytic pathway can damage the outer membrane of Gram-negative bacteria such as *Neisseria* spp.

4.2 There is a clear deficiency in C3 and components of the alternative pathway. Components of the classical pathway are on the lower end of normal. At first this looks surprising, because the initial assay for lytic complement required the activity of the classical and lytic pathways. Nevertheless, both the bacterial infections and the lack of total hemolytic complement can be explained by the very low levels of C3. Note that the genes for C3, fB, and fI are not genetically linked, so we cannot explain this apparent multiple deficiency of alternative pathway components by some multiple gene deletion. The explanation lies in the alternative pathway amplification loop. Because the children lack fI, they cannot break down the alternative pathway C3 convertase C3bBb. Therefore C3 is continuously activated and binds fB. All the fB is consumed, as is most of the free C3. The genetic deficiency of fI therefore leads to secondary deficiencies in the components of the alternative pathway and this then affects C3 and the function of the classical and lytic pathways.

4.3 The children have a homozygous fI deficiency – both copies of the gene are missing. Replacing fI, either by an infusion of normal serum or by providing pure fI, restores all the other components to normal levels and allows the children to clear bacterial infections. Antibiotic prophylaxis will help prevent bacterial infections.

Discussion point

What problem might occur if you inject a protein such as fI into an individual who lacks it due to a genetic deficiency?

5. SOMATIC HYPERMUTATION

5.1 There are at least three theories why TCRs do not undergo somatic hypermutation.

1. T cells control most antibody responses – they therefore represent an important mechanism for maintaining self tolerance. According to this view, the immune system can afford to let immunoglobulin genes undergo somatic hypermutation because (non-mutating) T cells retain control.

2. TCRs must retain the ability to recognize self (MHC), and therefore cannot be allowed to undergo somatic hypermutation.

3. The main purpose of somatic hypermutation of antibodies is to give a more robust secondary response.

In the case of T cells, as opposed to antibodies, it is possible to increase the efficacy/avidity of the memory T cell by affecting TCR density, presence of co-stimulatory/inhibitory molecules, or other aspects of the wiring of T cell signaling. Mutating the receptor is therefore simply not necessary because it is potentially dangerous as well. According to this theory, it is best avoided.

5. THE SPECIFICITY OF T CELLS

5.2 This is an example of genetic restriction in antigen presentation. The SM/J T cells are primed with antigen on MHC molecules of the SM/J haplotype and will only respond to this combination of antigen–MHC. They do not recognize the same antigen presented by other MHC molecules. Because MHC molecules are co-dominantly expressed, the H-2v MHC molecules are present on the APCs from the F1 animal and so they too stimulate the T cells.

5.3 The minimum peptide needed to activate the T cells appears to be 80–94, which is 15 residues long and therefore corresponds well to the expected size of antigen peptides that can fit into the MHC class II binding site. This peptide is included within peptide 80–102, which also stimulates strongly. Peptides 84–98 and 73–88 lack the N and C terminals of the antigenic peptide, respectively, and therefore lack some of the anchor residues needed to hold them in the MHC peptide-binding groove.

5.4 This is called a superagonist or a strong agonist peptide. Typically such a peptide will have a stronger binding affinity for the MHC molecule and/or the TCR.

6. THE ROLE OF ADHESION MOLECULES IN T CELL MIGRATION

6.1 IL-1 induces the expression of a number of adhesion molecules, including ICAM-1 and VCAM-1, both of which can potentially mediate leukocyte migration by their interaction with the integrins LFA-1 and VLA-4, respectively.

6.2 Because it takes several hours to increase migration, and ICAM-1 and VCAM-1 appear to be involved in the process, one can infer that their expression is increased as a result of protein synthesis (which takes several hours) rather than by a relatively rapid release from intracellular stores.

6.3 Antibodies to ICAM-1/LFA-1 reduce migration of cells across unstimulated endothelium. Therefore, this pair of adhesion molecules is required for migration across resting endothelium.

6.4 Antibodies to both ICAM-1/LFA-1 and VCAM-1/VLA-4 reduce migration across IL-1-activated cells, therefore both pairs of adhesion molecules control this event. In practice it is known that ICAM-1 is present on unstimulated brain endothelium and is increased by IL-1, whereas VCAM-1 is virtually absent from unstimulated brain endothelium, but may be synthesized following stimulation with inflammatory cytokines.

7. ANTIGEN PROCESSING AND PRESENTATION

7.1 Macrophages express both MHC class I and class II molecules, and can therefore present antigen to either of the clones. Fibroblasts do not generally express MHC class II molecules and one would not expect them to stimulate the MHC class II-restricted clone.

7.2 Live flu virus infects the macrophages and flu virus polypeptides are synthesized in the cytoplasm of the cell, so the viral antigens are presented by the internal (MHC class I) pathway as well as the external (MHC class II) pathway. Inactivated virus is taken up by the macrophage, processed and presented via the class II pathway only – because there is no viral protein synthesis there is no presentation via the MHC class I pathway.

7.3 Emetine blocks protein synthesis, so no protein fragments are fed into the MHC class I pathway by the proteasomes. Chloroquine prevents phagosome/lysosome fusion so endocytosed virus cannot be broken down into peptides. Consequently no peptides are available for the MHC class II pathway.

7.4 The MHC class I-restricted T cells express CD8 and the MHC class II-restricted cells express CD4 because CD8 and CD4 are co-receptors for MHC class I and class II molecules, respectively.

8. DEVELOPMENT OF THE ANTIBODY RESPONSE

8.1 In a developing immune response to a TD antigen, B cells will switch from IgM production to IgG. Because the antigen is continuously present as a depot, by day 14 the response has the characteristics of a secondary response – IgG antibody titers are climbing rapidly.

8.2 Perhaps the two mice have already been infected by mouse hepatitis virus. By day 5 they are already making a secondary IgG response. This could be a problem in the colony, though usually all animals housed together would become infected. If these mice have been naturally infected it would be through the gut (unlike the vaccine) and one would therefore expect a stronger IgA response.

8.3 IgA-producing clones tend to be located in the mucosa-associated lymphoid tissues (see Chapter 2) and it is not surprising that no IgA-producing clones were generated from the spleen.

8.4 IgG-producing clones at day 14 are likely to be of higher affinity than IgM producers.

9. THE ROLE OF MACROPHAGES IN TOXIC SHOCK SYNDROME

9.1 TNFα, IL-1, IL-6, IL-10.

9.2 Lack of activity, ruffling of fur, respiratory distress, possibly leading to death within 24 hours.

9.3 BCG activates macrophages via infection of APCs and induction of IFNγ by NK and CD4$^+$ T cells, which primes macrophages. LPS delivers stimulus via LPS binding protein, CD14, Toll-like receptors, and NFκB activation, to enhance proinflammatory cytokine release. TNFα and IL-1, especially, act locally and systemically on vascular endothelium, neutrophils, and central nervous centers, causing hypotension and circulatory collapse.

9.4 CD14 knockout mice are extremely resistant to septic shock. Scavenger receptor A knockout mice are more susceptible to septic shock. IFNγ knockout mice are relatively resistant to septic shock.

9.5 CD14 is central to the LPS recognition and signaling pathway. SR-A clears LPS from the circulation to protect the host. IFNγ is needed to prime macrophages.

9.6 Evaluate the kinetics of pro- and anti-inflammatory cytokine production to establish the endogenous regulation of macrophage activation. Use blocking antibodies for TNFα and other cytokines, and receptor knockout mice to establish the roles of each. Evaluate cytokine production by peritoneal macrophages taken from BCG-primed mice after LPS challenge in vitro.

9.7 Septic shock is a major complication of Gram-negative (e.g. *Neisseria meningitidis*) infection. Therapeutic approaches include circulatory support, antibiotics, and possibly combinations of cytokine and receptor antagonists (blocking antibodies, inhibitors of TNFα cleavage, soluble receptors).

Relevant references

Haworth R, Platt N, Keshav S, et al. The macrophage scavenger receptor type A (SR-A) is expressed by activated macrophages and protects the host against lethal endotoxic shock. J Exp Med 1997;186:1431–1439.

Haziot A, Ferrero E, Kontgen F, et al. Resistance to endotoxin shock and reduced dissemination of Gram-negative bacteria in CD14 deficient mice. Immunity 1996;4:407–414.

9. THE DISTINCTION BETWEEN INFLAMMATORY RESPONSES AND HOUSE-KEEPING OF APOPTOTIC CELLS

9.8 Use blocking antibodies for phagocytic receptors (e.g. vitronectin receptors) or cells from knockout mice, if available.

9.9 Ligation and cross-linking of phagocytic receptors by apoptotic cells induce signaling pathways resulting in suppression of inflammatory and antimicrobial responses.

9.10 Use antibodies and antagonists to receptors to study candidate inhibitory responses such as production of prostaglandin E$_2$ and TGFβ.

9.11 Pathogens can exploit and induce the downregulation of inflammation by apoptotic cells to evade killing by host cells. This may be counteracted by the use of drugs to prevent inhibitory pathways, even in vivo.

Relevant references

Stein M, Keshav S, Harris N, Gordon S. IL-4 potently enhances murine macrophage MR activity; a marker of alternative immunologic macrophage activation. J Exp Med 1992;176:287–292.

Freire-de-Lima CG, Nascimento DO, Soares MBP, et al. Nature 2000;403:199–203.

9. THE ROLE OF MACROPHAGES IN T$_H$1 AND T$_H$2 RESPONSES

9.12 Macrophage activation involves a complex pattern of altered gene expression, covering a spectrum of activities and not just polar opposites between activation (T$_H$1, IFNγ) and deactivation (T$_H$2, IL-10). IL-4 and IL-13, T$_H$2 cytokines, use common receptor chains to induce an alternative pathway of macrophage activation involved in humoral immunity and possibly repair (enhanced APC function via MHC class II expression and MRs, as well as other effects on B cell production of antibody). IFNγ and IL-10 regulate cellular immune effector functions.

9.13 Broaden the range of macrophage markers examined, ultimately by DNA gene chip analysis, and look for consistency and reproducibility of similar patterns of altered gene expression by the cytokines above. Analyze macrophage functions in mice with knockouts of cytokines or their receptors.

9.14 Find model antigens (e.g. parasites) that induce TH2 responses in vivo, and establish whether these are recognized by APC receptors that enhance IL-4/IL-13 or inhibit IFNγ production by appropriate cells.

10. MECHANISMS OF CYTOTOXICITY

10.1 CTLs kill their targets using granule-associated mechanisms such as perforin, and by activating pathways of apoptosis – hence they produce both cell lysis and DNA fragmentation. CTLs recognize allogeneic MHC class I molecules on the targets – the effectors and targets come from different individuals. Note that there is always a low level of cell damage in the controls that contain no effector cells.

10.2 Tumor cells typically show reduced expression of MHC molecules by comparison with normal cells, and as they do they become susceptible to damage mediated by NK cells. Because NK cells recognize several different types of MHC molecule, the fact that the targets are allogeneic is not so relevant. Antibody can cross-link the NK cells to their targets (K cell activity) via their Fc receptor (CD16). This moves the balance of activity towards activation of the NK cell. Note that antibody itself does not damage the targets in this type of assay because the culture medium does not contain functional complement.

10.3 Purified perforin is extremely efficient at causing cell lyis, but does not activate the pathways of apoptosis, so there is no DNA fragmentation.

11. REGULATION OF THE IMMUNE RESPONSE

11.1 Overexcessive immune activation is harmful to the host. An incorrect or excessive immune response can lead to autoimmunity or allergy. Anergy, cell death, and suppression by cytokines and regulatory cells are three ways of inducing tolerance and preventing this.

11.2 Antibody regulates the immune system through a number of feedback mechanisms. Antibodies can form immune complexes with antigen and these can lead to expansion or suppression of immune responses. Passive IgM can enhance an immune response, whereas passive IgG suppresses the response through antibody blocking or receptor cross-linking. In addition, some immunoglobulins are idiotypic and have an immunogenic sequence within them. During an immune response antibodies can be generated against this idiotypic sequence leading to downregulation of the response.

11.3 Transfer of regulatory T cells into mice with autoimmunity can cause a reduction in the disease, but it is not known how this would affect other immune responses if the system was used in the treatment of human autoimmunity. It is possible that there could be a decreased immune response to viral and bacterial infections leading to an increase in these diseases.

11.4 If lymphocytes did not senesce they might begin to proliferate in an uncontrolled manner – this could cause cancers of the immune system and also lead to exaggerated immune responses causing autoimmunity or allergy.

12. IMMUNE REACTIONS IN THE GUT

Oysters are a food item that is normally tolerated by the body. Eating an infected shellfish causes the antigens in the food to be presented in association with components of the pathogen that can activate PAMP receptors, induce co-stimulatory molecules, and break tolerance. Additionally bacterial toxins may damage the gut epithelium again, enhancing antigen presentation and allowing antigens to access the gut-associated lymphoid tissues more readily. Once tolerance is broken the TH2-type response, which is characteristic of the gut, will lead to production of antigen-specific IgE antibodies. Consequently, eating another oyster, even a good one, will lead to an allergic reaction to antigen in the food.

13. VIRUS–IMMUNE SYSTEM INTERACTIONS

13.1 Features of a virus that enable it to evade host defense mechanisms include the following.
- Antigenic variation, as seen for example in HIV and influenza virus. Evasion of antibody and T cell recognition by mutation arising in genes encoding major antigenic targets.
- Production of 'decoy' molecules that interfere with host immune defenses, in particular molecules targeting the interferon system, downregulating MHC class I expression, subverting the function of cytokines and chemokines, and the action of complement.
- Establishment of virus latency, thereby avoiding detection by the immune system (e.g. HSV-1 in sensory ganglia, EBV in B lymphocytes).

13.2 Non-neutralizing antibodies could function by mediating antibody-dependent complement-mediated lysis of infected cells, complement-mediated neutralization, antibody-dependent cellular cytotoxicity (ADCC), or antibody-enhanced phagocytosis by macrophages.

13.3 Experiments to support the conclusions could involve:
- examination in vitro of whether complement mediates neutralization of virus in the presence of non-neutralizing antibodies;
- use of mice deficient in late complement components (i.e. C5-deficient mice);
- analysis of whether IgG subclasses were able to mediate ADCC in vitro using virus-infected cells.

14. IMMUNOENDOCRINE INTERACTIONS IN THE RESPONSE TO INFECTION

14.1 The immune system cannot be understood in isolation from the rest of mammalian physiology. One of the many effects of stress is increased production of adrenocorticotropic hormone (ACTH) from the pituitary. This in turn drives increased production of cortisol by the adrenal. The proof is that, in the animal models mentioned, the stressor can be replaced by mimicking the stress-induced levels of cortisol (or the rodent equivalent, corticosterone) with implanted slow-release cortisol pellets. The cortisol downregulates cell-mediated immunity to tuberculosis.

14.2 These observations provide clues as to why increased cortisol levels can lead to reduced immunity to tuberculosis. Raised cortisol levels cause APCs to release more IL-10 and less IL-12, so newly recruited T cells tend to develop a TH2 cytokine profile. Moreover, cortisol actually synergizes with some functions of TH2 cytokines, and enhances the ability of IL-4 to drive IgE production. It is interesting that BCG vaccination does not lead to protective immunity if the BCG is given to animals bearing cortisol pellets that mimic stress levels of cortisol. Cortisol also reduces the antimycobacterial functions of macrophages.

These points emphasize the need for a physiological approach to the understanding of infection. A narrowly immunological approach has solved some infections, but global emergencies such as tuberculosis, HIV infection and septic shock may require integrated physiological thinking as well as pure immunology.

15. IMMUNITY TO PROTOZOA AND HELMINTHS

15.1 Protozoa replicate within the host, so there is usually a balance between the effectiveness of the immune response and the virulence of the parasite. With certain parasites the infections may be short-lived and may kill the host, but this may not be a disadvantage to the parasite if it has already been transmitted to a new host. A good example is falciparum malaria, which is potentially fatal, particularly in children in endemic areas who have not developed any immunity, but are likely to have been bitten during the course of the infection by mosquitos, which will ensure further transmission. Helminths, by contrast, do not replicate within the host and are generally long-lived chronic infections. Transmission is by the release of eggs and larvae from an adult parasite, which may be excreted or be taken up by a vector.

15.2 By adopting an intracellular mode of existence parasites may be able to 'hide' from the immune response. A good example is falciparum malaria, which lives in mature red blood cells. Because this cell type has no nucleus it cannot express MHC class I molecules on its surface, so the parasite is invisible to CD8⁺ cytotoxic T cells. Other parasites live in nucleated cells, which will express class I MHC molecules, but experiments have shown this to be downregulated in cells infected with some parasites. *T. gondii* avoids being killed by the macrophage by inhibiting the fusion of the lysosome with the phagosome; *T. cruzi* escapes from the phagosome into the cytoplasm of the cell; and *Leishmania* spp. can resist the low pH of the phagolysosomes and are resistant to lysosomal enzymes.

15.3 Extracellular parasites can adopt a number of ways of avoiding immune attack. Parasites may 'disguise' themselves, for example by undergoing antigenic variation (African trypanosomes) or by adsorbing host molecules or undergoing molecular mimicry of the host (schistosomes). Parasites may 'hide' from the host immune response by becoming cysts (*Entameba* spp.) or by living in an immunoprivileged location (*Toxoplasma* in brain). They

may 'resist' attack by having a physical barrier (helminths) or by producing enzymes that resist the oxidative burst or disable antibodies. Many parasites are able to 'modulate' the host immune response to their advantage.

16. HYPER-IgM IMMUNODEFICIENCY

16.1 Normal infants do not become infected with *Pneumocystis carinii*. The occurrence of this type of pneumonia suggests the presence of an immunodeficiency disorder. Her immunoglobulin levels point to an elevated IgM level whereas the IgG, IgA, and IgE levels are very low. These findings almost certainly rule out the diagnosis of X-linked agammaglobulinemia because in that case the IgM would be undetectable. The normal white blood cell count probably rules out severe combined immunodeficiency (SCID) because an infant with SCID would have a very low lymphocyte count (< 3000/mm³). Had the IgD level been measured it would probably also be high, as is found in males with hyper-IgM immunodeficiency.

16.2 A blood sample should be obtained to isolate the B lymphocytes. In hyper-IgM immunodeficiency the B cells would stain only with fluorescent anti-IgM and anti-IgD. In a normal infant B cells that stain with anti-IgA and anti-IgG would also be present in addition to IgM⁺ and IgD⁺ cells. Furthermore, the mononuclear cells from the blood sample should be stimulated with phytohemagglutinin. After several hours of stimulation, the cells should be stained with fluorescent anti-CD40 ligand. Some 50% of normal T cells would stain positively whereas none would be positive in hyper-IgM immunodeficiency.

16.3 Antibodies formed to tetanus toxoid immunization are of the IgG class. Because this child is incapable of undergoing isotype switching she cannot make IgG antibodies. However, antibodies to the blood group substances are predominantly of the IgM class, which this child can synthesize. Furthermore the isohemagglutinins are so called T-independent antibodies; their formation does not require T cell help. Isotype switching to IgG, IgA, or IgE requires that the CD40 ligand on activated T cells engages CD40 on B cells. This is a critical first step in providing T cell help to antibody formation by B cells. This infant with a genetic defect in the CD40 ligand cannot effect isotype switching.

16.4 The child should be given intravenous gamma-globulin at regular monthly intervals to protect her against pyogenic infections. Intravenous gamma-globulin is virtually pure IgG. As this child is incapable of making IgG she will need lifelong infusions for passive protection. Intravenous gamma-globulin does not protect against intracellular microorganisms such as *P. carinii*. These and other microorganisms that reside in macrophages are eliminated by activating macrophages. Macrophages, like B cells, express CD40 and require interaction with the CD40 ligand on activated T cells to become highly microbicidal. This child therefore remains susceptible to recurrent *P. carinii* infection despite the gamma-globulin therapy. If it recurs she would need treatment again with pentamidine.

16.5 A normal result. The mother would exhibit random inactivation of her X chromosomes. In X-linked agammaglobulinemia non-random inactivation of B cells is observed in females who carry this X-linked disorder because the B cells that have the mutated *btk* gene cannot expand clonally; only the B cells carrying the normal allele can. The same is true in X-linked severe combined immunodeficiency (SCID). The T cells of heterozygous females which have a mutation in the common gamma chain cannot expand clonally; only the T cells with the normal allele can. The CD40 ligand is not required for clonal expansion of T cells. This molecule is only expressed when T cells are activated. Thus females who must be heterozygous for hyper-IgM immunodeficiency are immunologically normal and the clonal expansion of T cells bearing the wild-type allele and the mutated allele is normal.

16.6 It depends on the severity of the mutation in the child. If she has a missense mutation and expresses some mutated CD40 ligand on her activated T cell the prognosis is good if she continues to receive intravenous gamma-globulin. However, if her mutation results in an inability to express any CD40 ligand, her future is uncertain because these affected females usually develop an extensive polyclonal expansion of IgM-producing B cells that invade the liver and other parts of the gastrointestinal tract and cause fatal complications (see Fig. 16.4). In this case a bone marrow transplant from a histoidentical donor should be recommended as this would have a favorable outcome and would essentially be a cure of the disease.

17. SECONDARY IMMUNODEFICIENCY

17.1 Approximately 95% of HIV-positive individuals seroconvert within 3 months of infection. ELISAs for antibodies to gp41, an HIV surface glycoprotein, and p24, a core protein, are the most widely used to detect HIV infection. Confirmation is obtained by Western blot analysis to decrease the rate of false-positive results. The Centres for Disease Control and Prevention recommends that the

blot should be positive for two of the p24, gp41, and gp120/160 markers (gp160 is the precursor form of gp41 and gp120, the envelope protein). ELISAs for p24 antigen can also be used, though the false-negative rate is higher. The PCR is a technique for amplifying specific sequences of DNA or RNA to produce quantities that are readily detectable. The test in the context of HIV is highly sensitive and specific, but is more costly than ELISA techniques.

17.2 The mother's serological state should be tested by ELISA and confirmed by Western blot if positive. Around 20–30% of infants born to HIV-positive mothers are infected with the virus. Transmission can occur in utero or very rarely by breastfeeding. Diagnosis presents a problem because maternal IgG specific for HIV antigens crosses the placenta and can be detected in the infant even if the infant has not become infected. The presence of HIV-specific antibodies of IgA and IgM classes in the infant should imply infection because they do not cross the placenta. Current tests lack sensitivity and remain in development. The method most widely used in the UK and USA is the PCR, which demonstrates the virus directly. Below the age of 1 month the PCR may be negative in infected children. It has been shown that, in many children, HIV is sequestered into regional lymph nodes at this age. After establishing infection at these sites a viremia follows.

17.3 The figure shows the change in a variety of indices of HIV infection over time. Acute seroconversion causes an infectious mononucleosis-like illness in up to 50% of those infected with HIV. Common symptoms are fever, lymphadenopathy, pharyngitis, rashes, and myalgia. At this point there is a drop in the CD4 (and also CD8) lymphocyte count and a rise in plasma viremia and p24 antigen concentration. Antibodies to HIV surface glycoproteins gp120 and gp41 are produced from approximately 6 weeks after infection and are initially of the IgM class. IgG antibodies of the same specificities follow the IgM response and persist during the latent phase. Viremia

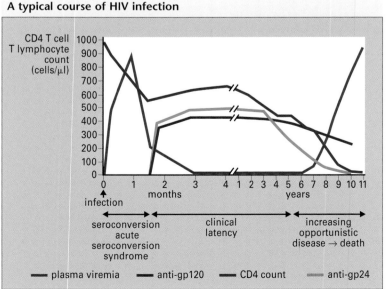

and p24 antigenemia are generally low during this period. Disease progression is heralded by a declining CD4 lymphocyte count and a rise in plasma viremia. Clinically, CD4 counts have become a widely used index of progression. Plasma viremia is the most accurate measure of disease progression, and is becoming a more commonly used method.

18. VACCINATION

18.1 Successful attenuation results in an organism still capable of generating an immune response against the wild-type virulent organism, but no longer capable of causing disease. This is a delicate balance to achieve. In some instances (e.g. hepatitis B and C viruses) the organisms cannot be cultured, so attenuation by repeated in-vitro passage is impossible.

18.2 There is no reason to believe that a vaccine cannot improve on nature. Many organisms express gene products that interfere with immune responses. Removal of these from the vaccine may allow protective responses to be generated.

18.3 Although smallpox was eliminated because there was no animal reservoir or carrier state, this is also the case for some other microorganisms and it should be possible to eliminate them. For other organisms, elimination will be difficult and maintenance of herd immunity will remain important.

18.4 Vaccines are unlikely ever to replace antibiotics completely. Microorganisms evolve very rapidly and vaccine production against complex organisms, such as mycobacteria, has proved very difficult. In addition, immunodeficient individuals and the elderly remain at risk even after vaccination.

18.5 BCG clearly has multiple effects. Specific immune responses to BCG antigens can be detected, but cell wall and other components of the bacterium have potent immunomodulatory effects. The efficacy of BCG as a vaccine has been suggested to depend on cross-reactions of BCG with environmental mycobacteria as well as *Mycobacterium tuberculosis* itself.

18.6 Strong immune responses may cause tissue damage in individuals with parasites already present. However, a vaccine that prevented establishment of infection would be unlikely to be damaging.

18.7 Antigens that induce T cell immunity may be useful vaccine antigens. Molecules that contribute to virulence, such as toxins, may be the best targets for vaccines. Because the genomes of many pathogens have been or are being sequenced, searching homologous gene products may identify potential targets.

19. TOLERANCE
Lineage commitment in thymocyte development

19.1 The presence of a constitutively active Lck molecule in developing thymocytes. This is revealed in the OT-1/dLGF experimental mouse.

19.2 The presence of a catalytically inactive Lck causes a massive reduction in the number of CD4 SP cells that are

selected in the AND mouse. There is a limited increase in the number of CD8 SP cells.

19.3 Yes, the results are consistent. Overexpression of Lck promotes CD4 cells and reduced expression of CD8 cells, regardless of the MHC restriction of the majority population of TCRs.

The molecular basis of activation-induced cell death (AICD)

19.4 AICD is mediated by signaling through the Fas pathway.

19.5 Activation of T cells with anti-CD3 fails to induce apoptosis in mice bearing defective Fas and FasL genes.

19.6 Despite having a defective FasL, the gld mouse has a normal Fas gene and ligation of this with the anti-Fas antibody is sufficient to cause apoptosis.

19.7 This is an important way of controlling immune homeostasis. If cells were to keep on proliferating after antigen encounter the lymph nodes would explode!

19.8 This is a good question! The answer is not yet known and obviously requires a lot more critical thinking.

The role of regulatory T cells in peripheral tolerance

19.9 This is because autoreactive lymphocytes exist as part of the normal T cell repertoire. CD25$^+$ cells clearly suppress these cells and prevent them from causing disease. Precisely how the CD25$^+$ cells work is not yet known.

19.10 It seems likely that these cells arise in the thymus. Comparison of groups A–D shows that CD25$^-$ thymocytes can cause disease and that their activity is normally regulated by CD25$^+$ thymocytes.

19.11 It looks like tissues such as the adrenal gland are relatively resistant to disease. This could be: (a) because the antigenic targets for autoimmune disease are more sequestered in these tissues; (b) because mechanisms that create immunologically privileged sites operate in these tissues to some extent.

20. AUTOIMMUNITY AND AUTOIMMUNE DISEASE

20.1 It is thought that free DNA filtered in the kidney fixes to the glomerular basement membrane and can then bind anti-DNA antibodies, which then form an immune complex in situ. Complement is then fixed, resulting in local damage.

20.2 This is a vexed question. Although DNA–anti-DNA complexes are found in tissues, efforts to find these complexes in the serum have failed. In addition, immunizing lupus-prone animals with DNA does not produce clinical lupus. However, introduction of transgenes encoding anti-ds DNA in mice can produce lupus.

20.3 A possible explanation is that the mononuclear–phagocyte system becomes saturated and is therefore unable to clear the soluble complexes, which are thought to be most likely pathogenic. It is also possible that the reduction in the complement receptors on red cells (complement receptor-1, CR1) might also predispose to poor clearance of complexes.

20.4 Over 95% of patients with SLE have ANA as the major autoantibody. Antibodies to extractable nuclear antigens are also seen, but much less frequently. Anti-dsDNA antibodies are the most specific to SLE because anti-single-stranded antibodies are found in a variety of other situations, such as other autoimmune disease, a variety of infections, and inflammatory conditions.

21. KIDNEY TRANSPLANTATION

21.1 There is a great shortage of donor organs. The supply of cadaveric organs depends on the deaths of healthy individuals and the willingness of their relatives to allow donation. In addition, the available organs are given to recipients with the best HLA tissue match. At random there is less than a 1 in 20 000 chance of finding a perfect match. In the case of kidney transplantation the blood group antigens must be taken into account. Mrs X is blood group B, which is uncommon (<10%), and will therefore have antibodies to tissues from blood group A donors. Blood group A is the most common blood group (about 45% of individuals).

21.2 Mrs X is HLA identical to her brother Fred and shares one HLA haplotype with her brother Gary. There is a 1 in 4 chance of siblings inheriting the same mendelian characteristics from their parents.

21.3 Like Mrs X and her brother Fred, Bert and Edna are HLA identical to each other. Of the five children of Mrs X, four have Mr X as their biological father. However, it is clear that Dave was fathered by a man other than Mr X! This is not uncommon. Approximately 5–10% of children may be like Dave!

21.4 HLA identical: Fred; HLA haplotype match: Anne, Bert, Chas, Dave, Gary; complete HLA mismatch: Mr X.

21.5 If only HLA matching is considered, Fred would be the best donor because there would be no HLA mismatch between the donor and recipient.

21.6 Mrs X is blood group B, and therefore has antibodies to blood group A, thus excluding Mr X, Anne, Bert, Edna, and Fred. Only Chas, Dave, and Gary would be suitable. Because Mrs X is Rhesus positive (has antigen D) she will not have anti-Rh antibodies, so typing for this blood group can be ignored in this instance.

21.7 Chas is first choice. He is HLA haplotype matched, he is ABO compatible, and is a young man. In general, younger kidneys last for longer than older kidneys, and younger people respond better to surgery. Gary might be considered. He too is haplotype identical and ABO compatible. In fact, in terms of his ABO blood group, being blood group O he is the 'universal donor', having no A or B blood group antigens on his tissues. However, he is older and therefore not an ideal donor. Dave is like his brother Chas, HLA haplotype identical and ABO compatible with his mother. However, he is only 15 years of age and minors are generally excluded from this kind of surgery.

21.8 The organ from Chas suffered hyperacute rejection. This is mediated by preformed antibodies in the recipient binding to antigens in the graft. The antibodies fix complement and initiate the process of graft thrombosis. Platelet aggregation in the blood vessels blocks blood flow and the graft dies from lack of oxygen (ischemia).

21.9 The main stimuli for antibodies that cause hyperacute rejection are rejection of a previous graft, blood transfusions, and multiple pregnancies by the same partner. Mrs X has had four children by the same father, Mr X, and is likely to have become sensitized towards class I HLA antigens that Mr X has but Mrs X does not possess. In this case antibodies to either HLA-A3 or HLA-B7 could have been responsible for the hyperacute rejection.

21.10 Cross-match tests are used to detect anti-donor antibodies before transplantation. These tests are becoming more and more sensitive, but occasionally an antibody in low titer may go undetected. It appears that the cross-match test used at the time of the transplantation failed to detect an antibody to a HLA class I antigen. Fortunately this seldom happens today and hyperacute rejection is now very rare.

21.11 There were three family members who were originally suitable for donation, Chas, Dave, and Gary. The kidney from Chas was transplanted and rejected by Mrs X. Gary is now 60 and is less attractive as a donor. In any case he shares the HLA-B14 antigen with Mr X, which, because Mrs X is sensitized to Mr X, may be a target for hyperacute rejection. The possibility that Mrs X has an antibody to HLA-B14 would have to be investigated very carefully! Dave has by now reached the age of majority and could be considered as a donor. He is HLA haplotype identical to his mother, and is ABO compatible. Furthermore, because he has a different father, Dave is less likely to express antigens that might be the target of hyperacute rejection. It seems that Dave would be the most suitable donor. You might like to consider the emotional pressure this puts on Dave, given the seriousness of his mother's condition and how his family are likely to react if he wants to change his mind about donation.

21.12 Triple immunosuppression is standard in most transplant centers. It consists of corticosteroids plus either ciclosporin or tacrolimus and either azathioprine or mycophenolate. Some centers add other agents such as anti-lymphocyte serum or a monoclonal antibody to T cells (OKT3).

21.13 About one-third of all transplant recipients suffer an episode of acute rejection in the first few weeks. This is mainly a cell-mediated immune response.

21.14 The anti-rejection therapy often used is to give three large doses of corticosteroid on three consecutive days (totaling 2–3 g of corticosteroid). This causes apoptosis (programmed cell death) of activated lymphocytes and stops the rejection episode very effectively. Other anti-rejection therapies are used, such as OKT3 anti-T cell monoclonal antibody.

21.15 Because of the immunosuppression, patients are more prone to infection. The immunosuppressive drugs used can be toxic, so a dose reduction or a change in medication may be required. In addition, transplant patients on high doses of immunosuppression may develop a post-transplant lymphoproliferative disorder caused by Epstein–Barr virus infection. Reduction of the dose usually helps. In the longer term transplant patients have a higher risk of cancer because of depressed immune surveillance.

21.16 Mrs X finally lost her kidney transplant to chronic rejection. This may involve both immunological and non-immunological damage. The damage initiates a repair process involving the production of growth factors in the graft. None of the drugs in current use controls this process very well, so although the doctors change drugs and doses it is very difficult to control chronic rejection.

22. IMMUNITY TO CANCERS

22.1 When animals are immunized prophylactically, an adaptive immune response to the tumors is generated. When the same animal is challenged with live cancer cells later, the pre-existing immune response is amplified rapidly and can eliminate the tumor challenge. In contrast, when a naive animal is challenged, the tumor has generally already grown to a considerable size by the time an immune response to it is generated. At the same time, this developing immune response is compromised by a number of immune downregulatory mechanisms (immunosuppressive cytokines, CD4$^+$ suppressor T cells, etc.) that get activated in a host with a growing tumor. Thus, even as the tumor keeps growing, the immune response to it is compromised, and the host succumbs to the tumor.

22.2 The immunity elicited by HSP preparations does not derive from the HSP molecules per se, but from the antigenic peptides chaperoned by them. The HSPs isolated from tumors are associated with antigenic tumor-specific peptides in addition to the normal non-immunogenic peptides. In contrast, HSPs isolated from normal tissues are associated with only the non-immunogenic, normal peptides. This difference accounts for the lack of immunogenicity of normal tissue-derived HSPs and immunogenicity of tumor-derived HSPs.

22.3 Tumor antigens have been defined by a number of methods, such as by their ability to elicit tumor rejection in animal models or by recognition by T cells or antibodies in animals or in patients with cancer. Altogether, tumor antigens may be classified into the following classes:
- differentiation antigens;
- cancer testes antigens;
- unique mutated antigens;
- common mutated antigens (including oncogene-encoded antigens);
- viral antigens; and
- heat-shock proteins (which act as carriers of all of the above categories of antigen).

22.4 Concomitant immunity is defined as the presence in a host of an anti-tumor immune response that is able to successfully eradicate a tumor at one site in the concomitant presence of another tumor, which is apparently unresponsive to it. This phenomenon is a dramatic demonstration of the two opposing forces in cancer immunity – the immune response to a growing cancer, and the subversion of that response.

22.5 Several observations can be cited in support of down-regulation of immune response in the tumor-bearing state, as follows:

(a) The phenomenon of concomitant immunity is clear evidence in this regard. Tumor-reactive and tumor-protective T cells can be isolated early during tumor growth. At a later stage, one can show the presence of immune-suppressive T cells in the same animal. The CD4$^+$CD25$^+$ regulatory T cells have also been shown to play a downregulatory influence on the anti-cancer immune response.

(b) The phenomenon that the same animal can reject a skin allograft while not rejecting a tumor expressing the same allo-MHC shows that there are local factors that make the tumor apparently resistant to the existing systemic anti-tumor immune response.

(c) The extensive murine and emerging clinical data that blocking of the CTLA-4 molecule (which transmits an inhibitory signal to activated T cells) leads to tumor regression or other forms of protection from tumor growth suggest strongly that the anti-tumor immune response in a cancer-bearing host is downregulated.

23. SEVERE ANAPHYLACTIC SHOCK

23.1 Traditionally, the term anaphylaxis has been used to describe a systemic clinical syndrome caused by IgE-mediated degranulation of mast cells and basophils. Susceptible individuals exposed to a sensitizing antigen produce specific IgE antibodies, which bind to high-affinity IgE receptors (FcεRI) found on mast cells and basophils. The receptor binds the Fc portion of the antibody, leaving the Fab binding sites available to interact with antigen. The avidity of this Fc binding reaction is high and therefore the dissociation of IgE from the receptors is slow, with a long half-life. On subsequent exposure, the antigen is bound by the IgE-receptor complexes, which causes receptor-mediated activation of the cells with release of preformed and de-novo synthesized mediators. Degranulation is rapid and completed within 30 minutes. These mediators, released on a large scale, are responsible for the clinical manifestations of anaphylaxis. The IgE-mediated mechanism of mast cell degranulation has been implicated in the pathogenesis of anaphylaxis triggered by a variety of agents. These include antibiotics (e.g. penicillins, cephalosporins), foods (e.g. milk, nuts, shellfish), foreign proteins (e.g. insulin, bee venom, latex), and pharmacological agents (e.g. streptokinase, vaccines). Patients who have anaphylaxis may or may not have a history of atopy. Natural exposure to common allergens such as pollen or dust mites is only very rarely a cause of anaphylaxis. However, when patients who also have asthma develop anaphylaxis due to venom, penicillin, or food antigens, the reactions are more dangerous because they can include rapid onset of bronchospasm.

Mast cell degranulation can occur by IgE-independent pathways. In these cases prior exposure is not a prerequisite because specific IgE antibodies are not involved. Three putative mechanisms of anaphylactoid reactions are given below.

- Blood, blood products, and immunoglobulins can cause an anaphylactoid reaction. The suggested mechanism is the formation of immune complexes with subsequent complement activation and production of C3a and C5a. Both of these complement components (anaphylatoxins) are capable of degranulating mast cells directly. In addition, both components increase vasopermeability and may induce hypotension.
- Certain therapeutic and diagnostic agents such as opiates, muscle relaxants, and contrast media are also capable of directly causing mast cell degranulation and anaphylaxis.
- 5–10% of asthmatic subjects produce a reaction to non-steroidal anti-inflammatory drugs (NSAIDs), such as aspirin or indometacin. Symptoms commonly include bronchospasm, rhinorrhea, and, rarely, vascular collapse. The ability of these agents to cause anaphylaxis appears to correlate with their effectiveness in inhibiting prostaglandin synthesis. The mechanism of this sensitivity is unknown, but increased leukotriene production occurs, which suggests that triggering of mast cells is part of the reaction.

23.2 There is a great variation in the timing and nature of anaphylactic symptoms. The onset is usually within seconds or minutes of exposure, though delays of an hour have been reported. The following are common presentations, which may occur singly or in combination:

- cutaneous – erythema, pruritus of hands, feet, and abdomen, urticaria, angioedema;
- respiratory – laryngeal edema causing hoarseness, which may progress to asphyxia, bronchoconstriction causing wheezing, rhinorrhea;
- cardiovascular – hypotension, arrhythmias, tachycardia, vascular collapse;
- gastrointestinal – cramping abdominal pain, nausea, vomiting, diarrhea.

The majority of cases of anaphylactic reaction are not fatal. It has been estimated that 1–2% of courses of penicillin therapy are complicated by systemic reactions, but only 10% of these are serious. In the USA some 400–800 people die annually from penicillin anaphylaxis, with a similar figure for contrast media – 70% of deaths result from respiratory complications (laryngeal edema and/or bronchospasm) with 25% resulting from cardiovascular dysfunction. Prompt treatment of anaphylaxis is essential because death may occur rapidly. The patient is placed in the recovery position, oxygen is given by mask, and 0.5–1.0 ml epinephrine 1:1000 w/v is injected intramuscularly. This has the effect of raising the blood pressure, relaxing bronchial smooth muscle, and preventing further mediator release. Intravenous antihistamines (e.g. 10 mg chlorpheniramine) can be useful because histamine can cause vasodilation, cardiac arrhythmias, and bronchospasm. Corticosteroids (e.g. 100 mg hydrocortisone) intravenously may help to reduce any late-phase response.

23.3 The first step is to obtain a thorough history of previous adverse reactions. The timing and nature of such reactions should be noted. Skin prick testing with insect venom is a fast and sensitive method of detecting anti-venom IgE. Radioallergosorbent tests can detect venom-specific IgE, but are positive in only 80% of those with significant reactions to venom skin prick tests. Immunotherapy is best reserved for those with life-threatening systemic reactions to insect venom. The patient is given increasing subcutaneous dosages and then a monthly maintenance dose of 100 μg. The clinical protection rate is in the order of 98% for both adults and children.

24. BLOOD GROUPS AND HEMOLYTIC DISEASE OF THE NEWBORN

24.1 Because Mrs Chareston has clearly becomed sensitized to Rhesus D, it is most likely that her first child is RhD⁺. The alternative explanation, that she has become sensitized by a blood transfusion, is highly unlikely, because of the routine matching of this blood group when carrying out transfusions.

24.2 HDNB usually becomes more serious with successive pregnancies because the mother has become sensitized to the fetal red cells and successive sensitizations produce progressively stronger responses in the mother, and more serious disease in susceptible children.

24.3 Anti-Rhesus D antibodies are given to the mother to clear the fetal RhD⁺ erythrocytes before they have a chance to sensitize the mother's immune system.

24.4 If the antibodies are given pre-partum, they would cross the placenta and produce or exacerbate HDNB in the fetus.

24.5 Rhesus prophylaxis is not always successful, but in this case there was no treatment after the first pregnancy and Mrs Chareston was already sensitized to RhD. Preventing further responses in an individual who is already sensitized is less likely to succeed because of the nature of secondary immune responses – less antigen is required to trigger the response.

24.6 The most likely explanation is that the child is Rh⁻. Indeed this turns out to be the case. A Rh⁻ child must have received a Rh⁻ gene from both parents. Assuming that Mr Chareston is the father of the fourth child, we can say that his genotype is RhD⁺/RhD⁻ (heterozygote), and that the child received RhD⁻ genes from both parents.

24.7 Antigens of the ABO blood group are carbohydrates and tend to induce IgM antibodies, which do not undergo affinity maturation or class switching (see Chapter 8). IgM does not cross the placenta (see Chapter 3) and so does not produce HDNB.

24.8 The second child was definitely not fathered by Mr Chareston because ABO blood groups are co-dominantly expressed. For a child to have the blood group B, one or both parents must have blood group B. As neither Mr or Mrs Chareston has this blood group, the B gene must have come from someone else.

24. TYPE II AHA OR AHA PLUS ITP WITH LUPUS

24.9 There is clinical evidence for a systemic disease, with arthritis, thrombocytopenia, anemia, and dermatitis. The positive Coombs' test indicates that there are serum antibodies to RBCs, and she also has anti-platelet antibodies. These circulating antibodies bind to cell surface antigens. When autoantibody–RBCs and autoantibody–platelets enter the liver and spleen, their Fc regions engage FcRs on resident macrophages, and are removed. This is a consuming process, which is accelerated by complement activation on the surface of RBCs and platelets, so that erythropoiesis and thrombopoiesis do not keep up with consumption, thus lowering the RBC and platelet counts.

Immune complex formation in the joints results from deposition of autoantibody–autoantigen complexes (e.g. anti-DNA antibody–nucleosome complexes). This is facilitated by altered vascular permeability. In-situ immune complex formation may also be operative, with free nucleosomes entering the joint space and binding to cell surface antigens or matrix components through charge–charge interactions. In either case the tissue-fixed immune complexes engage activating FcR (e.g. FcγIII) to initiate inflammation.

24.10 Because local vascular permeability in other tissues was not altered, so immune complexes and activated inflammatory cells could not traverse vessels walls (because of size restriction). Alternatively, because autoantibodies specific for either cell surface antigens or matrix components were not present, inflammation was not observed within them. In some cases immune deposits may form in tissues, but, because vascular permeability is not altered or/and inflammatory cells are not stimulated, inflammation is not observed.

24.11 Ideally one could target only those B cells that produce the autoantibodies, using therapy directed at the antigen binding regions of the antibodies. However, because the antigen-binding regions are likely to vary from patient to patient, designing therapy for each individual is impractical. More general immunosuppression (e.g. against B cells) is reasonable and should be initiated. Using drugs that alter the clearance of RBCs and platelets is also a good strategy and this could be accomplished by either enhancing the expression of the inhibitory FcRs or decreasing the clearance of the activating FcR. Intravenous immunoglobulin (IVIg) works through this mechanism and would be a reasonable therapeutic choice.

25. TYPE III SERUM SICKNESS AFTER FACTOR IX ADMINISTRATION

25.1 This is a classic example of serum sickness induced by a 'foreign protein' factor IX because the boy does not produce it.

25.2 Corticosteroids were prescribed to decrease inflammation and for immunosuppression.

25.3 The likelihood that this type of reaction will develop again is relatively high because a memory response will be produced; T cells and plasma cells will respond more rapidly during re-exposure to the same foreign antigen (i.e. factor IX).

25.4 Short courses of corticosteroids with/without transient immunosuppression.

25.5 In this case, the clinical presentation is associated with an apparent non-inflammatory process (inferred because there is only proteinuria and inflammation has not reduced the glomerular filtration rate). Although the precise pathogenesis is uncertain, it is thought that the administered factor IX gets modified (becomes more positively charged) in the circulation. Because of its charge, it becomes trapped during normal filtration between the negatively charged glomerular basement membrane and glomerular epithelial cells, where it serves as a 'planted antigen' for circulating anti-factor IX antibodies. The Fc regions of local or 'in-situ' formed immune complexes activate the classical complement system, whereby C5b–9 causes sublytic injury to the epithelial cells, leading to their detachment. Because these cells normally participate in maintaining the glomerular integrity and limiting protein filtration, this pathologic process causes loss of large amounts of protein in the urine. Inflammation is not observed because FcR engagement on circulating inflammatory cells is prevented by the intact basement membrane. Pathologically there is epithelial cell 'effacement' from the basement membrane, but a conspicuous absence of inflammation. By contrast, in acute serum sickness, when immune deposits form between the endothelium and the basement membrane (or on the basement membrane), the deposited IgG engages FcR on circulating cells, and inflammation (with cellular infiltration) is the predominant feature.

25.6 The likelihood that this type reaction will develop again is relatively high because a memory response will be produced; T cells and plasma cells will respond more rapidly during re-exposure to the same foreign antigen (i.e. factor IX).

25.7 Immunosuppression until the proteinuria resolves to treat the present episode. Because the probability of immunologic recall is high, transient immunosuppression with each factor IX therapy is indicated to reduce the production of antibodies to factor IX.

26. A HYPERSENSITIVITY TYPE IV REACTION

26.1 Granulomas are composed of lymphocytes, macrophages, and epithelioid cells. The latter develop from macrophages following chronic antigenic stimulation and may fuse to form multinucleate giant cells, typical of granulomas. Cytokines involved in this process include T cell-derived IFNγ and TNF, both for the activation of macrophages and for the organization of the granuloma.

26.2 Histological examination at the site of a DTH reaction reveals edema of the dermis with an infiltrate of monocytes and lymphocytes. This resolves over 1–2 weeks. Granulomas do not form at the sites of DTH reactions if soluble antigen, such as tuberculin, is used. By contrast, in the lymph node a chronic granulomatous response develops as the mycobacteria survive within macrophages, leading to persistent stimulation of T cells and chronic inflammation.

26.3 CD4 T lymphocytes are the major cells responsible for the recognition of soluble recall antigens and the stimulation of DTH reactions.

503

26.4 Other infections, such as cat scratch fever due to *Bartonella henselae*, histoplasmosis, and tularemia, may cause granulomas in lymph nodes. These are diagnosed by the clinical pattern and microbial cultures. Sarcoidosis causes non-caseating granulomas and is diagnosed by clinical features, histology, and the absence of an infectious cause. Granulomas may also develop in response to foreign bodies, such as talc and silica, or exposure to beryllium.

26.5 The brother's DTH reaction is evidence of a strong T cell response to soluble antigens from *M. tuberculosis*. This indicates that he has been infected with *M. tuberculosis*, but does not mean that he has active tuberculosis disease at present. Normally he would have investigations to exclude active tuberculosis, and if this is not present he would be considered for chemoprophylaxis to eradicate the infection and prevent progression to disease in later life.

Appendix

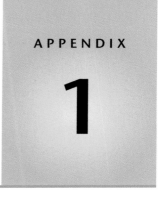
Major Histocompatibility Complex

The major histocompatibility complex (MHC) is the most polymorphic gene locus known in humans.

Originally the MHC class I and class II molecules from the principal loci (HLA-A, HLA-B, HLA-C, and HLA-D) were distinguished using specific antibodies, which could recognize polymorphic variants at these loci. For example, HLA-A2 identifies a particular variant at the HLA-A locus. These are termed serological HLA specificities.

Later it became clear that the HLA-D region contained several class II loci (HLA-DP, HLA-DQ, and HLA-DR), and that some serological specificities were specific for variants at these loci.

As serological analysis became more refined, it was found that some specificities could be subdivided into two or more types, using newer antibodies. For example, HLA-A9 is made up of two subgroups, HLA-A23 and HLA-A24.

In some cases the designation of the serologically defined MHC molecules was not fully certain, so they were given provisional or workshop designations 'w' (e.g. HLA-DPw1).

Later, sequence analysis of MHC genes was undertaken and the sequences could be related to the serological specificities. For example, the sequences termed HLA-B*1301, HLA-B*1302, HLA-B*1303, HLA-B*1304, HLA-B*1305, and HLA-B*1306 are six different sequences, all of which encode HLA-B molecules, which can be serologically defined by anti-HLA-B13 antibody.

Following the '*', the first two digits indicate the serological specificity, and the subsequent digits the sequence number associated with that specificity. Hence several genetic variants can have the same serological specificity.

Finally, an additional two-digit figure may be added to identify different alleles that generate synonymous variants.

The number of genetic variants is very large. A current list (January 2006) can be viewed at http://www.anthonynolan.com/HIG/lists. This site also gives information on the relationship of serological specificities and genetically defined variants.

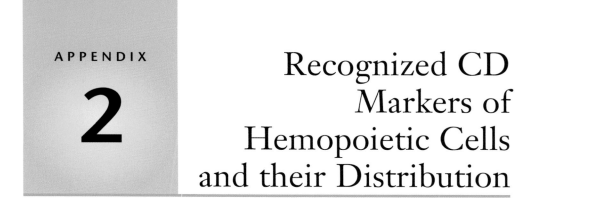

APPENDIX
2

Recognized CD Markers of Hemopoietic Cells and their Distribution

Filled box, molecule is expressed; open box, molecule not expressed or not determined yet; half-filled box, sub-population only

★, activated cells only

B, basophil; G, granulocyte; B, B cell; Carb, carbo-hydrate; CCP, complement control protein domains; Clec, C-type lectin; CytR, hemopoietic cytokine receptor family; DC, dendritic cell; Ect, ectoenzyme; End, endothelium; Eo, eosinophil; IgSF, immunoglobulin supergene family; Intα, integrin alpha chain; Intβ, integrin beta chain; LC, Langerhans' cell; LSC, lymphoid stem cell; M, mononuclear phagocyte lineage; MC, mast cell; MSC, myeloid stem cell; Muc, mucin; N, neutrophil; FDC, follicular dendritic cell; NK, natural killer cell; P, platelet; Thy, thymocyte; p, precursor; RBC, red blood cell; RTK, receptor tyrosine kinase; TM4, tetramembrane pass family; PC, plasma cell; TM7, seven- transmembrane pass; G protein- coupled receptor; SC, stem cell; TNF, TNF-like; Scav, scavenger receptors; TNFR, TNF receptor/NGF receptor family; Sial, sialoglycan; T, T cell; ZnMP, zinc metalloproteinase.

This gives principal family relationships only. Some molecules are composite. The designation 'w' (workshop) indicates a provisional assignment. Detailed information on many of the CD molecules is distributed as 'CD guides' from http://www.ncbi.nlm.nih.gov/prow. A further set of CD numbers were assigned at the 7th International Workshop in June 2000, numbered CD167–CD247. Minor refinements and corrections were also made to existing designations. The new designations can be seen at http://gryphon.jr2.ox.ac.uk/.

Recognized CD markers of hemopoietic cells and their distribution

CD	identity/function	family	mol. wt (kDa)	T cell	B cell	NK cell	monocyte/macrophage	granulocyte	platelet	dendritic cell	other
CD1a	presentation of lipids/glycolipids	IgSF	49	Thy						LC	
CD1b	presentation of lipids/glycolipids	IgSF	45	Thy						LC	
CD1c	presentation of lipids/glycolipids	IgSF	43	Thy						DC	
CD1d	presentation of lipids/glycolipids	IgSF	55	Thy							
CD1e	presentation of lipids/glycolipids	IgSF	50								
CD2	LFA-3 receptor (adhesion)	IgSF	50								
CD3	TCR signaling complex (γ,δ,ε) (ζ,υ)	IgSF IgSF	25,20,19, 16,22								
CD4	MHC class II receptor	IgSF	55								
CD5	co-stimulator (activation)	Scav	67								
CD6	co-stimulator (activation)	Scav	105								
CD7	signal transduction	IgSF	40								
CD8	MHC class I receptor	IgSF	36,32								
CD9	platelet activation	TM4	24		p			Eo, B			LSC
CD10	neutral endopeptidase	ZnMP	100	p	p						
CD11a	LFA-1	Intα	180								
CD11b	CR3	Intα	165								

Continued

509

Listing of all recognized serological and cellular HLA specificities—cont'd

CD	identity/function	family	mol. wt (kDa)	T cell	B cell	NK cell	monocyte/ macrophage	granulocyte	platelet	dendritic cell	other
CD11c	CR4	Intα	150								
CDw12		P-prot	120					Eo, N			
CD13	aminopeptidase N	ZnMP	150								End
CD14	LPS-binding protein receptor		53–55								
CD15	sialyl Lewis	Carb									
CD16	FcγRIIIA/FcγRIIIB	IgSF	50–65								
CD16b	FcγRIIIB	IgSF	48								
CDw17	lactosyl ceramide	Carb	120								
CD18	LFA-1/CR3/CR4	Intβ	95								
CD19	B cell co-receptor subunit	IgSF	95								FDC
CD20	Ca²⁺ channel	TM4	33–37								
CD21	CR2 B cell co-receptor subunit	CCP	140								FDC
CD22	adhesion molecule	IgSF	130–140								
CD23	FcεRII	Clec	45		★		★	Eo			
CD24	co-stimulator (activation)		41,38								
CD25	IL-2R	CytR	55	★	★						
CD26	dipeptidyl peptidase IV		120	★	★						
CD27	binds CD70	TNFR	55								
CD28	binds CD80, CD86	IgSF	44								
CD29	VLA-1–VLA-6	Intβ	130								

CD	Function	Family	MW	Expression/notes
CD30	signal transduction (apoptosis)	TNFR	120	★ ★ ★
CD31	PECAM-1	IgSF	140	End
CD32	FcγRII	IgSF	40	
CD33		IgSF	67	MSC
CD34	binds L-selectin	Muc	105–120	End MSC
CD35	CR1	CCP	160–260	Eo N; FDC
CD36	adhesion molecule	Scav	88	End
CD37	signal transduction (activation)	TM4	40–52	
CD38	ribosyl cyclase	Ect	45	PC; ★ ★; LSC
CD39	ecto-apyrose	Ect	70–100	★ ★; FDC
CD40	binds CD154, co-stimulatory	TNFR	48	FDC
CD41	GPIIb adhesion to matrix	Intα	120,25	
CD42a	GPIX adhesion		23	
CD42b	GPIbα adhesion		135,23	
CD42c	GPIbβ adhesion		22	
CD42d	GPV adhesion	85		
CD43	leukosialin (anti-adhesive)	Muc	95	
CD44	Pgp-1 adhesion to matrix		80–95	
CD45	leukocyte common antigen (LCA)		200	

Continued

511

Listing of all recognized serological and cellular HLA specificities—*cont'd*

CD	identity/function	family	mol. wt (kDa)	T cell	B cell	NK cell	monocyte/ macrophage	granulocyte	platelet	dendritic cell	other
CD45RA	restricted LCA		220								
CD45RB	restricted LCA		190,205								
CD45RO	restricted LCA		190								
CD46	MCP (membrane cofactor protein)	CCP	66,56								
CD47		IgSF	47–52								
CD48	binds CD2 (rodents)	IgSF	41								
CD49a	VLA-1 adhesion to matrix	Intα	210	★							
CD49b	VLA-2 adhesion to matrix	Intα	160								
CD49c	VLA-3 adhesion to matrix	Intα	125								
CD49d	VLA-4 adhesion	Intα	150,80,70							LC	
CD49e	VLA-5 adhesion to matrix	Intα	135,25								
CD49f	VLA-6 adhesion to matrix	Intα	120,25								
CD50	ICAM-3	IgSF	124								
CD51	vitronectin receptor α	Intα	120,24								
CD52	Campath-1		21–28								
CD53	signal transduction	TM4	32–40								
CD54	ICAM-1	IgSF	75–115							LC	
CD55	DAF (decay accelerating factor)	CCP	70								

CD	Description	Family	MW (kDa)	Notes
CD56	NCAM (neural cell adhesion molecule)	IgSF	220,135	
CD57	HNK-1	Carb	110	
CD58	LFA-3 binds CD2	IgSF	40–65	
CD59	protectin inhibits MAC		19	
CDw60	NeuAc-NeuAc-Gal	Carb		
CD61	vitronectin receptor subunit	Intβ	105	End
CD62E	E-selectin	Clec	115	★End
CD62L	L-selectin	Clec	75–80	
CD62P	P-selectin	Clec	150	★End
CD63	adapter	TM4	53	End
CD64	FcγRI	IgSF	70	
CD65	ceramide dodecasaccharide	Carb		
CD66a	BGB-1 adhesion	IgSF	180–200	
CD66b	was CD67 adhesion	IgSF	95–100	
CD66c	NCA adhesion	IgSF	90–95	
CD66d	CGM1	IgSF	30	
CD66e	CEA (carcinoembryonic antigen)	IgSF	180–200	
CD66f	pregnancy-specific glycoprotein	IgSF	54–72	
CD68	macrosialin	Scav	110	N, B; MC Sav
CD69	activation induction	Clec	32,28	Thy

Continued

Listing of all recognized serological and cellular HLA specificities—cont'd

CD	identity/function	family	mol. wt (kDa)	T cell	B cell	NK cell	monocyte/ macrophage	granulocyte	platelet	dendritic cell	other
CD70	binds CD27	TNF	175,95,75	★	★		★				
CD71	transferrin receptor		95	★	★	★	★				★
CD72		Clec	43,39								
CD73	ecto-5′-nucleotidase	Ect	69								End FDC
CD74	Ii (MHC class II invariant chain)		41,35,33								
CD75	Lactosamine	Carb									
CD75s	α-2,6 sialyl lactosamine	Carb									
CD77	globotriaosylceramide	Carb									
CD79a	Igα	IgSF	33								
CD79b	Igβ	IgSF	39								
CD80	B7-1, binds CD28 and CD152	IgSF	60	★	★						
CD81	TAPA B cell co-receptor unit	TM4	26								End
CD82	signal transduction	TM4	60								
CD83	? antigen presentation	IgSF	43								
CDw84	? co-stimulation	IgSF	74								
CD85											
CD86	B7-2 binds CD28 and CD152	IgSF	80		★						
CD87	urokinase plasminogen activator		35–39								

CD	Description	Family	MW (kDa)								MC
CD88	C5αR	TM7	43								
CD89	FcαR	IgSF	50–70								
CD90	Thy-1	IgSF	25–35	Thy							
CD91	α2-macroglobulin receptor	LDLR	515,85								
CD92			70					N			End
CD93			120					N			End
CD94	binds MHC class I	Clec	70								
CD95	Fas signal transduction (apoptosis)	TNFR	43	★	★						
CD96		IgSF	160	★							
CD97	binds CD55	EGFR	75–85	★	★						
CD98	modulates intracellular Ca²⁺		80,45								
CD99		Muc	32								
CD100	? proliferation	IgSF	150	★							
CD101		IgSF	120								
CD102	ICAM-2 binds LFA-1	IgSF	55,65								End
CD103	αEb7 integrin	Intα	150,25								
CD104	β4 integrins	Intβ	220								End
CD105	endoglin binds TGFβ		90				★				End
CD106	VCAM-1 binds VLA-4	IgSF	90–110								End
CD107a	LAMP-1		110	★				★	★		★End
CD107b	LAMP-2		120	★				★	★		★End

Continued

515

Listing of all recognized serological and cellular HLA specificities—cont'd

CD	identity/function	family	mol. wt (kDa)	T cell	B cell	NK cell	monocyte/ macrophage	granulocyte	platelet	dendritic cell	other
CD108	? adhesion		80								
CD109	platelet activation factor		170	★					★		End
CD114	G-CSFR		110–130					N			
CD115	M-CSFR	IgSF	150–130								
CD116	GM-CSFR α chain	CytR	60					N, Eo			
CD117	c-kit stem cell factor receptor	IgSF	145	Thy							SC
CD118	IFNα/β receptor										
CD119	IFNγ receptor		90–100								
CD120a	TNFR-I	TNFR	60								
CD120b	TNFR-II	TNFR	75–85								
CD121a	IL-1R type I	IgSF	80								End
CDw121b	IL-1R type II	IgSF	60–70								
CD122	IL-2R β chain	CytR	75								
CD123	IL-3R	CytR	70								SC
CD124	IL-4R	CytR	130–150								
CD125	IL-5R	CytR	55–60		★			Eo, B			
CD126	IL-6R	IgSF	80		★						End
CD127	IL-7R		68–80		Pre B						LSC
CD128	IL-8R chemokine receptor CXCR1	TM7	58								
CD130	IL-6R, IL-11R common subunit	IgSF	130		★						

CD	Description	Family	MW							Expr
CDw131	IL-3R, IL-5R common subunit	CytR	140							SC
CD132	IL-2R, IL-4R, IL-7R, IL-4R, IL-15R common subunit	CytR	64							
CD133	AC133		120							SC
CD134	? adhesion molecule	TNFR	50	★						
CD135	growth factor receptor		155,130		p		p			SC
CDw136	macrophage-stimulating protein receptor	180								
CDw137	co-stimulatory (activation)	TNFR	30							
CD138	syndecan binds type I collagen									
CD139			228,209							FDC
CD140	PDGF receptor		180,180							End
CD141	thrombomodulin	Clec	105			N				End
CD142	tissue factor procoagulant		46							
CD143	ACE (angiotensin converting enzyme)	ZnMP	170–180	★				★		End
CD144	VE-cadherin adhesion		135							End
CDw145			110,90,25							End
CD146	? adhesion	IgSF	130	★						End
CD147	neurothelin, basigin ? adhesion	IgSF	55–65							End
CD148	contact inhibition		250							

Continued

Listing of all recognized serological and cellular HLA specificities—cont'd

CD	identity/function	family	mol. wt (kDa)	T cell	B cell	NK cell	monocyte/ macrophage	granulocyte	platelet	dendritic cell	other
CDw149	≡ CD47	IgSF	47–52								
CDw150	SLAM ? co-stimulation		75–95	Thy							End
CD151	PETA3 ? signaling (adhesion)	TM4	32								End
CD152	CTLA-4 binds CD80 and CD86	IgSF	33	★							
CD153	CD30L binds CD30	TNF	38–40	★			★				
CD154	CD40L binds CD40	TNF	32–39	★							
CD155	polio virus receptor	IgSF	80–90	Thy							
CD156	ADAM8	ZnMP	60–70					N			
CD157	ADP-ribosyl cyclase	Ect	42–50		p						FDC End
CD158a	p58.1,p50.1 binds MHC class I (KIR)	IgSF	58,50								
CD158b	p58.2,p50.2 binds MHC class I (KIR)	IgSF	58,50								
CD159			43								
CD160			26								
CD161	NKRP-1 modulates cytotoxicity	Clec	44								
CD162	PSGL-1 binds selectins	Muc	240								
CD163	M130	Scav	130								
CD164	MGC-24 adhesion to stromal cells	Muc	80								
CD165	AD2 adhesion to thymic epithelium		37	Thy							SC
CD166	ALCAM binds CD6	IgSF	100	★			★				

CD	Name	Family	MW							
CD167a	DDR1	RTK	120							
CD168	RHAMM		84–88	Thy			N			
CD169	Sialoadhesin	Siglec	185							
CD170	Siglec-5	Siglec	140							
CD171	L1	FN/IgSF	200							
CD172a			110							SC
CD173	Blood gr. H (2)	Carb								
CD174	Lewis Y	Carb								SC
CD175	TN	Carb								SC
CD175s	Sialyl-TN	Carb								RBC
CD176	Thomson-Fr. Antigen	Carb								RBC
CD177	NB1		56–62							
CD178	Fas ligand	TNF	38–42	★	p		N			
CD179a	V pre beta	IgSF	16		p					
CD179b	Lambda-5	IgSF	22							
CD180	Rp105/Bgp95	TLR	95–105							
CD183	CXCR3	TM7	40	★		★				End
CD184	CXCR4	TM7	45							
CD195	CCR5	TM7	45							
CDw197	CCR7	TM7	45							
CD200	Ox-2		45–50	★						
CD201	EPCR	Ect	50							End

Continued

Listing of all recognized serological and cellular HLA specificities—cont'd

CD	identity/function	family	mol. wt (kDa)	T cell	B cell	NK cell	monocyte/ macrophage	granulocyte	platelet	dendritic cell	other
CD202b	TEL/Tie2	RTK	150								SC, End
CD203c	E-NPP3	Ect	130–150					B	MegaK		
CD204	Macrophage Scavenger R.	Scav	220								
CD205	DEC205	Clec	205								
CD206	Macrophage mannose R.	Clec	180								
CD207	Langerin	Clec	40							LC	
CD208	DC-LAMP	Clec	70–90								
CD209	DC-SIGN		44								
CD210	IL-10R		90–110								
CD212	IL-12R		100	★		★					
CD213a1	IL-13R A1		65								
CD213a2	IL-13R A2		65								
CD217	IL-17R		120								
CD220	Insulin receptor	RTK	140 + 70								
CD221	IgF1 receptor	RTK	140 + 70								
CD222	IgF2 receptor		250								
CD223	LAG3	IgSF	70	★		★					
CD224	γ-glutamyl transferase	Ect	27, 68								
CD225	Leu13		17								
CD226	DNAM-1	IgSF	65								
CD227	MUC1	Muc	300								
CD228	Melanotransferrin		80–95								SC

CD	Name	Family	MW	Cell
CD229	Ly-9	IgSF	95, 110	
CD230	PrPc		35	
CD231	TALLA-1	TM4	30–45	
CD232	VESPR		200	
CD233	Band3		90	RBC
CD234	Duffy	TM7	35–45	RBC
CD235a	Glycophorin-A		36	RBC
CD235b	Glycophorin-B		20	RBC
CD236	Glycophorin-CD		32/23	RBC
CD236R	Glycophoein-X		32	RBC
CD238	Kell		93	RBC
CD239	Lutheran		78–85	RBC
CD240CE	Rhesus CE		30–32	RBC
CD240D	Rhesus D		30–32	RBC
CD241	Rhesus 50gp		50	RBC
CD242	ICAM-4	IgSF	42	RBC
CD243	MDR1		180	RBC
CD244	2B4	IgSF	70	SC
CD245	P220/240		220–240	
CD246		RTK	80	
CD247			16	

For the most recent additions to the list of recognized CD markers, see Protein Reviews on the Web at http://mpr.nci.nih.gov/prow.

The Major Cytokines

cytokine	immune system source	other cells	principal targets	principal effects
IL-1α IL-1β	macrophages, LGLs, B cells	endothelium, fibroblasts, astrocytes, etc.	T cells, B cells, macrophages, endothelium, tissue cells	lymphocyte activation, macrophage stimulation, ↑ leukocyte/endothelial adhesion, pyrexia, acute phase proteins
IL-2	T cells		T cells	T cell proliferation and differentiation, activation of cytotoxic lymphocytes and macrophages
IL-3	T cells	stem cells		multilineage colony stimulating factor
IL-4	T cells		B cells, T cells	B cell growth factor, isotype selection, IgE, IgG1
IL-5	T cells		B cells	B cell growth and differentiation, IgA selection
IL-6	T cells, B cells	fibroblasts, macrophages	B cells, hepatocytes	B cell differentiation, induces acute phase proteins
IL-7		bone marrow stromal cells	pre-B cells, T cells	B cell and T cell proliferation
IL-8	monocytes	fibroblasts	neutrophils, basophils, T cells, keratinocytes	chemotaxis, angiogenesis, superoxide release, granule release
IL-9	T cells			enhances T cell survival, mast cell activation, synergy with erythropoietin
IL-10	T cells		TH1 cells	inhibition of cytokine synthesis
IL-11		bone marrow stromal cells, fibroblasts	hemopoietic progenitors, osteoclasts	osteoclast formation, colony stimulating factor, elevates platelet count in vivo, inhibits proinflammatory cytokine production
IL-12		monocytes	T cells	induction of TH1 cells
IL-13	activated T cells		monocytes, B cells	B cell growth and differentiation, inhibits proinflammatory cytokine production
IL-14	T cells			stimulates proliferation of activated B cells, inhibits Ig secretion
IL-15	monocytes	epithelium, muscle	T cells, activated B cells	proliferation

cytokine	immune system source	other cells	principal targets	principal effects
IL-16	eosinophils, CD8$^+$ T cells		CD4$^+$ T cells	chemoattraction of CD4$^+$ cells
IL-17	CD4$^+$ T lymphocytes		epithelium, fibroblasts, endothelium	release of IL-6, IL-8, G-CSF, PGE$_2$, enhances ICAM-1, stimulates fibroblasts to sustain CD34$^+$ progenitors
IL-18	macrophages	hepatocytes, keratinocytes	PBMC, co-factor in TH1 induction	induces IFNγ production, enhances NK activity
IL-21	T cells, mast cells		T cells, B cells, mast cells, eosinophils, hepatocytes	induces acute phase reactants, levels raised after LPS
IL-22	activated T cells		TH2 cells	inhibits IL-4 production
TGFβ1			most cell types	downregulates inflammatory cytokine production, promotes wound healing responses and scar tissue, growth inhibition
TNFα	macrophages, mast cells, lymphocytes		macrophages, granulocytes, tissue cells	activation of macrophages, granulocytes and cytotoxic cells, leukocyte/endothelial cell adhesion, cachexia, pyrexia, induction of acute phase protein, stimulation of angiogenesis, enhanced MHC class I production
TNFβ (LT)	lymphocytes			as for TNFα
IFNα	leukocytes	epithelia, fibroblasts	tissue cells	MHC class I induction, antiviral state, stimulation of NK cells, antiproliferative, stimulates IL-12 production and TH1 cells
IFNβ	fibroblasts, epithelia		tissue cells, leukocytes	MHC class I induction, antiviral state, antiproliferative
IFNγ	T cells, NK cells	epithelia, fibroblasts	leukocytes, tissue cells, TH2 cells	MHC class I and II induction, macrophage activation, $\uparrow$ endothelial cell/lymphocyte adhesion, MØ cytokine synthesis, antiviral state, antiproliferative (TH1 cells)
M-CSF	monocytes	endothelium, fibroblasts		proliferation of macrophage precursors
G-CSF	macrophages	fibroblasts	stem cells	stimulates division and differentiation
GM-CSF	T cells, macrophages	endothelium, fibroblasts		proliferation of granulocyte and macrophage precursors and activators
MIF	T cells, macrophages		macrophages	migration inhibition, macrophage activation, enhances T cell activation

Human Chemokines and their Receptors

The table below lists the major human chemokine receptors and their principal ligands. Individual chemokines (e.g. CCL5, RANTES) often bind to more than one receptor. Similarly, individual receptors (e.g. CXCL1) often bind to more than one chemokine. The systematic nomenclature has now superceded the descriptive names, although the older names are widespread in the scientific literature and are still sometimes encountered in recent papers. The table lists only the most-frequently used names; some chemokines have several names.

BCA, B cell attracting chemokine; BRAK, breast and kidney expressed chemokine; CTACK, cutaneous T cell attracting chemokine; ENA, epithelial-cell derived neutrophil activating protein; GCP, granulocyte chemotactic protein; Gro, growth related oncogene; HCC, hemofiltrate CC-chemokine; I-309, inducible protein-309; IL-8, interleukin-8; IP-10, inducible protein-10; I-TAC, inducible T cell α chemoattractant; LARC, liver and activation regulated chemokine; MCP, monocyte chemotactic protein; MDC, macrophage-derived chemokine; MEC, mammary enriched chemokine; Mig, monokine induced by interferon-γ; MIP, macrophage inflammatory protein; NAP, neutrophil activating peptide; MPIF, myeloid progenitor inhibitory factor; PARC, pulmonary and activation regulated chemokine; PF4, platelet factor-4; RANTES, regulated on activation, normal T cell expressed and secreted; SCM, single-C-motif; SDF, stromal cell-derived factor; SLC, secondary lymphoid tissue chemokine; TARC, thymus and activation regulated chemokine; TECK, thymus-expressed chemokine.

Chemokine	Name	Receptors, CCL1–CCL10									
		1	2	3	4	5	6	7	8	9	10
CCL1	I-309								∎		
CCL2	MCP-1	∎	∎								
CCL3	MIP-1α				∎						
CCL4	MIP-1β								∎		
CCL5	RANTES			∎	∎						
CCL7	MCP-3		∎								
CCL8	MCP-2		∎								
CCL11	Eotaxin	∎									
CCL13	MCP-4	∎									
CCL14	HCC-1	∎									
CCL15	MIP-1δ	∎									
CCL16	HCC-4	∎	∎								
CCL17	TARC				∎						
CCL18	PARC			∎					∎		
CCL19	MIP-3β							∎			

Chemokine	Name	Receptors, CCL1–CCL10									
		1	2	3	4	5	6	7	8	9	10
CCL20	MIP-3α						X				
CCL21	6Ckine							X			
CCL22	MDC										
CCL23	MPIF-1	X									
CCL24	Eotaxin-2			X							
CCL25	TECK									X	
CCL26	Eotaxin-3		X	X							X
CCL27	CTACK										
CCL28	MEC			X							X

Chemokine	Name	Receptors CXCR1-6					
		1	2	3	4	5	6
CXCL1	Groα		X				
CXCL2	Groβ		X				
CXCL3	Groγ		X				
CXCL4	PF4			X			
CXCL5	ENA-78	X					
CXCL6	GCP-2	X					
CXCL7	NAP-2		X				
CXCL8	IL-8	X	X				
CXCL9	Mig			X			
CXCL10	IP-10			X			
CXCL11	ITAC			X			
CXCL12	SDF-1				X		
CXCL13	BCA-1					X	
CXCL14	BRAK						
CXCL16	–						X

Chemokine	Name	Receptor
XCL1	Lymphotactin	XCR1
XC:2	SCM-1b	XCR1
CX3CL1	Fractalkine	CX3CR1

Glossary

Acquired immune deficiency syndrome (AIDS). A progressive immune deficiency caused by infection of CD4 T cells with the human retrovirus HIV.

Activation-induced cytidine deaminase (AID). An enzyme expressed in activated B cells that causes somatic mutation in the immunoglobulin gene locus.

Acute phase proteins. Serum proteins whose levels increase during infection or inflammatory reactions.

ADCC (antibody-dependent cell-mediated cytotoxicity). A cytotoxic reaction in which Fc receptor-bearing killer cells recognize target cells via specific antibodies.

Adhesion molecules. Cell surface molecules involved in the binding of cells to extracellular matrix or to neighboring cells, where the principal function is adhesion rather than cell activation (e.g. integrins and selectins).

Adjuvant. A substance that non-specifically enhances the immune response to an antigen.

AFCs (antibody-forming cells). Functionally equivalent to plasma cells.

Affinity. A measure of the binding strength between an antigenic determinant (epitope) and an antibody-combining site.

Affinity maturation. The increase in average antibody affinity frequently seen during a secondary immune response.

Allelic exclusion. Occurs when the use of a gene from the maternal or paternal chromosome prevents the use of the other. This is seen with antibody and T cell receptor genes.

Allergen. An agent (e.g. pollen, dust, animal dander) that causes IgE-mediated hypersensitivity reactions.

Allergy. Originally defined as altered reactivity on second contact with antigen; now usually refers to a type I hypersensitivity reaction.

Allotype. The protein of an allele that may be detectable as an antigen by another member of the same species.

Alternative pathway. The activation pathways of the complement system involving C3 and factors B, D, P, H, and I, which interact in the vicinity of an activator surface to form an alternative pathway C3 convertase.

Amplification loop. The alternative complement activation pathway that acts as a positive feedback loop when C3 is split in the presence of an activator surface.

Anaphylatoxins. Complement peptides (C3a and C5a) that cause mast cell degranulation and smooth muscle contraction.

Anaphylaxis. An antigen-specific immune reaction mediated primarily by IgE that results in vasodilation and constriction of smooth muscle, including those of the bronchus, and may result in death.

Anergy. Failure to make an immune response following stimulation with a potential antigen.

Antagonist peptides. Analogs of antigenic peptides that bind to MHC molecules and prevent stimulation of specific clones of T cells.

Antibody. A molecule produced by animals in response to antigen that has the particular property of combining specifically with the antigen that induced its formation.

Antigen. A molecule that reacts with preformed antibody and the specific receptors on T and B cells.

Antigen receptors. The lymphocyte receptors for antigens including the T cell receptor (TCR) and surface immuno-globulin on B cells, which acts as the B cell's antigen receptor (BCR).

Antigen presentation. The process by which certain cells in the body (antigen-presenting cells) express antigen on their cell surface in a form recognizable by lymphocytes.

Antigen processing. The conversion of an antigen into a form in which it can be recognized by lymphocytes.

Antigenic determinants. See 'epitopes'.

Antigenic peptides. Peptide fragments of proteins that bind to MHC molecules and induce T cell activation.

Antiviral proteins. Proteins whose synthesis is induced by interferons. They become activated if the cell is infected by virus and limit viral replication.

APCs (antigen-presenting cells). A variety of cell types that carry antigen in a form that can stimulate lymphocytes.

Apoptosis. Programmed cell death that involves nuclear fragmentation and condensation of cytoplasm, plasma membranes, and organelles into apoptotic bodies.

Arthus reaction. Inflammation seen in the skin some hours following injection of antigen. It is a manifestation of a type III hypersensitivity reaction.

Atopy. The clinical manifestation of type I hypersensitivity reactions, including eczema, asthma, rhinitis, and food allergy.

Autocrine. This refers to the ability of a cytokine to act on the cell that produced it.

Autoimmunity. Immune recognition and reaction against the individual's own tissue.

Avidity. The functional combining strength of an antibody with its antigen, which is related to both the affinity of the reaction between the epitopes and paratopes, and the valencies of the antibody and antigen.

β_2-Microglobulin. A polypeptide that constitutes part of some membrane proteins including the class I MHC molecules.

B7-1 (CD80), B7-2 (CD86). Two molecules that are present on antigen-presenting cells. They ligate CD28 on T cells and act as powerful co-stimulatory signals.

B cells. Lymphocytes that develop in the bone marrow in adults and produce antibody. They can be subdivided into two groups, B1 and B2. B1 cells use minimally mutated receptors, which are close to the germline immunoglobulin sequences, whereas B2 cells are the major responding population in conventional immune responses to protein antigens.

B cell co-receptor complex. A group of cell surface molecules consisting of complement receptor type 2 (CD21), CD81, and CD19, which act as a co-stimulatory receptor on mature B cells.

B cell receptor complex (BCR). B cell surface immunoglobulin and its associated signaling molecules, CD79a and CD79b.

Basophil. A population of polymorphonuclear leukocytes that stain with basic dyes and have important roles in the control of inflammation.

BCG (bacille Calmette–Guérin). An attenuated strain of *Mycobacterium tuberculosis* used as a vaccine, an adjuvant, or a biological response modifier in different circumstances.

Bcl-2. A molecule expressed transiently on activated B cells that have been rescued from apoptosis.

Biozzi mice. Lines of mice bidirectionally bred to produce low or high antibody responses to a variety of antigens (originally sheep erythrocytes).

Blood groups. Sets of allelically variable molecules expressed on red cells and sometimes other tissues that may be the target of transfusion reactions.

Bradykinin. A vasoactive nonapeptide that is the most important mediator generated by the kinin system.

Bursa of Fabricius. A lymphoepithelial organ that is the site of B cell maturation and is found at the junction of the hindgut and cloaca in birds.

Bystander lysis. Complement-mediated lysis of cells in the immediate vicinity of a complement activation site that are not themselves responsible for the activation.

C domains. The constant domains of antibody and the T cell receptor. These domains do not contribute to the antigen-binding site and show relatively little variability between receptor molecules.

C genes. The gene segments that encode the constant portion of the immunoglobulin heavy and light chains and the α, β, γ, and δ chains of the T cell antigen receptor.

c-Kit (CD117). A receptor for stem cell factor, which is required for the early development of leukocytes.

C1–C9. The components of the complement classical and lytic pathways, which are responsible for mediating inflammatory reactions, opsonization of particles, and lysis of cell membranes.

C3 convertases. The enzyme complexes C3b,Bb and C4b2a that cleave complement C3.

Capping. A process by which cell surface molecules are caused to aggregate (usually using antibody) on the cell membrane.

Carrier. An immunogenic molecule or part of a molecule that is recognized by T cells in an antibody response.

Caspases. A group of enzymes that are particularly involved in the transduction of signals for apoptosis.

Cathelicidins. A group of cytotoxic peptides produced by granulocytes.

CD markers. Cell surface molecules of leukocytes and platelets that are distinguishable with monoclonal antibodies and may be used to differentiate different cell populations.

CDRs (complementarity determining regions). The sections of an antibody or T cell receptor V region responsible for antigen or antigen–MHC molecule binding.

Cell adhesion molecules (CAMs). A group of proteins of the immunoglobulin supergene family involved in intercellular adhesion, including ICAM-1, ICAM-2, ICAM-3, vascular cell adhesion molecule-1 (VCAM-1), mucosal addressin cell adhesion molecule-1 (MAdCAM-1), and platelet endothelial cell adhesion molecule (PECAM).

Central tolerance. Tolerance of T cells or B cells induced during their development in the thymus or bone marrow.

Chemokines. A large group of cytokines falling into four families, of which the main families are the CC and the CXC group. Chemokines are designated as ligands belonging to a particular family (e.g. CCL2). Many chemokines have older descriptive names, for example CCL2 is macrophage chemotactic protein-1 (MCP-1). They act on G protein-linked, seven-transmembrane pass receptors and have a variety of chemotactic and cell-activating properties.

Chemokinesis. Increased random migratory activity of cells.

Chemotaxis. Increased directional migration of cells, particularly in response to concentration gradients of certain chemotactic factors.

Ciclosporin. A T cell suppressive drug that is particularly useful in suppression of graft rejection.

Class I/II/III MHC molecules. Three major classes of molecule are coded within the MHC. Class I molecules have one MHC-encoded peptide complexed with β_2-microglobulin, class II molecules have two MHC-encoded peptides which are non-covalently associated, and class III molecules are other molecules including complement components.

Class I/II restriction. The observation that immunologically active cells will cooperate effectively only when they share MHC haplotypes at either the class I or class II loci.

Class switching. The process by which an individual B cell can link immunoglobulin heavy chain C genes to its recombined V gene to produce a different class of antibody with the same specificity. This process is also reflected in the overall class switch seen during the maturation of an immune response.

Classical pathway. The pathway by which antigen–antibody complexes can activate the complement system, involving components C1, C2, and C4, and generating a classical pathway C3 convertase.

Clonal selection. The fundamental basis of lymphocyte activation in which antigen selectively causes activation, division, and differentiation only in those cells that express receptors with which it can combine.

CMI (cell-mediated immunity). A term used to refer to immune reactions that are mediated by cells rather than by antibody or other humoral factors.

Collectins. A group of large polymeric proteins, including conglutinin and mannan-binding lectin (MBL), that can opsonize microbial pathogens.

Complement. A group of serum proteins involved in control of inflammation, activation of phagocytes, and lytic attack on cell membranes. The system can be activated by interaction with the antibodies of the immune system (classical pathway).

Complement control protein (CCP) domains (also called **short consensus repeats**). A domain structure found in many proteins of the complement classical and alternative pathways and in some complement receptors and control proteins.

Complement receptors (CR1–CR4 and C1qR). A set of four cell surface receptors for fragments of complement C3. CR1 and CR2 have numerous complement control protein (CCP) domains, and CR3 and CR4 are integrins. C1qR binds C1q.

ConA (concanavalin A). A mitogen for T cells.

Congenic. Animals that are genetically constructed to differ at one particular locus.

Conjugate. A reagent that is formed by covalently coupling two molecules together, such as fluorescein coupled to an immunoglobulin molecule.

Constant regions. The relatively invariant parts of immunoglobulin heavy and light chains, and the α, β, γ, and δ chains of the T cell receptor.

Contact hypersensitivity. A delayed inflammatory reaction on the skin seen in type IV hypersensitivity.

Co-stimulation. The signals required for the activation of a lymphocyte, in addition to the antigen-specific signal delivered via their antigen receptors. CD28 is an important co-stimulatory molecule for T cells and CD40 for B cells.

Cross-reaction. The sharing of antigenic determinants by two different antigens.

CSFs (colony stimulating factors). A group of cytokines that control the differentiation of hematopoietic stem cells.

CTLA-4 (CD152). A downregulatory signaling molecule of T cells that competes with CD28 for ligation by B7 on antigen-presenting cells.

Cytokines. A generic term for soluble molecules that mediate interactions between cells.

Cytotoxic T cells. Cells that can kill virally infected targets expressing antigenic peptides presented by MHC class I molecules.

D genes. Sets of gene segments lying between the V and J genes in the immunoglobulin heavy chain genes, and in the T cell receptor β and δ chain genes, which are recombined with V and J genes during ontogeny.

Decay accelerating factor (DAF). A cell surface molecule on mammalian cells that limits activation and deposition of complement C3b.

Defensins. A group of small antibacterial proteins produced by neutrophils.

Degranulation. Exocytosis of granules from cells such as mast cells and basophils.

Dendritic cells. A set of cells present in tissues that capture antigens and migrate to the lymph nodes and spleen, where they are particularly active in presenting the processed antigen to T cells. Dendritic cells can be derived from either the lymphoid or mononuclear phagocyte lineages.

DM molecules. Molecules related to MHC class II molecules that are required for loading antigenic peptides onto class II molecules.

Domain. A region of a peptide having a coherent tertiary structure. Both immunoglobulins and MHC class I and II molecules have immunoglobulin supergene family domains.

Dominant idiotypes. Individual idiotypes that are present on a large proportion of the antibodies generated by a particular antigen.

DTH (delayed-type hypersensitivity). This term includes the delayed skin reactions associated with type IV hypersensitivity.

Education of T cells. The process by which developing thymocytes are selected for those that recognize peptides on self MHC molecules, but not for those that recognize self antigenic peptides.

Effector cells. A functional concept, which in context means those lymphocytes or phagocytes that produce an end effect.

Eicosanoids. Products of arachidonic acid metabolism including prostaglandins, leukotrienes, and thromboxanes.

Endocytosis. Internalization of material by a cell by phagocytosis or pinocytosis.

Endothelium. Cells lining blood vessels and lymphatics.

Endotoxin. Lipolysaccharide produced by Gram-negative bacteria that activates B cells and macrophages.

Enhancement. Prolongation of graft survival by treatment with antibodies directed towards the graft alloantigens.

Eosinophils. A population of polymorphonuclear granulocytes that stain with acidic dyes and are particularly involved in reactions against parasitic worms and in some hypersensitivity reactions.

Epithelioid cells. A population of activated mononuclear phagocytes present in granulomatous reactions.

Epitopes. The parts of an antigen that contact the antigen-binding sites of an antibody or the T cell receptor.

Epstein–Barr virus (EBV). Causal agent of Burkitt's lymphoma and infectious mononucleosis that has the ability to transform human B cells into stable cell lines.

Fab. The part of an antibody molecule that contains the antigen-combining site consisting of a light chain and part of the heavy chain; it is produced by enzymatic digestion.

Factors B, P, D, H, and I. Components of the alternative complement pathway.

Fas (CD95). A molecule expressed on a variety of cells that acts as a target for ligation by Fas ligand (FasL) on the surface of cytotoxic lymphocytes.

Fc. The portion of an antibody that is responsible for binding to antibody receptors on cells and the C1q component of complement.

Fc receptors. Surface molecules on a variety of cells that bind to the Fc regions of immunoglobulins. They are antibody class specific and isotype selective.

Ficolins. A group of opsonins that recognize carbohydrate PAMPs.

Flow cytometry. Analysis of cell populations in suspension according to each individual cell's expression of selected surface markers.

Fluorescence-activated cell sorter (FACS). A machine that analyzes cells by flow cytometry and then allows them to be sorted into different populations and collected separately.

Follicular dendritic cells (FDCs). Antigen-presenting cells in the B cell areas of lymphoid tissues that retain stores of antigen.

Formyl-methionyl peptides. Prokaryotes initiate protein synthesis with f-Met. Peptides such as f-Met-Leu-Phe are highly chemotactic for mononuclear phagocytes and neutrophils.

Framework segments. Sections of antibody V regions that lie between the hypervariable regions.

Freund's adjuvant. An emulsion of aqueous antigen in oil. Complete Freund's adjuvant contains killed *Mycobacterium tuberculosis,* whereas incomplete Freund's adjuvant does not.

Frustrated phagocytosis. A term to describe the events that occur when a phagocyte attempts to internalize an antigen or antigenic particle, but is unable to do so (e.g. because of its size).

γδ T cells. The minor subset of T cells that express the γδ form of the T cell receptor.

GALT (gut-associated lymphoid tissue). The accumulation of lymphoid tissue associated with the gastrointestinal tract.

Genetic association. The condition where particular genotypes are associated with other phenomena, such as particular diseases.

Genetic restriction. The term used to describe the observation that lymphocytes and antigen-presenting cells cooperate most effectively when they share particular MHC haplotypes.

Genome. The total genetic material contained within the cell.

Genotype. The genetic material inherited from parents; not all of it is necessarily expressed in the individual.

Germinal centers. Areas of secondary lymphoid tissue in which B cell differentiation and antibody class switching occur.

Germline. The genetic material that is passed down through the gametes before it is modified by somatic recombination or maturation.

Giant cells. Large multinucleated cells sometimes seen in granulomatous reactions and thought to result from the fusion of macrophages.

GPI (glycosylphosphatidylinositol) – linkage. A way in which proteins become attached to the outer leaflet of the phospholipid bilayer that forms the plasma membrane.

Granulocytes. Neutrophils, eosinophils, and basophils.

Granulomatous reactions. Chronic inflammatory reactions (often a manifestation of type IV hypersensitivity) caused by a failure to clear antigen.

Granzymes. Granule-associated enzymes of cytotoxic T cells and large granular lymphocytes.

GVHD (graft versus host disease). A condition caused by allogeneic donor lymphocytes reacting against host tissue in an immunologically compromised recipient.

H-2. The mouse major histocompatibility complex.

Hemagglutination. Clumping of erythrocytes caused by antibody. This forms the basis of a number of immunoassays and blood group typing.

Haplotype. A set of genetic determinants located on a single chromosome.

Hapten. A small molecule that can act as an epitope, but is incapable by itself of eliciting an antibody response.

Helper (TH) cells. A functional subclass of T cells that can help to generate cytotoxic T cells and cooperate with B cells in the production of antibody responses. Helper cells recognize antigen in association with MHC class II molecules.

Heterologous. Refers to interspecies antigenic differences.

HEV (high endothelial venule). An area of venule from which lymphocytes migrate into lymph nodes.

Hinge. The portion of an immunoglobulin heavy chain between the Fc and Fab regions that permits flexibility within the molecule and allows the two combining sites to operate independently. The hinge region is usually encoded by a separate exon.

Histamine. A major vasoactive amine released from mast cell and basophil granules.

Histocompatibility. The ability to accept grafts between individuals.

HIV (human immunodeficiency virus). The causative agent of acquired immune deficiency syndrome (AIDS).

HLA. The human major histocompatibility complex.

Homologous restriction factors. Complement components that restrict the action of the membrane attack complex on cells of the host.

Humoral. Pertaining to the extracellular fluids, including the serum and lymph.

Hybridoma. Cell line created in vitro by fusing two different cell types, usually lymphocytes, one of which is a tumor cell.

5-Hydroxytryptamine (serotonin). A vasoactive amine present in platelets and a major mediator of inflammation in rodents.

Hypersensitivity. An inordinately strong immune response that causes more damage than the antigen or pathogen that induced the response.

Hypervariable region. The most variable areas of the V domains of immunoglobulin and T cell receptor chains. These regions are clustered at the distal portion of the V domain and contribute to the antigen-binding site.

ICAM-1 (CD54), ICAM-2 (CD102), and ICAM-3 (CD50) (intercellular adhesion molecules). Cell surface molecules found on a variety of leukocytes and non-hematogenous cells that interact with leukocyte functional antigen-1 (LFA-1).

Iccosomes. Immune complexes in the form of small inclusion bodies found in follicular dendritic cells.

Idiotope. A single antigenic determinant on an antibody V region.

Idiotype. The antigenic characteristic of the V region of an antibody.

IELs (intraepithelial lymphocytes). A population of lymphocytes defined according to location in which γδ T cells are strongly represented.

Immune complex. The product of an antigen–antibody reaction that may also contain components of the complement system.

Immune response (Ir) genes. Genes that affect the level of immune responses. MHC class II genes are very important in controlling responses to specific antigens.

Immunoblotting (Western blotting). A technique for identifying and characterizing proteins using antibodies.

Immunofluorescence. A technique used to identify particular antigens microscopically in tissues or on cells by the binding of a fluorescent antibody conjugate.

Immunogenic. Having the ability to evoke B cell- and/or T cell-mediated immune reactions.

Immunoglobulins. The serum antibodies, including IgG, IgM, IgA, IgE, and IgD.

Immunoglobulin supergene family (IgSF). Molecules that have domains homologous to those seen in immunoglobulins, including MHC class I and II molecules, the T cell receptor, CD2, CD3, CD4, CD8, ICAMs, VCAM, and some of the Fc receptors.

Immunological synapse. The closely apposed region plasma membrane in the interaction between T cells and antigen-presenting cells, centered on interacting TCRs and MHC–peptide complexes.

Induced fit. A description of the way in which an antigen can alter the normal tertiary structure of the binding site on a receptor following binding, by displacing amino acids.

Inducible nitric oxide synthase (iNOS). An enzyme induced by inflammatory cytokines in macrophages that catalyzes the synthesis of nitric oxide (NO).

Inflammation. A series of reactions that bring cells and molecules of the immune system to sites of infection or damage. This appears as an increase in blood supply, increased vascular permeability, and increased transendothelial migration of leukocytes.

Integrins. A large family of cell surface adhesion molecules, some of which interact with cell adhesion molecules (CAMs), others with complement fragments, and others with components of the extracellular matrix.

Interferons (IFNs). A group of molecules involved in signaling between cells of the immune system and in protection against viral infections.

Interleukins (IL-1–IL-22). A group of molecules involved in signaling between cells of the immune system.

Ir gene. A group of immune response (Ir) genes determining the level of an immune response to a particular antigen or foreign stimulus. A number of them are found in the major histocompatibility complex.

Isotype. Refers to genetic variation within a family of proteins or peptides such that every member of the species will have each isotype of the family represented in its genome (e.g. immunoglobulin classes).

ITAMs (immunoreceptor tyrosine activation motifs) and ITIMs (immunoreceptor tyrosine inhibitory motifs). These are target sequences for phosphorylation by kinases involved in cell activation or inhibition.

JAKs (Janus kinases). A group of enzymes with two catalytic domains. They activate by cross-phosphorylation and are particularly involved in signaling from type I and II cytokine receptors.

J chain. A monomorphic polypeptide present in polymeric IgA and IgM, and essential to their formation.

J genes. Sets of gene segments in the immunoglobulin heavy and light chain genes and in the genes for the chains of the T cell receptor, which are recombined during lymphocyte ontogeny and contribute toward the genes for variable domains.

K cells. A group of lymphocytes that are able to destroy their target by antibody-dependent cell-mediated cytotoxicity. They have Fc receptors.

κ (kappa) chains. One of the immunoglobulin light chain isotypes.

Karyotype. The chromosomal constitution of a cell that may vary between individuals of a single species depending on the presence or absence of particular sex chromosomes or on the incidence of translocations between sections of different chromosomes.

Killer immunoglobulin-like receptors (KIRs). Receptors on NK cells that belong to the Ig superfamily, having either two or three extracellular domains. They may either inhibit or activate cytotoxicity, depending on their intracellular domains.

Kinins. A group of vasoactive mediators produced following tissue injury.

Knockout. An animal whose endogenous gene for a particular protein has been deleted or mutated to be non-functional.

Kupffer cells. Phagocytic cells that line the liver sinusoids.

λ (lambda) chains. One of the immunoglobulin light chain isotypes.

Langerhans' cells. Antigen-presenting cells of the skin that emigrate to local lymph nodes to become dendritic cells; they are very active in presenting antigen to T cells.

Large granular lymphocytes (LGLs). A group of morphologically defined lymphocytes containing the majority of K cell and NK cell activity. They have both lymphocyte and monocyte/macrophage markers.

Lectin pathway. A pathway of complement activation initiated by mannan-binding lectin (MBL) that intersects the classical pathway.

Leukotrienes. A collection of metabolites of arachidonic acid that have powerful pharmacological effects.

LFAs (leukocyte functional antigens). A group of three molecules that mediate intercellular adhesion between leukocytes and other cells in an antigen non-specific fashion. LFA-1 is CD11a/CD18, LFA-2 is CD2, and LFA-3 is CD58.

Ligand. A linking (or binding) molecule.

Line. A collection of cells produced by continuous growth of a particular cell culture in vitro. Such a cell line will usually contain a number of individual clones.

Linkage. The condition where two genes are both present in close proximity on a single chromosome and are usually inherited together.

Linkage disequilibrium. A condition where two genes are found together in a population at a greater frequency than that predicted simply by the product of their individual gene frequencies.

LPS (lipopolysaccharide). A product of some Gram-negative bacterial cell walls that can act as a B cell mitogen.

Ly antigens. A group of cell surface markers found on murine T cells that relate to the differentiation of T cell subpopulations. Many are now assigned to the CD system.

Lymphokines. A generic term for molecules other than antibodies that are involved in signaling between cells of the immune system and are produced by lymphocytes (cf. interleukins).

Lymphokine activated killer cells (LAKs). Cytotoxic cells generated ex vivo by stimulation with interleukin-2 (IL-2) and possibly other cytokines.

Lymphotoxins. A group of cytokines, related to tumor necrosis factors, that act on TNF receptors and mediate inflammatory reactions and leukocyte activation.

Lysosomes. Intracellular vesicles containing stored enzymes, adhesion molecules, or toxic molecules depending on the cell type.

Lysozyme. An enzyme secreted by mononuclear phagocytes that hydrolyzes bonds present in bacterial cell walls.

Lytic pathway. The complement pathway effected by components C5–C9 that is responsible for lysis of sensitized cell plasma membranes.

MALT (mucosa-associated lymphoid tissue). Generic term for lymphoid tissue associated with the gastrointestinal tract, bronchial tree, and other mucosas.

Mannose receptor (MR). A lectin-like receptor found on mononuclear phagocytes.

MAP kinases. A group of intracellular enzymes involved in signaling cascades that lead to the activation of transcription factors.

Marginal zone. An area surrounding the splenic white pulp that separates the lymphoid areas from the surrounding red pulp.

Mast cells. Cells found distributed near blood vessels in most tissues. These cells are full of granules containing inflammatory mediators.

Matrix metalloproteases. A group of zinc-containing degradative enzymes that can break down components of the extracellular matrix (e.g. collagenase).

MCPs (macrophage chemotactic proteins). A group of chemokines.

Membrane attack complex (MAC). The assembled terminal complement components C5b–C9 of the lytic pathway that becomes inserted into cell membranes.

Memory cells. Long-lived lymphocytes that have already been primed with their antigen, but have not undergone terminal differentiation into effector cells. They react more readily than naive lymphocytes when restimulated with the same antigen.

MHC (major histocompatibility complex). A genetic region found in all mammals, the products of which are primarily responsible for the rapid rejection of grafts between individuals and function in signaling between lymphocytes and cells expressing antigen.

MHC restriction. A characteristic of many immune reactions in which cells cooperate most effectively with other cells that share a MHC haplotype.

Microglia. Mononuclear phagocytes resident in the brain and spinal cord. Microglial precursors colonize the human central nervous system early in gestation.

MIF (migration inhibition factor). A group of peptides produced by lymphocytes that are capable of inhibiting macrophage migration.

MIIC compartment. An endosomal compartment where MHC class II molecules are loaded with antigenic peptides.

MIPs (macrophage inflammatory proteins). A group of chemokines.

Mitogens. Substances that cause cells, particularly lymphocytes, to undergo cell division.

MLR/MLC (mixed lymphocyte reaction/mixed lymphocyte culture). Assay system for T cell recognition of allogeneic cells in which response is measured by proliferation in the presence of the stimulating cells.

Mononuclear phagocyte system. The lineage of fixed and mobile long-lived phagocytic cells related to blood monocytes and tissue macrophages.

Myeloid cells. The lineages of bone marrow-derived phagocytes, including neutrophils, eosinophils, and monocytes.

Myeloma. A lymphoma produced from cells of the B cell lineage that can invade bone.

N regions. Gene segments present in recombined antigen receptor genes that are not present in the germline DNA.

Neoplasm. A synonym for cancerous tissue.

Neutrophils. Polymorphonuclear granulocytes, which form the major population of blood leukocytes.

NF-κB. A transcription factor that is widely used by different leukocyte populations to signal activation – sometimes called the master-switch of the immune system.

NK (natural killer) cells. A group of lymphocytes that have the intrinsic ability to recognize and destroy some virally infected cells and some tumor cells.

Nucleotide oligomerization domains (NODs). Domains in intracellular receptors for pathogen-associated molecular patterns.

Nude mouse. A genetically athymic mouse that lacks a transcription factor, which is also required for hair production.

Opsonization. A process by which phagocytosis is facilitated by the deposition of opsonins (e.g. antibody and C3b) on the antigen.

PAF (platelet activating factor). A factor released by basophils that causes platelets to aggregate.

PALS (periarteriolar lymphatic sheath). The accumulations of lymphoid tissue constituting the white pulp of the spleen.

Paneth cells. Cells present in the crypts of the small intestine that secrete antimicrobial peptides.

Paracrine. The action of a cytokine on a cell distinct from the cell that produced it.

Passenger cells. Donor leukocytes present in a tissue graft that may sensitize the recipient to the graft.

Patch test. Application of antigen to skin on a patch to test for type IV hypersensitivity reactions.

Pathogen. An organism that causes disease.

Pathogen-associated molecular patterns (PAMPs). Biological macromolecules produced by microbial pathogens that are recognized by receptors on mononuclear phagocytes and some opsonins in serum and tissue fluids.

PC (phosphorylcholine). A commonly used hapten that is also found on the surface of a number of microorganisms.

PCA (passive cutaneous anaphylaxis). The technique used to detect antigen-specific IgE, in which the test animal is injected intravenously with the antigen and dye, the skin having previously been sensitized with IgE antibody.

Pentraxins. A group of acute-phase pentameric molecules present in serum that recognize PAMPs and opsonize bacteria for phagocytosis.

Perforin. A granule-associated molecule of cytotoxic cells, homologous to complement C9. It can form pores on the membrane of a target cell.

Peyer's patches. Collections of lymphoid cells in the wall of the gut that form a secondary lymphoid tissue.

PFC (plaque forming cell). An antibody-producing cell detected in vitro by its ability to lyze antigen-sensitized erythrocytes in the presence of complement.

PHA (phytohemagglutin). A mitogen for T cells.

Phagocytosis. The process by which cells engulf material and enclose it within a vacuole (phagosome) in the cytoplasm.

Phenotype. The expressed characteristics of an individual (cf. genotype).

Plasma cell. An antibody-producing B cell that has reached the end of its differentiation pathway.

Plasmin system. One of the plasma enzyme systems that generates the fibrinolytic enzyme, plasmin, and also contributes to inflammation and tissue remodeling.

Pokeweed mitogen. A mitogen for B and T cells.

Polymorphs. A common acronym for polymorphonuclear leukocytes, including basophils, neutrophils, and eosinophils.

Prick test. Introduction of minute quantities of antigen into the skin to test for type I hypersensitivity.

Primary lymphoid tissues. Lymphoid organs in which lymphocytes complete their initial maturation steps; they include the fetal liver, adult bone marrow, and thymus, and bursa of Fabricius in birds.

Primary response. The immune response (cellular or humoral) following an initial encounter with a particular antigen.

Prime. To induce an initial sensitization to antigen.

Privileged tissues/sites. In the context of transplantation these are tissues that induce weak immune responses or sites of the body that are partly shielded from graft rejection reactions.

Prostaglandins. Pharmacologically active derivatives of arachidonic acid. Different prostaglandins are capable of modulating cell mobility and immune responses.

Proteasomes. Organelles that degrade cellular proteins tagged for breakdown by ubiquitination.

Protein A and protein G. Components of the cell wall of some strains of staphylococci that bind to Fc of most IgG isotypes.

Pseudoalleles. Tandem variants of a gene: they do not occupy a homologous position on the chromosome (e.g. C4).

Pseudogenes. Genes that have homologous structures to other genes, but are incapable of being expressed (e.g. *Jk3* in the mouse).

Radioimmunoassay (RIA). A number of different sensitive techniques for measuring antigen or antibody titers using radiolabeled reagents.

RAG-1 and RAG-2. Recombination activating genes required for recombination of V, D, and J gene segments during generation of functional antigen receptor genes.

Receptor. A cell surface molecule that binds specifically to particular extracellular molecules.

Receptor editing. A process by which immunoglobulin genes can undergo a secondary recombination event, in order to rescue B cells that are producing non-functional or autoreactive antibodies.

Recombination. A process by which genetic information is rearranged during meiosis. This process also occurs during the somatic rearrangements of DNA, which occur in the formation of genes encoding antibody molecules and T cell antigen receptors.

Recurrent idiotype. An idiotype present in the immune response of different animals or strains to a particular antigen.

Relative risk. A number that expresses how much more likely (>1) or less likely (<1) an individual is to develop a particular disease if they possess a particular genotype.

Respiratory burst. Increase in oxidative metabolism of phagocytes following uptake of opsonized particles.

Reticuloendothelial system. A diffuse system of phagocytic cells derived from the bone marrow stem cells that are associated with the connective tissue framework of the liver, spleen, lymph nodes, and other serous cavities. An old-fashioned term that is rarely used – mononuclear phagocyte system is the preferred term.

ROIs/RNIs (reactive oxygen intermediates/reactive nitrogen intermediates). Bactericidal metabolites produced by phagocytic cells, including hydrogen peroxide, hypohalites, and nitric oxide.

Rosetting. A technique for identifying or isolating cells by mixing them with particles or cells to which they bind (e.g. sheep erythrocytes to human T cells). The rosettes consist of a central cell surrounded by bound cells.

Scavenger receptors. A group of receptors that recognize cell debris and are involved in the phagocytosis of apoptotic cells and some pathogens.

SCID (severe combined immunodeficiency). A group of genetic conditions leading to major deficiencies or absence of both B cells and T cells.

Secondary response. The immune response that follows a second or subsequent encounter with a particular antigen.

Secretory component. A polypeptide produced by cells of some secretory epithelia that is involved in transporting secreted polymeric IgA across the cell and protecting it from digestion in the gastrointestinal tract.

Selectins. Three adhesion molecules – P-selectin (CD62P), E-selectin (CD62E), and L-selectin (CD62L) – involved in slowing leukocytes during their transit through venules.

Serotonin. 5-Hydroxytryptamine.

SLE (systemic lupus erythematosus). An autoimmune disease (non-organ specific) of humans usually involving anti-nuclear antibodies.

Somatic mutation. A process occurring during B cell maturation and affecting the antibody gene region that permits refinement of antibody specificity.

Spleen. A major secondary lymphoid organ in the peritoneal cavity next to the stomach.

STATs. A group of proteins that form components of transcription factors following activation by kinases.

Stem cell factor (SCF). Also called Steel factor. A cytokine required for the earliest stages of leukocyte development in bone marrow.

Superantigens. Antigens that stimulate clones of T cells with different antigen specificity but using the same TCR V genes.

Suppressor (Ts) cell. Functionally defined populations of T cells that reduce the immune responses of other T cells or B cells, or switch the response into a different pathway to that under investigation.

Surface plasmon resonance. A biophysical phenomenon that can be used to measure the association and binding constants of proteins in solution interacting with bound ligands.

Synergism. Cooperative interaction.

Syngeneic. Strains of animals produced by repeated inbreeding so that each pair of autosomes within an individual is identical.

T cells. Lymphocytes that differentiate primarily in the thymus and are central to the control and development of immune responses. The principal subgroups are cytotoxic T cells (CTLs) and T helper cells (TH0, TH1, and TH2).

TAP transporters. A group of molecules that transport proteins and peptides between intracellular compartments.

TCR (T cell receptor). The T cell antigen receptor consisting of either an αβ dimer (TCR-2) or a γδ dimer (TCR-1) associated with the CD3 molecular complex.

T-dependent/T-independent antigens. T-dependent antigens require immune recognition by both T and B cells to produce an immune response. T-independent antigens can directly stimulate B cells to produce specific antibody.

TGFs (transforming growth factors). A group of cytokines identified by their ability to promote fibroblast growth; they are also generally immunosuppressive.

Thoracic duct. Drains efferent lymph into the venous system.

Thromboxanes. Products of arachidonic acid metabolism, some of which are involved in inflammation.

Thymus. A primary lymphoid organ in the thoracic cavity over the heart.

Tissue inhibitors of matrix metalloproteases (TIMPs). A group of proteins released by cells in tissues, that limit the activity of matrix metalloproteases.

Tissue typing. Determination of an individual's allotypic variants of MHC molecules.

TNF (tumor necrosis factor). A cytokine released by activated macrophages that is structurally related to lymphotoxin released by activated T cells.

Tolerance. A state of specific immunological unresponsiveness.

Toll-like receptors (TLRs). A group of cell surface receptors that recognize molecules from pathogens (e.g. LPS). Some TLRs transduce signals for inflammation.

Tonsils. Paired lymphoid organs in the throat that form part of the mucosa-associated lymphoid tissue (MALT).

Transformation. Morphological changes in a lymphocyte associated with the onset of division. Also used to denote the change to the autonomously dividing state of a cancer cell.

Transgenic animal. An animal in which one or more new genes have been incorporated. These are often placed under specific promoters so that they are expressed only in particular tissues for limited periods.

Tumor necrosis factors (TNFs). A group of proinflammatory cytokines encoded within the MHC.

V domains. The N terminal domains of antibody heavy and light chains and the α, β, γ, and δ chains of the T cell receptor that become recombined with appropriate sets of D and J genes during lymphocyte ontogeny.

Vaccination. A general term for immunization against infectious disease, originally derived from immunization against smallpox, which uses the vaccinia virus.

Vasoactive amines. Products such as histamine and 5-hydroxytryptamine (serotonin) released by basophils, mast cells, and platelets that act on the endothelium and smooth muscle of the local vasculature.

Veiled cells. Cells of the dendritic cell lineage as seen in afferent lymph. They may be derived from Langerhans' cells or other dendritic cell types.

VLA-1–VLA-6 (very late antigens). The set of integrins that share a common β1 chain (CD29).

Waldeyer's ring. The secondary lymphoid tissues of the nasopharynx that includes the tonsils and adenoids.

Western blotting. A technique for identifying and characterizing proteins using antibodies. Synonymous with immunoblotting.

White pulp. The lymphoid component of spleen consisting of periarteriolar sheaths of lymphocytes and antigen-presenting cells.

Xenogeneic. Refers to interspecies antigenic differences.

Index